CLINICAL SURGE

CLINICAL SURGERY PEARLS

SECOND EDITION

R Dayananda Babu MS MNAMS
Professor and Head
Department of Surgery
Sree Gokulam Medical College and Research Foundation
Venjaramoodu, Thiruvananthapuram, Kerala, India

Foreword
Mathew Varghese

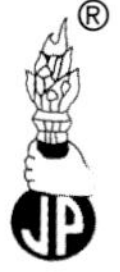

JAYPEE BROTHERS MEDICAL PUBLISHERS (P) LTD.

New Delhi • London • Philadelphia • Panama

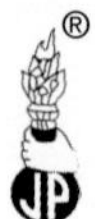

Jaypee Brothers Medical Publishers (P) Ltd

Headquarters

Jaypee Brothers Medical Publishers (P) Ltd
4838/24, Ansari Road, Daryaganj
New Delhi 110 002, India
Phone: +91-11-43574357
Fax: +91-11-43574314
Email: jaypee@jaypeebrothers.com

Overseas Offices

J.P. Medical Ltd
83, Victoria Street, London
SW1H 0HW (UK)
Phone: +44-2031708910
Fax: +02-03-0086180
Email: info@jpmedpub.com

Jaypee-Highlights Medical Publishers Inc.
City of Knowledge, Bld. 237, Clayton
Panama City, Panama
Phone: +507-301-0496
Fax: +507-301-0499
Email: cservice@jphmedical.com

Jaypee Brothers Medical Publishers, Ltd
The Bourse
111 South Independence Mall East
Suite 835, Philadelphia, PA 19106, USA
Phone: + 267-519-9789
Email: joe.rusko@jaypeebrothers.com

Jaypee Brothers Medical Publishers (P) Ltd
17/1-B Babar Road, Block-B, Shaymali
Mohammadpur, Dhaka-1207
Bangladesh
Mobile: +08801912003485
Email: jaypeedhaka@gmail.com

Jaypee Brothers Medical Publishers (P) Ltd
Shorakhute, Kathmandu
Nepal
Phone: +00977-9841528578
Email: jaypee.nepal@gmail.com

Website: www.jaypeebrothers.com
Website: www.jaypeedigital.com

Inquiries for bulk sales may be solicited at: jaypee@jaypeebrothers.com

Clinical Surgery Pearls

First Edition: 2010

Second Edition: **2013**

ISBN 978-93-5090-396-4

Printed at: Ajanta Offset & Packagings Ltd., New Delhi

Dedicated to

My late parents for their love and affection –
Mr Raghavan and Mrs Mallakshy
My only sister – late Ms Damayanthy
My wife – Professor (Dr) Geetha Bhai and
to my beloved son Deepak D Babu
for their moral support
My teachers for their wisdom
My patients for their trust and support
My students for their assistance

Foreword

Professor R Dayananda Babu is known to me for the past forty years. I have great admiration for his wealth of knowledge in the subject of surgery.

He has written the book *Clinical Surgery Pearls* with careful and persistent effort. The overriding goal has been the mobilization of information relative to the science and skills of surgery. In addition to defining the frontiers of surgical knowledge, it affords the student to assimilate the fundamentals in an easy way.

This book will be an enormous help to those who are studying surgery at both undergraduate and postgraduate levels.

I wish the book a great success.

Professor (Dr) Mathew Varghese
MS FRCS Ed
Emeritus Professor of Surgery
Government Medical College
Kottayam, Kerala, India

Preface to the Second Edition

The first edition of this book was published in 2010. It is gratifying to note the wide acceptance of this book as an exam cracker by undergraduates and postgraduates alike; and, therefore, I was forced to bring out the second edition within 2 years of the initial publication. I am happy to note that now this book is recommended by many universities.

There is no need to stress the importance of refreshing a book like this. I was forced to spend many hours in rectifying the errors which have crept up in the first edition. The old chapters have been thoroughly revised and updated. The new American Joint Committee on Cancer (AJCC), 7th edition, has been used for staging and management, instead of the 6th edition of AJCC as used in the first edition. At the end of some of the important cases, colored boxes have been used under the title "What is new—For postgraduates, the unique unorthodox style, the student-oriented approach and the question-answer format are still retained."

I am grateful to Professor John S Kurian, who is Professor of Surgery at Government Medical College, Kottayam, Kerala, India, for the effort he has taken to find out the errors and for coming up with suggestions for improvement. I also thank Dr Deepak George, for his valuable suggestions for improvement of many of the chapters.

I also thank the publisher M/s Jaypee Brothers Medical Publishers (P) Ltd, New Delhi, India, for bringing out a high-quality second edition book quickly.

R Dayananda Babu

Preface to the First Edition

This book is the final result of my continuous teaching and learning process with my undergraduate and postgraduate students in surgery. Whenever I interact with my students, I realize their problems and deficiencies and find out the solutions, so that it reaches them. Whenever I read a chapter, a series of questions will come to my mind and then I will try to answer those questions. That is exactly the reason why this book is in question-answer format. The flow charts and tables in this book are evolved in the classrooms and bedside teaching area.

Whenever I read a topic, I try to define the condition. I feel that when you define something, half the problem is solved; and, therefore, the first chapter is devoted to definitions. There are more than 100 definitions in this book.

Another important aspect of any learning process is to find out the concepts behind the disease process and management. These concepts are converted to an easily digestible capsule form in this book for the students. As an examiner at undergraduate and postgraduate levels, I realized that most of the time the students miss many important clinical points during case presentation, not because they do not know them but because they do not have a checklist. Therefore, I have given the checklist for all clinical cases. The questions for the postgraduate (PG) students are marked as PG in brackets so that the undergraduate students can skip them if they feel so.

More than 50 clinical cases are discussed in this book (both long ones and short ones). Each case starts with a clinical capsule and questions are formulated based on the clinical capsule. There is a separate chapter for radiology and imaging and about 32 skiagrams are discussed. Important tables and charts are included as a separate chapter for ready reference.

This is a clinical book of definitions, checklists, tables, flow charts, questions and answers. All my classes are distilled into a book and the title is *Clinical Surgery Pearls*. The preparation of this book took seven long years of hard work, and I completed this book single handedly. All the clinical photographs are taken by me with a small Kodak digital camera. The highlighted boxes and charts in this book will make it easily readable. I am sure, the unique style and the student-oriented approach will make the learning process a pleasant experience.

R Dayananda Babu

Acknowledgments

I am grateful to:

- All my patients, for permitting me to take clinical photographs.
- My favorite student Dr Suraj Rajan, who has drawn the medical illustrations in Adobe photoshop and who is now working in the US. He also read the first "raw copy" and gave suggestions from the "student point of view", which is incorporated as student review. I am short of words to thank him.
- All my Professors and teachers in surgery. I remember my great teachers like Professor CKP Menon, Professor KJ Jacob, Professor Mathew Varghese, Professor Balsalam, Professor Mohankumar, Professor KY Roy and Professor CK Bahuleyan.
- My wife Dr Geetha Bhai, who helped me in proofreading and editing this book and without her help this could not have been possible.
- All my postgraduate and undergraduate students in surgery.
- Shri Jitendar P Vij (Group Chairman), Mr Ankit Vij (Managing Director) and Mr Tarun Duneja (Director-Publishing) of M/s Jaypee Brothers Medical Publishers (P) Ltd, New Delhi, India.
- Mr PM Sebastian (Branch Manager, Jaypee Brothers, Kochi) and Mr Arun Kumar (Senior Sales Executive, Jaypee Brothers, Kochi) and all the staff of Kochi Branch for bringing out this book in time.
- Finally, Mr Subramanian, for spending time with me and doing the DTP work of this book.

Contents

SECTION 1: Definitions

SECTION 2: Long Cases

SECTION 3: Short Cases

SECTION 4: Radiology and Imaging

SECTION 5: Important Tables and Charts

Sayings of the Great

1. *Take up one idea*
   Make that one idea your life
   Think of it, dream of it, live on it
   Let the brain, muscle, nerves and every part of your body be full of that idea
   Leave the other ideas alone.

   —Swami Vivekananda

2. *Give the best you have and the best shall come back to you.*

   —Holy Bible

3. *Reading maketh a full man, conference a ready man and writing an exact man.*

   —Francis Bacon

4. *All truth passes through three stages*
   First, it is ridiculed
   Second, it is violently opposed
   Third, it is accepted as being self-evident.

   —Schopenhauer

5. *The world is not divided into the rich and poor, the successes and failures,*
   but into learners and non-learners.

   —Benjamin Barber

1 SECTION

Definitions

Definitions

1. Abdominal Apoplexy

Spontaneous hemorrhage into the peritoneal cavity.
Causes:

a. *Tumors*
   - Hepatoma
   - Spleen
   - Other organs

b. *Arteriosclerotic lesion* in older individuals
   - Superior mesenteric artery: **Mesenteric apoplexy** (spontaneous rupture)
   - Right colic artery
   - Branches of celiac.

c. *Hemorrhage* from congenital aneurysm in young patients — bleeding from **splenic artery aneurysm in pregnancy.**

2. Abscess, Cold Abscess

Abscess: It is a localized collection of pus in a **pathological space lined by granulation tissue.**

Cold Abscess: Soft fluctuant swelling without signs of inflammation, which is mistaken for a cyst. This is lined by granulation tissue and caseous material. It is due to **tuberculous infection** and **contains tubercle bacilli.** It is not hot. Brawny induration, edema and tenderness are absent.

3. Acute Abdomen

Any sudden spontaneous nontraumatic disorder affecting the abdomen for which urgent operation may be necessary and undue delay in diagnosis may adversely affect the outcome.

4. Activities of Daily Living (ADL)

It is critical to assess the functional status of the prospective older candidate for surgery prior to scheduling an operation.

The activities are:

1. Feeding oneself
2. Bathing
3. Toileting (continence)
4. Transferring from bed to chair
5. Dressing
6. Grooming.

Instrumental ADLs are more complex:

a. Food preparation
b. Shopping
c. Blanching.

5. Agenesis/Atresia

Agenesis: Failure of the development of an organ or structure.

Atresia: Failure to canalize viscera.

6. Amylase

A serum amylase level four times above the normal is indicative of acute pancreatitis.

7. Ankyloglossia

Inability to protrude the tongue due to involvement of the muscles of tongue by carcinoma. The tongue deviates to the affected side.

8. Apathetic Hyperthyroidism

Asymptomatic mild hyperthyroidism occurring in the elderly recognized only by laboratory findings.

9. Arc of Riolan (Meandering Mesenteric Artery)

The left colic artery near the splenic flexure bifurcates; one of the branches passes to the right in the transverse mesocolon to anastomose with a similar branch of middle colic artery to form the Arc of Riolan. This has got important role in supplementing the marginal artery (Fig. 10.1).

10. Bacteremia, Pyemia, Septicemia

Bacteremia: Circulating bacteria in the blood without producing disease.

Pyemia: Circulating infective emboli composed of masses of organisms, vegetations and infected clots in the bloodstream.

Septicemia: Circulation of bacteria in blood producing disease.

11. Barrett's Esophagus

It is a metaplasia of the lower esophageal mucosa due to replacement of the squamous epithelium, by columnar epithelium, endoscopically having salmon pink appearance replacing the whitish squamous epithelium pathologically showing intestinal type of epithelium with goblet cells.

12. Biliary Colic, Cholecystitis

The term colic is inaccurate for gallbladder. It produces constant pain in most cases as a result of obstruction to cystic duct. The pain last for 1–5 hours, and rarely shorter than 1 hour duration (Right upper quadrant pain radiating to right upper back, right scapula or between the scapulas). Pain lasting beyond 24 hours suggests acute inflammation—Cholecystitis.

13. Boil, Furuncle, Furunculosis, Folliculitis, Carbuncle

Folliculitis: Affection of the root of one hair follicle alone by *Staphylococcus* is called folliculitis.

Boil/Furuncle: Infection of the root of the hair follicle with perifolliculitis caused by *Staphylococcus* is called Boil/Furuncle.

Furunculosis: Multiple boils with intervening normal tissue is called furunculosis.

Carbuncle: Infective gangrene of skin and subcutaneous tissue caused by *Staphylococcus* (multiple boils with involvement of intervening tissue also).

14. Breast Carcinoma—Definitions

Skin tethering and fixity: The skin tethering is due to early involvement of ligaments of Cooper.

Manifested as puckering of the skin. The underlying lump can be moved independently of the skin to some extent.

Skin fixity: It is because of invasion of carcinoma along the ligaments of Cooper to the skin.

The lump and the skin cannot be moved separately.

Retraction (Recent) of nipple: Extension of growth along the lactiferous duct and subsequent fibrosis.

Peau d' Orange appearance is due to blockage of the lymphatics draining the skin—cutaneous lymphedema. The hair follicles are more firmly fixed to the subcutaneous tissue than the rest of the skin. The hair follicles appear to be retracted and the between areas swell giving the orange peel appearance.

Terminal Duct Lobular Unit (TDLU): The functional unit of the breast is the terminal duct lobular unit. All cancers of the breast and most benign conditions arise within TDLU (Fig. 5.4).

Skin Involvement: T4b

Edema (including *peau d' orange*) or ulceration of the skin of the breast or satellite skin nodules confined to the breast. Dimpling of the skin and nipple retraction is not considered skin involvement.

Inflammatory carcinoma breast: It is a clinicopathological entity characterized by diffuse erythema and edema (peau d' orange) of the breast **without an underlying palpable mass,** involving the **majority of the skin of the breast.** This is due to tumor emboli within dermal lymphatics. The biopsy should demonstrate cancer within the **dermal lymphatic** or in breast parenchyma itself. Neglected LABC (locally advanced breast cancer) is not inflammatory Ca.

Extensive in situ component: If more than 25% of the main tumor mass contains in situ disease and there is in situ cancer in the surrounding breast tissue, the cancer is classified as having an extensive in situ component.

Chest wall infiltration: Chest wall includes **ribs, intercostal muscles and serratus anterior muscle** but not the pectoral muscle.

Supraclavicular nodes: These are seen in a triangle defined by the omohyoid muscle and tendon, internal jugular vein (medial border) and the clavicle and subclavian vein (lower border). Adjacent nodes outside this triangle are considered to be lower cervical nodes (M1).

Multifocal: Tumor foci in the same quadrant are called multifocal.

Multicentric: Tumor foci in different quadrants are called multicentric.

Microinvasion: (Ti mic): Microinvasion of 0.1 cm or less in greatest dimension.

Micrometastasis: Tumor deposits **greater than 0.2 mm,** but not greater than 2 mm in largest dimension having histologic evidence of malignant activity namely proliferation or stromal reaction.

Isolated tumor cells: Single cell or small clusters of cells not greater than 0.2 mm in largest dimension with no histologic evidence of malignant activity.

15. Bruit

It is the sound produced by the turbulent blood flow through a stenotic arterial segment which is **transmitted distally** along the course of the artery. When a bruit is heard over the peripheral vessel, stenosis is present at or proximal to that level.

It is heard **loudest during systole** and with greater stenosis may extend into diastole. The pitch of the bruit rises as the stenosis becomes more marked. **Absence of bruit does not indicated absence of occlusion.**

When the vessel becomes completely occluded, the bruit may disappear.

16. Burns, Scald, Fat Burn

Burns: Injury by dry heat.

Scald: Injury by moist heat.

Fat burn: Injury by boiling oil.

17. Bursae: Bunion, Clergyman's Knee, Golfer's Elbow, Students Elbow, Housemaid's Knee, Tennis Elbow

Bursae: These are fluid-filled cavities lined with flattened endothelium similar to synovium. Usually seen in relation to joints. When they develop **over pressure points,** they are called **adventitious bursae** (see examples). They prevent friction during movement. **Fluctuation, fluid thrill and transillumination are positive.**

Housemaid's knee: It is a subcutaneous bursa between patella and skin.

Clergyman's knee: It is a subcutaneous bursa between skin and ligamentum patella.

Students elbow: It is a subcutaneous bursa between skin and olecranon.

Golfer's elbow: It is medial epicondylitis Tenderness can be elicited at the medial epicondyle at the common flexor origin.

Tennis elbow: It is lateral epicondylitis (Common extensor origin at the lateral epicondyle is affected).

Bunion: It is a subcutaneous bursa between skin and head of 1st metatarsal bone.

18. Carbuncle

Read boil.

19. Cellulitis, Erysipelas

Cellulitis: **Spreading inflammation of subcutaneous** and fascial tissue caused by *Streptococcus pyogenes.* Commences in a trivial infected wound. It has "*No edge, No fluctuation, No pus and No limit*".

Morison's aphorism: Cellulitis occurring in children is never primary in the cellular tissue, but **secondary to an underlying bone infection.**

Cellulitis of the scrotum: Always rule out extravasation of urine.

Erysipelas: It is cuticular lymphangitis.

Milian's ear sign: Facial erysipelas spreads and involves the pinna because it is cuticular lymphangitis. Subcutaneous inflammations stop short for the pinna because of close adherence of the skin to the cartilage.

20. Claudication, Rest Pain

Claudication: (I limp). Claudication is the **cramp like muscle pain** which appears following exercise when there is an inadequate arterial blood flow.

It must fulfil three criteria

1. It is a cramp like muscle pain (usually the calf)
2. Pain develops only when the muscle is exercised
3. The pain disappears when the exercise stops.

Rest pain: It is the **continuous pain** caused by severe ischemia. This pain is present at rest **throughout the day and the night.** The pain is relieved by putting the leg below the level of the heart.

21. Clergyman's Knee

Read bursae.

22. Cold Abscess

Read abscess.

23. Compressibility, Reducibility

Compressibility: When the contents of a swelling can be emptied by squeezing but the swelling reappear spontaneously on release of pressure.

Reducibility: When the contents of a swelling can be emptied by squeezing but does not return spontaneously. This requires additional force such as cough or effect of gravity. For example, Hernia.

24. Compound Palmar Ganglion

Compound palmar ganglion: It is a **tuberculous affection** of ulnar bursae, with a swelling in the hollow of the palm, extending to the lower forearm. Cross fluctuation can be elicited between the palm and lower forearm.

25. Constipation, Obstipation

Constipation: A bowel frequency of less than one every 3 days. *(Fewer than two per week).*

Obstipation: (Absolute constipation): Absence of passage of both stool and flatus.

26. Cough Impulse

Cough Impulse: Expansile impulse seen or felt over a swelling when the patient coughs, cries or strains.

27. Crepitus

Crepitus: (Grating or crackling sensation imparted to the examining fingers) may be present when the joint contain loose bodies. May communicate with joint. It is also seen in the following conditions:

- Subcutaneous emphysema **(surgical emphysema)**—gas is present in the subcutaneous tissue. Four types:
  a. Traumatic: Fracture ribs, injury to nasal fossa, breach of continuity of larynx, tracheostomy, fracture skull involving sinuses
  b. Infective: Gas gangrene
  c. Extraneous: After fluid administration, closure of surgical wound, etc.
  d. Complicating rupture of esophagus
- Fracture of bones
- Extravasation of gas in pneumoperitoneum
- Pseudo gas gangrene (air entrapped in the subcutaneous tissue after laparotomy).

28. Cyst

Cyst: It is a pathological fluid-filled sac bound by a wall. It may be **true or false, congenital or acquired**.

True cyst: It is one in which the sac is **lined with cells of epithelial origin.**

False cyst: It is a walled off fluid collection **not lined by epithelium.** False cyst may be inflammatory or degenerative.

Examples of false cyst

- Dental/Radicular cyst
- Encysted pleural effusion
- Pseudocyst of pancreas
- Cystic degeneration of tumors
- Brain cyst.

29. Dermoid

Dermoid: Cyst formation due to sequestration of epithelium deep to the skin surface.

30. Dietl's Crises

Dietl's crisis: This is because of **intermittent hydronephrosis.** After an attack of acute renal pain, a swelling is found in the loin due to the hydronephrosis. Following the passage of large volume of urine some hours later, the pain is relieved and the swelling will disappear.

31. Diverticulum, Diverticulosis

Diverticulum: Abnormal external projection from a hollow viscus external to the serosa is called diverticulum. **It may be true or false, congenital or acquired.** Congenital is true and acquired is false (one meaning of diverticulum is a **wayside house of ill-fame).**

True diverticulum: Containing all the layers of the bowel wall.

False diverticulum: There is no muscle coat, but all other layers (herniation of mucosa or submucosa through the muscular coat).

Pulsion diverticulum: The diverticulum is pushed out by intraluminal pressure.

Traction diverticulum: Diverticulum develops as a result of external traction.

Diverticulosis: Presence of multiple false diverticulae.

32. Diarrhea

Diarrhea: If stools contain **more than 300 mL** fluid daily.

33. Edema

Edema: It is an **imbalance between capillary filtration and lymphatic drainage** (this does not mean that all edemas are lymphedemas). This will occur only when the lymphatic system fails to drain the tissue fluid produced by normal capillary filtration.

34. Empyema

Empyema: It is collection of pus in a physiological space.

35. Erysipelas (Read Cellulitis)

Erysipelas: Spreading cuticular lymphangitis caused by *Streptococcus pyogenes.* It has a sharply defined margin unlike cellulitis. The vesicles contain serum. Milian's ear sign—Erysipelas can spread to the pinna.

36. Erythroplakia, Leukoplakia

Erythroplakia: Any lesion of the oral mucosa that presents as **bright red velvety plaques** that cannot be characterized clinically or pathologically as any other recognizable condition.

Leukoplakia: Any **white patch or plaque** that cannot be characterized clinically or pathologically as any other disease.

37. Exotoxin, Endotoxin

Exotoxin: Toxin liberated by living bacteria.

Endotoxin: Toxin liberated after death of bacteria, being a part of the organism itself.

38. Evidence—Levels

Levels of evidences: Agency for health care policy and research grading system for evidence and recommendation.

Evidence	*Description*
I a	Evidence from **meta-analysis** of randomized controlled trials *RCT*
I b	Evidence from **at least one RCT**
II a	Evidence from at least **one controlled study without randomization**
II b	Evidence from at least **one other type of quasi-experimental study**
III	Evidence from nonexperimental descriptive studies, such as c**omparative studies and case control studies**
IV	Evidence from expert committee reports or opinions or clinical experience of **respected authorities or both.**

Recommendation of Strength:

A – Directly based on category I evidence.

B – Directly based on category II evidence or extrapolated recommendation from category I evidence.

C – Directly based on category III evidence or extrapolated recommendation from category I or II evidence.

D – Directly based on category IV evidence or extrapolated recommendation from category I, II, or III evidence.

Levels of evidences: Pragmatic grading (only three grades).

39. Fistula, Sinus

Fistula: It is a communicating tract between two epithelial surfaces lined with granulation tissue. It may be a communication between the skin and hollow viscera or between two hollow viscerae (Internal fistula).

Sinus: Sinus is a blind track leading from the surface down to the tissue lined by granulation tissue/epithelium.

Fistula-in-ano: The pathology of fistula-in-ano is 'cryptoglandular infection' (Infection of the anal glands in the crypt).

	Levels of Evidences		*Recommendations*
I.	Beyond reasonable doubt, high quality RCT, systematic reviews, high quality synthesized evidence	A.	Strong recommendations which should be followed
II.	**On the balance of probabilities** Evidence of best practice from high quality review of literature	B.	Based on evidence of effectiveness that may need interpretation in the light of other factors like local facilities, audit, etc.
III.	**Unproven** in sufficient evidence upon which to base a decision or contradictory evidence	C.	When there is inadequate evidence

40. Flail Chest

Flail chest: Three or more ribs fractured in 2 or more places.

Bilateral costochondral separation will result in **flail sternum**.

41. Folliculitis

Read boil.

42. Ganglion

Ganglion: Cystic, myxomatous degeneration of fibrous tissue. They are not pockets of synovium protruding from joints. It may be multilocular occasionally.

Content—Viscous gelatinous material.

Disappear underneath adjacent structure during certain movements.

Fluctuation is present if not tense.

43. Gangrene, Necrosis, Infarction, Slough

Gangrene: Macroscopic death of tissue with putrefaction.

Necrosis: Microscopic death of tissue.

Infarction: Ischemic necrosis is called infarction.

Slough: A piece of dead tissue separated from living tissue.

44. Early Gastric Cancer

Early gastric cancer: Cancer of the stomach confined to the mucosa and submucosa irrespective of the nodal status.

45. Gastrinoma

Gastrinoma: A basal gastric acid output more than 15 mmol/HR and a fasting gastrin level of more than 200 pg/mL is strongly supporting the diagnosis.

46. Gastrinoma Triangle (Passaro's Triangle)

Gastrinoma triangle: The three points forming the triangle are:

1. Junction between the head and neck of the pancreas.
2. Junction of cystic duct with CBD.
3. Junction between 2nd and 3rd parts of the duodenum.

47. Goiter

Goiter: Any enlargement of thyroid gland is called goiter.

Grading of goiter:

WHO (1990) Perez Classification

Grade 0	No goiter
Grade I a	Not visible, but palpable
Grade I b	Visible with neck extended and palpable
Grade II	Visible with neck in normal position and palpable
Grade III	Large gland evident from a distance.

WHO classification (1994)

Grade 0 – No palpable or visible swelling

Grade 1 – A mass in the neck that is consistent with an enlarged thyroid that is palpable, but not visible when neck is in normal position. It moves upwards in the neck as the subject swallows

Grade 2 – A swelling in the neck that is visible when the neck is in a normal position and is consistent with an enlarged thyroid when neck is palpated.

Large goiter:
- Protrusion of goiter beyond chin or jaw.
- Goiter which weighs 80 g or more after excision.
- Largest neck circumference crossing the goiter being 40 cm or more.
- Stage III—WHO classification.

48. Granuloma

Granuloma: Tumor-like mass formed in chronic inflammatory tissue.

49. Hamartoma, Teratoma

Hamartoma: A tumor-like formation of tissues indigenous to the site due to developmental aberration.

Teratoma: Tumor-like proliferation of tissues, not indigenous in origin, containing more than one germinal layer.

50. Hematemesis, Melemesis, Melena, Hematochezia

Hematemesis: Vomiting of bright red or dark blood.

Melemesis: Vomiting of altered blood is called melemesis. Coffee ground vomitus is due to vomiting of blood that has been in the stomach long enough for gastric acid to convert Hb to methemoglobin.

Melena: Passage of black or tarry sticky, semisolid, stools because of the presence of altered blood. It can be produced by blood entering the bowel at any point from mouth to cecum. The black color is due the **Hematin** (from Heme). **50 to 100 ml** of blood in stomach can produce melena. 1 liter of blood in stomach will produce melena for **3–5 days**.

Hematochezia: Passage of bright red blood from the rectum (Colon, rectum and anus) is called hematochezia. Brisk bleeding from upper intestine with rapid transit can also produce it.

51. Hernia, Prolapse

Hernia: Abnormal protrusion of a viscus or part of a viscus **lined by a sac** through a normal or abnormal opening in the abdominal wall.

Prolapse: Abnormal protrusion of a viscus through a normal or abnormal opening not lined by a sac.

52. Hurthle Cell Tumor

Hurthle cell tumor: Presence of more than 75% follicular cells having oncocytic features in thyroid histology is called Hurthle cell tumor.

53. Hydronephrosis, Dietl's Crisis (Read Above)

Hydronephrosis: Aseptic dilatation of pelvicalyceal system due to partial or intermittent obstruction.

54. Hyperparathyroidism

Hyperparathyroidism: The combinations of increased PTH levels and hypercalcemia without hypocalciuria (Hypercalciuria of more than 400 mg/24 hour is diagnostic).

55. Incontinence of Urine

Incontinence of urine: Involuntary evacuation of urine.

56. Incontinence of Stool

Incontinence of stool: Involuntary evacuation of stool.

Three Types

a. Incontinence for solid feces
b. Incontinence for liquid feces
c. Incontinence for gas.

57. Infarction

Read gangrene.

58. Inguinal Canal

Inguinal canal: It is an **intermuscular slit** situated between the superficial inguinal ring and deep inguinal ring.

59. Intussusception

Intussusception: Telescoping of proximal intestine to the distal intestine.

Retrograde intussusception: Telescoping of distal intestine into the proximal intestine (e.g. jejuno-gastric intussusception) after gastrojeunostomy).

60. Jaundice

Jaundice: Yellowish discoloration of skin and mucous membrane due to excessive circulating bile.

61. Karnofsky Performance Status (KPS)

Karnofsky performance status (KPS): The KPS is reliable independent predictor of survival of outcome for patients with **solid tumors**. It is a required baseline assessment in clinical protocols in **head and neck and other cancers**.

The American joint committee on cancer (AJCC) strongly recommends recording of KPS along with standard staging information (TNM). It is a method of measuring **co-morbidity.** It provides a uniform objective assessment of an individuals functional status. The **scale** in **ten** point increments from **zero (Dead)** to **100 (Normal, no complaints, no evidence of disease)** was devised in 1948 by **David A Karnofsky.**

Karnofsky Performance Status (KPS)

100 – Normal; no complaints; no evidence of disease. 90 – Able to carry on normal activity; minor signs or symptoms of disease. 80 – Able to carry on normal activity with effort; some signs or symptoms of disease. 70 – Care for self; unable to carry on normal activity or do active work. 60 – Requires occasional assistance, but is able to care for most of own needs. 50 – Requires considerable assistance and frequent medical care. 40 – Disabled; requires special care and assistance. 30 – Severely disabled, hospitalization is indicated by although death is not imminent. 20 – Very sick. Hospitalization necessary. Active supportive treatment is needed. 10 – Moribund. Fatal process rapidly progressing. 0 – Dead.

A. Able to carry on normal activity. No special care is needed (scale 80–100).
B. **Unable to work**, able to live at home, cares for most personal needs; a varying amount of assistance is needed (50–70).
C. **Unable to take care of self**; requires the equivalent of institutional or hospital care; disease may be progressing rapidly (scale 10–40).

62. Line of Demarcation

Line of demarcation: Zone of demarcation between viable and gangrenous tissue indicated by a band of **hyperemia and hyperesthesia** on the surface and separation is achieved by a **layer of granulation tissue.**

In dry gangrene the line of demarcation appears in a matter of days without infection and this is called "**separation** by **aseptic ulceration**".

In moist gangrene the line of demarcation is more proximal than dry gangrene and the process is called "**separation by septic ulceration**".

63. Lipoma (Universal Tumor)

Lipoma: It is benign tumor from "**adult fat cell**" It is called "universal tumor" or "**ubiquitous tumor**" and hence the aphorism: "**when in doubt hedge on fat**".

64. Lower GI Bleed, Upper GI Bleed

Lower GI bleed: It is a bleeding from distal to the ligament of Treitz.

Upper GI bleed: It is a bleeding from proximal to the ligament of Treitz.

65. Marginal Artery of Drummond, Arc of Riolan (Read Above)

Marginal artery of Drummond: It is the paracolic vessel of anastomosis between the superior mesenteric and inferior mesenteric arterial system.

66. Massive Hemothorax

Massive hemothorax: When **1500 mL** or more of blood is acutely removed from the pleural space, then it is called massive hemothorax.

67. Massive Blood Transfusion

Massive blood transfusion: The term massive transfusion implies a single transfusion greater than **2500 mL** or **5000 mL** transfused over a period of 24 hours.

68. Melena, Melemesis

Read hematemesis.

69. Menarche—Early

Early menarche: Age of menarche before 12 years.

70. Menopause—Late

Late menopause: Menopause after 50 years.

71. Mesentery of Small Intestine — Attachment

Mesentery of small intestine—attachment: The base of the mesentery attaches to the posterior abdominal wall to the left of the second lumbar vertebra and passes obliquely to the right and inferiorly to the right sacroiliac joint crossing 3rd part of the duodenum, aorta, IVC and right ureter. It is **6 inches (15 cm)** in length. Remember the small intestine has got **6 meters length** (Fig. 2.1).

72. Mesentery of Sigmoid — Attachment

Mesentery of sigmoid—attachment: It is shaped like an inverted V. The apex of the V is at the bifurcation of left common iliac artery crossing the brim. The right limb descends to the third piece of the sacrum. The left limb runs along the brim of left side of pelvis (Fig. 10.2).

73. Mesentery of The Transverse Colon

Mesentery of the transverse colon: It is attached to the descending part of duodenum to the head and lower aspect of the body of the pancreas and placed horizontally to the anterior surface of the left kidney.

74. Necrosis

Read gangrene.

75. Old Age

Old age: Above 65 years is old age and above 85 years is very old age.

76. Oral Cavity, Buccal Mucosa, Retromolar Trigone, Trismus, Ankyloglossia

Oral cavity: Starts at **skin vermilion junction** of lip **anteriorly** to circumvallate papillae of tongue, posterior part of the hard palate, and anterior pillar of tonsil **posteriorly.** Oral cavity includes the following.

- Lips
- Buccal mucosa
- Upper and lower alveolar ridge
- Retromolar trigone
- Floor of the mouth
- Hard palate
- Oral tongue.

Buccal mucosa: Extends from the upper alveolar ridge down to the lower alveolar ridge, and from the commissure anteriorly to the mandibular ramus and retromolar region posteriorly.

Retromolar trigone: It is defined as the anterior surface of the ascending ramus of the mandible. It is **triangular in shape** with the base being superior **behind the third upper molar** tooth and the apex inferior behind the 3rd lower molar.

Trismus: (Spasmodic clenching) is inability to open the mouth.

Causes for Trismus

- Oral carcinoma—Involvement of pterygoid, masseter, temporalis and buccinator muscle.
- Inflammatory—Parotitis
- Tooth abscess (Dental)
- Erupting wisdom tooth
- Peritonsillar abscess (Quinsy)
- Tetanus — (Painful smiling risus sardonicus).

Ankyloglossia (Read above).

77. Pancreatitis, Pancreatic Necrosis, Pancreatic Abscess, Pancreatic Ascites, Pancreatic Effusion, Pseudocyst, Pancreatic Necrosis, Acute Fluid Collection

Chronic pancreatitis: It is a disease in which there is **irreversible progressive destruction of pancreatic tissue.** Its clinical course is characterized by **dynamic progressive fibrosis** of the pancreas.

Acute Pancreatitis

Acute fluid collection: It is fluid collection in or near the pancreas with ill defined wall occurring early in acute pancreatitis.

Pancreatitis acute pseudocyst: It is a collection of pancreatic juice enclosed in a wall of fibrous or granulation tissue (Requires **4 weeks**).

Pancreatic necrosis: Diffuse or focal area of non-viable pancreatic parenchyma. Associated peri-pancreatic fat necrosis is present.

Infected pancreatic necrosis: Same as above with infection.

Pancreatic abscess: Circumscribed intra-abdominal collection of pus in proximity to pancreas. There is no pancreatic necrosis.

Pancreatic ascites: Chronic generalized peritoneal enzyme rich effusion associated with pancreatic ductal disruption.

Pancreatic effusion: Encapsulated collection of fluid in the pleural cavity.

78. Papilloma (Benign Papilloma), Polyp, Polyposis

Benign papillomas: These are hamartomas consisting of an **overgrowth of all skin layers and its appendages** having a central core and normal sensation. They are well-defined, usually, pedunculated ranging from few millimeters to a few centimeters in size, commonly 5 mm across. The surface may be grooved or deeply fissured. The complications of papilloma are **inflammation, bleeding ulceration, pigmentation and keratosis.**

Polyp: It is a morphological term and no histologic diagnosis is implied. They are masses of tissue that project into the lumen of viscera. When the base is broader than the head, it is called **sessile**. When the base is narrower than head, it is called **pedunculated**. It may be benign or malignant, mucosal or sub-mucosal or muscular.

Polyposis: Presence of many polyps.

Classification of polyp

a. Neoplastic
   - Adenoma
     - Tubular adenoma,
     - Tubulovillous
     - Villous adenoma
   - Carcinoid
   - Adenocarcinoma

b. Hamartomatous
   - Juvenile polyp (associated with malrotation or Meckel's diverticulum)
   - Peutz–Jeghers polyps

Contd...

Contd...

c. Inflammatory (Pseudo-polyp)
   - Benign lymphoid polyp

d. Hyperplastic polyp (Metaplastic polyp)
   - Diminutive lesions most often found in left side of the colon

e. Miscellaneous
   - Lipoma
   - Leiomyoma.

79. Paralytic Ileus

Paralytic ileus: Defined as a state in which there is failure of transmission of peristaltic waves in the intestine secondary to **neuromuscular failure [in the myenteric (Auerbach) and the submucous (Meissner) plexuses.**

80. Paraphimosis, Phimosis

Phimosis: Inability to retract the foreskin to expose the glans.

Paraphimosis: Inability to reduce a previously retracted foreskin.

81. Peau D' Orange

Read breast

82. Perfusion, Transfusion

Perfusion: Artificial passage of fluid through blood vessel (usually veins).

Transfusion: Intravenous administration of blood or its components.

83. Prolapse—Read Hernia

Abnormal protrusion of a viscus through a normal or abnormal opening not lined by a sac.

84. Pseudo Thyrotoxicosis

Seen in **critically ill patients** characterized by increased levels of T_4 and decreased levels of T_3 due to failure of conversion of T_4 to T_3.

85. Pus

Pus: It is a fluid composed of **living and dead bacteria,** dead fixed and **free cells** (the latter representing body's phagocytic response) and **foreign material** such as sutures, implants and splinters.

Color of the pus may give a clue regarding the organism.

- Creamy yellow—Staphylococci
- Watery opalescent—*Streptococcus*
- Blue/Green—*Pseudomonas*
- Purplish brown—Amebic liver abscess
- Yellow granules—Actinomycosis.

86. Renal Angle

Renal angle: Angle between the 12th rib and the edge of the erectorspinae muscle. Normally this is empty and resonant. There should not be any tenderness.

Rest pain: It is the continuous pain caused by severe ischemia. This pain is present at rest throughout the day and the night. The pain is relieved by putting the leg below the level of the heart.

87. Retention of Urine

Retention of urine: Accumulation of urine in the bladder with inability to void.

Acute retention: Sudden inability to pass urine with a **painful bladder**.

Chronic retention: Retention with a **painless bladder**.

Size of Urinary Catheter
French or Charriere's scale
Fr or Ch
3 Fr = 1 mm outer diameter of catheter

Recall Shakespeare's 'Seven Ages of Man' from As You Like It.

The entire World is a stage
And all the men and women merely players;
They have their exits and their entrances;
And one man in his time plays many parts,
His acts being seven ages. At first the infant,
Mewling and puking in the nurse's arms.
And then the whining school boy, with his satchel,
And shining morning face, creeping like snail,
Unwillingly to school. And then the lover,
Sighing like furnace, with a woeful ballad
Made to his mistress' eyebrow. Then a solider,
Full of strange oaths and bearded like the pard,
Jealous in honor, sudden and quick in quarrel,
Seeking the bubble reputation
Even in the cannon's mouth. And then the justice,
In fair round belly with good capon lin'd,
With eyes severe, and beard of formal cut,
Full of wise saws and modern instances;
And so he plays his part. The sixth age shifts
Into the lean and slipper'd pantaloon,
With spectacles on nose and pouch on side;
His youthful hose well say'd a world too wide
For his shrunk shank; and his big manly voice,
Turning again towards childish treble, pipes
And whistle in his sound. Last scene of all,
That ends this strange eventful history,
Is second childishness, and mere oblivion
Sans teeth, sans eyes, sans taste, sans everything

Important causes for retention of urine as per the seven ages are:

1. The infant – Posterior urethral valve
2. The school boy – Enlarged bladder neck (Marion's disease)
   – Obturation by stone
3. The "lover age" – Retention following acute urethritis
4. The soldier – Urethral stricture
5. The justice – Benign enlargement of the prostate
6. The sixth age – Carcinoma of the prostate
7. The last age – Carcinoma of the prostate
   – Benign enlargement of the prostate

Three most important causes for acute retention in **female:**

- Retroverted gravid uterus (Do bimanual palpation of uterus)
- Disseminated sclerosis (CNS examination).
- Hysteria.

"Bashful bladder"—Cannot pass urine when another person is in the vicinity.

88. Retromolar Trigone

Read oral cavity

89. Rigidity, Guarding

Reflex contraction of the abdominal wall muscles secondary to intraperitoneal inflammation.

Rigidity: In rigidity there is contraction even at rest.

Guarding: In guarding it is secondary to provocation from the examining hand of the physician.

90. Run in, Distal Run off

Distal run off: Patency of the main vessel beyond an arterial occlusion seen in angiogram.

Run in: Patency of the main vessel proximal to the site of occlusion in angiogram.

91. Scoliosis

Scoliosis: Rotatolateral deformity of the spine.

92. Screening, Surveillance

Screening: It is defined as testing a group of people considered to be **at normal risk for a disease**, to discover those at increased risk.

Surveillance: It is defined as testing of a group known to be **at increased risk for a disease.**

93. Sinus

Read fistula

94. Stricture, Stenosis

Stricture: Narrowing of a length of canal or hollow organ.

Stenosis: Narrowing of a segment of canal or orifice.

95. Strangury, Tenesmus

Strangury: Painful, frequent, ineffective attempts at micturition.

Tenesmus: Painful, frequent, ineffective attempts at defecation.

96. Tension Pneumothorax

Tension pneumothorax: Presence of air in the pleural cavity with signs of mediastinal shift like: Tracheal shift or and Shift of Apex beat.

Differences between simple pneumothorax and tension pneumothorax

	Simple	Tension
Tracheal position	Normal	Displaced
Percussion note	Normal	Increased
Jugular pressure	Normal	Elevated (unless hypovolemic)
Breath sounds	Normal	Decreased
Pulse	Normal	Weak
BP	Normal	Low

A tension pneumothorax impairs venous return by caval distortion from mediastinal shift and raised intrathoracic pressure with compression of the contralateral lung.

Radiological signs of tension pneumothorax:
1. Tracheal shift
2. Spreading of the ribs (Space between ribs increased)
3. Lowering of hemidiaphragm.

97. Third Day Fever

Third day fever: If a patient is developing fever on the third postoperative day of surgery, suspect septic foci in the IV cannula.

98. Tubercle, Caseous Material, Tuberculous Pus

Tubercle: Microscopically consists of an area of caseation surrounded by:

a. Giant cells (having 20 or more peripherally arranged nuclei)
b. Zone of epithelioid cells around giant cells
c. Zone of inflammatory cells—lymphocytes and plasma cells.

Tubercle is visible to the naked eye towards the end of second week.

Caseous material: It is a dry, granular and cheese like material (Granular structureless material microscopically).

Tuberculous pus: Softening and **liquefaction of the caseous material** result in a thick creamy fluid called tuberculous pus. Liquefaction is associated with **multiplication of bacteria.** It is **highly infective.** It contains fatty debris in serous fluid with a few necrotic cells (It is **usually sterile**).

99. Ulcer

Ulcer: Abnormal breach in the continuity of the skin or mucous membrane due to molecular death of tissue.

100. Upper GI Bleed

Read Lower GI.

101. Varicose Vein

Varicose vein: (WHO Definition) Abnormally dilated saccular or cylindrical superficial veins which can be circumscribed or segmental.

102. Volvulus

Volvulus: Axial rotation of a portion of bowel about its mesentery. Volvulus can occur in the cecum, sigmoidcolon and in the stomach.

In the stomach, there are two types of volvulus.
- Organoaxial—rotation of stomach in horizontal direction (common).
- Mesenteroaxial—rotation of the stomach in the vertical direction.

103. WEIGHT LOSS

Weight loss: Loss of more than 10% body weight over a period of 6 month.

2

SECTION

Long Cases

Case 1 Toxic Goiter

Case Capsule

A 30-year-old female patient with a thin build has presented with **diffuse enlargement of the thyroid** and palpitation of 6 months duration. She complains of increased appetite and **loss of weight.** She is apparently **irritable** and says, she is intolerant to hot weather with excessive sweating. She has a preference for cold weather. She also complains of **insomnia** and loss of concentration ability. She has **diarrhea** in addition. She is married and has a baby of 6 months old. She complains of **amenorrhea** for the last 3 months. On examination, patient is **agitated and nervous.** Examination of the palms revealed that they are **moist and sweaty**. She has **tachycardia, fine and fast tremor and protruded eyeballs.** There is visible **diffuse enlargement** of the thyroid. On auscultation, there is a **systolic bruit** heard in the upper pole of the thyroid. The carotids are felt in the normal position. The trachea is central. There is no evidence of retrosternal extension. The cervical lymph nodes are not enlarged.

In all goiters or swelling in the neck assess the following:

1. What is the anatomical diagnosis—by assessing the plane—deep to the deep fascia and deep to the sternomastoid?
2. What is the pathological diagnosis, e.g. nodular goiter, solitary thyroid nodule, carcinoma, etc.
3. What is the functional diagnosis—whether the patient is euthyroid, hyperthyroid, hypothyroid?

Checklist for history

- Onset related to **puberty, pregnancy**
- Residence: Endemic area or not
- Ingestion of **goitrogens**
- **Intolerance to hot/cold** temperature
- **Increased appetite with loss of weight** (Hyperthyroidism)
- Gain in weight (Hypothyroidism)
- **Change in menstrual cycle**
- Bowel habit—**diarrhea (hyper), constipation (hypo)**
- Difficulty in swallowing
- Difficulty in breathing
- Hoarseness of voice
- **Postural cough** during sleeping (retrosternal extension)
- History of palpitation/shortness of breath on exertion
- **Insomnia,** loss of concentration (hyper)
- **Irritability/nervousness** (hyper).

Checklist for examination of thyroid

- Always **check the pulse** for tachycardia before examining the thyroid
- Look for **tremor** of hands and tongue before examining the thyroid
- Ask the patient to take a **sip of water and to hold it in his/her mouth.** Then ask the patient to swallow (goiter moves on swallowing)
- Ask the patient to **put out the tongue** (thyroglossal cyst moves up)
- **Stand behind** the patient and palpate the thyroid (ask the patient to take another sip of water)
- Decide whether it is diffuse enlargement, single nodule, multiple nodules and the nature of the surface
- Decide the **consistency**
- Look over the top of the head for **exophthalmos** (look for lid lag, lid retraction and other eye signs)
- Check the eye movements, double vision
- Now stand in front of the patient for palpation of the trachea for deviation, for assessing the lower limit by **'getting below'**
- Assess the **plane** of the swelling (stretch the deep fascia by extending the neck and see whether it becomes less prominent, contract the sternomastoid muscle against resistance and see whether it becomes less prominent
- Do **Pemberton's test** for retrosternal extension
- **Percuss the manubrium sterni** for dullness (seen in retrosternal extension)
- Palpate the carotids on both sides
- Examine the **regional lymph nodes**
- Feel the skin (dry in hypothyroidism, shiny skin in hyperthyroidism)
- Look for pretibial myxedema (hyperthyroidism)
- Assess the **build of the patient** (Thin—hyperthyroidism, obese—hypothyroidism)
- Examine the palms—warm, moist and changes of acropachy in hyperthyroidism
- Assess the **behavior of the patient** (agitated in toxic, lethargic in hypothyroidism)
- Ask the patient to rise from squatting position without using hands for support (proximal myopathy in hyperthyroidism)
- **Test the biceps reflex and look for slow relaxing reflex suggestive of hypothyroidism.**

Final checklist for clinical examination of thyroid

1. Look for signs of toxicity
2. Look for signs of malignancy
3. Look for signs of retrosternal extension
4. Look for position of carotid artery
5. Look for position of trachea
6. Look for cervical lymph nodes
7. Look for bony swellings especially in the scalp.

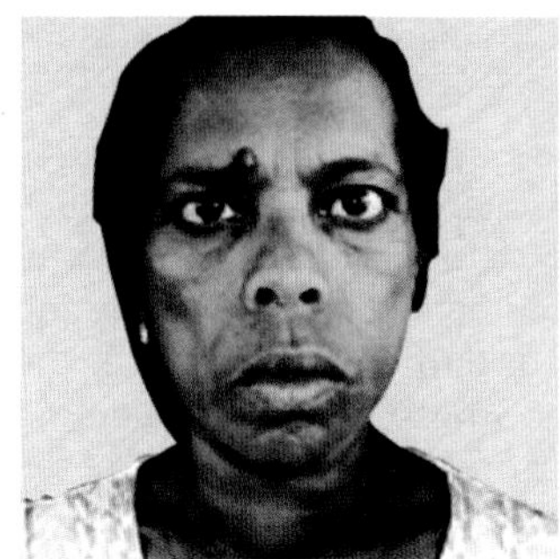
Early exophthalmos

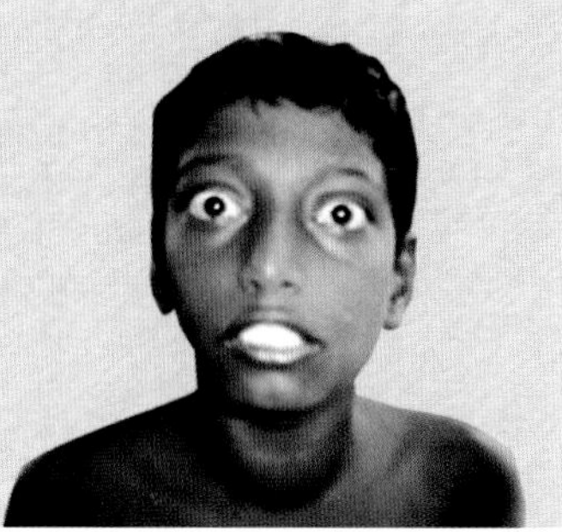
Exophthalmos of graves

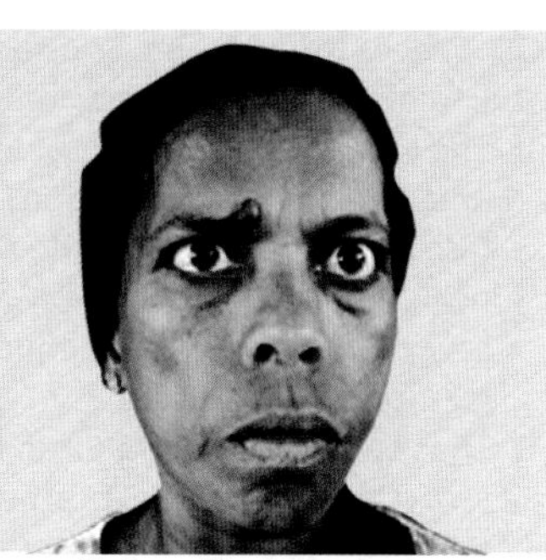
Goiter with staring look

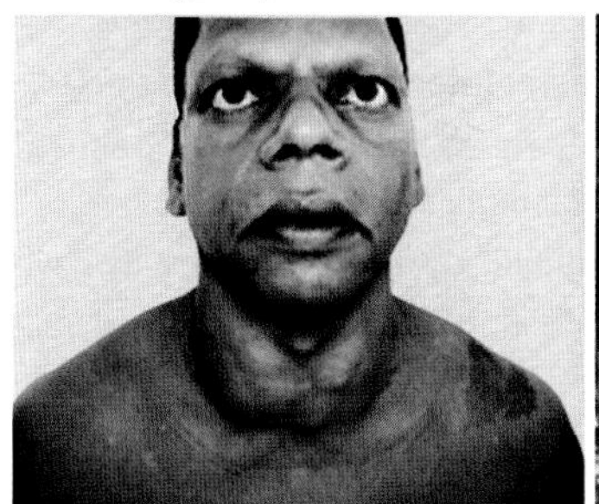
Multinodular goiter with toxicity

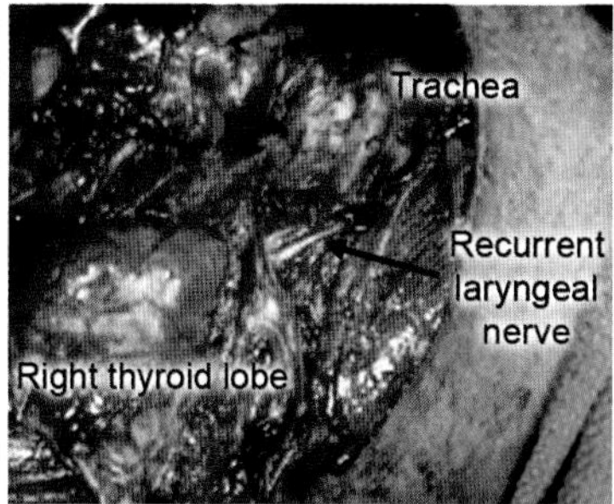

Recurrent laryngeal nerve

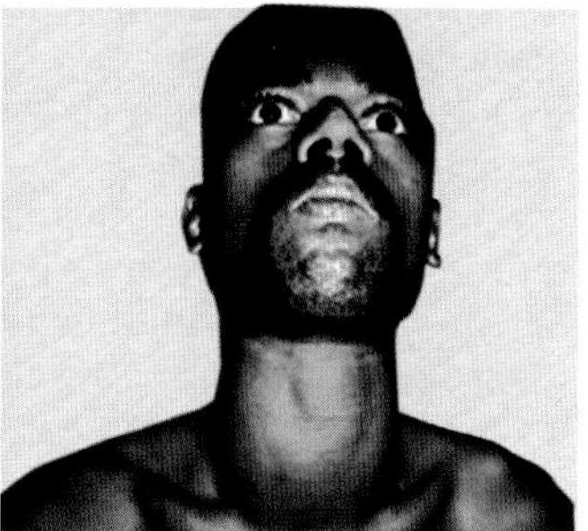
Diffuse toxic goiter

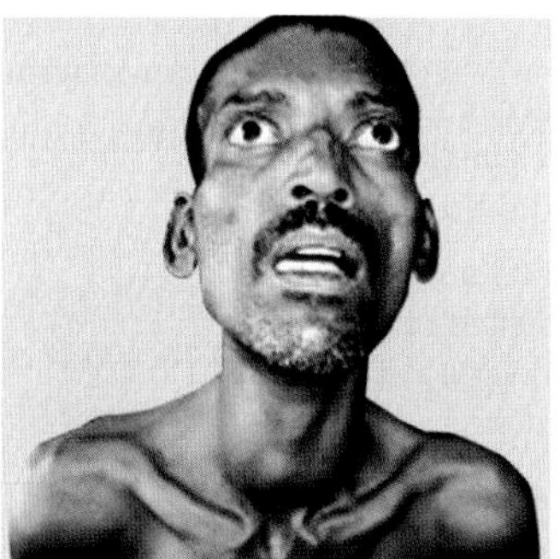
Primary thyrotoxicosis with staring look

Q 1. Why is the swelling a goiter?

The points in favor of goiter are:

1. The plane of the swelling is deep to deep fascia and deep to sternocleidomastoid (the deep fascia of the neck is stretched by extending the neck and sees whether the swelling is becoming less prominent or not, similarly contracts the sternomastoid muscles.
2. The swelling moves up and down with deglutition.
3. It occupies the normal position of thyroid.
4. It is having the shape of thyroid.

Q 2. Why does the thyroid gland move up and down with deglutition?

The inferior constrictor muscle has two parts namely, thyropharyngeus and cricopharyngeus and they are attached respectively to thyroid cartilage and cricoid cartilage. Therefore, when the patient swallows this muscle will contract and the thyroid and cricoid cartilage will move up. The thyroid gland is attached to the cricoid by means of the suspensory ligament of Berry that is nothing but a condensation of pretracheal fascia. Therefore, the thyroid gland will move up and down with deglutition.

Q 3. What is goiter?

Any enlargement of thyroid gland is called goiter. Even though for neoplasms we call it malignancy and for inflammation we call it thyroiditis.

Q 4. Can the normal thyroid be felt on palpation?

In a reasonably slender person it can be felt as a smooth firm structure that moves upwards during deglutition.

Q 5. How do you grade a goiter?

WHO grading (1994) of goiter		
Grade 0	:	**No palpable/visible** goiter
Grade 1	:	A thyroid that is **palpable** but **not visible** when the neck is in normal position
Grade 2	:	An enlarged thyroid that is **visible with** the neck in normal position.

Q 6. What are the signs of retrosternal extension?

1. Cannot 'get below' the swelling.
2. Pemberton's test positive (arm raising test)—when both arms are elevated so as to touch the sides of the face, after a few moments there will be congestion of face, some cyanosis and distress. This is due to the narrowing of the thoracic inlet and when the arms are elevated this results in obstruction of great veins of the neck.
3. On percussion over the manubrium sterni there will be dullness (normally this is resonant).
4. Radiological assessment.

Q 7. How will you assess the position of trachea?

The position of trachea can be assessed by:

1. Palpation of trachea by three finger test (this will be difficult in case of large goiter).
2. Auscultation to detect the position of trachea.
3. Radiological.

Q 8. In which position you normally palpate a patient with thyroid?

The examiner stands behind the patient and will do the palpation.

Q 9. What is Kocher's test?

Slight compression on the lateral lobes of thyroid produces stridor. If this test is positive it signifies that the patient has an obstructed trachea.

Q 10. What are the conditions in which you get narrowing of the trachea?

Narrowing of trachea is found in:

1. Carcinoma of the thyroid
2. Retrosternal goiters
3. "Scabbard" trachea of long standing multinodular goiter
4. Riedel's thyroiditis.

Q 11. What is plunging goiter?

In this condition, the whole of the enlarged thyroid lies in the superior mediastinum and there is no palpable thyroid gland in the neck. When the intrathoracic pressure rises as in coughing, the goiter will be seen in the neck, this is called plunging goiter.

Q 12. What is Berry's sign?

In goiter, the carotid artery may be pushed posteriorly by the enlarging thyroid and this is called displacement. When there is infiltration of the carotid by tumor the **carotid pulse on that side will be absent.** This absent carotid pulse is called Berry's sign.

Q 13. What are the signs of malignancy in a goiter?

Signs of malignancy in a goiter

1. Rapidly enlarging thyroid
2. Hard consistency (unripe apple)
3. Fixity of the thyroid (the lateral mobility becomes restricted before there is noticeable movement on deglutition
4. Regional lymph nodes (the first lymph node to be involved in carcinoma is called Delphic lymph node which is nothing but prelaryngeal lymph node). This is also called the Delphian lymph node
5. Berry's sign (absent carotid pulse)
6. Horner's syndrome
7. Hoarseness of voice
8. Stridor due to tracheal obstruction
9. Distant metastases (pulsatile, bony swelling from the scalp).

Q 14. Where will you auscultate for thyroid bruit?

The usual position to look for thyroid bruit is at the upper pole where the superior thyroid artery enters the thyroid gland.

Q 15. What are your points in favor of toxicity in this patient?

The toxicity is diagnosed on the basis of symptoms and signs in this patient. The symptoms of toxicity are:

Symptoms of toxicity

System	*Symptoms*
• *Nervous system,*	Nervousness agitation, irritability, insomnia, nervous instability, tremor of the hands and tongue
• *Cardiovascular system*	Palpitation, dyspnea on system exertion, chest pain, etc.
• *Metabolic and alimentary system*	Increase in appetite and loss of weight, change in bowel habit, usually diarrhea; preference for cold weather; excessive sweating; intolerance to hot weather
Menstrual changes	Usually amenorrhea or oligo-menorrhea
• *Musculoskeletal*	Generalized weight loss; wasting and weakness of small muscles of the hand, shoulder and face.
• *Skin*	Pretibial myxedema
• *Nail*	Onycholysis—Plummer's nail.

Signs of toxicity

1. Uniform, smooth, soft or firm enlargement of thyroid in Graves' disease (primary) bosselated swelling or solitary nodule in case of secondary
2. The gland is vascular as evidenced by bruit
3. Tremor of the outstretched hands (fine, fast) and tongue
4. Warm and moist hands
5. Tachycardia
6. Extra systoles, atrial fibrillation, and cardiac failure
7. Eye signs
8. Myopathy — weakness of the proximal limb muscle is commonly found. Severe muscular weakness resembling myasthenia gravis occurs occasionally. Inability to get up from chair is called **Plummer's sign.**

Q 16. What are the eye signs of thyrotoxicosis?

Eye signs

1. *Lid retraction*—this sign is caused by over activity of involuntary smooth muscle part of the levator palpebrae superior is muscle. If the upper eye lid is higher than normal and the lower lid is in correct position, the patient has lid retraction (this is not exophthalmos)
2. *Lid lag (Von Graefe's sign)*—when the upper lid does not keep pace with the eyeball as it follows a finger moving from above downwards, it is lid lag
3. *Exophthalmos*—here both the eyelids are moved away from center with sclera visible below or all around. Here the eyeball is pushed forwards by increase in retro-orbital fat, edema, and cellular infiltration (sclera should be always visible below the lower edge of eyes in exophthalmos)
4. *The other eye signs are*:
   a. Widening of the palpebral fissure **(Stellwag's sign)** this is due to lid retraction
   b. **Joffroy's sign**—absence of wrinkling of the forehead when the head is bent down
   c. **Möbius's sign**—difficulty in convergence when the patient is asked to look at near objects
5. *Severe exophthalmos*—Intraorbital edema is super added to the increased deposition of intraorbital fat. It comprises of:
   a. **Intraorbital congestion**—watering of eyes, dilated blood vessels in lateral conjunctiva
   b. Increased intraocular tension
   c. Muscle paralysis **(Ophthalmoplegia)**—evidenced by double vision, especially when eye is moved upward end and outwards (muscles of elevation and abduction namely, superior rectus and inferior oblique muscles are affected)
   d. **Chemosis.**

Q 17. What is pretibial myxedema?

This is a misnomer and it is seen in primary toxicosis (In Graves' disease with exophthalmos only). It is usually symmetrical. The earliest stage is a shiny red plaque of thickened skin with coarse hair, which may be cyanotic when cold. In severe cases the skin of the whole leg below knee is involved, together with that of foot and the ankle and there may be clubbing of the fingers and toes **(Thyroid acropachy)**.

Q 18. What are the three most important clinical types of toxicity?

Clinical types of thyrotoxicosis

1. Primary thyrotoxicosis/Graves/diffuse toxic goiter
2. Secondary thyrotoxicosis/Plummer's disease/toxic nodular goiter
3. Toxic nodule/adenoma/autonomous nodule.

Q 19. What is the difference between thyrotoxicosis and hyperthyroidism?

Thyrotoxicosis refers to the biochemical and physiological manifestations of excessive thyroid hormone. Hyperthyroidism is a term reserved for disorders that result in the over production of hormone by the thyroid gland. Thyrotoxicosis need not be due to hyperthyroidism. In short in hyperthyroidism the pathology is in the thyroid gland itself. The causes for hyperthyroidism and toxicosis without hyperthyroidism are shown below.

Hyperthyroidism	*Toxicosis without hyperthyroidism*
1. Graves's disease	1. Subacute thyroiditis*
2. Toxic nodular goiter	2. Ectopic functioning thyroid tissue
3. Toxic adenoma	3. Silent thyroiditis
4. Jod-Basedow's disease	4. Struma ovarii
	5. Metastatic follicular carcinoma (functioning)
	6. Trophoblastic tumors
	7. Postpartum thyroiditis
	8. Thyrotoxicosis factitia

*Note: In thyroiditis, inflammation of thyroid causes release of already formed thyroid hormones into the circulation, resulting in toxicosis. In other conditions such as struma ovarii, trophoblastic tumors, etc., there is extrathyroid production of thyroxin from these tissues.

Q 20. What is Graves' disease?

The essential components of Graves' disease are:

- Diffuse goiter
- Thyrotoxicosis
- Autoimmune manifestations like:
  - Infiltrative ophthalmopathy
  - Dermatopathy
  - Myopathy.

Q 21. What is the essential etiology of Graves' disease?

Graves' disease is an autoimmune disorder caused by thyroid stimulating immunoglobulins **(TSIs)** that have been produced against an antigen in the thyroid. This is directed to the thyroid stimulating hormone receptors **(TSHR - Ab).** This acts like TSH agonist. TSH-Ab is found only in Graves' disease.

Q 22. What are the precipitating factors for primary thyrotoxicosis?

Remember 3 - S

- Sex (puberty, pregnancy)
- Sepsis
- Psyche (sudden emotional upset).

Q 23. What are the differences between primary thyrotoxicosis and secondary thyrotoxicosi?

Primary	*Secondary*
1. Etiology—Autoimmune	Not autoimmune
2. Enlargement of goiter is diffuse, firm or soft	Bosselated or nodular not uniform
3. Onset is abrupt	Insidious
4. Hyperthyroidism is usually severe	Hyperthyroidism usually mild
5. Cardiac failure is rare	Cardiac failure or multiple extrasystole, paroxysmal atrial tachycardia, paroxysmal atrial fibrillation, or persistent atrial fibrillation
6. Eye signs common	Except lid lag and retraction other eye signs are not seen
7. No pre-existing goiter	Pre-existing nodular goiter for a long duration
8. Usually younger women	Usually middle aged or elderly
9. The entire gland is overactive	Internodular thyroid tissue is overactive, rarely one or more nodules also may be overactive
10. Presence of bruit	Bruit need not be present
11. It is due to abnormal thyroid stimulating antibodies (TSAb)	No such antibodies (it is due to over activity of nodules)
12. Can be managed by, drugs, radioiodine, and surgery	Surgery is the treatment of choice after control of the toxicity
13. Manifestations not due to hyperthyroidism pretibial myxedema may occur	Not seen

Q 24. How will you confirm your diagnosis of toxicity?

Confirmation by:

- **Thyroid Function Test** – **T_3, T_4** and **TSH** (Immunochemiluminometric assay is the current method).
- **Free T_3, T_4** are more significant and meaningful. The T_3 and T_4 are raised and TSH is lowered in hyperthyroidism.

  Normal values are total **Free T_3** 3.5 – 7.5 μol/L
  Free T_4 10 – 30 nmol/L
  TSH 0.3 – 3.3 mU/L

Note: The total T_3 and T_4 hormone level will vary depending upon the amount of thyroid binding globulin **(TBG).**

Q 25. What are the other investigations required?

- *Antithyroglobulin antibody:* More than 1:100.
- *Thyroid peroxidase (TPO):* > 25 units (TPO and TSH antibodies are increased in autoimmune thyroiditis).
- TSH receptor antibodies are difficult to estimate.
- Radioisotope scintigraphy (radionuclide scan).

Q 26. What is the role of isotope scanning in thyroid?

- The only absolute indication in thyrotoxicosis for isotope scanning is for the diagnosis of **Autonomous Toxic Nodules.**
- Toxicity with nodularity is an indication. It can identify hypofunctioning nodule (cold). Cold nodule in Graves' is likely to be malignant.
- It is the only method by which one can definitely differentiate **primary, secondary** and **toxic nodules.**
- Isotope scan can also differentiate hyperthyroidism from toxicosis due to other causes. (**To differentiate hyperthyroid thyrotoxicosis from non-hyperthyroid thyrotoxicosis**). The radioactive iodine uptake (RAIU) is increased in hyperthyroidism whereas toxicosis because of **extrathyroidal** causes the RAIU is decreased (e.g. **thyroiditis**).

Other indications for isotope scan are:

- To identify ectopic thyroid tissue.
- To identify recurrence and metastases in thyroid carcinoma.

Q 27. What is the isotope of choice for diagnostic scanning of the thyroid?

- **^{99m}Tc** is the isotope of choice for diagnostic purposes. It is cheap and the radiation is less than radioiodine. Twenty minutes after intravenous injection of ^{99m}Tc, scanning is done over the thyroid.
- If radioactive iodine is used ^{123}I is the isotope of choice for diagnostic purposes.

Q 28. What is the half-life of the various radioisotopes used in thyroid?

Isotope	*Half life*	*Route*	*Rays*	*Comment*
^{123}I	13 hours	Oral	Gamma rays	Will not detect nodules < 1 cm size
^{131}I	8 days	Oral	Gamma and beta rays	**Too much irradiation if used for diagnostic scanning**
^{132}I	2.3 hours	Oral	Gamma and beta rays	Not used for clinical purposes
^{99}Tc	6 hours	IV	Gamma rays	Commonly used for diagnostic scanning of thyroid

Q 29. What is the problem with technetium scanning?

Carcinoma concentrates technetium and therefore a hot nodule need not necessarily be benign.

Q 30. What is discordant scan?

A nodule which is warm on technetium scanning and cold on radioiodine scanning is called discordant scan. This is suggestive of malignancy.

Q 31. Why technetium is preferred over radio-iodine for diagnostic scanning?

It gives small amount of radiation and you get the image within minutes.

Q 32. What will be the appearance in scintigraphy in primary, secondary and toxic nodule?

- *Primary*: Uniform diffuse increased uptake (Fig. 1.1).
- *Secondary:* Heterogeneous pattern with some focal areas of enhanced uptake (Fig. 1.2).
- *Toxic nodule:* Increased uptake only in the nodule, with no uptake in the surrounding thyroid tissue (Fig. 1.3).

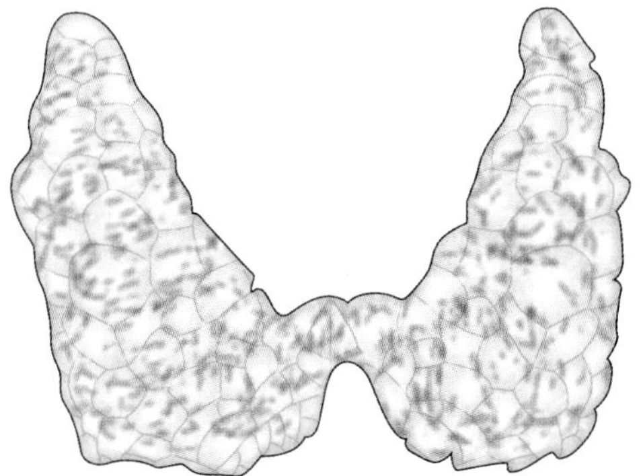

Fig. 1.1: Primary toxicosis

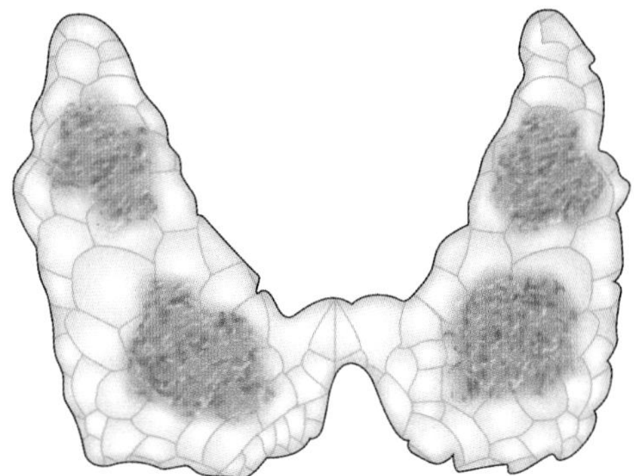

Fig. 1.2: Secondary toxicosis

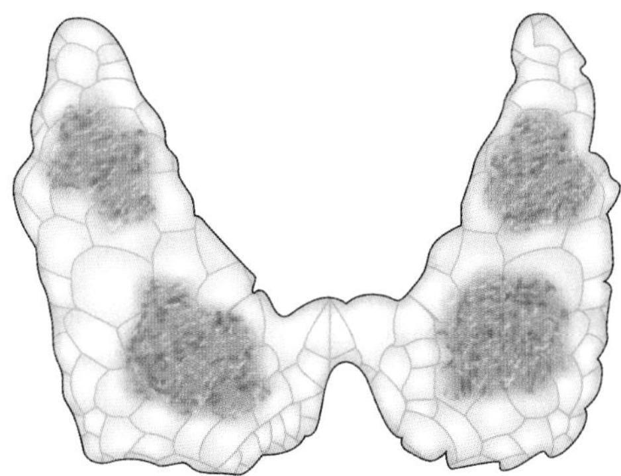

Fig. 1.3: Toxic nodule

Q 33. What are the toxic situations where there is decreased uptake of isotope in thyroid gland?

Low uptake is seen in:

- Thyroiditis
- Postpartum thyrotoxicosis
- Struma ovarii
- Factitious thyrotoxicosis
- Jod-Basedow thyrotoxicosis.

Q 34. What are the features of toxic adenoma?

Toxic Adenoma

- These are: Benign, monoclonal thyroid tumors of more than 3 cm size
- Are autonomous rather than responding to TSH stimulation
- Eye signs and other stigmata of Graves' are absent
- Somatic mutation of **TSH receptor gene** or **G protein gene** is present
- T_4 may be normal (hence check T_3 levels).

Q 35. What are the conditions in which Thyroid Binding Globulins (TBG) are increased?

The concentrations of TBG are increased in pregnancy, liver diseases and where there is hyperestrogenism. The levels of free T_3 and T_4 in these conditions are normal despite high TBG.

Q 36. What are the conditions in which the TBG levels are decreased?

High androgens, severe hypoproteinemia, chronic liver disease and acromegaly.

Q 37. What is the problem with the measurement of free T_3 and T_4?

The method usually used is radioimmunoassay and it is costly.

Q 38. What is the normal free T_3 and T_4 value?

Free T_3—3.5 to 7.5 pmol/L

Free T_4—10 – 30 nmol/L

It is to be noted that 0.3% of the total T_3 and 0.03% of the total T_4 are free and physiologically active.

Q 39. What is T_3 Thyrotoxicosis?

T_3 alone is raised and TSH is decreased in this condition.

Q 40. What is subclinical hyperthyroidism?

- Seen in 1% of hyperthyroids
- Serum TSH is low but the free T_4 is normal
- Symptoms are absent and hence called 'sub-clinical'.

Q 41. What is apathetic hyperthyroidism (masked)? (PG)

Apathetic hyperthyroidism

- Lack almost all of the clinical manifestations
- Presents as behavior problems
- May end up at the psychiatrist's
- Thyroid gland is not usually enlarged
- Commonly seen in elderly patients
- Decreased appetite and lethargy
- New onset of atrial fibrillation and increased angina.

Q 42. Is there any role for FNAC in thyrotoxicosis?

Yes. Sometimes the thyrotoxicosis may be associated with a papillary carcinoma of the thyroid. It is better to do after controlling toxicosis because of the increased vascularity of the gland.

Q 43. How you will manage thyrotoxicosis?

In primary thyrotoxicosis we have 3 options.

1. Antithyroid drugs
2. Radioiodine therapy
3. Surgery.

Q 44. What will be the choice of therapeutic agent in thyrotoxicosis?

We have some **broad guidelines.** This must be modified according to the facilities available and wishes of the patient.

Age over 25 years – Radioiodine therapy (when development is complete)

Under 25 years – Surgery for large goiter
– **Antithyroid drugs for the small goiter**

Toxic nodular goiter usually will not respond very well to radioiodine and antithyroid drugs. **Therefore, surgery is the treatment of choice.**

Q 45. What are the drugs available for the treatment?

Drugs available for the treatment of thyrotoxicosis
a. *Thionamides* • Carbimazole (Neomercazole) Dose 40 – 60 mg daily for first 3 weeks, 20 – 40 mg daily for 4 – 8 weeks, Maintenance of 5 – 20 mg/daily for 18 – 24 months (each tablet is 5 mg) • Propylthiouracil **(PTU)** • Methimazole 20 – 30 mg daily (single dose) b. *Beta blockers* c. *Potassium per chlorate* inhibits iodide transport d. *Lugol's iodine* e. *Iopanoic acid*—500 mg bid *Severe cases unresponsive to conventional therapy* f. *Lithium carbonate* – 300 mg 6th hourly g. *Guanethidine* 30 – 40 mg oral 6th hourly h. *Reserpine* 2.5 – 5 mg IM 4th hourly i. *Glucocorticoids:* **dexamethasone** 2 mg oral 6th hourly.

Q 46. What is the dose of Propylthiouracil?

About 100 to 300 mg 3 times daily orally initially for 4 to 6 weeks followed by 100 mg 3 times daily.

Q 47. What is the action of Propylthiouracil?

a. PTU blocks conversion of T_4 to T_3 in periphery (liver)
b. Inhibits iodine organification and coupling of iodotyrosines
c. Immunomodulatory effects that reduces thyroid stimulating antibodies.

Q 48. What are the advantages of PTU?

a. PTU may be given during **pregnancy** at reduced doses.
b. If thyroidectomy is required in **second trimester,** the patient can be prepared with PTU.
c. Useful for the treatment of **thyroid storm** (multiple doses needed).

Q 49. What are the adverse effects of PTU? (PG)

Adverse effects of PTU
• Hepatotoxicity which is not dose related • Mild transaminase elevation in 30% • Agranulocytosis • Minor side effects as seen in carbimazole therapy • Antineutrophilic cytoplasmic antibody (ANCA) in 20% especially with long-term treatment.

Q 50. What is the action of carbimazole?

Carbimazole acts by the following methods:

a. Blockage of organic binding and oxidation of iodine
b. Immunosuppression (decreases thyroid antigen, prostaglandin and cytokine release)
c. Reduction of thyroid autoantibody titers.

Q 51. What are the side effects of carbimazole?

Side effects of carbimazole
• Fever, rash, urticaria and arthralgia (**minor side effects**) • Liver dysfunction • Neuritis • Myalgia • Lymphadenopathy • Psychosis • Occasional agranulocytosis (< 1 in 200 cases).

Q 52. What is the clinical manifestation of agranulocytosis?

Agranulocytosis presents as sore throat, which warrants immediate cessation of the drug.

Q 53. Can the thyroid be enlarged during medical treatment?

Yes. During treatment in 1/3rd to half of the patients, the thyroid will shrink. Enlargement usually occurs because of commencement of hypothyroidism, which should be avoided.

Q 54. What is "block and replacement" regime?

The thyroid enlargement because of the development of hypothyroidism during medical treatment is prevented by supplementing **low dose of levothyroxine (0.1 mg) along with the antithyroid drugs.**

Q 55. In what percentage of patients is medical treatment effective?

Permanent remission is possible only in a small minority of adults and 20% of children.

Q 56. What is the dose of beta blocker?

Propranolol is the drug of choice for initial control of adrenergic symptoms.

- The dose is 20 – 80 mg every 6 – 8 hours orally.
- 1 – 2 mg IV propranolol for thyroid storm.

Q 57. What is the action of propranolol?

a. Peripheral conversion of $T_4 - T_3$ is blocked
b. Adrenergic antagonistic action helps to alleviate cardiac symptoms, tremor, etc.

Contraindications for propranolol

- Bronchial asthma
- COPD
- Heart block
- CCF.

Q 58. Is propranolol indicated in all patients with toxicity?

No;

- It is given for emergency surgical management of toxicity
- It is also used for control of the adrenergic symptoms.

Q 59. If the patient was prepared using propranolol before thyroid surgery, how long should it be continued postoperatively?

Propranolol should be given over a period of 1 week and preferably tapered over a period of 2 weeks after surgery.

Q 60. What are the drugs inhibiting peripheral conversion of T_4-T_3? (PG)

Drugs inhibiting peripheral conversion of T_4-T_3

- Beta blockers
- PTU
- Glucocorticoids
- Iopanoic acid.

Q 61. What is the minimum duration of medical treatment required before surgery?

Thyroidectomy performed immediately after control of thyrotoxicosis is associated with risk of thyroid crisis and it is preferable to wait approximately **two months until after a patient is euthyroid.**

Q 62. Is there any role for Dexamethasone in the management of thyrotoxicosis? (PG)

- It is used for the management of thyrotoxic crisis
- Dose is 2 mg every 6th hourly (injection)
- The actions are:
  a. Inhibits glandular secretion of hormone
  b. Inhibits peripheral conversion of T_4 to T_3
  c. Immunosuppression.

Q 63. What is Lugol's iodine and what is its dose?

Five percent iodine in 10% potassium iodide is called Lugol's iodine.

The dose is 10 drops in a glass of water 3 times daily for 10 days.

Q 64. What are the actions of Lugol's iodine?

a. Decreases the vascularity of the gland
b. Makes the thyroid firm and less friable (helps in surgical removal)
c. Prevents the release of hormone from the gland—**thyroid constipation.**

Q 65. What will happen if Lugol's iodine is given for more than 10 days?

After 2 weeks the effect of **Lugol's iodine** therapy is lost due to the so called **thyroid escape** from iodine control.

Q 66. What are the indications for radioiodine therapy?

- Radioiodine (**^{131}I**) is usually given to patients above 45 years for primary thyrotoxicosis.
- Isotope facility must be available.

Q 67. What are the problems of radioiodine therapy? (PG)

Problems of radioiodine therapy
a. Indefinite follow-up is essential as the patient may develop hypothyroidism (75%)
b. Chance of permanent thyroid failure – 90% (hypo is more because of failure of cellular reproduction)
c. Theoretical possibility of genetic damage, leukemia, damage to fetus and carcinoma (no convincing evidence)
d. Takes 2 – 3 months for control of symptoms
e. Worsening of ophthalmopathy (especially in smokers) and dermatopathy
f. Mild anterior neck pain
g. Increased risk of benign tumors
h. Malignant transformation in young patients
i. May induced hyperparathyroidism.

Q 68. What are the contraindications of radio-iodine therapy?

Contraindications of radioiodine therapy
• Pregnancy
• Lactating mothers
• Women desiring pregnancy within 1 year
• Children/adolescents (relative).

Q 69. What is the dose of radioiodine? (PG)

300 to 600 MBq, if there is no clinical improvement after 12 weeks further dose is given. Two or more doses are necessary in 20 to 30% of cases.

Q 70. What is the method of radioiodine treatment for toxicity? (PG)

a. Make the patient euthyroid with drugs
b. Discontinue drugs for 5 days
c. Administer ^{131}I 300–600 MBq (5–10 mCi)
d. Start antithyroid drugs after 1 week and continue for 6 to 8 weeks
e. After 12 weeks, if there is no improvement, give another dose of radioiodine
f. Two or more doses of radioiodine may be required.

Q 71. What are the indications for surgery in thyrotoxicosis? (PG)

a. Intolerance or non-compliance with antithyroid drugs
b. Contraindications to radioiodine therapy
c. Graves' disease in children, adolescents and those who are under the age of 25 years
d. In women who are potential mothers
e. Large goiter
f. Persistent thyromegaly

Contd...

Contd...

g. If antithyroid medication is required for more than 2 years
h. Graves' with nodules
i. Ophthalmopathy
j. Pressure symptoms
k. Toxic MNG
l. Substernal goiter
m. Amiodarone induced thyrotoxicosis.

Q 72. What are the drugs used for preparation of a patient for "urgent thyroidectomy"? (PG)

Combination of oral iopanoic acid 500 mg bid and dexamethasone 1 mg bid and PTU or MMI and beta blockers for 5 to 7 days.

Q 73. What are the advantages of surgery? (PG)

Advantages of surgery

a. Surgery is effective in achieving euthyroid status in 95–97% of patients
b. Controls hyperthyroidism immediately
c. Hazards associated with radioiodine therapy are avoided
d. Surgery will provide **tissue for histology**
e. Surgery will remove **occult foci of malignancy**
f. Childbearing is immediately possible
g. Coexisting parathyroid carcinoma can be removed
h. Is a better treatment for **toxicity with ophthalmopathy**
i. No need for follow up because nodules are not left behind.

Q 74. What is the surgical treatment of primary thyrotoxicosis?

Near total thyroidectomy is now recommended as the treatment of choice.

Q 75. What is the recommended treatment for secondary thyrotoxicosis?

Surgery is preferred over radioiodine for secondary thyrotoxicosis because:

- It will not respond to radioiodine as most of the nodules may not take up radioiodine.
- Large and repeated doses of radioiodine may be required.

Q 76. What is the recommended treatment of toxic nodule?

Once the patient is made euthyroid, surgery in the form of **Hemithyroidectomy** will give permanent relief.

Q 77. What is subtotal (bilateral) thyroidectomy?

Two grams of thyroid remnant is kept on both sides and the rest of thyroid gland is removed in subtotal thyroidectomy.

Q 78. What is Hartley-Dunhill procedure?

Total lobectomy and isthmectomy on the affected side and 4 g remnant left on the contralateral (normal) side. This form of surgery is recommended by some authorities for the surgical management of toxic goiter.

Operation	*Part of thyroid removed*	*Indications*
Lobectomy	Removal of one lobe of thyroid	Solitary thyroid nodule
Hemithyroidectomy	Removal of one lobe and isthmus	• STN • Toxic nodule • Follicular neoplasm

Contd...

Contd...

Bilateral subtotal thyroidectomy (Fig. 1.4)	2 g of thyroid remnant is kept on both sides and the rest of the thyroid gland is removed	• Toxic goiter • Toxic nodular goiter • Multi nodular goiter (**Near total** is the preferred treatment for these conditions now)
Hartley-Dunhill procedure (Fig. 1.5)	Total lobectomy and isthmectomy on the affected side and 4 g remnant left on the contralateral side	Toxic goiter
Near total thyroidectomy	1 to 2 g remnant is left on the contralateral side of the lesion and the rest of the thyroid is removed	• Toxic goiter • MNG • Papillary carcinoma • Follicular carcinoma • Medullary carcinoma, etc.
Total thyroidectomy isthmusectomy/ isthmectomy	Entire gland is removed Removal of isthmus alone	Thyroid malignancy • Emergency decompression of trachea for anaplastic carcinoma • Biopsy for anaplastic carcinoma

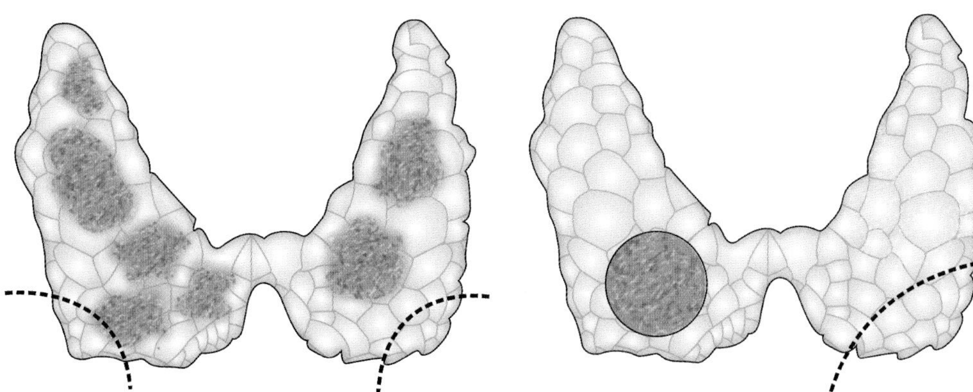

Fig. 1.4: Subtotal thyroidectomy

Fig. 1.5: Hartley-Dunhill procedure

Q 79. What is the management of intrathoracic goiter with toxicity? (PG)

- **Antithyroid drugs will increase the size** of the retrosternal and intrathoracic goiter and therefore dosage should be carefully adjusted.
- Surgery is the treatment of choice for intrathoracic goiter with toxicity.

Q 80. What is the management of intrathoracic toxic goiter in pregnancy? (PG)

- **Antithyroid drugs are given in small doses** in first trimester to prevent fetal goiter and airway obstruction
- Antithyroid drugs may be combined with propranolol and **surgery is done in the second trimester.**

Q 81. What is the treatment for recurrent toxicity? (PG)

Radioiodine/medical treatment.

Q 82. What are the preoperative preparations for thyroid surgery?

- Thyroidectomy is done only after making the patient euthyroid
- Lugol's iodine is given for a period of 10 days for reducing the vascularity and making the gland firm (for toxic cases only)
- Always send the patient for preoperative **indirect laryngoscopy (or video laryngoscopy)** to rule out occult vocal cord palsy and document for medicolegal purposes
- Arrange cross matched blood for vascular thyroids
- Assessment of the cardiac status by ECG
- Assessment of the chest by an **X-ray chest and X-ray neck AP view** (for **detecting tracheal displacement**) and lateral view (for detecting **luminal narrowing**). X-ray neck will also reveal **soft tissue shadows and calcifications.** X-ray chest may reveal the presence of **retrosternal extension**
- Rule out hypertension and diabetes mellitus.

Q 83. What are the preliminary steps of thyroid surgery?

- Surgery is done under general anesthesia using endotracheal intubation (preoperative X-ray neck to rule out displacement of the trachea and luminal narrowing).
- Position of the patient: Supine with sand bag behind the shoulders and head ring for adequate neck extension.
- Skin is painted with antiseptics and proper draping with sterile towels and head cover.
- **Kocher's collar incision** is used for incising the skin (1 to 2 cm above the manubrium sternum). Incision is deepened up to the deep fascia by incising the platysma.
- **Anterior jugular veins** seen on the surface of the investing layer, may be ligated (communicating vein seen connecting the two anterior jugulars requires ligation).
- **Investing layer** is opened vertically in the midline.
- The **strap muscles** are retracted laterally (in big thyroids, they may be divided either on one side or bilaterally in the upper part to save the Ansa hypoglossi nerves entering the strap muscles in the lower part)
- The **Pretracheal fascia** is incised vertically and the **thyroid gland is mobilized** by ligating the **middle thyroid vein** (this is the first vessel to be ligated).

Q 84. What are the essential steps of thyroidectomy?

A. *Identification of parathyroid glands:*
   - Identify the parathyroids before ligating the vessels.
   - Parathyroids have the color of peanut butter, each of 6 × 3 × 3 mm size and less than 40 mg weight.
   - The recurrent laryngeal nerve (RLN)—**Inferior thyroid artery junction** is critical in

identifying the parathyroids (this is a critical area of RLN injury as well).

- The superior parathyroid glands are **above and behind** this junction.
- The inferior parathyroid glands are **below and anterior to** this junction having variable positions. The inferior glands may be situated on the inferior pole of the thyroid, thyrothymic ligament, in the thymus or in the perithymic fat.

B. *Identification of the recurrent laryngeal nerve:*

- It is preferable to identify the entire course of the nerve in thyroid surgery.
- There is **no role** for the old axiom "nerve seen is nerve injured", which is called the 'ostrich philosophy'.
- The first identification is at the so-called **Riddle's triangle,** which is bound by **inferior thyroid artery** above, the **carotid artery** laterally and the trachea medially.
- From there, the **nerve is traced upwards** to the point of its entry into the larynx at the greater cornu of the thyroid cartilage.
- Before entry, the nerve may divide into two or more extralaryngeal branches.
- When there is difficulty in identifying the RLN, the entry point of the nerve can be located by identifying Zuckerkandl's tubercle.
- The nerve may cross the inferior thyroid artery usually deep to the artery, sometimes superficial or may even pass through the fork of the branches of the artery.

C. *Ligation of vessels:*

- The branches of the **superior thyroid vessels** are individually **skeletonized** and ligated as close to the superior pole as possible after identifying the external branch of the **superior laryngeal nerve.**
- A medial approach to the superior pole via the **avascular space** between the cricothyroid muscle and the upper pole of the gland is ideal.
- **"Mass Ligation"** of the superior pole is to be avoided.
- *Capsular ligation of the inferior thyroid artery:*
  a. Inferior thyroid artery is an end artery to the parathyroids and hence ligation of the trunk of the inferior thyroid artery is not recommended.
  b. The small branches entering the capsule of the gland alone are ligated, thereby preserving the blood supply to the parathyroids.
  c. These small branches are therefore situated between the parathyroid and the thyroid gland
     - Finally, the lower pole veins are ligated. Blind "mass ligation" of the lower pole may injure the RLN in this situation.

D. *Removal of the gland:*

- The gland is now free for removal. Depending on the type of surgery, the extent of removal and the amount of remainder may be decided (see box on various operations of thyroid gland in page 38).
- Beware of the **suspensory ligament of Berry,** which is the last attachment of the gland to the cricoid cartilage.
- The RLN may pass through the substance, superficial or deep to the Berry's ligament.
- **Take care of the nerve** before the final removal of the gland.

Q 85. What are the critical areas of recurrent laryngeal nerve injury? (PG)

There are 3 critical areas of RLN injury:

- At the site of where the inferior thyroid artery crosses the RLN.

- At the region of the suspensory ligament of Berry.
- At the lower pole of the gland during 'mass ligation' of the vessels of the inferior pole, especially on the right side (Fig. 1.6).

Q 86. What is Zuckerkandl's tubercle? PG)

- It is the posterior extension of the lateral lobes of the thyroid gland near the ligament of Berry.
- It is found in 14–55% of cases.

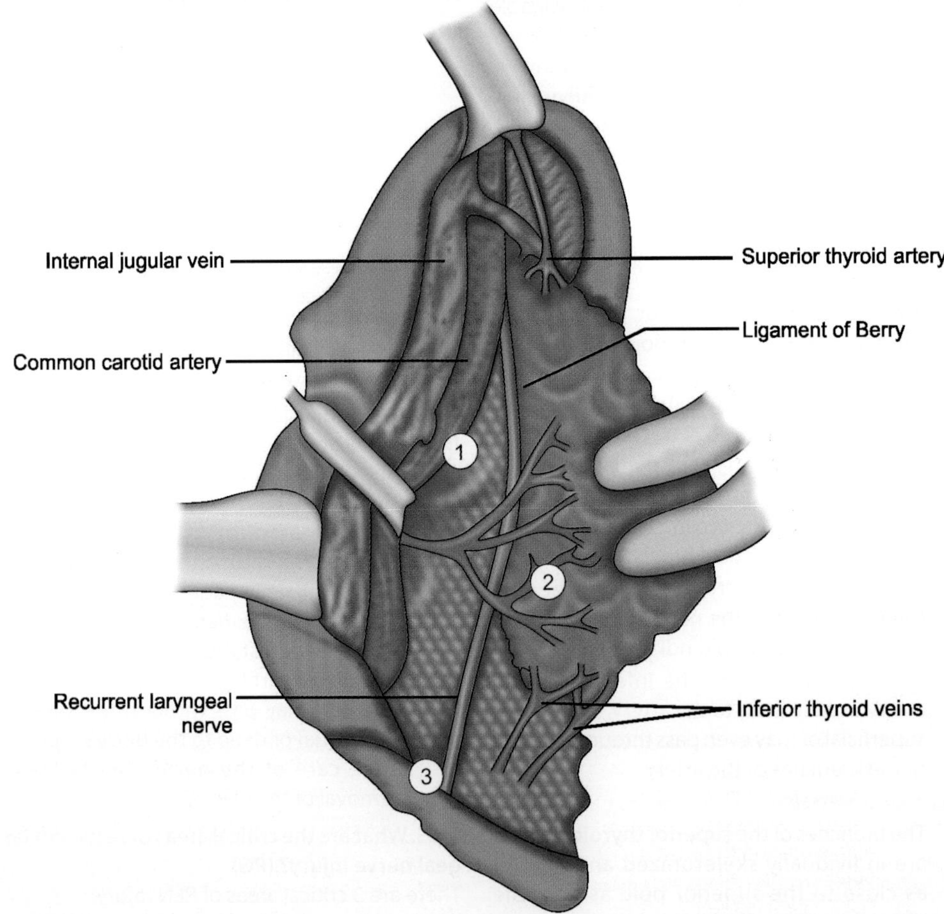

Fig. 1.6: Recurrent laryngeal nerve injury—critical sites

- The RLN runs cranially in a fissure between the Zuckerkandl's tubercle and the main body of the gland or the tracheal surface.
- The RLN may have a sharp angle beneath the tubercle.
- The nerve is so constantly related to this tubercle, that it is often called "**an arrow pointing to the RLN.**"

Q 87. What is non-recurrent laryngeal nerve?

- This is seen on the right side as a result of failure of development of the 4th aortic arch.
- The RLN here may arise as a branch from the vagus at the level of the inferior horn of the thyroid cartilage (instead of going down, curving around the subclavian artery and coming up).
- The incidence is **0.2 – 0.5%**.

Q 88. What is suspensory ligament of Berry?

- It is nothing but a condensation of the pretracheal fascia attaching the thyroid gland to the cricoid.
- The two ligaments on either side form a sling anchoring the gland to the larynx.
- It must be severed before the gland can be removed.
- The RLN is in immediate contact with the back of the ligament.

Q 89. What are the complications of thyroidectomy?

Complications of thyroidectomy can be classified as

A. *Metabolic*
   1. *Hypoparathyroidism*
      - Temporary Hypoparathyroidism
      - Temporary hypocalcemia without hypoparathyroidism (**'hungry bone' syndrome**)
      - Permanent hypoparathyroidism (ischemia and removal of the gland)
      - Spurious hypoparathyroidism (total calcium is decreased but ionized calcium is normal)

Contd...

Contd...

   2. *Thyroid storm (thyrotoxic crisis)*
   3. *Hypothyroidism* (20 – 40%)

B. *Non metabolic*
   1. *Neural:*
      - RLN injuries
      - External laryngeal nerve injuries
   2. *Nonneural:*
      - Hemorrhage
      - Hematoma
      - Stridor and airway obstruction
      - Skin flap necrosis
      - Compromise of tracheoesophageal blood supply
      - Horner's syndrome (sympathetic nerve injury)
      - Chylous fistula (extremely rare).

Q 90. What are the two most important complications of thyroidectomy?

1. Hypoparathyroidism
2. Recurrent laryngeal nerve injury.

Note: The incidence of both should be less than 1% for an experienced thyroid surgeon.

Q 91. What are the clinical manifestations of hypoparathyroidism?

Clinical manifestations of hypoparathyroidism

- Acral paresthesia
- Circumoral tingling numbness and paresthesia
- Anxiety
- Carpopedal spasm
- Laryngeal stridor
- Spasm of respiratory muscles: dread of suffocation
- Convulsions in later stages
- Blurring of vision due to spasm of intraocular muscles
- Prolonged unrectified tetany can give rise to cataracts.

Note: These clinical manifestations can occur on the same day of surgery or may be noticed later on.

Q 92. What will be the biochemical finding in hypoparathyroidism?

- Decrease in calcium and increase in phosphorus is the feature of hypoparathyroidism.
- Decrease in calcium with a decrease in phosphorus is suggestive of "hungry bone" syndrome.

Q 93. What is Chvostek sign?

With a **knee hammer,** gently tap the **facial nerve** as it courses in front of the external auditory meatus. When tetany (as a result of hyperparathyroidism) exists, the tapping of the hyperexcitable nerve provokes a **brisk muscular** twitch on the same side of the face.

Q 94. What is Trousseau's sign?

A **sphygmomanometer** cuff is placed around the arm and the pressure is raised to **200 mm of Hg**. If tetany is present, in **5 minutes**, typical contractions of the hand are seen: the fingers are extended except at the metacarpophalangeal joints and the thumb is strongly adducted, the combined effect of which is to produce the so-called **obstetrician's hand (accoucheur's hand).**

Note: The migratory superficial thrombophlebitis is also called **Trousseau's sign** (seen in visceral malignancies and TAO).

Q 95. What is carpopedal spasm?

Strong adduction of the thumb is always present in tetany and this when coupled with extension of the feet is called "**Carpopedal spasm**".

Q 96. What is spurious hypocalcemia? (PG)

- Decrease in **total calcium, albumin** and **hematocrit** are seen in first two postoperative days following any surgery including nonthyroid.
- This is as a result of **antidiuretic hormone release** from general stress of the surgery and the consequent **water retention** by kidneys and **hemodilution.**
- The **albumin-bound total calcium** is decreased as a result of this.
- The **nonprotein bound free (ionized) calcium** will be normal in this situation and therefore estimation of the **free calcium** is important to distinguish spurious hypocalcemia from true hypocalcemia.

Q 97. How can you prevent hypoparathyroidism?

It is prevented by taking the following precautions during surgery:

- Identification of parathyroids preoperatively
- Protection of blood supply to parathyroid glands
- Capsular ligation of inferior thyroid vessels
- Autotransplantation of parathyroids in an event of inadvertent removal.

Q 98. What is the treatment of hypoparathyroidism? (PG)

A. *Emergency:* 20 mL of 10% **calcium gluconate** IV in 100 mL of D5W over 10 – 15 minutes

B. *Chronic Patient:*
   - **Calcium alone is not enough for the management of** hypoparathyroidism.
   - **Calcium carbonate** 500 mg oral tablets (1.5 to 2.5 g per day).
   - **Vitamin D** (ergocalciferol) 50 – 100,000 units per day or **dihydrotachysterol** (DHT) 250 – 1000 micrograms daily.
   - **Magnesium** parenteral IV/IM 0.5g (4 mEq) and 2 to 4 mEq per Kg body weight over 3–5 days. **Magnesium gluconate** oral 500 mg tablets.

Note: If true hypocalcemia is identified, it is better to treat it pre-emptively rather than to wait for the symptoms.

Q 99. Can the patient get recurrent thyrotoxicosis after surgery? (PG)

Yes, in 5% of cases. Cure is possible if the thyroid tissue can be reduced below a critical mass. This will result in reduction of TSAb. When the mass of thyroid tissue is small it can produce only limited hypertrophy and hyperplasia even if the circulating TSAb is high.

Q 100. What are the causes for stridor post-operatively?

Causes of post-thyroidectomy stridor

a. Hematoma (rule out hematoma first by change of dressing)
b. Laryngeal edema—three causes
   1. Edema because of intubation
   2. Edema because of hematoma
   3. Edema because of hypothyroidism as a result of aggressive antithyroid drug therapy
c. Recurrent laryngeal nerve injury.

Q 101. What are the clinical manifestations of RLN injury?

The most common manifestation is **hoarseness.** The other manifestations are:

- Dysphonia
- Paralytic aphonia
- Periodic aspiration
- Ineffective cough.

Note:

- Unilateral RLN palsy is well-compensated normally
- Normal voice does not mean that the nerve is intact
- All hoarseness are not because of nerve injury either.

Q 102. What is the indirect laryngoscopy finding in unilateral RLN palsy? (PG)

- Paramedian position of the paralyzed cord
- Hyperadduction of the normal cord during phonation as compensation.

Q 103. Is there any role for routine post-operative indirect laryngoscopy? (PG)

- **Early routine indirect laryngoscopy** is done on fourth or fifth day.
- Cord paralysis is more common than supposed.
- Asymptomatic bilateral vocal cord paralysis is possible.

Q 104. What is the treatment of unilateral RLN palsy? (PG)

- Symptomatic improvement is seen within 6 weeks.
- Perioperative steroids are given to reduce the incidence of temporary RLN palsy resulting from edema or contusion.
- **Steroids should be started within 7 days** of surgery.
- **Prednisolone** 15 mg tid for 10 days is given.
- Gradually taper the dose to zero over the next 10 days.
- If there is not any recovery within 6 months, degeneration is to be suspected (recovery may be delayed for 6 – 12 months; no regeneration after 18 months).
- **Speech therapy** is instituted if there is no recovery.
- **Medialization of the cord** by Teflon injection or some other technique.

Q 105. What are the clinical presentations and treatment of bilateral RLN palsy? (PG)

- This will cause paralysis in adduction
- Clinically this may go undetected for long periods.
- Patient may tolerate minimal airway for many years.
- May present as inspiratory stridor, dyspnea, or minimal dysphonia.
- Emergency **endotracheal intubation** may be required.
- It is better to do **tracheostomy** and wait for **1 year** (valved tracheostomy tubes are available).
- **Arytenoidopexy, cordectomy or endoscopic laser treatment** is done after 18 months.

Q 106. What is the innervation of external laryngeal nerve (a branch of superior laryngeal nerve)?

The nerve supplies the **cricothyroid muscle,** which is a **tensor of the vocal cord.**

Q 107. What is the clinical presentation of unilateral external laryngeal nerve injury?

Clinical presentation:

- Loss of high pitch for the voice
- Voice fatigue
- Breathy voice
- Frequent throat clearing.

Indirect laryngoscopy will reveal:

- Shorter and hyperemic vocal cord
- The affected vocal cord will be at a lower level
- The glottic chink is oblique (rotation of the posterior commissure to the paralyzed side).

Q 108. What is thyrotoxic crisis (thyroid storm)?

It is a sudden life-threatening exacerbation of thyrotoxicosis seen in 1 to 2% of patients. This is a syndrome manifested by high grade fever, sweating, tachypnea, hyperventilation, tachycardia, palpitation, restlessness, tremor, psychosis, delirium, diarrhea, dehydration, nausea, vomiting, hypotension and end-stage coma. The causes for crisis are:

a. Inadequate preparation prior to surgery
b. Infection in thyrotoxicosis
c. Trauma in thyrotoxicosis
d. Pre-eclampsia
e. Diabetic ketoacidosis
f. Surgical emergency
g. Emotional stress
h. Vigorous palpation of the gland.

Q 109. What is Bayley's symptom complex?

Bayley's symptom complex of thyroid storm

a. Insomnia
b. Anorexia
c. Vomiting
d. Diarrhea
e. Diaphoresis
f. Emotional instability
g. Temperature > 38°C
h. Tachycardia
i. Accentuated symptoms and signs of toxicosis
j. System dysfunction.

Q 110. What is the treatment of thyroid storm?

Treatment of thyroid storm

1. *To control fever:*
   - Acetaminophen is used
   - Aspirin is never used as it can elevate the free thyroid hormones
   - Tepid sponging
   - Cooling blankets
2. *To correct dehydration and electrolyte imbalance:*
   - IV fluids
3. *To control the heart rate:*
   a. Propranalol 1–2 mg IV 6th hourly (40–80 mg QID) orally)
   b. Esmolol 250 – 500 microgram per Kg body weight loading and 50 microgram/Kg/minute maintenance
4. *To inhibit hormone release:*
   a. Logols' iodine 10 drops 3 times
   b. Sodium iodide 1gm IV over 24 hours
   c. Super saturated potassium iodide (SSKI) 10 drops twice daily
5. *To inhibit new hormone synthesis:*
   a. Propylthiouracil (50–200 mg)
   b. Carbimazole (20 mg every 4 hours)

Contd...

Contd...

In case of adverse reaction to PTU or carbimazole, use lithium carbonate 300 mg every 6th hours

6. *To reduce systemic symptoms:*
   a. Hydrocortisone 100mg IV 6th hourly
   b. Dexamethasone injection 6–8 mg IV or 2 mg orally 6th hourly
7. *Treatment of CCF*
8. *Antibiotic coverage for infection*
9. *Sedation*
10. *Dialysis if required.*

Q 111. What are the methods available to remove T_3 and T_4 from serum? (PG)

a. Oral cholestyramine
b. Peritoneal dialysis
c. Hemoperfusion.

Q 112. What is the treatment of thyrotoxicosis in pregnancy? (PG)

- **Radioiodine is absolutely contraindicated** because of the risk to the fetus.
- The antithyroid drugs and TSH **cross the placenta** and therefore the baby is born goitrous and hypothyroid.
- Low dose antithyroid drugs, preferably **PTU is the ideal treatment** (to keep the free T_4 of pregnant women in the high normal.
- **Avoid methimazole:** Associated with cutis aplasia, and esophageal and choanal atresia.
- The danger of surgery is **miscarriage**.
- Surgery can be carried out in the **second trimester.**

Q 113. What is the treatment of hyperthyroidism during lactation? (PG)

- Thionamides are secreted in breast milk and this was once considered a contraindication.
- PTU at a dose of 750 mg is safe.

Q 114. What is postpartum hyperthyroidism?(PG)

Pregnancy will lead onto exacerbation of autoimmune diseases. This may occur with previously diagnosed or undiagnosed hyperthyroidism. There is a strong association with **HLA-DR3** and **HLA-DR5** haplotypes.

Q 115. What is thyrotoxicosis factitia?

This is usually seen in health cranks as a result of oral intake of thyroxine usually taken to reduce weight).

Q 116. What is Jod-Basedow thyrotoxicosis?

Large doses of iodide given to hyperplastic endemic goiter which is iodine avid may produce temporary hyperthyroidism. This is Jod-Basedow thyrotoxicosis.

Q 117. What is neonatal thyrotoxicosis?

This is seen in babies born to hyperthyroid mothers. TSAb can cross the placental barrier. The hyperthyroidism gradually subsides after 3 to 4 weeks.

Q 118. What is thyrocardiac?

Severe cardiac damage wholly or partly due to hyperthyroidism. This is usually because of secondary thyrotoxicosis and is mild. This must be rapidly controlled with propranolol to prevent further cardiac damage.

Q 119. What is struma ovarii?

Teratoma of the ovaries may differentiate into thyroid tissue. This thyroid tissue becomes hyperactive resulting in mild thyrotoxicosis. T_3 and T_4 are raised with suppressed TSH. Radioactive iodine uptake (RAIU) in neck is suppressed and higher intake is seen in the pelvis.

Q 120. What is Hashitoxicosis? (PG)

- This is because of painless thyroiditis.
- This is an early stage of **autoimmune thyroiditis.**
- FNAC picture is that of Hashimoto's thyroiditis.

- Thyrotoxicosis in this situation is mild.
- Glandular enlargement is seen only in 60% of cases.
- The inflamed gland releases the already formed thyroid hormones into the bloodstream resulting in toxicosis.

Q 121. What is trophoblastic thyrotoxicosis?(PG)

The hCG from hydatidiform mole, choriocarcinoma and metastatic embryonal carcinoma exhibit cross specificity to thyroid stimulating hormone receptor (TSHR). This results in thyroid overactivity.

Q 122. What is the histopathological appearance of hyperthyroidism?

a. There is hyperplasia of the acini lined by high columnar epithelium.
b. The acini are empty and some of them contain vacuolated colloid **(Scalloping).**
c. Pseudopapillary formation is seen.

Q 123. What will happen to exophthalmos after surgery or radioiodine therapy?

Both will worsen ophthalmopathy. Thionamides will alleviate the eye problem through immuno-suppression.

Q 124. What is the management of exophthalmos (Thyroid Associated Ophthalmopathy)?

Symptom control:

a. Sleeping with head end elevation.
b. 1% methylcellulose eye drops to prevent corneal ulceration.
c. High dose prednisolone orally or hydrocortisone IV.
d. Collimated super voltage radiation to retro orbital space (needs expertise).

Note: Radioiodine is avoided in ophthalmopathy.

Q 125. Is there any role for surgery in exophthalmos?

Surgical removal of lateral wall or roof of orbit is done for decompression when optic nerve is in danger.

FOR PG'S—WHAT IS NEW?

1. Thyrotoxic periodic paralysis
   It is common in Asian population with thyrotoxicosis. It is seen in 1.9% of hyperthyroidism. It is usually seen in the third decade. It is a condition where there is weakness of the proximal muscles in the form of mild weakness to generalized flaccid paralysis with loss of deep tendon reflexes. It is precipitated by trauma, exposure to cold and after excessive ingestion of carbohydrate. Attacks are usually seen in night after a carbohydrate rich food. During attack the serum potassium will be in the range of 2.2 to 3.2 mEq. It is a metabolic abnormality of the cell membrane in hyperthyroid state with resultant shift of potassium to the intracellular position. There is associated decreased serum phosphate and magnesium. The treatment is by administering potassium. Propranolol is given to prevent periodic paralysis. Patient is given low carbohydrate diet. If patient requires diuretics, potassium sparing diuretics are given. The EMG will show myopathic pattern during attack. The ECG will show sinus tachycardia, increased PR interval and prolonged QTu interval.
2. Severe thyrotoxicosis—T_4 more than 21 mu/dL.

Case 2 Solitary Thyroid Nodule (STN-Nontoxic)

Case Capsule

A **40-year old male** patient presents with a swelling in the lower part of right side of the neck. There are **no symptoms of toxicity or hypothyroidism**. On examination, the patient has a **pulse rate of 70/minute**. There is **no tremor**. The swelling is seen on the right side of the neck and **moves with deglutition** but **without** any **movement with protrusion of the tongue**. The swelling is of about **4 × 3 cm size, firm** in consistency. The surface of the swelling is smooth. There is **no fixity** of the swelling. The **lower limit of the swelling is visible and palpable**. The trachea is shifted to the left side. The **left lobe** of the thyroid is **not palpable.** The carotids are normally felt. There are **no regional nodes.** There is no clinical evidence of toxicity. Examination of the oral cavity is normal. Examination of the skull is normal.

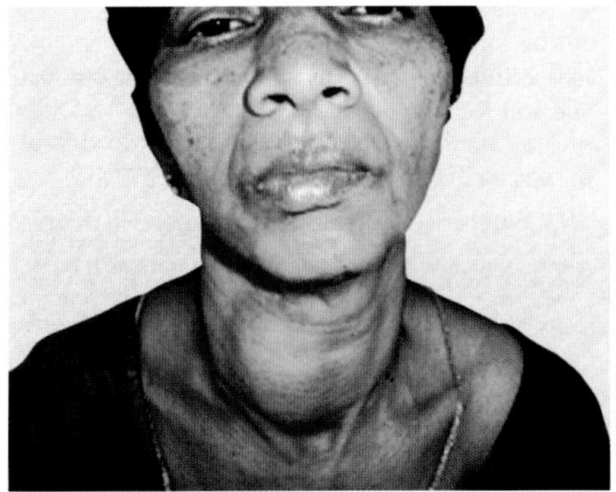

Dominant nodule

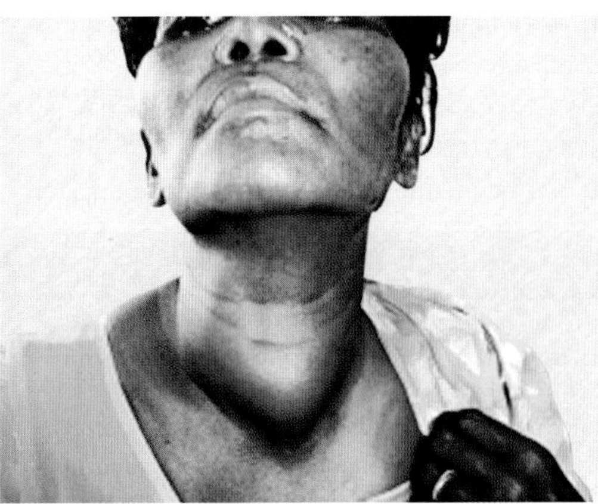

Solitary thyroid nodule

Q 1. What are your points in favor of solitary thyroid nodule?

Points in favor of Solitary Thyroid Nodule (STN):

a. There is only a single palpable thyroid nodule.
b. The rest of the gland is impalpable.

Q 2. What is the difference between a dominant nodule and solitary thyroid nodule?

A discrete swelling in a gland with clinical evidence of abnormality in the form of palpable contralateral lobe or generalized mild nodularity is called dominant nodule. As mentioned earlier, a discrete swelling in an otherwise impalpable gland is called **isolated or STN**. About 70% of the discrete thyroid swellings are STN and 30% are dominant nodules.

Q 3. What percentage of the so-called STN will ultimately become a dominant nodule of nodular goiter?

The true incidence of STN after USG/surgical exploration comes down to only 50%.

Q 4. What is the importance of STN?

The importance of STN lies in the risk of malignancy compared with other thyroid swellings.

Q 5. What percentages of STN prove to be malignant?

Twenty percent of STN prove to be malignant.

Q 6. What are the differential diagnoses of STN?

Differential diagnoses of STN		
a. Nodular goiter with dominant nodule	–	50%
b. Adenoma	–	20%
c. Cancer	–	20%
d. Thyroiditis	–	5%
e. Cyst	–	5%

Q 7. What is the most important single investigation for diagnosis in STN?

Because of the risk of neoplasia, the single most important investigation of choice is **fine needle aspiration cytology (FNAC)**.

Q 8. Can you differentiate a follicular carcinoma from follicular adenoma in FNAC?

FNAC cannot differentiate follicular adenoma from carcinoma. The distinction is dependent not on cytology but on histological criteria namely **capsular and vascular invasion.** The capsular and vascular invasion can only be identified on histology, which requires the thyroid tissue taken as paraffin block.

Q 9. What are the new techniques available for differentiating follicular carcinoma from adenoma in FNAC? (PG)

In future, FNAC differentiation may be possible by the following techniques:

a. Ploidy study of the DNA material: Polyploidy for benign and aneuploidy for carcinoma
b. Benign tumors are monoclonal and malignant tumors are polyclonal (monoclonal antibody **MOAB 47**)
c. Magnetic resonance spectroscopy
d. Thyroimmunoperoxidase estimation.

Q 10. What is the definition of 'adequate smear' in FNAC? (PG)

An adequate smear should have at least **six clusters** of cells each containing about **20 cells.**

Q 11. What are the possible FNAC reports in thyroid?

Possible FNAC reports in thyroid
a. Benign—abundant colloid and typical follicular cells.
b. Malignant
c. Indeterminate—little colloid and many follicular cells or Hurthle cells (Follicular neoplasm/ suspicious)
d. Inadequate—cystic lesions, degenerating adenomas.

Q 12. What is the classification of fine needle aspiration cytology?

Classification of fine needle aspiration cytology of thyroid	
Thy 1	Non-diagnostic
Thy 2	Non-neoplastic
Thy 3	Follicular
Thy 4	Suspicious of malignancy
Thy 5	Malignant

Q 13. What is the overall diagnostic accuracy of FNAC?

- The overall diagnostic accuracy is **about 95%**
- The diagnostic sensitivity of 83% and specificity of 92%.

Q 14. What are the conditions in which FNAC will give a definite diagnosis?

- Colloid nodule
- Thyroiditis
- Papillary carcinoma
- Medullary carcinoma
- Anaplastic carcinoma
- Lymphoma.

Q 15. Which institution was responsible for pioneering the technique of FNAC?

Karolinska Hospital, Sweden (they decide the Nobel Prize for Medicine).

Q 16. What is the minimum number of needle passes required in FNAC?

Minimum **6 passes**.

Q 17. What is the approach if the STN is cystic?

The FNAC is less reliable in cystic swellings. After aspirating cyst fluid, a further sample should be taken from the cyst wall for cytology.

Q 18. What will be the course of action if the cyst is recurring after aspiration?

A recurrent cyst should be removed surgically.

Q 19. What is the malignancy rate in cystic lesion?

Cystic lesions are less likely to be malignant. Malignancy rate in **complex cysts** is 72% and simple cyst is 7%.

Q 20. What are the indications for true cut (core) biopsy in thyroid?

It is useful in:

a. Anaplastic carcinoma
b. Lymphoma.

In these two situations, **true cut** biopsy can avoid an operation.

Q 21. What are the problems of a true cut (core) biopsy in thyroid?

- Poor patient compliance
- Pain
- Bleeding
- Tracheal injury
- Recurrent laryngeal nerve damage.

Q 22. What is the role of isotope scan in STN?

Routine isotope scanning has been abandoned in STN. When toxicity is associated with nodularity, isotope scanning is done to localize the area of hyperfunction.

Q 23. What are hot nodules, warm nodules and cold nodules?

A **hot nodule** 5% (**of which 5% of these are malignant**) is one that takes up isotope while the surrounding thyroid tissue does not. Here the surrounding thyroid tissue is inactive due to TSH suppression as a result of excess thyroid hormone (Fig. 2.1).

A **warm nodule** 10% (**of which 10% are malignant**) takes up isotopes along with normal thyroid tissue (Fig. 2.2).

A **cold nodule** 80% (**of which 20% are malignant**) is one where there is no isotope uptake (Fig. 2.3).

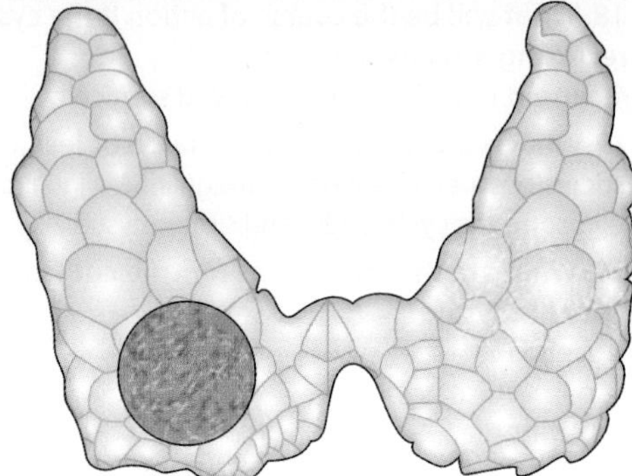

Fig. 2.1: Hot nodule

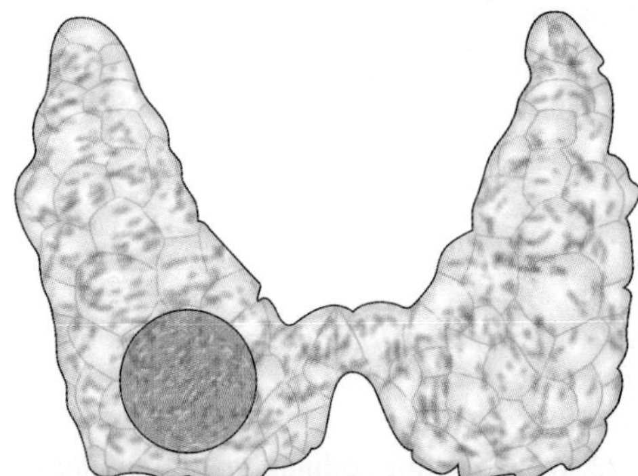

Fig. 2.2: Warm nodule

Q 24. What is the significance of a cold nodule and what are the differential diagnoses of cold nodule?

A **cold nodule** is more likely to be malignant. About 80% of the discrete nodules are cold but only 20% of the **cold nodules** are malignant. That means 80% of **cold nodules** are benign and therefore **cold nodule** as such is not an indication for surgery.

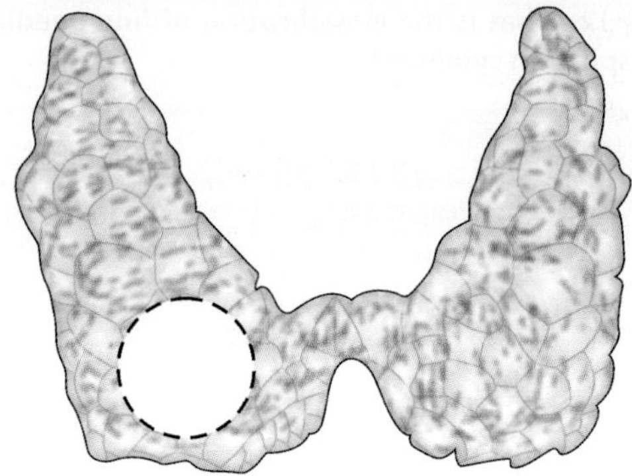

Fig. 2.3: Cold nodule

Differential diagnoses of cold nodule
1. Cyst
2. Hemorrhage
3. Benign adenomas
4. Malignancy
5. Thyroiditis.

Q 25. What is the role of ultrasonography in thyroid?

- Differentiate benign from malignant nodule
- The ultrasonography can demonstrate sub-clinical nodularity and identify deep non-palpable thyroid nodules
- Size of the nodule can be measured
- It can also differentiate solid from cystic swellings
- Sono guided FNAC can be done
- Identify cervical lymph nodes
- Identify multicentricity.

Q 26. Can you differentiate benign condition from malignancy in ultrasonography? (PG)

Yes, the differences between benign and malignant conditions in USG are given here in the table.

Benign	*Malignant*
1. Hyperechoic nodule	1. Hypoechoic
2. Significant cystic component	2. Need not be there
3. Peripheral egg shell like calcification	3. Microcalcifications inside
4. A sonolucent rim (halo) around the nodule	4. No halo
5. Well-defined nodule margin	5. Poorly defined margin
	6. Taller than wide lesion
	7. Increased central vascularity

Q 27. What are the differential diagnoses of thyroid cysts?

a. Colloid degeneration—50%
b. Involution of follicular adenoma
c. Malignancy—10–15%
d. Papillary carcinoma.

Q 28. What are the indications for surgery in STN?

Indications for surgery in STN
a. FNAC positive for malignancy
b. Follicular neoplasm
c. Clinical suspicion—hard texture, fixity, hoarseness, lymph node, male sex, etc.
d. Recurrence of a cyst after aspiration
e. Toxic adenoma
f. Pressure symptoms
g. Cosmesis

Q 29. When the FNAC report comes as follicular neoplasm. How will you proceed?

Follicular neoplasm may be **follicular adenoma** or **follicular carcinoma** and distinction is possible only on histology evidenced by **capsular** and **vascular invasion**. Majority (about 80%) of the follicular neoplasms are benign.

Q 30. What are the clinical situations in favor of malignancy?

Suspect malignancy in the following clinical situations
a. Discrete swelling in a **male** (more likely to be malignant)
b. **Child** with a thyroid nodule (50% malignant)
c. Extremes of age with discrete swelling (above 50 years and < 20 years teenagers)
d. **Hard** irregular swelling
e. **Fixity**
f. Recurrent laryngeal **nerve paralysis**
g. Lymph node
h. **Size > 4 cm**
i. History of **head and neck irradiation**
j. Association with other endocrine neoplasia (e.g. Multiple Endocrine Neoplasia—**MEN**).

Q 31. What are the causes for a hard thyroid nodule?

Causes of a hard thyroid nodule
a. Malignancy
b. Calcification—dystrophic
c. Thyroiditis
d. Hemorrhage into nodules.

Q 32. What is the meaning of follicular neoplasia?

- Follicular neoplasia **may be benign or malignant.**
- **80%** of follicular neoplasia are **benign** (20% are malignant) and therefore total thyroidectomy as a treatment is recommended only after getting the histopathology report.
- The pathologist can make a **cytological diagnosis** of a carcinoma only in the following situations:
  1. **Papillary thyroid carcinoma (PTC):** Orphan Annie eyed nucleus.
  2. **Medullary thyroid carcinoma (MTC):** Cell balls and amyloid stroma.
  3. Anaplastic carcinoma (difficulty in differentiating it from lymphoma) .
- Follicular carcinoma cannot be diagnosed by cytology.

Q 33. What is the minimum surgery for a case with FNAC report of follicular neoplasia when the STN is confined to one lobe of thyroid?

It is preferable to do a **hemithyroidectomy** on the side of the STN, i.e. removal of the affected lobe along with the isthmus. The minimum surgery should be a lobectomy.

Q 34. After hemithyroidectomy histopathology is reported as carcinoma (papillary carcinoma / follicular carcinoma), how will you proceed?

In this situation, **re-exploration** and **completion total thyroidectomy** is recommended in all patients so that further postoperative follow-up is possible.

Q 35. Why is re-exploration and completion thyroidectomy recommended in carcinoma thyroid?

a. In follicular carcinoma, the main **mode of spread** is by bloodstream. When a patient develops **metastases**, the treatment of **choice is radioiodine therapy**. If the remaining thyroid is not removed the iodine will be taken up by the remaining thyroid and metastases will not take up radioiodine. Therefore, it cannot be located and treated.

b. The **tumor marker** for **differentiated thyroid cancer** (Papillary and follicular carcinomas) is **thyroglobulin**. The thyroglobulin level as a tumor marker is significant only after total thyroidectomy. The thyroglobulin levels are elevated in **tumor bed recurrence** and **metastases** anywhere in the body.

c. **Multicentricity** and **intrathyroid spread** which are seen in papillary thyroid cancer can be tackled with re-exploration and completion thyroidectomy.

Q 36. What is the timing for completion thyroidectomy? **(PG)**

- It is better to do it as early as possible.
- The ideal timing would be **2 to 3 days** after the initial surgery.
- If this is not possible, do it after **12 weeks** of the initial surgery (it takes 12 weeks for the inflammatory response to settle).

Q 37. What is the treatment if the histopathology returns as papillary thyroid carcinoma (PTC)?

In this particular situation, patient may be categorized into low risk and high risk. In high risk group and in tumors of more than 1 cm, re-exploration and completion thyroidectomy is carried out. Tumor of less than 1cm is called **microcarcinoma** and follow-up is enough for such patients. Some surgeons routinely practice total thyroidectomy for such cases. (Please read the risk categorization in the topic carcinoma thyroid).

Flow chart for the management of solitary thyroid nodule depending on the four possible cytology reports

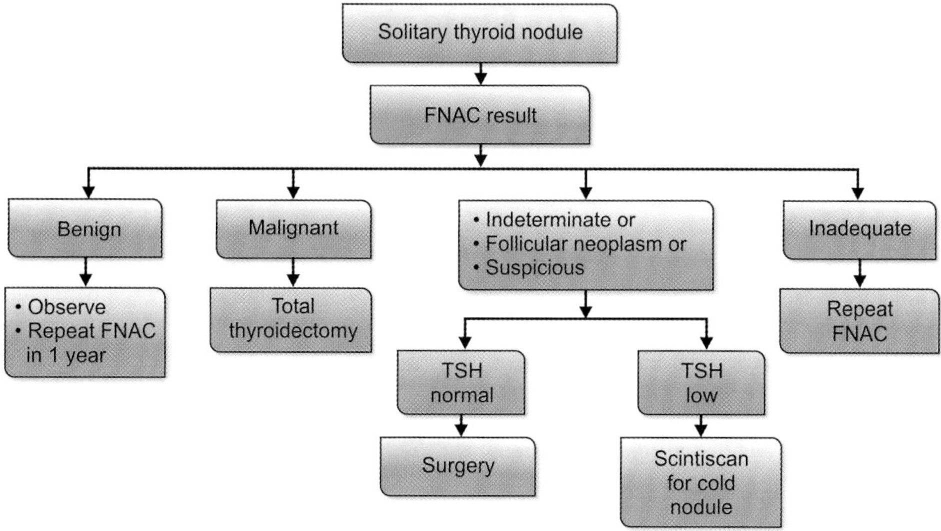

FOR PG'S—WHAT IS NEW?

- US guided FNAC is the most important investigation
- For indeterminate FNAC molecular markers are used to identify RAS and BRAF mutations, so also RET/PTC rearrangement
- More than 70% of papillary thyroid cancer have BRAF and RAS mutations
- Follicular lesion of undetermined significance (FLUS)—the risk of malignancy 10%.
- FLUS positive for BRAF or RAS—total thyroidectomy is indicated
- The immunohistochemical stains available for thyroid are:
  - Leukocyte common antigen (LCA)
  - HBME - 1
  - Galectin – III
  - Cytokeratin
  - Calcitonin—for medullary thyroid cancer
- The rate of cancer for 4 cm size nodule is 19%
- FDG PET avid thyroid nodule found incidentally deserves thorough work-up
- FNAC
  - Straw colored fluid—benign cyst
  - Clear watery fluid—parathyroid cyst
  - Hemorrhagic fluid—high risk of malignancy.

Case

3 Papillary Carcinoma Thyroid with Lymph Node Metastases

Case Capsule

A 45-year-old female patient **presents with a** swelling on the left side **of the front of the neck of** 5 years duration**. For the last 1 year there is** rapid increase in size. **There is** no history of radiation to the neck **or exposure to radiation in childhood. There is** no family history of goiter **or breast carcinoma. The patient is coming from an** endemic area. **There is** no history of hypertension, or diarrhea**. Patient complains of** hoarseness of voice **for the last 6 months. On examination there is a** hard irregular swelling **of about** 8 × 5 cm **size with distinct edges. It moves with deglutition, but not with protrusion of the tongue. There is** restriction of the lateral mobility **of the swelling. The** carotid arteries are displaced backwards **on the left side of the neck. There are** multiple lymph nodes **on the left side of the neck in the posterior triangle (Level 5). The lymph nodes move more easily in the transverse than vertical plane and do not move with swallowing.**

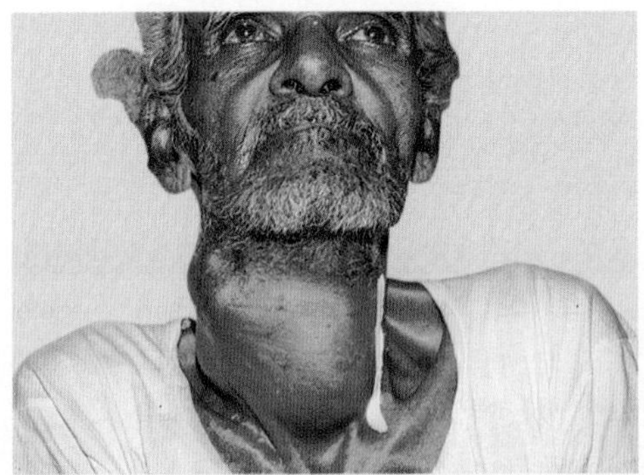

Anaplastic carcinoma thyroid

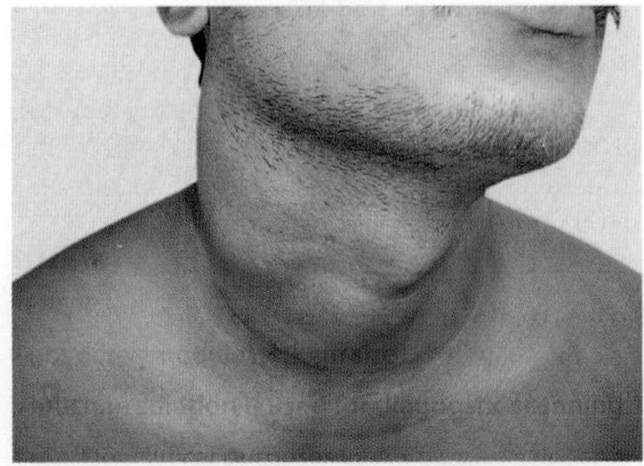

Carcinoma thyroid with metastatic node

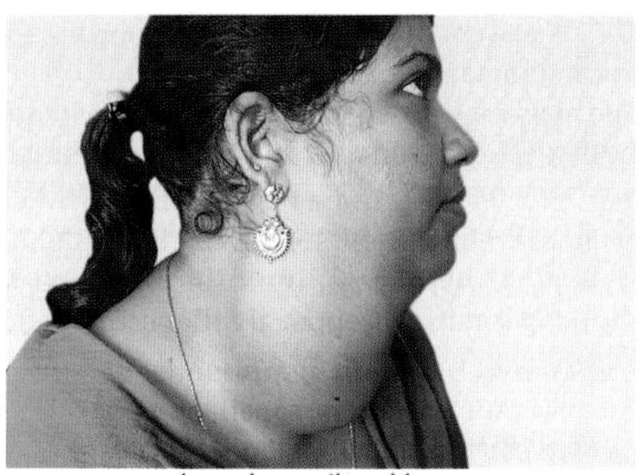
Lymphoma thyroid

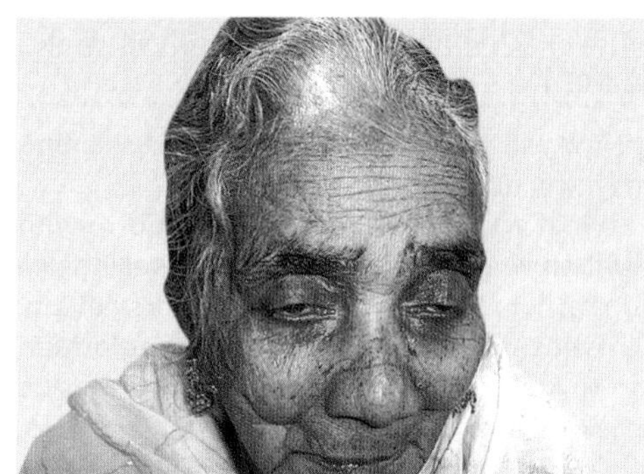
Metastases scalp from carcinoma thyroid

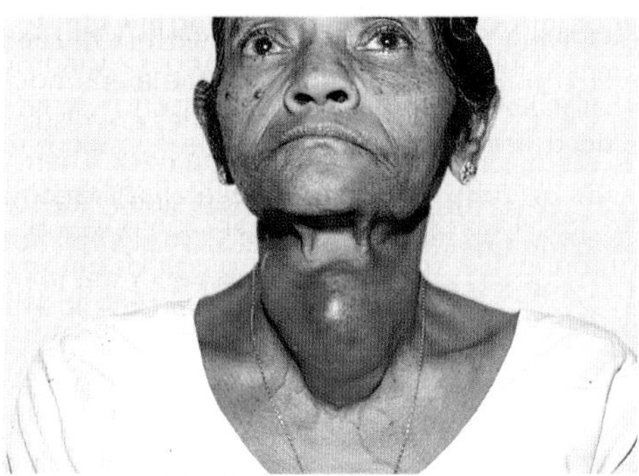
Papillary thyroid cancer

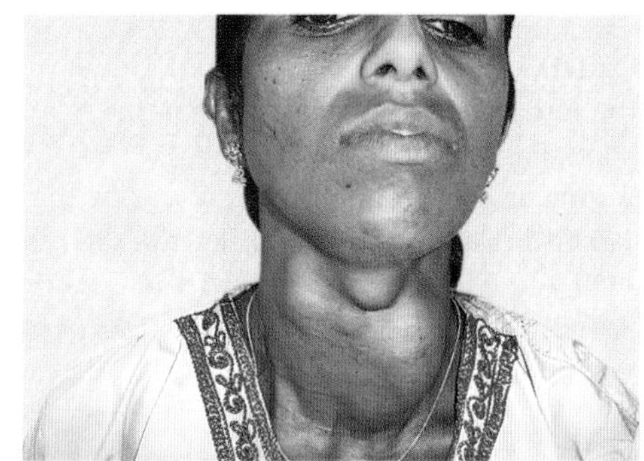
Recurrent carcinoma thyroid

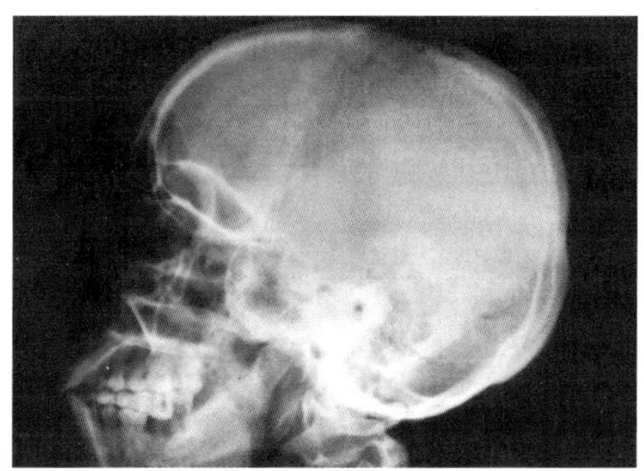
Skull metastases

Read the Preliminary Portion and Checklist of Case No: 1

Q 1. How will you differentiate thyroid swelling from lymph nodes of the neck?

The thyroid swelling will move up and down with deglutition whereas the lymph node swelling will not do so. **For all practical purposes any swelling, which is not moving up and down with deglutition is non-thyroidal, e.g. may be lymph nodes, may be neurofibroma or other solid and cystic swellings.**

Q 2. What are the diagnostic points favoring carcinoma thyroid in this case?

The diagnostic points are:

a. Hard thyroid nodule
b. The suspicious lymph nodes in the neck
c. Hoarseness of voice
d. Restriction of lateral mobility
e. Carotid displaced backwards on left side (Berry's Sign).

Q 3. What are the differential diagnoses of a hard thyroid nodule?

Differential diagnoses of a hard thyroid nodule are:

a. Calcification of a nodule of a nodular goiter
b. Carcinoma
c. Thyroiditis.

Q 4. How will you identify calcification of a thyroid nodule?

Simple plain X-ray of the neck will reveal calcification corresponding to the nodule.

Q 5. What type of calcification do you get in such cases?

The type of calcification is **dystrophic**.

Q 6. What is Delphic lymph node?

The **Delphic Lymph Node** is the first lymph node involved in carcinoma thyroid. It is nothing but the enlarged **prelaryngeal lymph node**.

Q 7. What is the importance of examining the scalp in carcinoma thyroid?

The main mode of spread of follicular carcinoma is by bloodstream and the most common metastases are bony metastases that are usually seen in the skull bone as a **pulsatile bony swelling**.

Q 8. What are the differential diagnoses of pulsatile bony swelling in the scalp?

The differential diagnoses are:

a. Primary malignancy—solitary plasmacytoma, telengiectatic variety of osteogenic sarcoma.
b. Metastases—from papillary carcinoma, renal cell carcinoma, etc.

Q 9. What are the types of carcinoma thyroid in which you get lymph node metastases?

1. Papillary carcinoma thyroid
2. Medullary carcinoma thyroid.

Q 10. What are the malignancies associated with autoimmune thyroiditis?

a. Lymphoma of thyroid
b. Papillary carcinoma thyroid.

Q 11. What is the most important investigation in this patient to confirm the diagnosis of carcinoma thyroid?

Fine needle aspiration cytology (FNAC) from thyroid nodule and FNAC or biopsy of the lymph node.

Q 12. Why FNAC or biopsy of lymph node?

The lymph node may harbor **another pathology like tuberculosis,** which can be proved or disproved by FNAC or lymph node biopsy. If the lymph node biopsy report is coming as metastases from papillary carcinoma, even if the thyroid is apparently normal one should carefully palpate the thyroid and **exclude a suspicious nodule.**

Q 13. What is the lymphatic drainage of thyroid?

The gland is drained by 2 sets of lymph vessels, ascending and descending. Each consists of medial and lateral channels (Fig. 3.1).

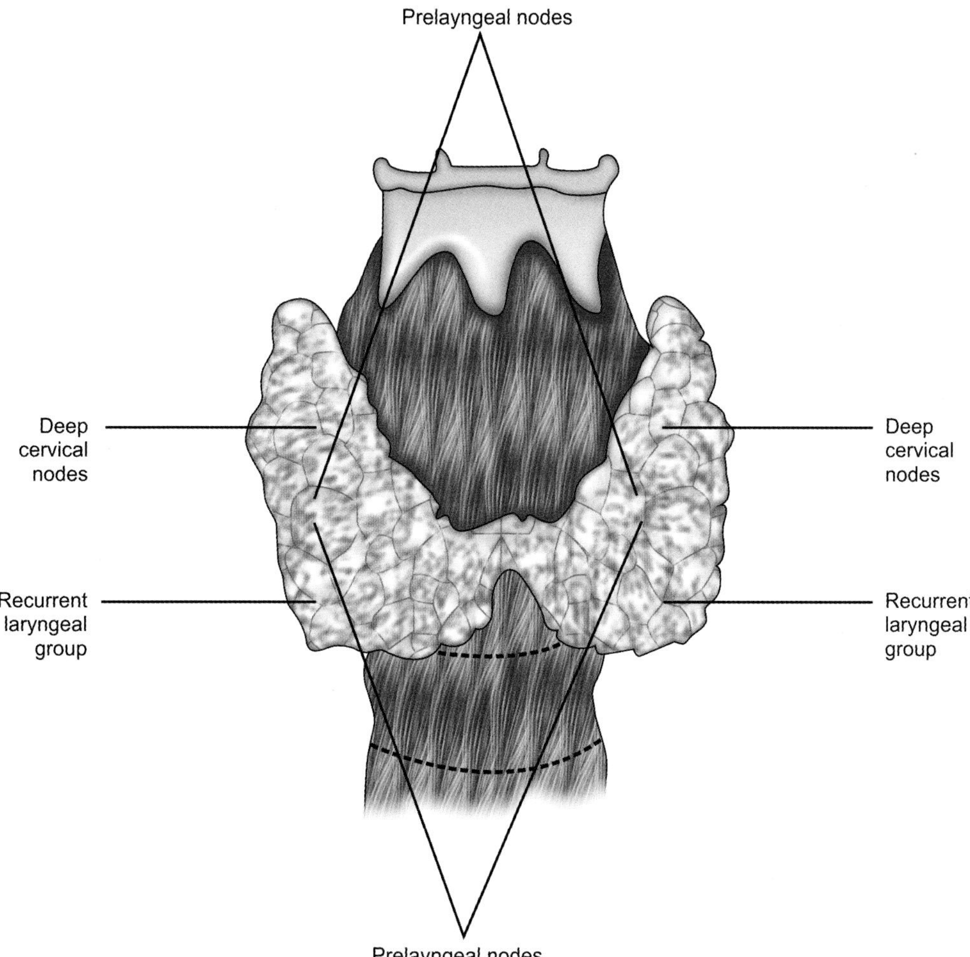

Fig. 3.1: Thyroid lymphatic drainage with arrows

- **Ascending vessels medial:** Leave the upper border of the isthmus and go to the nodes in the cricothyroid membrane, i.e. the **prelaryngeal node.**
- **Ascending vessels lateral:** Leave the upper pole of the gland along with the superior thyroid artery to the **deep cervical lymph nodes.**
- **Descending medial:** Pass from lower border of the isthmus to the **pretracheal group** of lymph nodes.
- **Descending lateral:** Pass from the deep surface of the thyroid to small nodes of the **recurrent laryngeal chain.**

Q 14. What is the classification of neoplasms of thyroid?

Classification of thyroid neoplasm is shown in Flow chart 3.1.

Flow chart 3.1: Classification of thyroid neoplasm

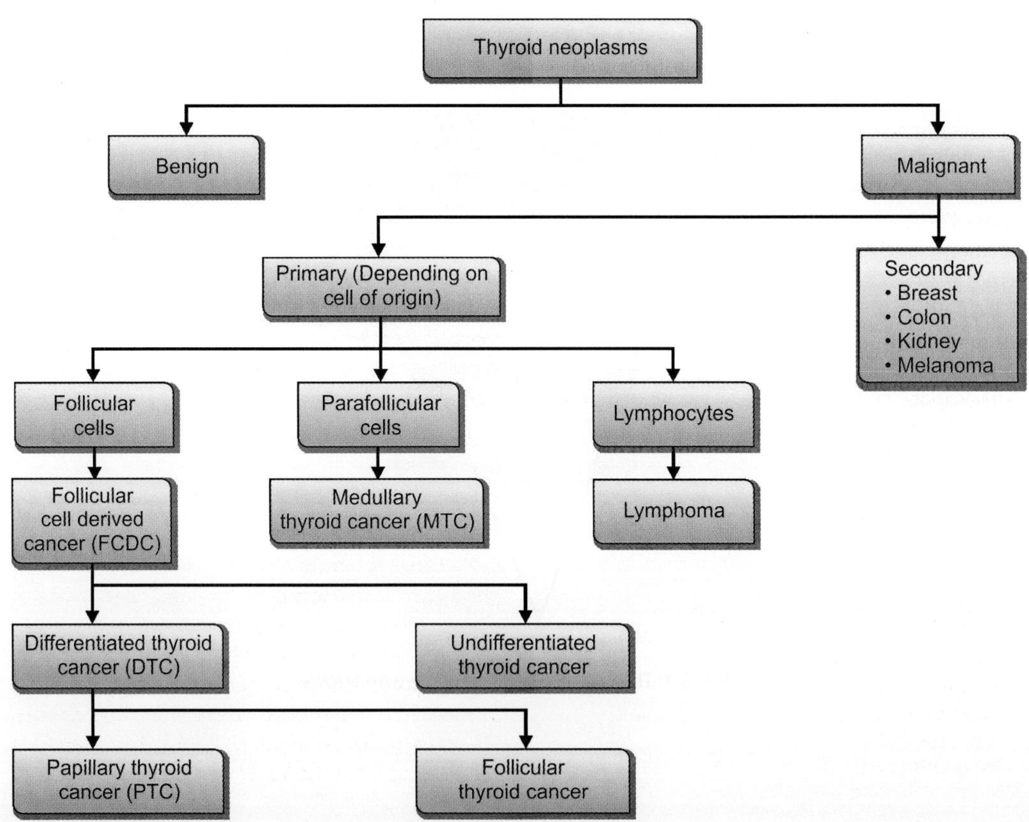

Q 15. What is the relative incidence of the various malignant tumors of thyroid gland?

Carcinoma of the thyroid forms less than 1% of human malignant tumors. It is the most common endocrine malignancy.

- About 90% are well differentiated (Papillary, follicular, Hurthle cell)
- About 10% are poorly differentiated (Anaplastic, medullary and Lymphoma).

Incidence of malignant tumors of thyroid		
1. Papillary carcinoma	–	60%
2. Follicular carcinoma	–	17%
3. Anaplastic carcinoma	–	13%
4. Medullary carcinoma	–	6%
5. Malignant lymphoma	–	4%

Q 16. What are the differences between the two types of differentiated carcinoma namely papillary carcinoma and follicular carcinoma?

Papillary carcinoma	*Follicular carcinoma*
• Multiple foci in the same lobe or on both lobes (21–46%)	Unifocal
• Main mode of spread – lymphatic	Main mode of spread bloodstream
• Blood borne metastases unusual	Common
• Intrathyroid lymphatic spread present	Absent
• Papillary structure present	Papillary structure absent
• Orphan Annie eyed nuclei	Absent
• Capsular and vascular invasion absent	Diagnostic
• Lymph node involvement common	Uncommon
• Prognosis good	Prognosis bad

Q 17. What are the indications for tru-cut biopsy in thyroid (core biopsy)?

a. Anaplastic carcinoma
b. Lymphoma.

Q 18. What are the complications of tru-cut biopsy?

a. Pain
b. Bleeding
c. Tracheal injury
d. Recurrent laryngeal nerve damage.

Q 19. What is the main mode of spread of various primary malignant tumors of thyroid?

The main mode of spread of papillary carcinoma is lymphatic.

The main mode of spread of follicular carcinoma is bloodstream.

The main mode of spread of anaplastic carcinoma is both bloodstream and lymphatic.

Q 20. Can you make a diagnosis of follicular carcinoma in FNAC?

No. The diagnosis of follicular carcinoma is by capsular and vascular invasion which is by histology (paraffin block).

Q 21. What is the FNAC appearance of papillary carcinoma?

In FNAC the cells will be having **Orphan Annie Eyed Nuclei (pale empty nuclei)**.

Q 22. What is lateral aberrant thyroid?

This is also called **occult carcinoma.** The term lateral aberrant thyroid is a misnomer because what we mean by lateral aberrant thyroid is a lymph node metastasis from an impalpable papillary tumor. The primary tumor may be a few millimeter in size only. The **term occult carcinoma** is applied to all papillary carcinomas less than 1.5 cm diameter.

Q 23. What is papillary microcarcinoma?

- Papillary cancer **less than 1cm** is called Microcarcinoma. This is also called **microscopic cancer** or **laboratory cancer**.
- This is unexpectedly detected after a **lobectomy** or **hemithyroidectomy** for a benign thyroid condition.
- Since recurrence and cancer-specific mortality rates are near zero, **no more surgery** or ^{131}I is **required** in this situation.
- Thyroid suppression therapy with thyroxine is instituted.

Q 24. What are the etiological factors for carcinoma thyroid?

1. *Ionizing radiation:* Accidental exposure to radiation in **less than 10 years of age** (**Chernobyl Nuclear disaster**). May produce **papillary carcinoma** and follicular variant of papillary carcinoma.
2. *Iodine deficiency and raised TSH:* Increased TSH stimulation (Follicular carcinoma in seen in iodine deficient areas and papillary thyroid cancer in iodine rich areas).
3. Radiotherapy to head and neck for lymphoma and thymoma in childhood will also lead on to carcinoma thyroid in later years.
4. *Autoimmune thyroiditis:* Hashimoto is associated with a 70-fold increase in lymphoma.
5. *Genetic:* Papillary carcinoma as a result of RET proto-oncogene rearrangement, Kindred's of PTC, **Cowden syndrome** (DTC and Breast carcinoma and Hamartomas), APC gene mutation, (associated with papillary carcinoma) and **BRAF** and **RAS mutations** are seen in papillary thyroid cancer. RET gene for familial medullary thyroid carcinoma.
6. *Oncogenes:* C-myc, C-erb, Ras Oncogene, etc. (associated with MEN).

Q 25. What is Cowden syndrome?

- The association of DTC with carcinoma breast and multiple hamartomas.
- The defect is because of a germ line mutation of PTEN tumor suppressor gene in chromosome 10.

Q 26. What is the pathology of papillary thyroid cancer (PTC)?

- Demonstration of true papillae
- Orphan Annie nuclei
- Nuclear pseudo inclusions
- Nuclear grooves
- Psammoma bodies in 50% of cases.

Q 27. What are the scoring systems available for categorization of patients into low risk and high risk in differentiated thyroid cancer?

Many scoring systems are available

1. AGES—Age, Grade, Extent and Size (Mayo clinic—Hay et al)
2. AMES—Age, Metastases, Extent and Size (Lahey clinic—Cady et al)
3. MACIS—Metastases, Age, Completeness of surgery, Invasion of extra- thyroidal tissue, Size (Hay et al)
4. Sloan—Kettering

In first 3 systems, patients are categorized into **low risk** and **high risk**. In **Sloan - Kettering,** patients are categorized into **3 groups** namely low risk, intermediate and high risk.

Low risk	Less than 45 years of age Less than 4 cm size Favorable tumor factors
Intermediate risk	Low risk patients with high risk tumors High risk patients with low risk tumors
High risk	More than 45 years of age More than 4 cm size Unfavorable tumor factors.

Q 28. What is logic behind considering papillary and follicular carcinoma together for management purposes?

They are considered together because, both of them are **Differentiated Thyroid Cancer Derived** from **follicular cells.** Differentiated Thyroid Cancer (**DTC**) is a spectrum of disease rather than a single disease entity. It is not a life-threatening disease and you can have near normal life-expectancy. It is a tumor with indolent biological behavior with variable aggressiveness.

Q 29. What do you mean by well-differentiated thyroid cancer?

They constitute 90% of the thyroid cancers:

- Papillary thyroid cancer
- Follicular cancer
- Hurthle cell tumors.

Note: 10% are poorly differentiated, comprising of anaplastic, medullary cancers and lymphomas.

Q 30. What is Hurthle cell neoplasm?

- It is a **variant of follicular neoplasm** in which **more than 75% of the follicles** have **oxyphil** (Asknazy or Hurthle) cells or oncocytic features.
- The cells are granular with acidophilic cytoplasm.
- Immunostaining for thyroglobulin is positive.
- **Mean age** of the disease is 60 years.
- It is **multicentric** in 33%.
- More likely to produce lymph node mets.
- It **will not take up radio iodine.**
- Distant metastases are seen in 18%.

Q 31. What are the types of follicular carcinoma ?

They are classified as **minimally invasive** and **widely invasive.**

Q 32. What are the peculiarities of follicular carcinoma?

- They do not invade the lymphatics and hence lack nodal mets.
- Immunostaining for thyroglobulin is positive.
- Seen predominantly in women.

Q 33. What is 'encapsulated variant' of papillary carcinoma? (PG)

- This tumor has a **capsule**-like adenoma but with local invasion.
- It may be associated with nodal metastases.
- There is problem in distinguishing this lesion from a hyperplastic nodule.
- The overall **prognosis is excellent.**

Q 34. What is 'diffuse sclerosing variant'? (PG)

- This is seen primarily in **children.**
- It is **highly aggressive** (often misdiagnosed as Hashimoto's).
- Prominent lymphocytic infiltration is present.
- Incidence of **lymph node mets is 100%.**
- **Prognosis is poor.**

Q 35. What is 'Lindsay tumor'? (PG)

It is a combination of the **encapsulated variant** and the **follicular variant** of papillary carcinoma. It behaves in a very indolent fashion and has good prognosis.

Q 36. What is extrathyroidal spread?

The term extrathyroidal indicates that the primary tumor has infiltrated through the capsule of the gland.

Q 37. What is the AJCC staging (postoperative) of differentiated thyroid carcinoma?

TNM classification for differentiated thyroid carcinoma	
T0	No primary
T1	Tumor diameter 2 cm or smaller
T1a	Tumor < 1 cm
T1b	Tumor > 1 cm, < 2 cm

Contd...

Contd...

T2	Tumor diameter > 2 to 4 cm
T3	Tumor diameter > 4 cm limited to the thyroid with **minimal extrathyroidal extension (extension to sternothyroid muscle or perithyroid soft tissue)**
T4a	**Moderately advanced disease;** Tumor of any size extending beyond the thyroid capsule to **invade subcutaneous soft tissue, larynx, trachea, esophagus or recurrent laryngeal nerve**
T4b	**Very advanced disease;** Tumor invades prevertebral fascia or encases the carotid artery or mediastinal vessels
Tx	Primary tumor size unknown, but without extrathyroidal invasion
N0	No metastatic nodes
N1a	Metastases to **level VI** (pretracheal, paratracheal, prelaryngeal/Delphian nodes)
N1b	Metastases to unilateral, bilateral, contralateral **cervical** or superior mediastinal node **metastases**
Nx	Nodes not assessed at surgery
M0	No distant metastases
M1	Distant metastases
Mx	Distant metastases not assessed

Q 38. What is the importance of age in differentiating thyroid cancer (DTC)?

This is the only human cancer where **age is included in staging**.

Q 39. What is the AJCC staging (postoperative) of differentiated thyroid carcinoma? (PG)

AJCC staging (postoperative) of differentiated thyroid carcinoma	
Age less than 45 years (only 2 stages)	
Stage I	: any T, any N and M0
Stage II	: any T, any N, M1
Age more than 45 years (4 stages)	
Stage I	: T1, N0 and M0
Stage II	: T2, N0 and M0
Stage III	: T3, N0, and M0
	: T1, N1a, M0
	: T2, N1a, M0
	: T3, N1a, M0
Stage IV A	: T4a, N0, M0 **(T4a/Lateral node is stage IVA)**
	: T4a, N1a, M0
	: T1, N1b, M0
	: T2, N1b, M0
	: T3, N1b, M0
	: T4a, N1b, M0
Stage IV B	: T4b, any N, M0 **(T4b is Stage IV B)**
Stage IV C	: any T, any N, M1 **(metastasis is Stage IV C)**

Contd...

Contd...

**Note*: *Stage III* constitutes minimal extrathyroid extension or level VI nodes.

All anaplastic carcinomas are considered stage IV.

The AJCC staging is for predicting the risk of death. For assessing the risk of recurrence, a three level stratification is recommended by the American Thyroid Association, which is as follows: (PG)

After initial surgery and remnant ablation:

1. *Low risk:*
   - No local/distant metastases.
   - All microscopic tumors resected
   - No tumor invasion of locoregional structures
   - No aggressive histology
   - No vascular invasion
   - No ^{131}I uptake outside thyroid bed.
2. *Intermediate risk:*
   - Microscopic invasion of tumor to perithyroid soft tissue
   - Tumor with aggressive histology
   - Vascular invasion
   - Cervical lymph node metastases
   - ^{131}I uptake outside the thyroid bed after remnant ablation
3. *High risk:*
   - Macroscopic tumor invasion
   - Incomplete tumor removal
   - Distant metastases.

Q 40. What is minimal extrathyroid extension? (PG)

Extension to **sternothyroid muscle** or **perithyroid soft tissue** is called minimal extrathyroid invasion.

Q 41. What is the prognosis of differentiated thyroid cancer (DTC)?

- The 25 year mortality rate of a **low-risk DTC is 2%. That means 98% of the patients will survive 25 years.**
- **For the high-risk group the 25 year mortality is 46%.**
- **80 to 90% of the patients come under the low-risk group**
- In short 80% of the patients **require lobectomy alone**
- **15% require aggressive treatment**
- **5% die regardless of a treatment.**

Q 42. What is the surgical treatment of choice for a preoperatively proven case of papillary carcinoma?

If the FNAC is diagnostic of **papillary thyroid cancer,** the treatment of choice is **near total** or **total thyroidectomy (TT)** with **central compartment dissection**. Lymph nodes in the jugular chain should be carefully looked for during surgery.

Q 43. What is the surgery for a non-diagnostic biopsy?

The surgery may be hemithyroidectomy or total thyroidectomy. Total thyroidectomy is indicated in the following situations.

- > 4 cm tumor size
- FNAC suspicious of PTC
- Family history of PTC
- History of radiation.

Q 44. What is the difference between near total and total thyroidectomy?

In near total thyroidectomy *1 to 2* g of thyroid tissue is preserved on the **contralateral side**, which preserves blood supply to one or both parathyroids.

Q 45. What is central compartment neck dissection?

- It extends from **hyoid bone** above to **innominate vein** below and **carotids** laterally.
- Thyroid and the thymus are removed en-bloc along with the paratracheal, tracheoesophageal, pretracheal and prelaryngeal nodes.

Q 46. What is the rationale for central compartment neck dissection and what are the problems associated? (PG)

- **Fifty percent node positivity** is seen in routine central compartment dissection.
- **Reoperation and nodal dissection** in the central compartment area are difficult.
- Thymus and thyroid are removed en-bloc in this dissection.
- Central compartment neck dissection is done as long as **low incidence of hypoparathyroidism** can be achieved.
- Lower parathyroids are a greater risk for damage in a central compartment neck dissection.

Q 47. What is the indication for central compartment dissection in DTC?

- Patients with clinically involved nodes **therapeutic central compartment dissection** done.
- Prophylactic central compartment dissection is recommended in DTC only for **T3 and T4 tumors.**

Q 48. What are the indications for completion thyroidectomy when there is histological surprise of carcinoma after a hemithyroidectomy?

Indications for completion thyroidectomy
1. History of radiation
2. High-risk factors
3. More than 1cm size
4. Contralateral thyroid nodule
5. Regional or distant metastases

Contd...

Contd...

6. Family history of DTC in first degree relatives
7. Age > 45 years
8. Multifocal tumor
9. Extrathyroid spread
10. Major vascular invasion
11. Major capsular invasion.

Q 49. Is there any role for lobectomy alone as a treatment for DTC?

Lobectomy is acceptable in *Low-risk* patients with

- Small intrathyroid tumor of < 1cm
- Node-negative
- Unifocal
- Intrathyroid.

Q 50. What are the indications for lateral neck node dissection (functional neck dissection)?

Indications for functional neck dissection
• Lymphadenopathy detected clinically • Node identified by imaging • Biopsy-proven metastatic nodes • Frozen-section node positivity during surgery.

Q 51. What are the bad histological subtypes of DTC?

Bad histological subtypes of DTC
• Tall cell variety • Columnar cell • Trabecular • Scirrhous • Solid • Oxyphilic subtype of follicular thyroid cancer • Insular type of follicular thyroid cancer.

Q 52. What are the features of tall cell variety of papillary cancer? **(PG)**

- This is an aggressive variant
- Seen in elderly
- Represents 10% of papillary tumors
- Extracapsular and vascular invasion in 30%
- Five-year survival rate is < 30%.

Q 53. What are the features of columnar cell variety of papillary cancer? **(PG)**

- This is seen only in men
- All patients will die within 5 years of diagnosis.

Q 54. What are the indications for total thyroidectomy in carcinoma?

Indications for total thyroidectomy in carcinoma
1. Primary thyroid cancer > 1cm 2. Contralateral thyroid nodule 3. Patients with regional or distant metastases 4. History of radiation 5. History of DTC in first degree relatives 6. Age > 45 years 7. High-risk category.

Q 55. What is the treatment of lymph node metastases in papillary thyroid cancer?

If lymph nodes are clinically present, a **functional neck dissection** (preserving the sternomastoid muscle, accessory nerve and internal jugular vein) is carried out along with total thyroidectomy. **Oncologically carcinoma thyroid is the only indication for a functional neck node dissection**. If clinically and peroperatively there are not any nodes, only **central compartment dissection** is done.

Q 56. What is the postoperative follow-up after total thyroidectomy?

All patients, after total thyroidectomy should receive the following:

a. **T_4 suppression** (300 microgram eltroxine daily) after scintigraphy for remnant thyroid tissue.
b. Look for thyroid remnant by scintigraphy at 6 weeks (1 mCi radioiodine for ^{131}I cervical scanning).

For optimal scanning, the **serum TSH level should be at least 30 mIU/L.** If the patient is on eltroxine, two injections of recombinant human TSH will give the desired effect.

c. If remnant is detected, Radio Remnant Ablation at a dose of 30 mCi **(RRA)** is given (^{131}I).
d. At 3 to 6 months, **whole body scan** with 3 mCi radioactive iodine for metastases and ultrasound examination is carried out.
e. If negative scanning is obtained, **follow-up with Thyroglobulin (Tg)** level. Upon detection of increased thyroglobulin level, further whole body scan is indicated.

Q 57. What is the rationale of RRA? (PG)

a. RRA will destroy occult **microscopic carcinoma.**
b. Later detection of persistent or recurrent disease is possible, after destruction of the thyroid remnant.
c. **Serum thyroglobulin as a tumor marker** is useful only after complete removal and destruction of the thyroid. (**Therefore, there is no role for thyroglobulin assay in the preoperative period**).

Q 58. What are the indications for radio remnant ablation?

- Tumor size > 4 cm
- Gross extrathyroid extension of tumor
- Distant metastases
- Less than 4 cm with lymph node metastases and high risk group.

Q 59. What is the upper limit of normal level of thyroglobulin (Tg)? (PG)

- When on suppressive therapy: **Above 2 ng/mL.**
- When the patient is hypothyroid: **more than 5 ng/mL.**

Increasing values are important and TG antibody should be quantitatively assessed.

These are indications of imaging for persistent, recurrent or metastatic disease.

Q 60. If thyroglobulin (Tg) measurement is high and total body scanning reveals metastases, what will be the course of action? (PG)

For metastases, 100 to 200 mCi radioiodine ^{131}I is given (**RAI**).

Q 61. What are the precautions to be taken before RAI therapy? (PG)

Precautions to be taken before RAI therapy

a. Low iodine diet for 10 days
b. Isolation of the patient (when dose is more than 30 mCi)
c. Oral fluid intake to increase urine output so that bladder injury is reduced
d. Lemon sucking to avoid sialadenitis
e. Avoid pregnancy for 6 months
f. Treat constipation with cathartics to reduce gonadal and colonic irradiation
g. Sperm count reduction is noticed for several months.

Note: Post-treatment whole body scan should be done 4 to10 days after RAI, which may detect new lesions that need further treatment.

Q 62. What is the dose for skeletal metastases? (PG)

250 to 300 mCi (milli Curie) of ^{131}I

Q 63. What is the role of WBS (Whole Body Scanning) and ultrasound in follow-up?

- **Low risk** patients with negative TG and negative cervical ultrasound no need for WBS
- **Intermediate and high risk**—6 to 12 months after ablation do diagnostic WBS

Cervical Ultrasound at 6 and 12 months and then annually for at least 3 to 5 years.

Q 64. What is the further follow?

a. Serum Tg level every 6 months along with TG antibody.

b. **Lifelong suppressive therapy with thyroxin** (the TSH should be monitored every 6 months and dose of thyroxin adjusted).

Q 65. What is the dosage of radio iodine?

Dose of radioiodine (^{131}I) in differentiated carcinoma thyroid		
• Cervical scan	–	1 mCi
• Total body scan	–	3 mCi
• Remnant ablation	–	30 mCi
• Treatment of metastases	–	100 – 250 mCi

Q 66. What is the treatment of a solitary metastasis in manubrium sterni from DTC?

- Solitary bone metastasis is ideally resected (the dosage of radio iodine required for treating bone metastases is very high and surgery gives lasting relief)
- Multiple bone metastases may be treated with radio iodine.

Flow chart for management of DTC

After total thyroidectomy and TSH suppression

↓

T_4 withdrawal for 3 weeks OR two IM injections of 0.9 mg of recombinant TSH

↓

Pre therapy low dose ^{131}I – scanning (1 to 3 mCi) before ablation

↓

Radio remnant ablation (30–100 mCi) **if indicated**

↓

Postablation whole body scan 5 to 8 days after RRA
If low-risk, negative thyroglobulin and normal neck USG, then no whole body scan

↓

If intermediate-risk and high-risk with persistent disease, then 6 to 12 months after RRA do diagnostic whole body scan

Contd...

Contd...

Further follow-up
- Thyroglobulin: 6 to 12 months
- Cervical US: 6 and 12 months, annually for 3 – 5 years

Q 67. What are the peculiarities of medullary thyroid carcinoma (MTC)?

a. They constitute **5 to 10%** of all thyroid cancers
b. Are derived from parafollicular cells (C-cells) developed from neural crests.
c. There is a characteristic **amyloid stroma.**
d. High levels of serum **calcitonin** are produced (more than 0.08 ng/mL); it is a **tumor marker** for medullary carcinoma
e. **Diarrhea** is a feature in 30% of cases
f. Some tumors are **familial** (~ 20%)
g. It may form part of **multiple endocrine neoplasia** (MEN) syndromes: IIa and IIb
h. Clinical course is **more aggressive** than differentiated thyroid cancers
i. Do not take up radioactive iodine
j. Higher recurrence rate and mortality
k. Radiation and chemotherapy are ineffective
l. This is perhaps the only situation where **a surgery based on genetic testing** is routinely done
m. Once the diagnosis of medullary thyroid cancer is suspected, all patients should be screened for mutation of the RET proto-oncogene to exclude familial disease
n. When a genetic defect is found, all family members should be screened.

Q. 68. What are the four clinical settings of MTC? (PG)

a. Sporadic medullary thyroid carcinoma (80%)
b. Familial MEN IIa
c. Familial MEN IIb
d. Familial non-MEN medullary thyroid carcinoma (FMTC).

Q 69. What are the features multiple endocrine neoplasia IIa ?

MEN IIa (Sipple's syndrome)
• *Pheochromocytoma:* frequently bilateral (may be extra-adrenal) • Hyperparathyroidism • Medullary thyroid cancer • Seen in late childhood and teenage • Amyloid deposits in the skin of upper back (Cutaneous Lichen Amyloidosis) • May be associated with Hirschsprung's disease • Autosomal dominant.

Q 70. What are the features of multiple endocrine neoplasia IIb?

Multiple endocrine neoplasia IIb
• Familial medullary thyroid cancer • *Mucosal neuromas* of lips, tongue, inner eyelid • *Marfanoid habitus* • *Pheochromocytomas* are common (40 – 50%) • Severe *gastrointestinal symptoms* of alternating diarrhea and constipation (because of the increased number of ganglion cells) • Toxic megacolon and pseudo-obstruction are seen

Note: MEN I (Wermer's syndrome) involves the parathyroids, pituitary and the pancreas.

Q 71. What is the hallmark of multiple endocrine neoplasia II?

- The hallmark of MEN II is **medullary thyroid carcinoma.**
- MTC in MEN II is bilateral, multifocal, and affects younger age group.

Q 72. What are the differences between MEN associated MTC and non-MEN MTC? (PG)

The MTC associated with MEN are **preceded by hyperplasia of C-cells**. It is possible to identify relatives of such patients at the stage of hyperplasia and operate before malignancy.

a. MTC with MEN are **more aggressive**
b. MTC with MEN is **multicentric,** (sporadic/non-MEN familial MTC is unicentric.
c. MTC with MEN occurs at a **younger age.**

Q 73. What are the features of familial non-MEN medullary thyroid carcinoma?

Features of familial non-MEN medullary thyroid carcinoma
• They are autosomal dominant (germ line mutation of RET gene) • *Indolent course* • *Least malignant* with very good prognosis • Mean age is 40 years • Occasion never manifests clinically • Extracellular/intracellular cysteine codon is seen.

Q 74. What are the features of medullary thyroid carcinoma in MEN IIb?

Medullary thyroid carcinoma in MEN IIb
• *Most aggressive* form of MTC is seen in this setting • *Rarely curable* • Affects very young age group: infancy and early childhood • Autosomal dominant: germ line mutation of RET gene • Typical phenotype: Marfanoid.

Q 75. What is the screening program for the family members of familial MTC? (PG)

- **Basal calcitonin** may be normal at the stage of hyperplasia but **stimulation by calcium or pentagastrin** will give high value.
- **Screening every 6 months from the age of 5 years up to 50 years** is useful.
- **Ultrasound** of the neck is also useful for identifying nodal metastases.

Q 76. Is there any role for prophylactic thyroidectomy in family members? If so, at what age?

- Yes. **Prophylactic thyroidectomy** can prevent tumor occurrence at the stage of C-cell hyperplasia.
- Surgery by **3 years** for MEN IIa.
- Surgery by **1 year** for MEN IIb.

Q 77. What are the clinical presentations of medullary thyroid carcinoma?

- Medullary thyroid carcinoma is a **great imitator**
- Lump in the neck
- Nodal metastases
- **Paraneoplastic syndromes:** Cushing and carcinoid
- Hoarseness, stridor and upper airway obstruction
- **Diarrhea** and flushing.

Q 78. How do you confirm the diagnosis of medullary thyroid carcinoma?

- FNAC
- **Calcitonin: unstimulated serum calcitonin** >100 pg/mL is suggestive of MTC
- **CEA:** 50% of medullary thyroid cancer
- USG/CT scan/MRI
- Screening for **pheochromocytoma** by 24 hours urinary catecholamines in all cases.

Note:

1. In all suspected MTCs, do USG abdomen and 24 hours urinary catecholamines to rule out **pheochromocytoma.**
2. Rule out MTC in all thyroid cases with **diarrhea.**
3. Rule out MTC in all thyroid cases with **hypertension.**

Q 79. What is the treatment of medullary thyroid carcinoma?

- Since they do not take up RAI, **surgery is the only curative treatment.**
- No role of anything less than total **thyroidectomy.**
- Routine **dissection of central compartment** is a must.
- **Sampling of the jugular nodes** are done (if positive, Modified Neck dissection is done).
- **Autotransplantation of parathyroid** is required (for completeness of thyroid resection): transplanted to the non-dominant forearm.
- Some centers do a thymectomy with these regularly (for fear of metastases in thymus).
- Postoperative stimulated calcitonin assay is done for assessment of the adequacy of surgical resection.

Q 80. What is the treatment of anaplastic carcinoma of the thyroid?

- It is very difficult to differentiate anaplastic carcinoma from **lymphoma of thyroid.**
- They are extremely **lethal tumors**
- The **treatment of choice** is not surgery but **radiotherapy.**
- The indication for surgery is to **relieve tracheal obstruction** by isthmusectomy. This will give tissue for histology.
- **Curative resection** is attempted when there is no infiltration through the thyroid capsule.

Q 81. What is the management of lymphoma?

- There is no role for surgery.
- Radiotherapy and chemotherapy are the treatment of choice.
- For low grade B cell MALT lymphoma, radiotherapy alone is enough.
- Tracheal obstruction requires urgent chemotherapy after intubation.
- The temptation for a tracheostomy must be resisted.

Q 82. What is incidentaloma?

When performing imaging for other head and neck problems, small nodule in the thyroid **less than 1 cm is identified by serendipity.** It is called incidentaloma. They are invariably benign and what is required is an ultrasound guided FNAC.

FOR PG'S—WHAT IS NEW?

1. *Insular Carcinoma*—It is otherwise called as Poorly Differentiated Thyroid Cancer (PDTC). It is having an intermediate position between differentiated thyroid cancer and anaplastic cancer. Histologically solid clusters of tumor cells are seen with variable number of small follicles. Capsular and vascular invasion are also seen. Sometimes peritheliomatous pattern is seen. Calcification and bone are seen in stroma. It is an example of De-differentiation theory of differentiated thyroid cancer. Metastasis are seen in bone and lungs. The 10-year survival is 42%. The differences between insular and anaplastic are given below.

Insular	*Anaplastic*
Younger – 45	Older – 70's
P 53 and P 21 – negative	P 53 and P 21–positive
Bone and lung metastasis	Metastasis in variety of organs
5-year survival – 46%, 10-year 42%	5-year 15%, 10-year 3%

   P53 ↓ (Well DTC → Insular); P53 ↓ (Insular → anaplastic)

   Well DTC → Insular → anaplastic

2. *Sonological findings of lymph node* metastasis
   - Loss of fatty hilus
   - Round shape of lymph node
   - Hypoechogenic
   - Cystic changes
   - Calcification
   - Peripheral vascularity
3. *Treatment of isolated bone metastasis from DTC*
   Wherever excision is possible e.g. Clavicle or sternum, surgery is preferred over radio iodine for therapy since a very high dose of radio iodine in the range of 200 to 300 mCi is required for bone metastasis with its side effects. The excisional surgery is more curative than radio iodine.

Case

4 Multinodular Goiter

Case Capsule

A **30-year-old female patient** comes from an endemic area for goiter and presents with painless swelling in front of the neck of **5-year duration**. She complains of **nocturnal dyspnea and discomfort.** In the recumbent position the patient gets **dyspnea when she is lying on the left side**. There are **no symptoms of toxicity**. On examination her **pulse rate is 72/min**. There is **no tremor** of the outstretched hands. The **jugular veins are distended.** A few dilated veins are seen over the swelling and upper chest. On **Pemberton's test there is congestion of the face and distress.** There is **asymmetrical nodular swelling** in the lower half of the neck with up and down movements on swallowing. The swelling has **irregular shape.** The **lower border** of the swelling is **not visible and palpable.** The nodules in the thyroid are having **varying consistency**, some are firm, some feel hard and some are soft in consistency. The nodules in the central part (isthmus) are more prominent. There is no fluctuation or transillumination. The **trachea is deviated to the right.** There is **no bruit** over the upper pole on auscultation. The **cervical lymph nodes are not enlarged.** There is no clinical evidence of toxicity or malignancy.

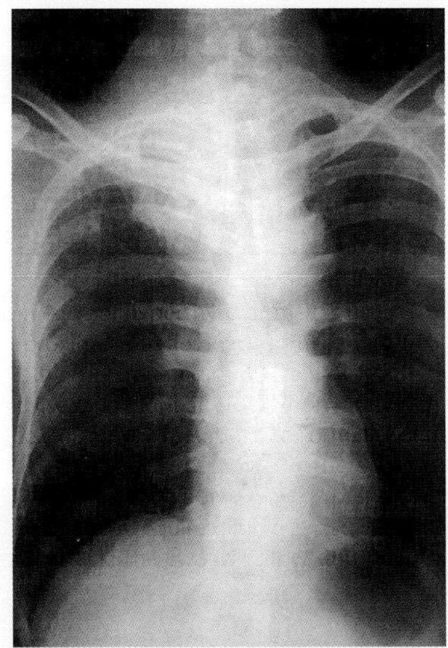

Nodular goiter

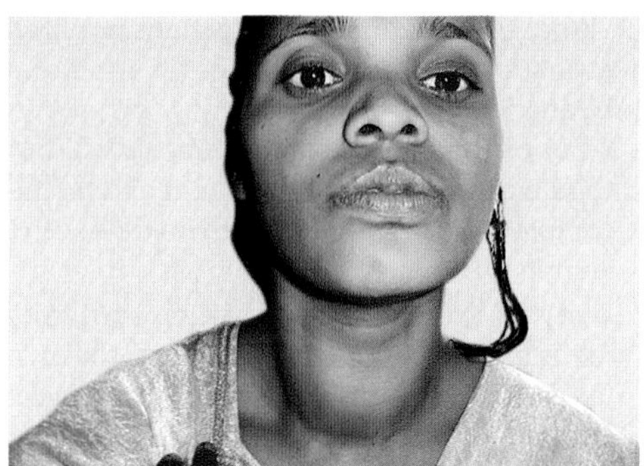

Recurrent goiter (MNG)

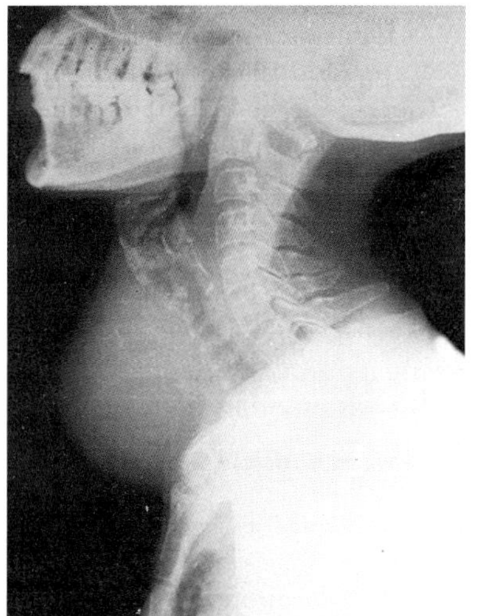

X-ray showing retrosternal extension of goiter

Read the Checklist and Preliminary Part of Clinical Examination in Case No: 1

Q 1. What are your points in favor of nodular goiter?

a. The swellings are arising from thyroid gland.

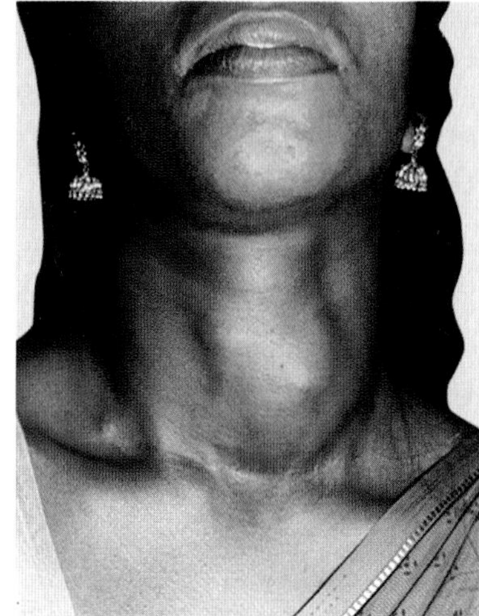

Multinodular goiter with tracheal compression

b. Both lobes and isthmus are studded with nodules of varying sizes.

c. There is no clinical evidence of malignancy or toxicity.

Q 2. What is the pathology in nodular goiter?

Multinodular goiter is defined as a thyroid enlargement with follicles that are morphologically and functionally altered (there is **structural and functional autonomy**). It is a **discordant growth of heterogeneous cell cohorts**.

The etiopathogenesis is enumerated below:

1. Increased TSH stimulation
2. Iodine deficiency
3. Other environmental factors
4. Goitrogens
5. Heredity
6. Dyshormonogenesis

7. Circulating growth factors like growth stimulating autoantibodies, thyroid stimulating peptides, immunoglobulin stimulating growth.

Q 3. What is the natural history of a nodule formation?

Increased TSH secretion acts as a goitrogen.

a. TSH stimulation will lead on to **diffuse hyperplasia** composed of active follicles. This is called diffuse hyperplastic goiter. At this stage it is reversible.
b. Later as a result of fluctuating TSH stimulation, mixed patterns of active and inactive lobules develop.
c. Active lobules become more vascular, hyperplastic followed by **hemorrhage and central necrosis.** The necrotic area is surrounded by rim of active follicles.
d. The necrotic lobules coalesce to **form a nodule** filled with either iodine-free colloid or inactive follicles.
e. Repetition of this process will result in a nodular goiter. Most nodules are inactive and active follicles are present only in the internodular tissue.

Q 4. Do you expect increased TSH in nodular goiter?

No. A plausible explanation for the growth promoting effects of TSH is the presence of a subset of thyroid follicular cells with an increased sensitivity to TSH.

Q 5. What are the investigations required in this case?

Most important investigations are **FNAC** and thyroid function test (**TFT**).

Q 6. Which nodule will you select for FNAC?

- The most **dominant** nodule
- The most **suspicious** nodule
- FNAC from more than one nodule may be required.

Q 7. What are the other investigations required?

Investigations for nodular goiter (In addition to FNAC and TFT).

- **X-ray of the neck** AP and lateral views. This is to rule out tracheal displacement and tracheal compression. Calcification of thyroid also can be identified.
- **X-ray of the chest** is also taken to rule out retrosternal extension. If the soft tissue shadow of the thyroid is coming down **beyond the clavicle,** it is radiologically suggestive of **retrosternal extension.**
- **Ultrasonography:** High resolution USG can identify clinically **impalpable nodules**. Expert sonologists can **differentiate benign from malignant nodule.** One can identify nodules as small as 0.3 cm size in USG.
- **USG guided FNAC** can also be done.
- **Indirect laryngoscopy:** In all cases of nodular goiter, it is important to have an indirect laryngoscopy done to rule out **occult recurrent laryngeal nerve palsy**, preoperatively.
- **Serum calcium:** The preoperative calcium assessment is important **to rule out parathyroid pathology** and it will act as a baseline value in the postoperative period.

Q 8. Is there any role for CT scan in a case of multinodular goiter?

Yes. The **only indication** for CT scan in nodular goiter is when you suspect **retrosternal extension**. MRI may also be useful in this situation.

Q 9. Is there any role for pulmonary function test (PFT) in MNG?

Clinically whenever there is **large/long-standing** goiter and **tracheal deviation** or **compression,** it is better to do a pulmonary function test so that one can identify a patient who is likely to develop **tracheomalacia/scabbard** trachea.

Q 10. How will you identify and tackle tracheomalacia (weakness of tracheal rings)?

After thyroidectomy, the surgeon should palpate for the tracheal rings for its strength. In case of doubt, **the anesthesiologist may withdraw the endotracheal tube** partially to check for weakness of tracheal rings. When there is suspicion of weakness of tracheal rings it is better to keep the tube as tracheal stent postoperatively for 24 hours. After 24 hours, extubate and see. If the patient is going for trouble, do a tracheostomy.

Q 11. Is there any role for thyroid scintigraphy?

It is not required routinely. It is useful in a **hyperthyroid patient with a dominant nodule** as it defines the area of hyperactivity, thereby choosing proper surgical therapy.

Q 12. What are the complications of nodular goiter?

Complications of nodular goiter
1. Toxicity 2. Malignancy 3. Retrosternal extension 4. Pressure effects 5. Calcification.

Q 13. What type of toxicity do you get in MNG?

1. When the patient develops **hypertrophy of the nodule** he/she gets **Plummer's disease,** (**secondary**).
2. When the **internodular tissue** is hypertrophied, patient will get **primary** thyrotoxicosis.

Q 14. What are the indications for surgery in MNG?

The indications for surgery are:

1. Complications (already mentioned)
2. Cosmesis.

Q 15. What is the role of suppressive levothyroxine therapy?

The results of T_4 suppression therapy are inconsistent and marginal. Only small goiter would respond and that too partially. Goiters that respond do so within a period of 6 **months.**

Q 16. What are the disadvantages of suppression therapy?

1. One should consistently suppress the TSH level to < **0.5 mIU/L**.
2. Periodic monitoring of TSH is required to rule out hyperthyroidism.
3. Large amounts of thyroid tissue are likely to be **hormone insensitive** in MNG.
4. **Variable TSH dependency by various thyrocytes** resulting in inconsistent response.
5. Indefinite treatment is required and most of the goiter recurs after cessation of therapy.

Q 17. Is there any role for radioiodine therapy in MNG?

Radioiodine therapy is of no value in large MNG with poorly functioning nodules. The efficacy of RAI depends on the presence of reasonable gland activity all over the thyroid that is not seen in large MNG. Radiation induced autoimmune thyroiditis and hypothyroidisms are other problems. It is of **limited value and useful only in two groups of patient**. Patients with small goiter with **reasonable gland function** and patients with substantially **increased operative risk**.

Q 18. What is the surgical option in a case of nodular goiter?

The conventional surgery is **subtotal thyroidectomy** that is not adequate in a case of nodular goiter that is involving both lobes of the gland. The ideal option will be to do a **total thyroidectomy**, with immediate and lifelong replacement of thyroid hormone.

When one lobe is more involved than the other lobe, total **lobectomy** on the more affected side with subtotal resection on the less affected side will be an ideal option. It is, therefore, ideal to have removal of the entire diseased gland, the so-called **adequate thyroidectomy**.

Q 19. What is the real problem if you leave behind diseased nodular portions?

1. It will produce enlargement and **recurrence** after 10–15 years.
2. **Reoperation** for recurrent nodular goiter is **more difficult** and hazardous because of altered anatomy and fibrosis. Therefore, it is better to favor total thyroidectomy in younger patients.

Q 20. What is the timing of recurrence?

It is seen usually after 10 to 15 years.

Q 21. Is there any role for TSH suppression in preventing recurrence?

If diseased nodules are left behind, **TSH suppression will not help in preventing recurrence.** At present its role is uncertain. However, once total thyroidectomy is done, patient needs replacement therapy to prevent hypothyroidism.

FOR PG'S—WHAT IS NEW?

Retrosternal Goiter

Definition: Goiter extending down to the level of the transverse process of the fourth thoracic vertebrae on chest radiograph or goiter extending down to the level of arch of aorta (Goldenberg) or more than 50% of the mass lying distal to the thoracic inlet (Katlic). 7 to 10% are bilateral, 7 to 10% are seen in posterior mediastinum.

Indications for surgery are:

1. Clinical symptoms (Stridor/dysphagia)—hoarseness, dyspnea, cough, etc.
2. Radiological evidence of tracheal narrowing
3. Esophageal compression
4. Superior venocaval syndrome
5. Malignancy
6. Toxicity.

Indications for sternotomy/thoracotomy

About 90% of the retrosternal goiters can be removed by cervical approach. Sternotomy is required in 2 – 8%.

The indications are:

The lower border below the level of aortic arch

More than 70% of the mass below the thoracic inlet

Posterior mediastinal mass (transthoracic approach through fourth space)

Malignancy technical tips for removal of retrosternal goiter

1. Division of strap muscles
2. Surgery on contralateral side first
3. Control of middle thyroid vein first
4. Ligation of superior thyroid pedicle initially

Contd...

Contd...

5. Identify RLN and stay anterior to the nerve
6. Pushing out rather than pulling out
7. In posterior mediastinal goiter, the nerve may be ventral to that:

Grading of intrathoracic goiter

Grade I 0 – 25% in chest

Grade II 26 – 50% in chest

Grade III 51 – 75% in chest

Grade IV > 75% in chest

Since evaluation of retrosternal goiter is not possible with ultrasound and FNAC, surgery is recommended for all.

Case

5 Early Breast Cancer

Case Capsule

A **40-year-old female patient** presents with a **painless lump** in the right breast of 6 months duration, which she noticed while washing. There is no history of backache, dyspnea, pleuritic pain or jaundice. There is **no family history of carcinoma breast.** The patient attained **menarche at the age of 13 years.** Her menstrual cycles are regular. Her first **child birth was at the age of 30-years**. She has two children and both were **breastfed.** On raising her hands above her head, there is **visible asymmetry** of the breast (right breast is more prominent and distorted). There is **retraction** of the nipple on right side and it is at a higher level. Areola is normal. There is no discharge from the nipple on right side and it is at a higher level. The skin overlying the breast is normal. There is no peau d' orange appearance or ulceration or edema. On palpation the lump is **4 × 3 cm** size, **stony hard in consistency** in the upper outer quadrant of right breast. The lump is **fixed to the breast**, but there is no fixity to the skin or pectoral muscles. There is a **mobile, firm pectoral node** palpable in the right axilla. Supraclavicular fossa and right arm are normal. Contralateral breast, axilla,

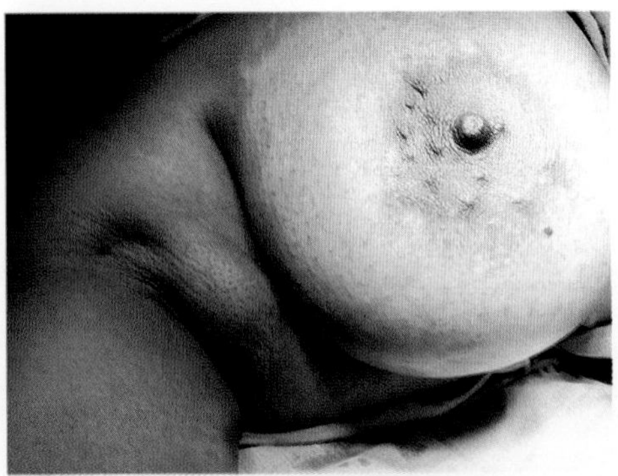

Axillary tail of Spence

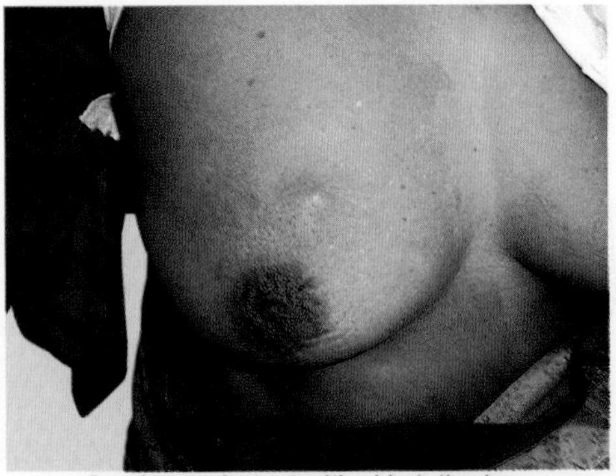

Carcinoma breast with skin tethering

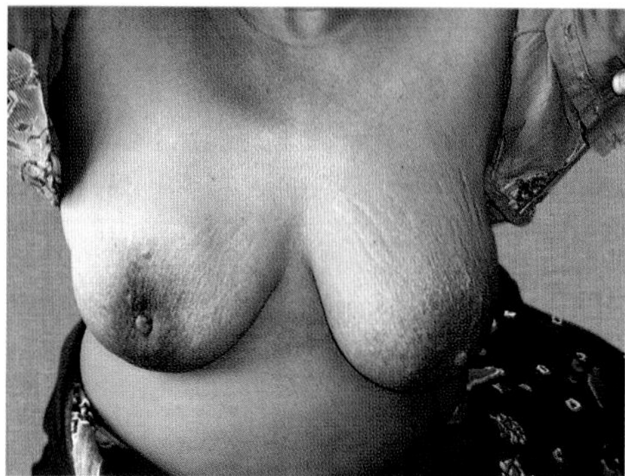

Carcinoma right breast, the entire right breast at a higher level

and supraclavicular fossa are normal. There is no evidence of hepatomegaly or ascites on examining the abdomen. There is no evidence of pleural effusion or consolidation on examining the chest. Skull and spine are normal. Pelvic examination is normal.

Checklist for Clinical Examination

1. Examine the patient in **supine** (45° semi-recumbent position is ideal), **sitting and arms by the side, arms raised,** hands **on the hip** and **leaning forward** positions (Figs 5.1A to C).
2. Inspect both breast simultaneously for **asymmetry,** look for visible lumps, and inspect the nipple areolar complex.
3. In nipple look for **6 Ds:**
   Discharge
   Destruction
   Depression (retraction)
   Discoloration
   Displacement
   Deviation.
4. Look for **peau d' orange**, skin tethering, skin fixity.
5. Check whether the lump is **freely mobile** within the breast (breast mouse), whether it is **fixed to the breast**, whether there is **fixity to pectoral** muscles or to chest wall.
6. Examine the **axilla for lymph nodes** (remember the various groups of lymph nodes). Examine the **supraclavicular area** for lymph nodes.
7. Always examine the **contralateral breast, axilla and supraclavicular area.**

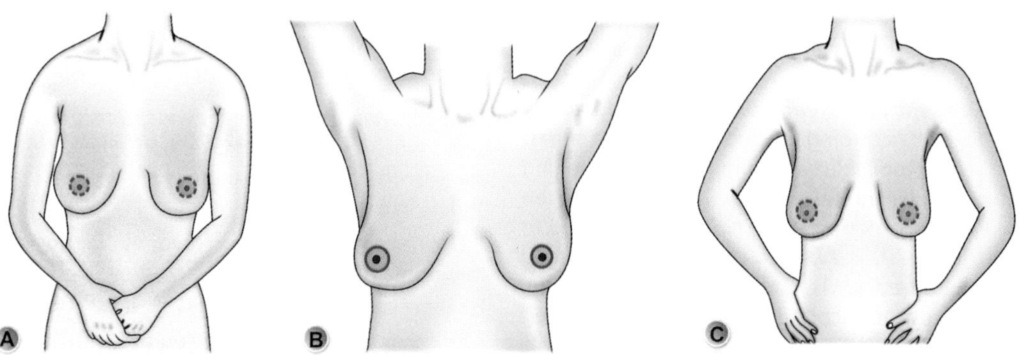

Figs 5.1A to C: Examination of the patient with arms by the side, arms raised and arms on the hip

8. Examine the **abdomen** for liver metastases and ovarian metastases (Krukenberg's tumor–ovarian metastases in premenopausal ovaries.
9. Always examine the **chest** for signs of metastases—pleural effusion, consolidation.
10. Look for bony tenderness—any evidence of **bony metastases** (examination of spine, long bones and skull).

Concepts in Breast Cancer

a. *Halstedian concept of spread of carcinoma breast*: The spread of carcinoma breast as per the Halstedian concept was that the tumor will remain localized to the breast for some time before spreading to the axillary nodes. The tumor will remain in the axillary nodes for some time before producing systemic spread and metastases. William Halstead believed that aggressively attacking the cancer when it is localized to the breast and lymph nodes can cure the cancer, i.e. the so-called **locoregional attack.** He, therefore, advocated **radical operations** in the form of removal of the entire breast, the pectoral muscles (both major and minor) and axillary nodes. Later it was found that this form of aggressive treatment will not change the final outcome and survival of the patient.
b. *Concept of systemic disease introduced by Fischer:* According to Fischer, carcinoma breast is a **systemic disease** from the very beginning and **micrometastases** may be present even when the tumor is very small and localized to the breast. The staged progression of spread described by Halstead is no longer true. Aggressive locoregional attack is not going tackle the micrometastases, which is possible in carcinoma breast. **Therefore, now we know that the surgical treatment alone is not enough for carcinoma breast.** The micrometastases must be managed by chemotherapy after the surgical removal of the cancer. Thus, the concept of **multimodality management** came into existence.
c. *Helman spectrum theory*
d. *Importance of axillary nodal status and dissection:* **The most important single prognostic factor** for carcinoma breast is the nodal status (whether the axillary nodes are involved or not). Four or more axillary node involvement is a **bad prognostic factor**. Therefore, axillary dissection has become a part of any form of surgical treatment including the conservative breast surgery.
e. *The concept of breast conservation:* This concept was initially introduced by **Veronessi** of Milan (Italy). He introduced the **QUART** regimen consisting of **Q**uadrantectomy, **A**xillary dissection and **R**adio**T**herapy for carcinoma breast and found that there is no difference in survival when this form of treatment is compared with radical operations. Finally the breast conservation therapy - **BCT** (consisting of wide local excision, axillary dissection and radiotherapy) is accepted as the treatment of choice for early breast cancer, world over.

Note: Always put elliptical for wide excision. If the lesion is nearer to the skin take more ellipse. When the growth is superficial there is more chance for nodal involvement.

Q 1. What are your points in favor of diagnosis of carcinoma breast?

1. There is a hard lump, which is fixed to the breast.
2. Hard mobile axillary lymph node.
3. The nipple is elevated and retracted.

Q 2. What are your differential diagnosis in this case?

1. Traumatic fat necrosis (It can present very similar to carcinoma breast, hence, it is the first differential diagnosis).
2. Antibioma.
3. Fibroadenosis (ANDI).
4. Fibroadenoma.

Note: Aberration in normal development and involution (ANDI).

Q 3. What is the order of palpation of axillary lymph nodes?

The examiner stands in front of the patient for examining the following axillary nodes:

1. Central group
2. Apical group
3. Brachial group (lateral)—near the insertion of pectoralis major muscle
4. Pectoral or anterior group.

Examiner stands behind the patient for palpation of the following group of nodes:

1. Subscapular or posterior group (anteroinferior to the latissimus dorsi muscle)
2. Supraclavicular nodes
3. Infraclavicular nodes.

Q 4. What is the incidence of carcinoma breast?

- In India—one in 100 to 120 women are affected.
- In Kerala—one in 50–60 women are affected.

Q 5. What are the predisposing factors for carcinoma breast (risk factors)?

Note: Normally 12% risk.

Two times risk means 25%.

1. The number of menstrual cycles between **menarche and first child birth** is the **most important predisposing factor** for carcinoma breast: If the number of cycles are more, there is more chance for carcinoma of the breast. When there is early menarche, which is seen in developed countries because of the good nutrition and the first pregnancy is delayed as is the usual practice there, there is more chance for carcinoma of the breast.
2. When the first **full-term pregnancy is after 35 years of age**, there is more chance for carcinoma of the breast.
3. Increased hormonal exposure as is seen in **early menarche and late menopause** (early menarche when the menarche occurs **before 12 years** and late menopause is when the menopause occurs **after 50 years**).
4. Patients who have had cancer in one breast are at increased risk of development of **cancer in the other breast at the rate of 1 to 2% per year.**
5. *Family history:* Carcinoma breast is more common in women with a family history of breast cancer than in the general population (they account for < **5% of all breast cancer**). If there is a history of a **first degree relative** (mother, daughter and sister) with carcinoma breast, there is more chance for carcinoma in others. Tamoxifen for 5 years appears to reduce the risk of carcinoma by 30 to 50% in this group.
6. *Genetic:*

   BRCA1 gene is seen in chromosome **17q**—it is associated with ovarian, colorectal and prostate cancer. If the gene is positive there is 50 to 80% risk of developing carcinoma breast (many will opt for prophylactic mastectomy).

   BRCA2 gene is seen in chromosome **13q**—is associated with familial **male breast cancer**.

   p53 is a tumor suppressor gene for carcinoma breast.

7. *A breast which is denied of its function (breastfeeding):* There is more chance for carcinoma.
8. Nulliparity is associated with increased chance of cancer of the breast.
9. Women with carcinoma of the endometrium is associated with increased risk of development of carcinoma of the breast.
10. *History of exposure to ionizing radiation*: History of **Mantle radiotherapy** for Hodgkin's disease in childhood is associated with increased incidence of carcinoma, especially when the breast is developing. But this will take at least 10 years.
11. *Postmenopausal obesity:* This is due to increased conversion of steroid hormones to estradiol in body fat.
12. *Diet:* Diets low in phytoestrogens and fatty food is associated with increased risk of developing breast carcinoma.
13. High intake of alcohol.
14. *Age:* Extremely rare below 20 years but there after the incidence steadily rises so that by the age of 90 years nearly 20% of women are affected.
15. *Geographical:* Common in the Western world, less common in developing countries and Japan.
16. History of benign proliferative breast disease is associated with increased chance so also a breast with previous scars.
17. *Environmental:* Pesticides, etc.
18. *Hormone replacement therapy:* Combination of **estrogen and progesterone** taken for a very long duration is associated with increased risk for carcinoma breast. Estrogen alone is associated with slightly increased risk for carcinoma.
19. *Sex:* Female breast is more prone for carcinoma than the male breast.
20. *Oral contraceptive pills:* Do not appear to increase the risk of carcinoma breast.

Note: The two protective factors are:
1. Breastfeeding for more than 2 years
2. First pregnancy less than 21 years of age.

Q 6. How will you proceed to investigate such a patient?

Triple assessment consisting of **clinical examination, imaging** (mammogram/ultrasound) and **FNAC/Core biopsy**. FNAC/Core biopsy is done first, after clinical examination.

Q 7. What is the first investigation of choice?

Imaging first - Mammogram/USG followed by FNAC/core biopsy. FNAC will give a cytological diagnosis of malignancy or benign nature. It is also cheap, simple and cost-effective.

Q 8. What are the different grades of cytological reporting?

Grade	*Result*
AC0 (Grade 0)	No epithelial cells present
AC1 (Grade 1)	Scanty benign cells
AC2 (Grade 2)	Benign cells
AC3 (Grade 3)	Atypical cells present—may need a biopsy if clinically or radiologically suspicious
AC4 (Grade 4)	Highly suspicious of malignancy
AC5 (Grade 5)	Definitely malignant

Q 9. What are the stains used for staining FNAC smears?

a. Giemsa
b. Papanicolaou
c. Hematoxylin and eosin.

Q 10. How many needle passes are required for FNAC and what is the needle size?

- Usually 23G needle is used.
- Minimum 6 needle passes are required.

Q 11. If the FNAC is inconclusive can you repeat the procedure?

Yes, you can repeat FNAC up to 3 times.

Q 12. Still FNAC is negative, how will you proceed?

Core biopsy is the investigation of choice in such a patient. Usually core biopsy is not recommended for lesions less than 2 cm because the small lesions can be easily excised under local anesthesia.

Q 13. How is core biopsy done?

After infiltrating 1% lignocaine anesthetic into the skin and down to around the lesion, a small incision is placed and the lesion is approached with the specific core biopsy needle at approximately 45° angle to the breast so that it will not damage the chest wall.

Q 14. What are the advantages of core biopsy (Tru-cut) over FNAC?

1. The FNAC cannot differentiate **in situ** carcinoma from infiltrating carcinoma.
2. Receptor assay (Estrogen receptor and progesterone receptor) can be done with core biopsy specimen.

Note: Therefore, core biopsy is the preferred method for diagnosis of suspicious breast lump.

Q 15. What are the indications for excision biopsy when FNAC is negative?

If a lesion is reported as malignant on cytology and is clinically and mammographically malignant, the patient does not require further confirmation.

Indications for excision biopsy

a. In lesions < **2 cm** where core biopsy is not possible without imaging.
b. In lesions between **2 and 4 cm where core biopsy is negative**
c. In **cystic lesions when the cyst recurs** or increases in size or there is residual mass after aspiration and FNAC is inconclusive twice
d. A **discrete breast lesion** even if it is considered benign by all investigation needs excision biopsy.

Q 16. Is there any role for incision biopsy?

For lesions **over 4 cm** in size where FNAC and core biopsy are negative, but the lesion is suspicious of malignancy on clinical examination and mammography, incision biopsy is done (excision biopsy of such a big lump will produce distortion of the breast).

Q 17. If the FNAC is inconclusive, what is the order of further investigations?

- Less than 2 cm size swelling—wide local excision
- 2–4 cm size swelling—core biopsy.

If core biopsy fails:

- Size of tumor < 4 cm—wide local excision
- Size of tumor > 4 cm—incisional biopsy.

Q 18. What is the incision planning for breast biopsy?

- Plan the incision in such a way that if the tumor turns out to be carcinoma, the biopsy scar can be included along with the nipple areolar complex within the future transverse elliptical incision of mastectomy.
- For lesions **within 5 cm** of areolar margin, cosmesis is better with **circum areolar** incision.
- There is **no role for radial incision** in breast except at 3 and 9 o'clock position.

- Prefer **curvi linear incisions.**
- Follow the lines of **resting skin tension/Langer's lines.**

Q 19. What are the modalities of imaging available for breast?

a. Mammography
b. Ultrasound
c. **MRI**—useful for differentiating **scar tissue from tumor recurrence**
   - Always use breast coil for MRI of breast
   - Always use contrast—type III enhancement is suggestive of malignancy
d. 18 FDG PET scan (not routinely done).

The most frequently used modalities are mammography and ultrasound. **Above 35 years of age, mammography** is preferred. In young patients **less than 35** years of age **ultrasound** is preferred.

Note:

1. Screening mammogram is ideally done 5 to 7 days postmenopausal.
2. Now a days **digital mammography** is favored.

Q 20. Is there any role for mammography in this patient if it is found to be positive for malignancy in FNAC?

Yes. Mammography is indicated for the same breast to rule out multicentricity. It is also indicated for the contralateral breast to rule out a non palpable lesion there.

Q 21. What are the mammography findings in a case of carcinoma breast?

Mammographic findings in carcinoma breast are:

Primary signs

a. Mass lesion with **clustered pleomorphic micro-calcification** (dense calcification is suggestive of benign disease).
b. Speckled mass lesion with ill defined margin.
c. Architectural distortion of the breast parenchyma (Stellate lesion).
d. Density of the lesion will be more than the rest of the breast.
e. Malignant lesions are **taller than wider.**

Secondary signs

a. Skin changes—retraction, thickening, dimpling.
b. Nipple changes—flattening, retraction, etc.
c. Increased vascularity.
d. Axillary lymphadenopathy.

Q 22. What is the commonest malignancy of the breast?

Infiltrating duct carcinoma.

Q 23. If the FNAC is reported as infiltrating duct carcinoma, what will be the further management?

One should proceed to **staging work up** in such a patient. Since this case clinically is an early breast cancer, the minimum investigations required in this patient are:

Staging work up in carcinoma breast

a. Mammography of the same breast and contralateral breast
b. Ultrasound of the abdomen to rule out metastasis in the liver and for Krukenberg's tumor
c. X-ray of the chest to rule out pulmonary metastasis
d. Liver function test (LFT).

Q 24. What is the staging of carcinoma breast?

It is divided into 4 stages by the AJCC 6th edition.

Stage I and II	are called early breast cancer (EBC).
Stage III	a, b, c are called locally advanced breast cancer (LABC).
Stage IV	is metastatic cancer.

Q 25. What is the TNM staging?

Primary tumor (T)

Tx—primary tumor cannot be assessed*
T 0—no evidence of primary
Tis—carcinoma in situ (Tis DCIS, Tis LCIS, Tis Paget's)
Tis (DCIS)—Ductal carcinoma **in situ**
Tis (LCIS)—Lobular carcinoma **in situ**
Tis (Paget's)—Paget's disease of the nipple with no tumor
T1— tumor **less than 2 cm**
T1 mi—Microinvasion **1 mm or less** in greatest dimension
T1a—Tumor more than **1 mm but not more than 5 mm** in greatest dimension
T1b—Tumor more than **5 mm but not more than 10 mm** in greatest dimension
T1c—Tumor more than **10 mm but not more than 20 mm** in greatest dimension
T2—Tumor **more than 20 mm but not more than 50 mm** in greatest dimension
T3—Tumor **more than 50 mm** in greatest dimension
T4—Tumor of any size with direct extension to the chest wall and or to the skin (**ulceration or skin nodule and peau d' orange**). Invasion of dermis alone does not qualify as T4
T4a—**Extension to chest wall, not including pectoralis muscle** adherence/invasion
T4b—Ulceration and or ipsilateral satellite nodules and or edema (including **peau d' orange**) of the skin which do not meet the criteria for inflammatory carcinoma
T4c—Both T4a and T4b
T4d—Inflammatory carcinoma

Note: **TX**-lump already excised, treated elsewhere without documentation of the size, or treated with chemotherapy.

The **chest wall** includes ribs, intercostal muscles and serratus anterior muscle, but not the pectoral muscles.

Regional nodes

Nx	Regional lymph nodes cannot be assessed (e.g. previously removed)
N0	No regional node metastases
N1	Metastases to movable **ipsilateral level 1 and 2 axillary** lymph nodes
N2	Metastases in **ipsilateral level 1 and 2 axillary lymph nodes that are clinically fixed or matted or in clinically detected ipsilateral internal mammary** nodes in the absence of clinically evident axillary lymph node metastases
N2a	Metastases in ipsilateral level 1 and 2 axillary lymph nodes fixed to one another (matted) or to other structures
N2b	Metastases only in clinically detected ipsilateral internal mammary nodes and in the absence of clinically evident level 1 and 2 axillary lymph node metastases
N3	Metastases in ipsilateral infraclavicular (level 3 axillary) lymph nodes with or without level 1, 2 axillary lymph node involvement or in clinically detected ipsilateral internal mammary lymph nodes with clinically evident level 1 and 2 axillary lymph node metastases or metastases in Ipsilateral supraclavicular lymph nodes with or without axillary or internal mammary lymph node involvement
N3a	Metastases in **ipsilateral infraclavicular** lymph nodes
N3b	Metastases in **ipsilateral internal mammary** lymph node(s) and **axillary** lymph node(s)
N3c	Metastases in **ipsilateral supraclavicular** lymph node(s)

Note: Clinically detected is defined as **detected by imaging studies** (excluding lymphoscintigraphy) or by **clinical examination** and having characteristics highly suspicious for malignancy or a presumed pathologic micrometastases based on fine needle aspiration biopsy with cytologic examination. Confirmation of clinically detected metastatic disease by fine needle aspiration without excision biopsy is designated with f suffix

Distant metastases	
Mx	Distant metastases cannot be assessed
M0	No distant metastases
M1	Distant metastases

Stage Grouping

Stage 0	Tis	N0	M0
Stage IA	T1	N0	M0
Stage IB	T0	N1mi	M0
	T1	N1mi	M0
Stage IIA	T0	N1	M0
	T1	N1	M0
	T2	N0	M0
Stage IIB	T2	N1	M0
	T3	N0	M0
Stage IIIA	Up to T3	Up to N2	M0
Stage IIIB	Any T4	N0/N1/N2	M0
Stage IIIC	Any T	N3	M0
Stage IV	Any T	Any N	M0

Note:

- T1 includes T1mi
- T0 and T1 tumors with nodal micrometastases only are excluded from Stage II A and classified as Stage IB.

  If a patient presents with MI prior to neoadjuvant systemic therapy, the stage is considered stage IV and remains Stage IV regardless of response to neoadjuvant therapy.

  Post-neoadjuvant therapy is designated with "yc" or "yp" prefix of note, no stage group is assigned if there is a complete pathologic response (CR) to neoadjuvant therapy.

Summary of Staging

- Early breast cancer – Stage I and II – T1N1, T2N1 and T3N0
- Locally advanced breast Cancer (**LABC**) – Stage IIIA and IIIB
- Metastatic breast cancer (**MBC**) – Stage IV

Q 26. What is the staging in this case?

Since the size of the tumor is T2 and patient is having a single clinically positive axillary lymph node the stage is IIB that is (T2, N1, M0).

Q 27. What is the origin of carcinoma breast?

The carcinoma breast originates from **TDLU** Terminal duct lobular unit (Fig. 5.2).

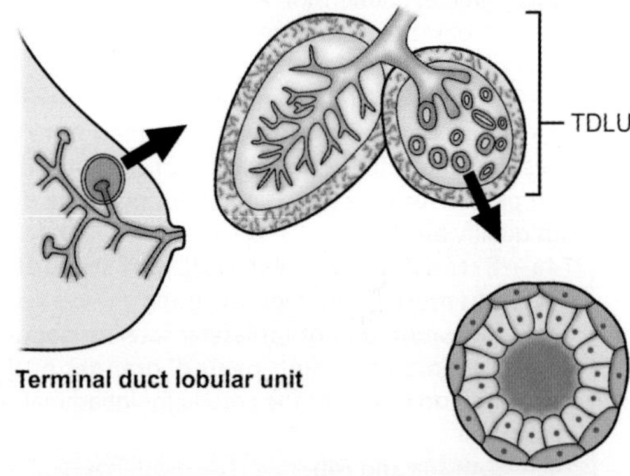

Fig. 5.2: Breast and terminal duct labular unit

Q 28. What is the new pathological classification?

It is classified into ductal carcinoma and lobular carcinoma depending on the origin from TDLU. Both may be in situ cancer or invasive cancer.

	In situ	*Invasive (infiltrating)*
Lobular carcinoma	LCIS (lobular carcinoma **in situ**)	Infiltrating lobular carcinoma
Ductal carcinoma	DCIS (ductal carcinoma **in situ**)	Infiltrating ductal carcinoma

The invasive carcinoma is classified into:
- **Special types (ST)**
- **No special type (NST)/not otherwise specified (NOS).**

Note:
- The special types are having **good prognosis** but forms only 15% of the total. The examples of special types are **tubular, mucinous, cribriform, medullary, etc.**
- NOS or NST is having bad prognosis (85%).

Q 29. What is the commonest pathological type of carcinoma breast?

Infiltrating carcinoma (NOS type is the commonest pathology).

Q 30. What is Gene array analysis?

There are two types:

a. Oncotype Dx—21 gene analysis
b. Mammoprint—17 gene

Five subtypes of carcinoma breast are identified

1. **Luminal A** (40–55%) – ER positive and HER 2 negative–. They are well or moderately differentiated. It occurs in postmenopausal women and is slow growing. They respond well to hormone treatment.
2. **Luminal B** (15–20%)—(**Triple positive** – ER, PR and HER2 positive) – they respond to chemotherapy.
3. **Triple negative** – ER, PR and HER2 negative (**Basal like**) (13–25%) They are high grade tumors with aggressive course and poor prognosis. Examples are medullary carcinoma and metaplastic carcinoma. There is high incidence of brain and lung metastases. It has got poor prognosis. It will affect younger patients often black races are affected. There is a chemosensitive subgroup of 15–20%. BRCA1 mutation is seen in this group.
4. **HER2 rich** (7–12%) They are ER negative and poorly differentiated with high proliferation rate and high frequency of brain metastases. Treatment of choice is chemotherapy and Trastuzamab/Herceptin. However Trastuzamab/Herceptin will not cross blood brain barrier in case of metastases. Lapatinab is the drug of choice when there is metastasis.
5. **Normal breast like** – (6–10%) ER positive and HER2 negative.

Q 31. What is the tumor doubling time for carcinoma breast?

- One doubling time takes 2–9 months.
- For reaching 1cm size of the tumor 30 doubling times are required.
- The minimum size required for clinical palpation of a tumor is 1cm.
- On an average, it takes five years for a tumor to become clinically palpable in the breast.

Q 32. What is the grading of the tumor?

The **Nottingham combined histological grade (Elston – Ellis modification of Scarff Bloom-Richardson grading system)** which is a modified **Bloom- Richardson** grading is used for grading. In this the **nuclear pleomorphism**, **mitotic count** and **tubule formation** are taken into account giving scores of 1 (favorable) 2–3 (unfavorable). A score of 3–5 is **grade I**, 6–7 is **grade II**, 8–9 is **grade III.**

Q 33. What is the surgical treatment of choice in this patient?

Now the gold standard surgical treatment option for stage I and II patients are **BCT (Breast conservation therapy). Modified radical mastectomy is another option** (Flow chart 5.1).

Flow chart 5.1: Management of early breast cancer

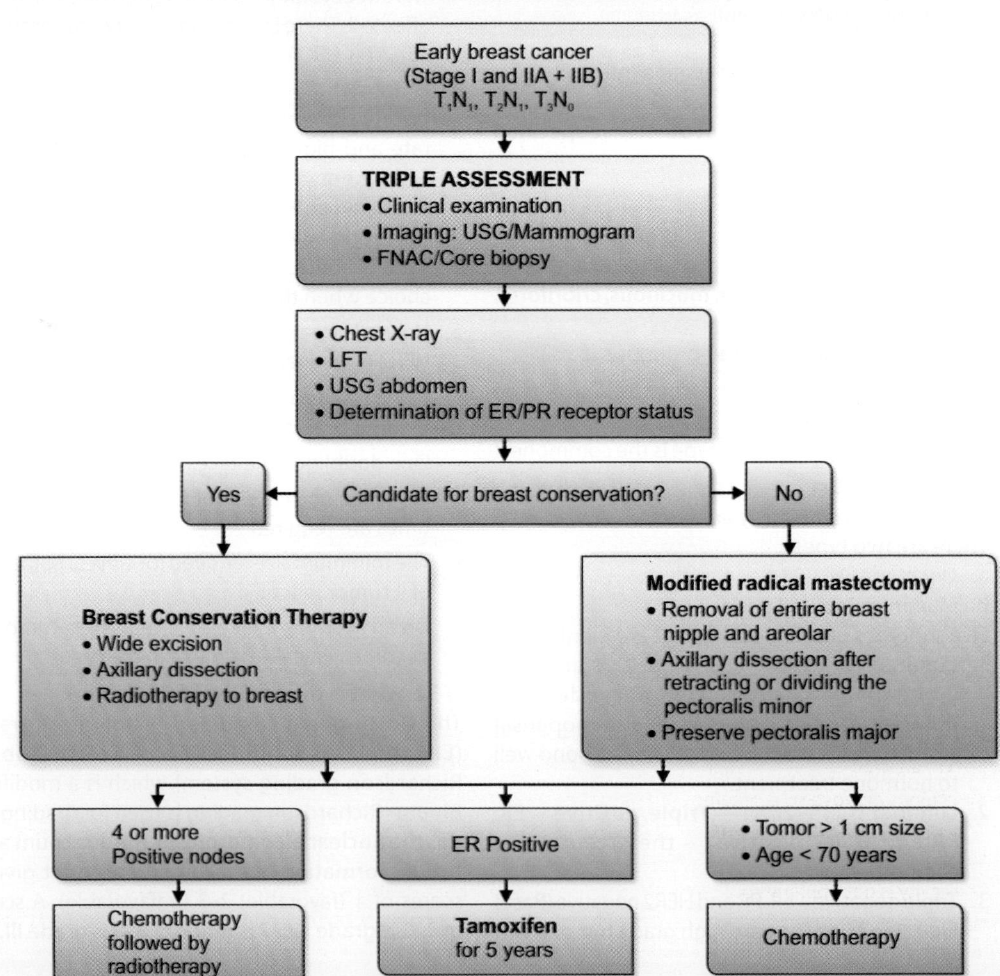

Q 34. What is breast conservation therapy?
Breast conservation consists of **wide excision** with 1 cm tumor clearance without excising the overlying skin, **axillary node dissection** through a separate incision in the axilla, followed by **radiotherapy** to the rest of the breast.

Components – of BCT
• Wide excision • Axillary node dissection • Radiotherapy to the remaining breast.

Note: Bilateral breast conservation surgery is not recommended because of the irradiation risk (bilateral).

Q 35. What are the precautions to be taken during wide excision in breast conservative surgery?

Important steps of wide excision for carcinoma breast
a. The incision should be curvilinear placed along the Langer's lines (skin tension lines) b. Removal of the skin overlying the lesion is unnecessary c. 1 cm tumor clearance is important (macroscopic) d. The skin flaps should not be undermined. e. Pectoral fascia is not excised unless involved f. If it is involving the muscle, a fillet of muscle should be removed g. Specimen should be oriented with sutures or clips h. Meticulous hemostasis is secured with diathermy i. The cavity is lavaged with dilute chlorhexidine solution and kept for 2 minutes j. The cavity is not obliterated k. No drain is put.

Q 36. What are the contraindication for breast conservation?

Contraindication for breast conservation
1. T3, T4 tumors, N2 or M1 2. Large or central tumors in small breast 3. Multifocal/multicentric disease 4. Collagen vascular disease 5. Extensive **in situ** component.

Consider MRM (Modified radical mastectomy) in these cases.

Q 37. What is the rationale for axillary dissection?
The **single most important prognostic factor** for carcinoma breast is **nodal status** (**4 or more pathologically positive** axillary node is prognostically bad). Therefore, axillary dissection will form part of the surgical management of all types procedures including breast conservation. **Minimum of 12 lymph nodes must be removed in axillary dissection.**

Q 38. What is the average number of axillary lymph nodes and internal mammary nodes?
- Average number of axillary nodes is 53
- Internal mammary nodes – 3 to 4.

Q 39. What is the rationale for radiotherapy in early breast cancer surgery?
Radiotherapy is given to tackle the multicentricity in the remaining breast.

The patient should be willing to undergo radiotherapy 5 days a week for 20 days and radiotherapy facility should be available.

The indications for radiotherapy in early breast cancer are:
1. Four or more positive axillary nodes
2. Lymphovascular invasion (1–3)—High grade tumors

3. Resection margin positive
4. Skin and chest wall involvement
5. Size more than 5 cm.

Q 40. What is the rationale for mastectomy in early breast cancer?

Mastectomy is recommended to remove the multicentricity seen in carcinoma breast.

Q 41. What is the difference between multicentricity and multifocality?

- When tumor foci are found in a different quadrant it is called **multicentricity**.
- When tumor foci are found in the same quadrant it is called multifocal.

Q 42. What is the type of mastectomy recommended for early breast cancer?

Modified radical mastectomy of **Auchincloss** is preferred (Case No 6).

Q 43. What is QUART Regimen of VERONESI (Contemporary Italian Surgeon Umbreto Veronesi from Milan)?

Veronesi of Milan is responsible for bringing a paradigm shift in surgical treatment of carcinoma breast from mastectomy to conservation. Now quart regimen is not followed. It consists of quadrantectomy, axillary dissection and radio therapy).

Q 44. What is extensive in situ component (EIC)?

The presence of EIC in an invasive cancer is defined as the presence of **more than 25% DCIS component** in the main tumor or if DCIS is present elsewhere in the surrounding tissue.

Q 45. What is inflammatory carcinoma?

Features of inflammatory carcinoma

- It is a rare and **most malignant** form of breast cancer, constituting less than 3% of cases.

Contd...

Contd...

- It is a **clinico pathological entity** characterized by **diffuse erythema and edema** (peau d' orange) of the breast, often **without underlying palpable mass** involving 1/3rd or more of the skin of the breast. Histologic presence of invasive carcinoma invading dermal lymphatic is supportive of diagnosis, it is not required nor is dermal lymphatic invasion without typical clinical findings sufficient for a diagnosis of inflammatory breast cancer.
- The clinical findings should involve the **majority of the skin of the breast.**
- The term **should not be applied** to a patient with neglected locally advanced cancer of the breast.
- The skin changes are due to lymphoedema caused by tumor emboli within dermal lymphatics
- On imaging there may be detectable mass and thickening of the skin over the breast.
- The clinical presentation is due to **tumor emboli within dermal lymphatics.**
- This is usually not associated with a palpable lump. It has a very bad prognosis and it is included under stage III (**classified as T4d**).

Q 46. Is there any role for chemotherapy in early breast cancer surgery?

Yes. **The indications for chemotherapy are:**

1. Node positive cases
2. HER2 positive cases
3. Triple negative
4. More than 0.5 cm size and less than 70 years of age

6 Cycles of **CMF** (Cyclophosphamide, Methotrexate, 5 FU) or **CAF** (**Adriamycin-based regimen**) (Flow chart 5.1). **It is important to remember that CMF regimen is not an adequate adjuvant therapy.** The new regimens are:

a. Adriamycin, Cyclophosphamide (AC) with Taxanes
b. AC followed by taxanes – 4 cycles of AC followed by 4 cycles of taxanes

Q 47. What is the rationale for chemotherapy?

The new concept about carcinoma breast is that it is a **systemic disease** from the very beginning. This is in contrast to the old Halstedian concept where a staged progression of the tumor from the breast to the axilla and from their to systemic dissemination was proposed. Therefore from the very beginning patient can have micrometastases, which cannot be detected. In order to tackle the micrometastases systemic chemotherapy is given.

Q 48. Is there any role for hormone therapy in this patient?

If the tumor is **ER and PR** (Estrogen receptor and progesterone receptor) **positive** the patient is given the antiestrogen called **Tamoxifen** 20 mg daily for five years (Flow chart 5.1).

Q 49. What are the actions of Tamoxifen?

Actions of Tamoxifen
a. It has **anti estrogenic action** on the breast and estrogenic action on other tissues
b. **Tumoricidal**
c. Prevent **recurrence in the contralateral breast.**

Note: Tamoxifen is a selective estrogen receptor modulator (**SERM**) that has antagonistic action on estrogen receptors in the breast and agonistic action on ER receptor elsewhere.

The **half-life of the drug is 7 days** and it takes **4 weeks for action**. The other **beneficial effects of tamoxifen** are:

a. Preservation of bone density in postmenopausal women
b. Decrease in cholesterol
c. Reduction in cardiovascular morbidity (These are due to the estrogenic effects of Tamoxifen on extra mammary tissues).

Q 50. What are the side effects of tamoxifen?

Side effects of tamoxifen
a. Hot flushes
b. Thromboembolic complications (deep vein thrombosis and pulmonary embolism) and stroke
c. Vaginal dryness and atrophy in premenopausal women
d. Vaginal discharge in postmenopausal women
e. Increase risk of endometrial cancer in post-menopausal women
f. Bone loss in premenopausal women
g. Weight gain.

Side effects in post-menopausal women	Side effects in pre-menopausal women
• Endometrial cancer	• Bone loss
• Pulmonary embolism	• Decreased vaginal secretion
• Stroke	• Atrophy of vaginal epithelium
• Vaginal discharge	

Q 51. What are the other hormones used in the treatment of carcinoma breast?

Aromatase inhibitors—the production of estrogen requires the activity of aromatase enzyme. Estrogen production in postmenopausal women is by **peripheral aromatization of androgens produced from the adrenal gland**. Aromatase inhibitors block estrogen production in postmenopausal women and therefore **they form adjuvant therapy for postmenopausal women**. A number of aromatase inhibitors are available like:

a. Aminoglutethimide—this also blocks cortisol.
b. **Newer aromatase inhibitors**, e.g. Anastrozole 1 mg daily, Letrozole, Exemestane
c. Raloxifene 60 mg daily (newer molecule of Tamoxifen
d. LHRH agonists—Goserelin, Buserelin,
e. Other LHRH agonists—Leuprolide
f. Antiestrogen—Fulvestrant
g. Progestational agents—Magestrol
h. Androgens—Fluoxymesterone.

Q 52. What is the source of estrogen in post-menopausal women?

- The circulating estrogen in postmenopausal women is **about 10%** of the level in premenopausal. They are synthesized peripherally **principally in fat including breastfat, skin, muscle and liver**.
- Adrenal gland.

Q 53. What is the timing of hormone therapy?

Hormone therapy is started after the completion of chemotherapy to reduce the side effects.

Q 54. What is the role of surgical oophorectomy?

Oophorectomy was the standard hormone treatment in the pre-tamoxifen era. Currently when patient compliant regarding tamoxifen intake is doubtful some centers are recommending oophorectomy. The other alternatives for oophorectomy are:

1. Medical oophorectomy with aminoglutethimide—suppress adrenal
2. High dose estrogen—diethyl stilbestrol
3. Radiation oophorectomy
4. Chemotherapy as such will produce temporary oophorectomy effect.

Q 55. Can you avoid axillary dissection in carcinoma breast?

Yes. Axillary dissection can be avoided by **sentinel node biopsy.**

Q 56. What is sentinel lymph node biopsy?

A sentinel node is a lymph node that primarily drains the tumor area. Sentinel node biopsy is done for **early breast cancer with clinically negative axillary nodes.** Injection of **radiolabeled (technetium) sulfur colloid** and or a **blue dye (methylene blue is acceptable)** into the **tumor or peri tumoral area** or the **skin overlying** before excision of the primary allows identification of the sentinel node in the axilla either by intraoperative visual inspection or with the help of **gamma probe**. The blue dye is injected intradermally during surgery and then wait for 10 minutes. The dye will spread along the lymphatics. 0.5 mL of the dye is used. The sulphur colloid is injected the day before surgery at **3 pm** at the areolar region (peri tumoral region also possible). Dissect out the axilla starting from axillary tail. Always remove the **blue node and hot node** (when radio labelled sulphur colloid is used). Do not remove nodes which are not blue and not hot. For patients with breast cancer one or two nodes are usually identified. The nodes are send for **frozen section** (– 21°C). 4 microns thick sections are taken.

The concept is that if the identified sentinel nodes are negative for malignancy in frozen section examination, the chances for a higher level node to be affected by skip metastases is remote and therefore an axillary clearance can be avoided with the consequent morbidity. **If the sentinel node is positive** the patient will go in for **formal axillary clearance. Node replaced completely by metastasis will not take up the dye.**

Note: Routinely as per NCCN guidelines level II dissection is adequate.

- There are two methods **level III lymph node dissection**—going between the sternal and clavicular fibres of pectoralis major from the breast side or through the axilla via the interpectoral route.

Q 57. What is axillary node sampling?

Removal of the nodes upto the intercostobrachial nerve is called axillary node sampling. Minimum 4 nodes are removed.

Q 58. What is the management of DCIS (Ductal carcinoma in situ)?

The DCIS can be classified into **widespread** type (i.e. more than 4 cm size) and **localized type.** For wide-spread type, the treatment of choice is **mastectomy.**

The **3 surgical options are**:

1. Simple mastectomy
2. Breast conservation surgery (Lumpectomy) and Radiotherapy to the breast and Tamoxifen for 5 years.
3. Lumpectomy alone (without radiotherapy).
   - There is **no need for axillary dissection** in DCIS because of the fact that chance for node involvement is negligible (4%).
   - There is no role for chemotherapy in DCIS.

Q 59. What are the indications for mastectomy in DCIS?

1. Women with multicentric DCIS
2. Extensive or diffused ductal carcinoma
3. Positive margins
4. Acceptable cosmesis cannot be achieved
5. Radiotherapy is contraindicated (Collagen vascular disease)
6. Pregnancy
7. Diffuse malignant appearing microcalcification
8. Patient preference.

Q 60. What is oncoplastic surgery?

Here immediate reconstruction is done after mastectomy of wide excision.

Q 61. What are the essential steps of lumpectomy?

Essential steps of lumpectomy
• Complete surgical excision • Careful orientation of the specimen • Negative margin of at least 1 mm width • There should be no tumor at the margin (optimal margin width not known) • Margin status is taken before closure of the wound • Radiography to confirm excision of micro-calcification • Postexcision breast imaging to confirm removal of suspicious areas • Re-excision as necessary to obtain negative margin.

Note: Lumpectomy is followed by radiotherapy in breast conservation treatment for DCIS.

Q 62. Is there any role for hormone therapy in DCIS?

Yes. If they are ER positive (Estrogen Receptor Positive), **Tamoxifen is given for 5 years.**

Q 63. What are the indications for lumpectomy alone

- Small lesions < 0.5 cm size
- Unicentric lesion
- Low grade lesion.

Q 64. What is the follow-up of DCIS after surgery?

- Physical examination every 6 months for 5 years
- **Mammogram every 12 months.**

Q 65. What is LCIS (Lobular carcinoma in situ)?

The present consensus regarding LCIS is that it is a marker of **subsequent development of invasive cancer** rather than a preinvasive cancerous lesion. (**It is not a precursor but a predictor for carcinoma. Hence it is called a bystander lesion**).

- **LCIS** is a rare form of non-invasive breast cancer. It **does not typically form micro- calcifications** and therefore not easily detectable on X-rays and is usually found incidentally on biopsy.

- Invasive ductal cancer develops in approximately 25% of patients, which may be delayed for 10–20 years
  - 45% develop ipsilateral carcinoma
  - 35% develop contralateral carcinoma
  - 15% develop bilateral carcinoma.
- The risk of development of invasive ductal cancer is equal for both breasts.
- LCIS tends to be multifocal in both breasts.
- The **contralateral breast is affected in 30%** of cases and in the residual breast in upto 70% of cases. The incidence of **nodal involvement is very low** in this cancer.

Q 66. What is the management of LCIS?

Management of LCIS
• History and physical examination every (6–12 months)
• Diagnostic bilateral mammogram (every 12 months)
• Pathology review
• **Observation** for the development of invasive cancer (ipsilateral and contralateral breast)
• **Risk reduction with Tamoxifen** for pre-menopausal women
• Risk reduction with **Raloxifen** for postmenopausal women
• **Bilateral mastectomy and reconstruction** in special circumstances.

Q 67. What are the indications for prophylactic mastectomy?

1. LCIS (Lobular carcinoma **in situ**)
2. BRCA1 and 2.

Q 68. What are the features of lobular carcinoma breast?

- Incidence is 15%
- Multifocal
- Bilateral
- The marker for lobular carcinoma is e-cadherin antibody.

Q 69. What are the bad prognostic factors for carcinoma breast?

Bad prognostic factors for carcinoma breast
1. Axillary nodal status is the most important single prognostic factor
2. Age < 35 years—bad prognosis
3. Grade of tumor (Bloom-Richardson grade)—higher the grade, bad the prognosis
4. Extensive **in situ** component – bad prognosis
5. Receptor status – ER negative and PR negative — bad prognosis
6. P^{53} status (Tumor suppressor gene called '**Guardian of Genome**') positive—bad prognosis
7. Presence of HER—2 (Tyrosine kinase receptor) — bad prognosis.

Q 70. What is Paget's disease of the breast?

It is nothing but a **ductal carcinoma with associated nipple destruction**, seen in **1–2%** of the patients. In **50%** there will be an underlying **mass lesion. 90%** of these patients will have **invasive carcinoma**. For the patients **without mass lesion 30%** will be later found to have an invasive carcinoma. It should be **differentiated from eczema.** Mammography is indicated in such patients and also imprint cytology of the lesion. **Incisional biopsy** is finally required.

- If a **mass lesion is present,** treatment is MRM (Modified Radical Mastectomy).
- Otherwise a wide local excision of the nipple areolar region, axillary dissection followed by radiotherapy and other adjuvant treatment is required.

Q 71. What are the difference between Paget's disease and eczema?

Difference between Paget's disease and eczema of the nipple	
Paget's disease	*Eczema*
1. Unilateral	Bilateral
2. Itching absent	Itching present
3. Absence of oozing	Presence of oozing
4. Scales and vesicles absent	Scales and vesicles present
5. Nipple destroyed	Nipple is intact
6. Underlying lump may be present	No underlying lump
7. Edges are distinct	Edges are indistinct
8. Will not respond to treatment	Will respond to treatment
9. Occurs at menopause (Old age)	Seen in lactating women (Young age)

Q 72. What are the causes for nipple discharge?

Causes for nipple discharge		
1. Bright red blood	Duct papilloma (commonest) Carcinoma in lactating breast	Duct carcinoma
2. Dark altered blood	Papilloma obstructing a duct (Discharge of blood is delayed)	
3. Blood stained fluid with sizeable cystic swelling	Intracystic papilliferous carcinoma (Disease of reclus)	
4. Clear serous fluid with a lumpy breast (Yellow)	ANDI In women taking OCP	
5. Green/Black discharge	Duct ectasia	
6. Milky discharge	Insufficient suppression of lactation after weaning Secreting prolactinoma of the Pituitary gland Hypothyroidism	
7. Purulent	Infection	

Pregnancy and Carcinoma Breast

Q 73. What is the management of carcinoma breast in pregnancy?

- It **behaves in similar way** to breast cancer in nonpregnant woman and treated accordingly.
- Breast cancer during pregnancy and lactation tends to be at a later stage because the symptoms are masked.
- **Radiotherapy is avoided** during pregnancy and therefore **mastectomy is preferred** over breast conservation, (causes death of embryo, intrauterine growth retardation, neurological anomalies, etc.).
- **Chemotherapy is avoided** during the first trimester but it is safe afterwards (CAF regimen is better. Breastfeeding is avoided while on chemotherapy).
- Most tumors are receptor negative and therefore hormone treatment is not required.

- Hormone treatment during pregnancy is **potentially teratogenic.**
- Lactation needs to be suppressed with bromocriptine if chemotherapy is instituted after delivery.

Q 74. What is the breast imaging of choice in pregnancy?

- MRI is the choice
- Ultrasound and mammogram are likely to yield more false-positive results because of increased parenchymal density, increased vascularity, water content and cellularity.

Q 75. What is the staging work up during pregnancy?

- There is no contraindication for X-ray chest. It can be done with abdominal shielding.
- Alkaline phosphatase is not dependable during pregnancy (It is elevated in pregnancy).
- Bone scan is delayed until after delivery (MRI is safe for metastasis).

Q 76. Can a patient become pregnant after treatment of carcinoma breast?

Women are usually advised to **wait for two years** for subsequent pregnancy since the maximum recurrences are seen during the first 2 years.

Q 77. What is the management of carcinoma breast during various trimesters of pregnancy?

First trimester

- Modified radical mastectomy and axillary dissection for the local disease
- If found to be node positive, terminate the pregnancy and give chemotherapy
- If it is locally advanced terminate the pregnancy and treat.

Second trimester

- The decision is based on the stage of the disease and the wish of the patient to continue pregnancy
- All stages surgery is recommended.

Third trimester

- Do surgery
- Wait till delivery and give adjuvant chemotherapy after delivery.

Q 78. What is the role of therapeutic abortion in carcinoma breast?

- It is indicated if radiotherapy and chemotherapy cannot be postponed due to the stage of the disease
- There is no advantage as such for therapeutic abortion, but the treatment is made easier.

Q 79. What is bilateral breast cancer?

- It means a separate primary cancer in each breast
- It can be synchronous or metachronous.

Q 80. How to differentiate whether the second tumor is primary or metastatic?

The **Choudary Millis criteria** used for calling the second tumor a primary are:

1. Demonstration of in situ change in the contralateral tumor.
2. If it is histologically different from the cancer in the first breast.
3. If the degree of histologic differentiation is distinctly greater than the lesion in the first breast.
4. In the absence of histologic difference, the contralateral is considered to be primary, provided there is no evidence of local, regional or distant metastases from the cancer in the ipsilateral breast.

Q 81. What are the risk factors for the development of a second primary?

- A woman who has had breast cancer has a **five fold increase in risk** for second breast cancer
- Multifocal cancer in the original breast
- Lobular carcinoma **in situ**
- Family history of breast cancer
- Diagnosis of original cancer at an early age.

Q 82. What is the treatment of second primary?

Give treatment appropriate for tumor depending on the stage of the disease.

Q 83. What is the mammographic findings in metastatic cancer of the breast?

Mammographic findings in metastatic cancer of the breast

- Metastatic cancer is less infiltrative (primary tumor is more infiltrative)
- More diffuse
- Fewer fine calcifications
- Presence of secondary edema.

Elegy for a Poor Breast

- For years and years they told me, be careful of your breasts. Do not ever squeeze or bruise them. And give them monthly tests
- So I heeded all their warnings, an protected them by law. Guarded them very carefully, and I always wore my bra
- After 30 years of astute care, my doctor found a lump
- She ordered up a mammogram
- To look inside that bump
- "Stand up very close" she said. As she got my boob in line, "And tell me when it hurts" she said. "Ah yes! There, that's fine
- She stepped upon a pedal. I could not believe my eyes! A plastic plate pressed down and down, my boob was in a vise!
- My skin was stretched and stretched, from way up under my chin. My poor boob was being squashed, to Swedish pancake thin
- Excruciating pain I felt, within it's vice—like grip. A prisoner in this viscous thing. My poor defense less tit!
- 'Take a deep breath' she said to me, who does she think she's kidding? My chest is mashed in her machine, and woozy I am getting
- 'There, that was good, "I heard her say as the room was slowly swaying. "Now, let's have a go at the other one," Lord have mercy I was praying
- It squeezed me from up and down. It squeezed me from both sides. I'll bet she's never had this done not to her tender little hide! If I had no problem when I came in, I surely have one now
- If there had been a cyst in there, it would have popped, "ker-pow!"
- This machine was created by a man, of this, I have no doubt. I'd like to stick his balls in there, and see how they come out!

FOR PG'S—WHAT IS NEW?

Paget's disease

- The MRI findings are type II or III contrast kinetics and nipple areolar complex flattening
- It is cytokeratin 7 positive
- The surgical treatment is central wide excision and breast conservation

MRI in breast cancer

- Indications are problem solving cases, equivocal cases and lobular lesions
- Silicone prosthesis will give snow storm appearance in mammogram

PET in breast cancer

- It is used for loco regional and distant metastasis
- PEM – PET Emission Mammography

Targeted therapy in breast cancer

- The oldest targeted therapy is ER and PR positive with tamoxifen
- 50% are ER positive and 20% HER2 new positive which is a human epidermal growth factor type IV
- Trastuzumab (Herceptin) for HER2 new positive (15 to 20%)—it will not cross blood brain barrier and therefore cannot be used for brain metastasis. This drug is used for adjuvant therapy concurrently with Taxane, as neoadjuvant therapy in LABC and in metastatic cancer. It is usually given weekly **(9 weeks upfront)** or three weekly regimen for 1year
- The complication of trastuzumab is heart failure
- Lapatinib is an EGF receptor antagonist it is an oral preparation and is available as tablets. It is used for stage IV disease in combination with traustuzumab—will cross blood brain barrier and used for HER2 positive metastasis
- Bevacizumab—VEGF blockade

Screening mammogram for non palpable lesions (not visualized in USG)

- The patient is kept in prone position (Swimmer's position)
- Stereo guided FNAC or core biopsy of the identified lesion is done and this is followed by specimen mammogram
- Another option is wire localization and excision (the localization is done by mammogram)
- Gene array (also called genetic profile) (please read the text)
- Two types are available: *Oncotype Dx*-21 genes (this is done in formalin fixed paraffin specimen
- **Mammaprint** - 17 gene analysis and is done in frozen section

Case

6 Advanced Breast Cancer

Case Capsule

A **55-year-old postmenopausal obese female** presents with a **swelling in the right breast**. Her elder **sister died of carcinoma breast** at the age of 40 years. There is no history of bony pain, no hemoptysis and dyspnea. There is no history of jaundice, headache and seizures. The patient attained **menarche at the age of 13 years.** She was married at the age of 25 years and her **first child birth** was at the age of **28 years**. She has got three children and **all were breastfed**. She gives **history of recent retraction** of the right nipple. There is **no history of discharge from the nipple**. On examination, the entire affected **breast is at a higher level** than the left breast. The breast as a whole is **pulled up and contracted** compared to the normal side. **Dilated veins are seen** in the skin overlying. There is **retraction and elevation of the right nipple**. There is a visible **lump of 6 × 7 cm size** occupying the upper and lower outer quadrants of right breast. There is **edema of the skin** over the mass with **peau d'orange appearance.** A few **satellite skin nodules** are seen but they are confined to the same breast. On palpation there is local rise of temperature and **fixity of the skin** overlying the mass. The lump is **hard in consistency** and **fixed to the breast**. It is also **fixed to the pectoral muscles** but there is no fixity to the chest wall. There is a visible axillary swelling on the right side. On palpation, there is **matted hard axillary lymph nodes of 5 × 3 cm size** involving both pectoral and central group. There are no infraclavicular nodes. The **supraclavicular fossa is empty** on both sides and no palpable nodes. There is **no edema of the right arm**. The contralateral breast and axilla are normal. There is no cervical lymph node enlargement. There is **no hepatomegaly and ascites** on abdominal examination. On chest examination there is **no evidence of consolidation or pleural effusion**. The lumbar spine is normal.

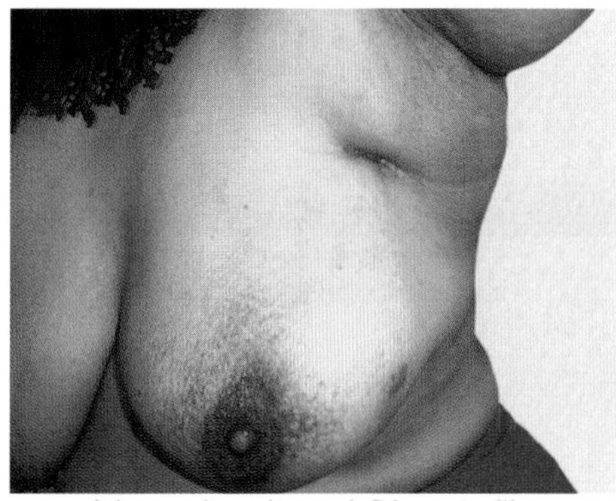

Advanced carcinoma left breast with skin ulceration

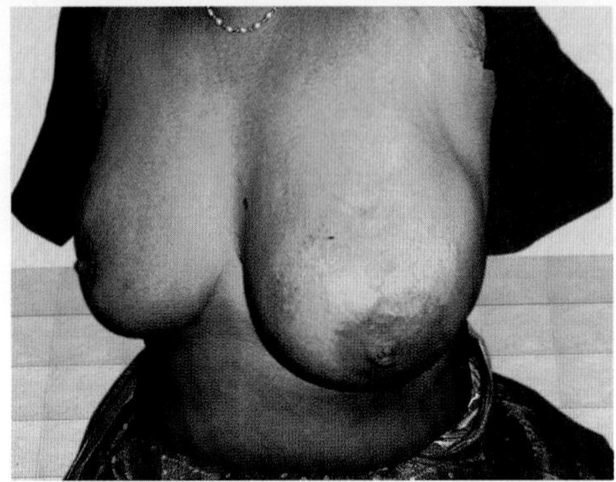
Big tumor in the left breast with skin overlying showing dilated veins

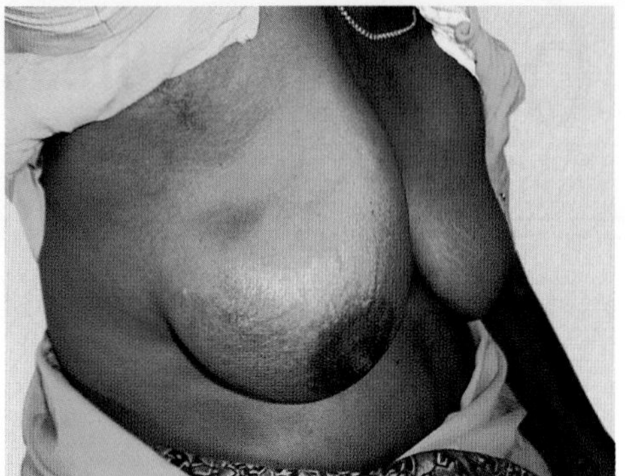
Carcinoma breast with big mass and peau d orange appearance

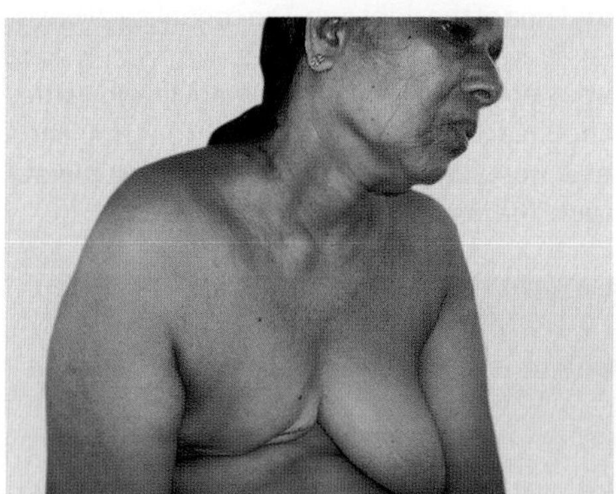
Post-mastectomy with supraclavicular lymph nodes

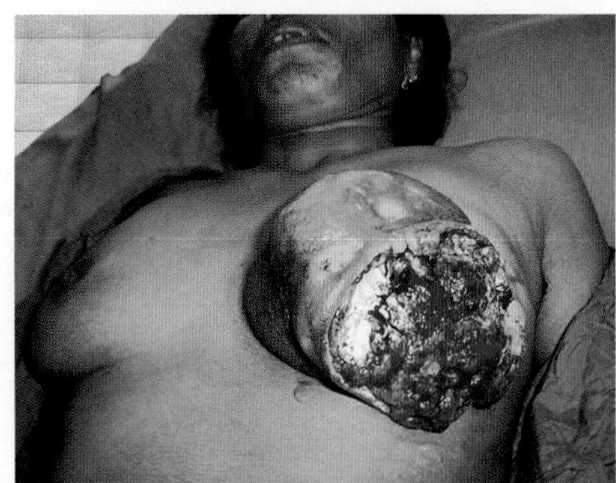
Carcinoma right breast with a big mass

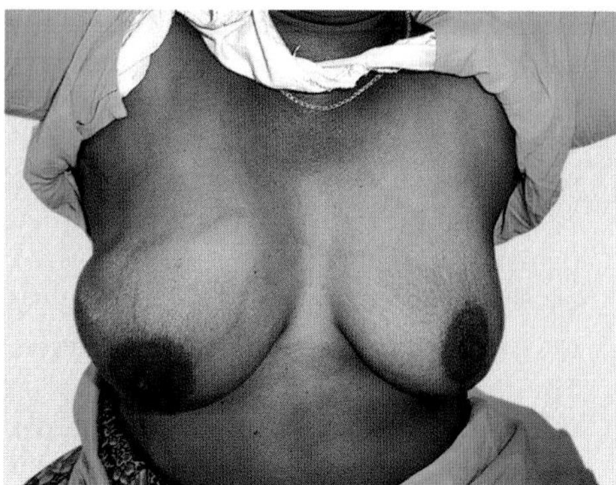

Advanced breast cancer with fungating mass

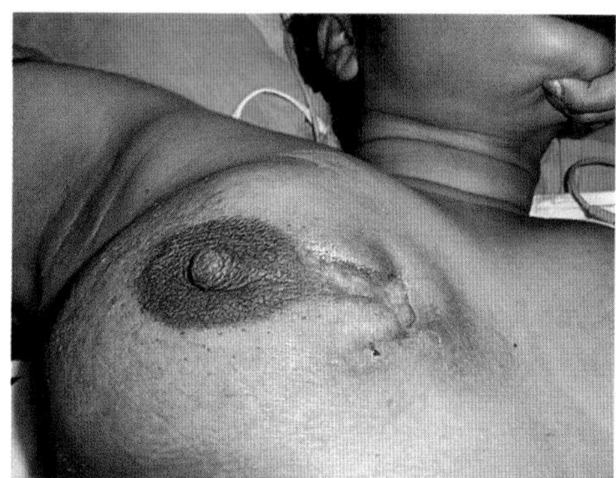

Tuberculosis of right breast

Read the Checklist of Case No. 5

Q 1. What is the probable diagnosis in this case?

The first diagnosis in this situation must be carcinoma breast because of the following reasons.

a. A hard lump which is fixed to the breast
b. Peau d' orange appearance
c. Nipple retraction and elevation
d. Presence of suspicious axillary nodes
e. Skin nodules
f. Skin fixity.

Q 2. What is the cause for peau d' orange appearance?

It is due to **cutaneous lymphedema** as a result of blockage of the lymphatics draining the skin. Here the pits of the hair follicles appear to be retracted beneath the skin. Wherever the hair follicles are anchored to the subcutaneous tissue, it cannot swell. In between the hair follicles the skin will swell like an orange peel.

Q 3. What is the cause for nipple retraction and elevation in malignancy?

Only recent retraction of nipple is of significance. It is due to the extension of growth **along the ducts and the periductal fibrosis.** This is responsible for nipple elevation also.

Q 4. What is the difference between skin tethering and skin fixity?

The breast is anchored to the underlying pectoral fascia by bands called ligaments of Cooper. The malignant cells invade these ligaments and reach the skin. In early stage, movement of the lump along the axis of the ligament of Cooper will not produce skin dimpling. The moment the axis is changed there will be dimpling. This is called skin tethering. In skin **fixity** there is extensive infiltration of the skin and skin cannot be pinched and there is no independent movement of lump.

Q 5. How is a skin nodule formed in carcinoma breast?

In carcinoma breast discrete nodules are formed. This is due to the fact that the lymphatic trunks from the skin drain separate portions of the skin. And there is no communication between adjacent territories. When cancer cells grow along these vessels it will result in small separate cutaneous nodules.

Q 6. What will be the staging in this case?

This patient has got a T4B N1 lesion and therefore it is **stage III B**. It is included in **LABC** (Locally Advanced Breast Cancer).

Q 7. What is LABC?

Stage IIIa and IIIb is called LABC.

Q 8. How will you proceed in such a case?

a. Confirm the diagnosis
b. Staging work up and investigation to exclude metastases
c. Other routine investigations and assessment of systems when surgery is considered.

Q 9. How to confirm the diagnosis?

a. FNAC of the lump breast and axillary node
b. If FNAC is inconclusive do core biopsy
c. If core biopsy is not feasible do incision biopsy (when the lump is more than 4 cm size it is preferable to do incision biopsy rather than excision biopsy).

Q 10. What are the investigations required to rule out metastases?

All investigations in early breast cancer including mammography:

a. FNAC of axillary lymph nodes
b. Ultrasound abdomen to rule out metastases liver
c. Bilateral mammography
d. A total body bone scan—If **bone scan is positive** it will alter the stage and it will become a stage IV disease (Metastatic breast cancer).

Q 11. Why mammography is required in LABC?

A **bilateral mammography is a must**. We can assess the tumor size and multicentricity. Tumor response to chemotherapy can be assessed if initial mammographic size is available. So also mammography of the contralateral breast is required.

Q 12. What is the purpose of total body bone scanning (if not available a skeletal survey)?

A routine X-ray will pick up metastatic lesion only when 60% of the bone is demineralized. Bone scanning will pick up metastases in about 20–30% of cases of stage III breast cancer and if metastases detected, it will become stage IV disease. A raised alkaline phosphatase will give a clue in this regard.

Q 13. How does metastatic lesion reach vertebrae?

The malignant cells from the breast reaches vertebrae via the **intercostal veins**.The intercostal vein will join the vertebral plexus of the veins. This is also called **Batson's plexus** of veins. The peculiarity of this plexus is that there are no valves and therefore the malignant cells can freely reach all the vertebrae from the base of the skull to the sacrum.

Q 14. What are the common sites of bone metastases?

Vertebrae, ribs, sternum, upper end of humerus and upper end of femur.

Q 15. How does a metastatic lesion reach the liver from a carcinoma breast?

The liver is involved **in 2 ways.** The most important route is **bloodstream** spread. The liver also can be involved by lymphatic route. The **lymphatics** from the lower inner quadrant of the breast traverse the plexus in the rectus sheath and reach the subperitoneal plexus. From their along the falciform ligament it will reach the liver.

Q 16. What are the common types of chest metastases?

a. Pulmonary metastases in the form of **"cannon balls"**
b. Pleural effusion
c. Consolidation
d. Chest wall metastases.

Q 17. What are the clinical features of brain metastases?

a. Headache
b. Vomiting
c. Signs of increased intracranial tension
d. Rarely seizures.

Q 18. What are the modes of spread of carcinoma breast?

1. Lymphatic
2. Local spread is responsible for the fixity of the lump to the breast tissue and it is also responsible for the increase in size of the tumor. Direct spread to the skin via the Cooper's ligament will result in skin tethering and fixity, direct extension to the pectoral muscle and chest wall.
3. Bloodstream spread—bloodstream spread along the draining intercostal veins will reach the vertebral plexus (**Batson's plexus**) which is a valveless system and result in **bone metastases** in the vertebrae. In order of frequency the lumbar vertebrae, femur, thoracic vertebrae, rib and skull are affected. Generally they are **osteolytic** metastases. Bloodstream spread is also responsible for liver, lung and brain metastases. It can produce metastases in most of the body sites including adrenal.

Q 19. What is the lymphatic drainage of the breast?

The lymphatics of the breast drain into the **axillary and internal mammary** nodes. The axillary nodes receive **85%** of the lymphatics and the axillary nodes are arranged as the **anterior (pectoral), posterior (subscapular), central, interpectoral** (Rotters—between the pectoralis major and minor), **lateral (brachial)** along the axillary vein and **apical nodes** which lie above the level of pectoralis minor. The apical nodes are in continuity with the **supraclavicular nodes**. From the supraclavicular nodes they drain to the thoracic duct or jugular trunk.

There are 2 plexus in the breast and they communicate freely.

a. Subareolar plexus of Sappey
b. A plexus over the pectoral sheath.

The subareolar plexus of **Sappey** and the upper outer quadrant of the breast drain to the **pectoral**, then to the **central** and to the **apical** axillary nodes. The subscapular and the lateral (brachial) are involved rarely and in a retrograde way. Part of the upper quadrant will also drain to the **deltopectoral** and apical nodes directly. From the inner quadrants the lymph spread occurs to the **internal mammary** group of nodes and also to the contralateral breast. From the lower inner quadrant the lymph will traverse through the plexus in rectus sheath and communicate with the **subperitoneal plexus. Tumors in the posterior 1/3rd of the breast generally drain to the internal mammary nodes.**

Q 20. What are the levels of axillary lymph nodes?

The division is by the pectoralis minor muscle.
There are III levels of axillary lymph nodes.

Level I – The axillary lymph nodes below and lateral to the lateral margin of the pectoralis minor muscle.

Level II – The nodes situated behind the pectoralis minor and **Rotter's nodes** (Interpectoral)

Level III – The nodes above and medial to the medial border of pectoralis minor and inferior to the clavicle these are also known as **apical or infraclavicular nodes.** Metastases to these nodes portend a worse prognosis.

Therefore, the infraclavicular designation is to differentiate it from the remaining level 1 and 2 nodes.

Note:

Supraclavicular lymph nodes—they are seen in the supraclavicular fossa a triangle defined by omohyoid muscle and tendon (lateral and superior border), the internal jugular vein (medial border) and the clavicle and subclavian vein (lower border). Adjacent lymph nodes **outside this triangle** are considered to be lower cervical nodes and hence **M1**.

Internal mammary lymph nodes are seen in the intercostal spaces along the edge of the sternum in the endothoracic fascia in 2nd, 3rd and 4th spaces. They lie along the internal mammary vessels.

Intramammary lymph nodes—the lymph nodes within the breast. These are considered axillary lymph nodes for purpose of N classification and staging.

Q 21. How many lymph nodes are there in the axilla?

There are about 20–25 lymph nodes in the axilla.

Level I - 15

Level II - 4–5

Level III - 2–3

Total - 25

Minimum of 10 nodes are necessary for adequate staging.

Q 22. What is Krukenberg's tumor?

This is nothing but the transcelomic spread of malignant cells from the subperitoneal plexus to the surface of the functioning ovaries in premenopausal women. If the ovaries are not functioning as in the case of postmenopausal group, the malignant cells cannot get implanted because of the absence of raw area on the surface of ovaries.

Q 23. What are the predisposing factors for carcinoma breast?

Read early breast cancer.

Q 24. What are the bad prognostic factors for carcinoma breast?

a. *Nodal status*—**The most important single prognostic factor is nodal status** more than 3 histologically positive node is prognostically bad.
b. *Age of the patient*—Less than 35 years has got bad prognosis.
c. *The size of tumor*—Tumors less than 1 cm size has excellent prognosis.
d. *Tumor grade*—Grade III Bloom Richardson grade is associated with bad prognosis.
e. *Nottingham prognostic index (NPI)*—NPI = [0.2 × size in cm] × grade + stage. The stage was based on nodal status and was the combination of triple node biopsy (the low axilla, high axilla and internal mammary chain).
f. *Histology*—Certain special types like classical lobular, tubular, cribriform, medullary, mucinous, papillary and adenoid cystic are having better prognosis than NST.
g. *ER and PR status*—Approximately 60% of the tumours contain detectable estrogen receptor (ER). ER and progesterone receptor (PR) positive patients having better prognosis. *It is a relatively weak prognostic factor.*
h. *Ploidy*—Ploidy is a measurement of the relative proportion of DNA in each cell. Anuploidy is associated with bad prognosis. Diploid tumors have a lower risk of relapse. The cells in active

cell division (S-phase) can be determined by floor cytometry. S-phase is better predictor of relapse and survival than ploidy. Low S-phase tumors have a more favorable prognosis. The use of antibody Ki-67 allows an easier estimation of proliferation.

i. *c-erb B2 (HER 2/neu)*—This is a cell membrane receptor protein and is the product of **neu** oncogene. Even though it should be done routinely to predict the likelihood of their response to **Herceptin** its prognostic significance is doubtful.

j. *p53*—The abnormality of p53 expression is seen in **breast, ovarian and bowel** cancer. The abnormality is associated with bad prognosis.

k. *Epidermal growth factor receptor (EGF)*—has got bad prognosis.

Q 25. If there is no evidence of metastases this case will be LABC and what will be the line of management?

The LABC may be **operable or inoperable**. T3 N1 is operable as per NCCN guidelines 2012. Operable lesions are subjected for surgery first. Multimodal treatment is the therapeutic option for inoperable LABC. It is an indication for **anterior chemotherapy,** i.e. chemotherapy given prior to surgery (**neoadjuvant**). Start the patient with CAF/CMF regimen. 2 cycles of chemotherapy are given first (5FU-600 mg/m^2, Adriamycin 50 mg/m^2, Cyclophosphamide 600 mg/m^2). After 2 cycles the patient is evaluated for response (Flow chart 6.1).

Q 26. How to assess response?

The response is assessed by mammography and clinical assessment. The patient is categorized into the following:

a. Complete responder (CR)—no palpable tumor after chemotherapy (absence of invasive carcinoma in breast and axillary nodes).
b. Partial responder—any decrease in size of tumor or node compared to pre-treatment T/N
c. Non responder—Less than 50% decrease in size to up to 25% increase in size
d. Progressive disease
   - More than 25% increase in size
   - New lesions appear
   - Depth of patient.

Q 27. Why chemotherapy is given first?

a. Down staging is possible with chemotherapy
b. Surgery is possible after cytoreduction
c. Local control is not the issue in LABC
d. LABC patients are likely to harbor micrometastases
e. The policy of hitting the micrometastases first
f. Systemic therapy is a must in all patients
g. Allows assessment of chemosensitivity.

Q 28. What are the options for non-responders/ progressive disease?

a. If operable, surgery is done
b. Otherwise, XRT (radiotherapy), hormone therapy are the options.
   - Small percentage will respond to the drug Taxol (only 15% of the chemoresistant will respond.
   - Radiotherapy is given to the chest, axilla and supraclavicular region
     5000 cGy in fractions—200 cGy over 5 weeks.

Q 29. If the patient is responding what surgery is done?

The surgeons who prefer breast conservation therapy will do **breast conservation surgery**. Some surgeons perform **MRM** (**modified radical mastectomy**) in this setting.

Flow chart 6.1: Locally advanced breast cancer management

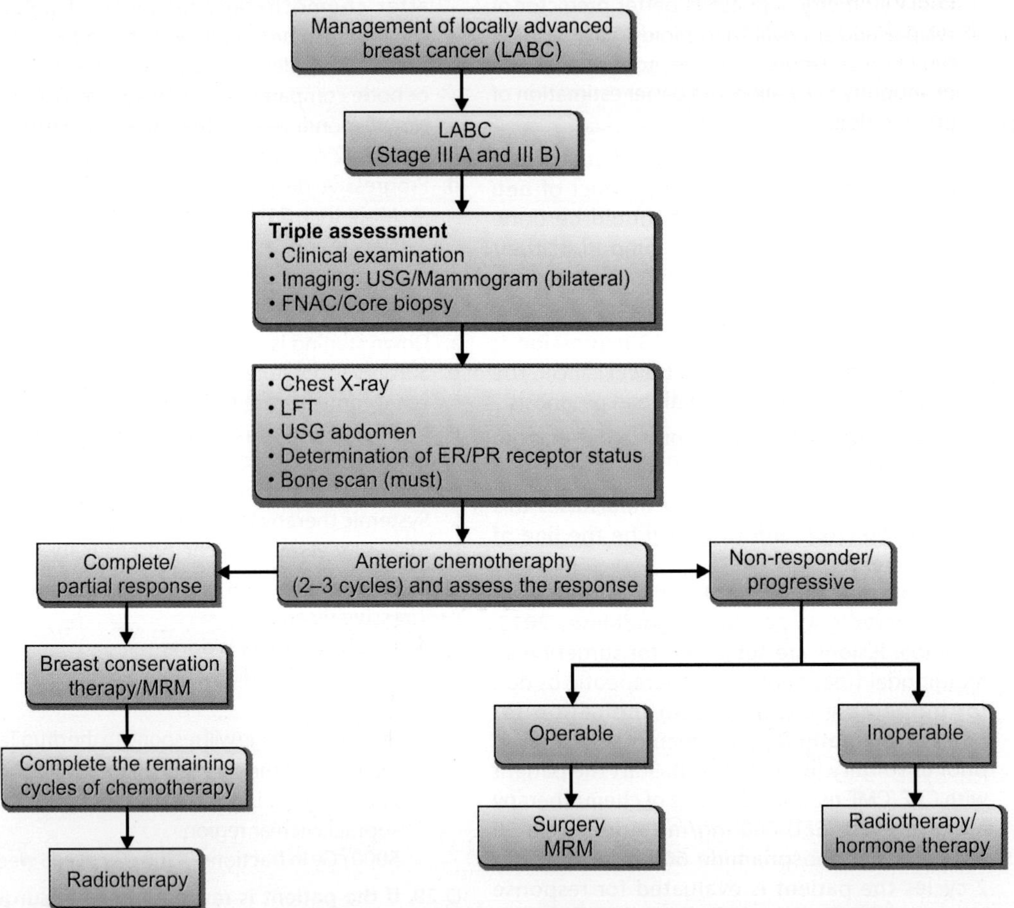

Q 30. After the breast conservation/mastectomy what is the sequencing of therapy?

For all those who undergo MRM the remaining 4 cycles of chemotherapy is given first. Those who undergo breast conservation and those with positive resection margin, radiotherapy is given first, followed by subsequent chemotherapy.

- Delaying **chemotherapy** beyond 12 weeks after mastectomy is not good. Usually chemotherapy is started within 6 weeks after mastectomy (for early breast cancer)
- **Tamoxifen** is given only after chemotherapy
- **Radiotherapy** is started within 4 to 6 months.

Q 31. What are the side effects of chemotherapy?

a. Bone marrow depression
b. Gastrointestinal (nausea and vomiting)
c. Alopecia.

The patient is monitored by Hb, TLC before therapy and after the cycle on day 21. If abnormal, do platelet count also. Serum albumin, SGOT, SGPT are done before and after therapy.

Q 32. Is there any use of cyto protective agents for chemotherapy induced hematological toxicity? (PG)

The GMCF—**Filgrastim** granulocyte macrophage colony stimulating factor, (GCSF) (Granulocyte Colony Stimulating Factor) are useful for reducing the severity and duration of neutropenia. They are given either before **or** upto 24 hours after chemotherapy. **Dose:** 30 million units. But it is costly.

Q 33. What is Trastuzamab/Herceptin?

It is a new biological agent used as a molecular target acting against the growth receptor HER2 (c-erb B2). It costs about 1 Lakh for a vial. It is given once in three weeks into 6 months to 1 year.

The other agents currently available include **Bevacizumab** which is a vascular growth factor receptor inhibitor and Lapitinab which is a combined growth factor receptor inhibitor.

Q 34. What is the role of hormone therapy in LABC?

It should be started in all patients from day 1 irrespective of menopausal status and carried on for 5 years.

Q 35. What is the cut off value of the ER for considering it as positive?

There is no cut off value but more than **10 fmol/mg** is considered positive. **About 2/3**rd **of post-menopausal** and **half of premenopausal** are positive. ER value more than 30 fmol/mg response rate for hormone therapy is 75%. ER value 3 to 10 fmol/mg the response rate is 20%.

Q 36. What type of MRM is done in carcinoma breast?

Three types of MRM are available.

a. The classical **Patey's** mastectomy where the pectoralis minor is removed and level III axillary dissection is done (after putting a transverse elliptical incision enclosing the nipple areolar complex and the skin overlying the tumor, the entire breast is removed initially). The pectoralis major is preserved.
b. The second modification is by **'Scanlon'** where the pectoralis minor muscle is divided, not removed and thereby a level III dissection is done.
c. **Auchincloss** modification. This differs from the Patey procedure by not removing or dividing the pectoralis minor muscle but by simply retracting the pectoralis minor. This modification limits a level III dissection. But only 2% of the patients will potentially benefit by removal of the highest level of nodes and therefore it is justified.

Q 37. What is the difference between axillary clearance and axillary sampling?

The **axillary sampling** is usually performed through a separate axillary incision and should ideally be undertaken immediately prior to the wide local excision. Starting from the lower axilla at least 4 palpable nodes are excised and sent separately for histological examination. If 4 nodes are not palpable in level I then higher palpable nodes from level II, level III, interpectoral region nodes are excised. Therefore, axillary sampling is not merely a level I dissection but samples of palpable nodes from any level of the axilla. This will allow detection of the so-called **skip metastases**, i.e. level II and III involvement without involvement of level I.

In **axillary clearance** the contents of axilla below the axillary vein are cleared upto the apex of the axilla preserving the long thoracic nerve, thoracodorsal nerve and vessels and if possible the intercostobrachial nerve.

Q 38. What is the important complication of level III dissection?

Lymphedema. The incidence of lymphedema rises with amount of axillary surgery. The combination of lymph node dissection and radiotherapy gives higher incidence.

Q 39. What are the two most important common myocutaneous flaps available for the reconstruction of breast after mastectomy?

a. *TRAM FLAP (transverse rectus abdominis myocutaneous flap)*
b. *Latissimus dorsi myocutaneous flap*

The tram flap may be carried out as a rotational flap based on the superior epigastric artery or as free flap using microvascular anastomosis of the inferior epigastric vessel to the subscapular or thoracodorsal vessels. Both these flap procedures can be carried out as an immediate procedure or delayed procedure. Immediate reconstruction is less time consuming for the patient.

Q 40. What is the other option for reconstruction after mastectomy?

Immediate placement of a prosthesis in the subpectoral position with the help of a **tissue expander** and later replacement of the expander with a **prosthesis.**

Q 41. What are the organs/tissues involved in stage IV disease (metastatic breast cancer)?

Sites of Metastases in Breast Cancer

a. Bone
b. Lung with or without pleural effusion
c. Pericardial effusion
d. Brain
e. Lymph nodes
f. Skin, soft tissues of chest wall, and axilla
g. Metabolic complications like hypercalcemia.

Q 42. What is the median survival of MBC (metastatic breast cancer)?

Two years.

Q 43. What are the treatment options in MBC?

Treatment options in MBC

H – Hormone therapy
E – Endocrine manipulation
R – Radiotherapy
O – Oestrogen blockers
I – Immunotherapy
C – Chemotherapy

(*Source:* Mnemonic by Dr Selvakumar)

Q 44. Which metastasis is prognostically better?

Soft tissue metastasis has better prognosis. Visceral metastasis has worst prognosis. Response to treatment decreases when the number of organs involved increases. Generally receptor negative tumors are aggressive and receptor positive are indolent.

Q 45. What is the basis for the selection of chemo/endocrine therapy?

Endocrine therapy is preferred for the following situations:

a. Slow growing soft tissue/**bone metastases** (only 30% will be hormone response)
b. Disease-free survival of more than two years
c. Age more than 35 years
d. Objective response to first line hormone therapy

Chemotherapy is preferred in following situations:

a. Rapidly growing **visceral,** skin metastases and lymphangitis
b. Disease free survival less than two years
c. Negative response to first line hormones
d. Receptor negative.

Q 46. What is the choice of drugs in MBC?

The CAF regime provides better response than CMF. Taxanes are used for anthracycline resistant cases. Combination of taxanes and anthracycline regimes are becoming gold standard.

Q 47. What are the indications for surgery in MBC?

Indications for surgery in MBC:

a. Locoregional control (**Toilet mastectomy**)
b. Spinal cord compression (Laminectomy)
c. CNS or choroidal metastases
d. Bone fractures (**Internal fixation + radiotherapy**)
e. Oophorectomy
f. Localized chest wall lesions.

Q 48. What are the indications for radiotherapy in MBC?

a. Pain relief in skeletal metastases
b. Spinal cord compression
c. CNS diseases
d. Tumor recurrence in chest wall
e. Ovarian ablation.

Q 49. What is biological therapy?

The **HER 2/neu**oncogene amplification and over expression is found in about 25–30% of patients with CA breast. Recombinant humanized monoclonal antibody against this oncogene is now available as **HERCEPTIN.** The response rate is around 15%. The drug is very costly. The combination of herceptin and chemotherapy may improve the results. Breast cancer vaccines, inhibitors of protein kinases and antiangiogenesis factors are also included in this category.

Q 50. What is the treatment of pleural effusion in CA breast?

After draining pleural fluid through intercostal drain, pleurodesis with tetracycline 1.5 g will give symptomatic relief. Pleurodesis with Bleomycin 30–60 units is also being tried.

Q 51. What is the treatment of hypercalcemia due to metastases?

This may sometimes be fatal. The treatment is hydration and steroids. **Bisphosphonates** (**pamidronate, clodronate**) in the dose of 90 mg IV once a month may be useful which will arrest demineralization and decrease the incidence of pathological fracture and vertebral collapse. It will also decrease the pain from bone metastases.

FOR PG'S—WHAT IS NEW?

Oligometastatic disease—Isolated single metastasis is called Oligometastatic
For a triple negative cases—Chemotherapy is given as first line treatment (for early breast cancer)
MRI is done before and after chemotherapy in LABC—(Titanium Clips are put in the periphery of the mass or tattooing before chemotherapy)
Sentinel node biopsy is discouraged in LABC
Multifocal pattern of residual disease is a contraindication for breast conservation, so also positive axillary nodes
Full course of chemotherapy is given instead of sandwich surgery for *complete pathological response*

Case

7 Epigastric Lump

Case Capsule

A 60-year-old male patient presents with **epigastric pain, discomfort, distension** of abdomen and **loss of appetite** of **8 months duration.** The patient has **lost 15 kg** in the last two months. He **vomits large quantities of undigested food.** His pain is not relieved by vomiting or eating. On examination there is **gross wasting** and **extreme pallor** visible in face and hands. Inspection of the abdomen revealed epigastric distension and **visible peristalsis.** The visible peristalsis is seen starting in the left upper quadrant and moving towards the right side. **Succussion splash** is heard. There is a **hard irregular massfelt in the epigastrium** extending to the right hypochondrium beneath the costal margin of **10 × 7 cm** size. The mass **moves with respiration** and one **cannot get above it**; however, **fingers can be insinuated** between the costal margin and the lump. All the borders except upper border are well made out. The lump is **resonant on percussion.** There is no shifting dullness and no ascites demonstrated. There is no other palpable lump. The liver is not palpable. The left supraclavicular nodes are not enlarged. Digital rectal examination revealed absence of Blumer's shelf. On chest examination, there is no evidence of pleural effusion. There is no evidence of superficial thrombophlebitis. (Fig. 7.2)

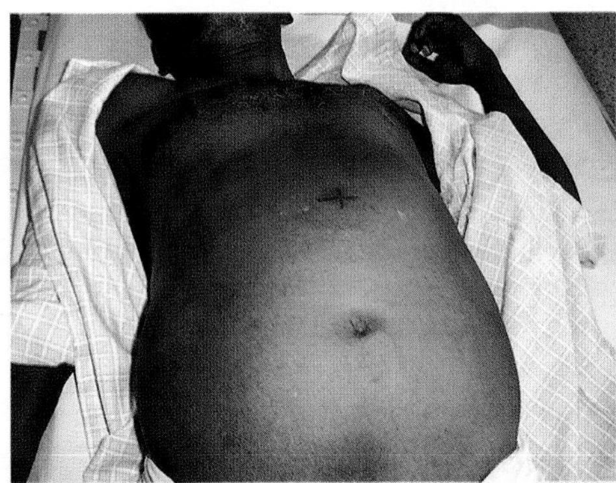

Advanced carcinoma:Stomach with ascites

Checklist for Examination

1. Remember the **9 areas of the abdomen.** (Fig. 7.1)
2. Remember that there is a large area called **retroperitoneum** in addition to these 9 areas.
3. **Pelvic organs** can also come and occupy the lower abdomen.
4. Look for **visible lumps** and visible **peristalsis** (left to right upper abdominal visible peristalsis is suggestive of gastric outlet obstruction and right to left visible peristalsis is suggestive of left sided colonic obstruction)

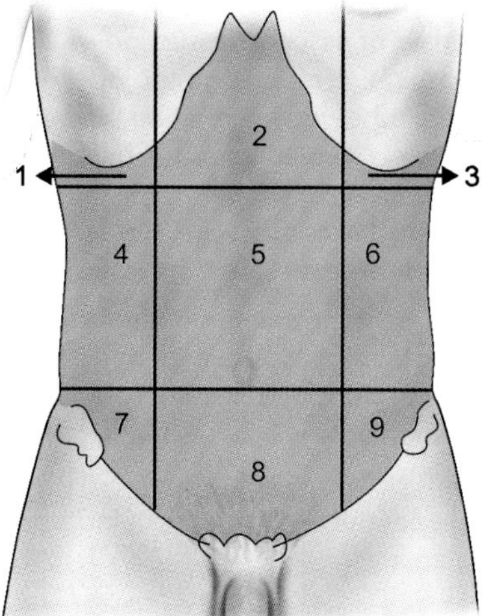

1. Right hypochondrium, 2. Epigastrium, 3. Left hypochondrium, 4. Right lumbar, 5. Umbilical, 6. Left lumbar, 7. Right iliac, 8. Hypogastrium, 9. Left iliac

Fig. 7.1: Nine areas of the abdomen

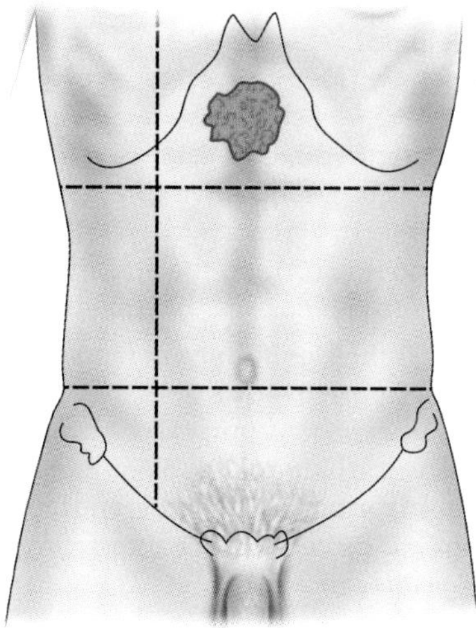

Fig. 7.2: Epigastric mass

5. Always assess the **plane of the lump** (Carnett's test, cough test, examination in knee elbow position.
6. Always check for **movement with respiration** and intrinsic mobility of the lump.
7. In upper abdominal lumps look for **finger insinuation between the lump** and **costal margin.**
8. Remember the causes for **disappearing mass** — intussusception and Dietl's crisis.
9. In suspected renal mass always look for **contralateral kidney**.
10. **Bimanual palpability** will be positive for all big lumps. Carefully palpate and decide with which hand it is better felt.
11. **Ballotability** is a sign specific for kidney.
12. **Percussion over the lump** to see whether it is dull or resonant and check whether the dullness is continuous with liver dullness/splenic dullness.
13. Palpate for nodules in the umbilicus (**Sister Joseph's nodule**).
14. Examine the **hernial orifices.**
15. Always examine the **genitalia** in males.
16. Do a per rectal examination (**Blumer's shelf**).
17. Examine the **renal angle** for fullness, tenderness and dullness.
18. Look for **supraclavicular lymph nodes** (especially on left side between the two heads of sternomastoid) – Troisier's sign.

Q 1. What is the most probable diagnosis in this case?

A distal gastric cancer with gastric outlet obstruction.

Q 2. What are the reasons for diagnosing a stomach lump?

a. Symptoms of loss of appetite, loss of weight and vomiting.
b. The type of visible peristalsis is from left to right which is suggestive of a gastric outlet obstruction by a tumor.
c. The lump is occupying the epigastrium and is moving up and down with respiration.

Q 3. What is the significance of family history in carcinoma stomach?

Gastric cancer can occur in families. A famous gastric cancer patient in history is **Napoleon Bonaparte.** He died of gastric cancer (?). His father and grandfather died of gastric cancer. His three sisters and a brother died of gastric cancer.

Q 4. What are the causes for gastric outlet obstruction?

Causes for gastric outlet obstruction

1. Duodenal ulcer with pyloric stenosis
2. Distal gastric malignancy with outlet obstruction
3. Congenital hypertrophic pyloric stenosis
4. Adult type of hypertrophic pyloric stenosis
5. Acid poisoning with stenosis.

Q 5. What are the signs other than visible gastric peristalsis (VGP) to diagnose gastric outlet obstruction?

1. The dilated and distended stomach can be palpated sometimes.
2. The succussion splash can be elicited.

Q 6. What is the objective evidence for gastric outlet obstruction?

The objective evidence for gastric outlet obstruction is **saline load test**. This is a simple means of assessing the degree of pyloric obstruction and is useful in following the patient's progress during the first few days of nasogastric suction.

After aspirating residual gastric juice through the nasogastric tube, 700 mL of normal saline at room temperature is infused over 3–5 minutes and the tube is clamped. 30 minutes later the stomach is aspirated and the residual volume of saline recorded. Recovery of more than 350 mL indicates obstruction.

Q 7. What are the other abdominal clinical signs, one should look for ascertaining that it is stomach?

a. May or may not be able to get above the lump
b. Percussion note will be resonant, may be some times impaired.

Q 8. What are the clinical signs of inoperability in such a patient?

Signs of inoperability in carcinoma stomach

a. The presence of **ascites** suggesting peritoneal metastases
b. The presence of **Blumer's shelf** which is nothing but a peritoneal metastasis in the rectovesical/rectouterine pouch
c. The presence of a **metastatic liver**
d. The presence of left supraclavicular lymph nodes (**Virchow's, Troisier's sign**)
e. The presence of a cutaneous nodule in the umbilicus (**Sister Mary Joseph's** nodule)
f. Presence of jaundice
g. Fixity of mass
h. Irish nodule (**Enlarged left axillary node**)
i. Pleural effusion
j. **Krukenberg's tumor** (enlarged ovaries in pelvic examination).

Q 9. In the absence of these signs can you say that it is an early gastric cancer?

No. By the time a lump is clinically palpable it will be advanced gastric cancer.

Q 10. What is the cause for jaundice in carcinoma stomach?

- Infiltration of the growth engulfing the *CBD* (common bile duct)
- Diffuse involvement of the **hepatoduodenal** ligament.

Q 11. What is the pathway for umbilical nodule formation (Sister Mary Joseph's Nodule)?

Growth in lesser curvature
↓
Involvement of lesser omentum
↓
Involvement of ligamentum teres
↓
Umbilicus

Note: Sister Mary Joseph was Nurse to Sir William Mayo.

Q 12. What is early gastric cancer (EGC)?

Early gastric cancer is a cancer confined to the mucosa and submucosa of the stomach irrespective of the nodal status (T_1 any N).

- EGC with nodes surgery is recommended
- EGC without nodes endoscopic surgery.

Q 13. What are the clinical manifestations of carcinoma stomach?

The pneumonic **STOMACH** helps in memorizing the clinical features.

- **S**ilent (No symptoms)
- **T**umor (Lump)
- **O**bstruction
- **M**elena
- **A**chlorhydria
  - Anemia
  - Asthenia
- **C**achexia
- **H**emtemesis.

Q 14. How will you proceed to investigate such a patient?

The most important investigation in this particular situation will be an upper GI endoscopy.

Q 15. Why upper GI endoscopy is preferred over a Barium meal examination?

- By **Upper GI endoscopy**, we can see the growth, assess the type and extent of growth, and also take **biopsy** for confirmation.
- In **Barium meal examination,** we will only see the shadow of the lesion in the form of **persistent irregular filling defect, persistent mucosal irregularity and persistent loss of peristalsis** in a particular segment.

Q 16. In which situation Barium meal examination is superior to upper GI endoscopy?

Barium meal examination is superior in the following situations:

- Barium meal is useful for the diagnosis of Linitis Plastica (endoscopic biopsy confirmation may be difficult because the mucosa is normal)
- Lesions in the cardiac.
- Lesions causing obstruction.
- For early gastric cancer lesions.

Q 17. How many endoscopic biopsies will you take from a suspected lesion in the stomach?

Minimum **Six biopsies** from different parts of the identified lesion (Diagnostic accuracy reaches 100% if **10 biopsy** samples are taken).

Q 18. What are the types of biopsies available endoscopically?

a. Biopsy with the help of a biopsy forceps
b. Punch biopsy
c. Brush biopsy
d. Gastric lavage and cytology.

Q 19. If the biopsy is being reported as adenocarcinoma (the most common carcinoma in stomach), how will you proceed?

In the order of priority, the following investigations are done to stage the disease and rule out metastases.

Staging investigations

a. Ultrasound abdomen to rule out metastases and assess the extent of the disease
b. X-ray chest to rule pulmonary metastases
c. CT abdomen if required to stage the disease
d. Liver function test (LFT) to rule out metastases
e. Hemogram to rule out anemia.

Q 20. In what way does the ultrasound examination help in evaluating this patient?

a. The presence of liver metastases can be assessed and if required a **sono guided FNAC** can be done
b. The **tumor thickness** can be assessed with the help of a high resolution probe
c. The presence or absence of **regional lymph node** and adjacent organ involvement
d. The presence of **free fluid** can be ascertained.

Q 21. Is there any role for endoscopic ultrasound (EUS)?

By ordinary abdominal ultrasound one may not be able to ascertain the tumor thickness and serosal involvement which is possible with **EUS**. To some extent the presence of nodes can be also assessed by endoscopic ultrasound.

Q 22. Why is CT required in addition to ultrasound examination?

The gastric carcinoma appear as areas of mural thickening. The measurement of the thickness of the wall will give an idea of transmural extension, when the thickness is more than 2 cm. In addition, a blurred serosal contour or strand like densities that extend into the perigastic fat may be seen. Direct invasion of the adjacent structures like pancreas, diaphragm, transverse colon, spleen or left lobe of liver can be ascertained by CT scan.

Q 23. Is there any role for laparoscopy in such a patient?

Yes.

Role of laparoscopy in carcinoma stomach

- Diagnostic laparoscopy is useful for **staging the disease**
- Pick up **peritoneal metastases** (CT will miss peritoneal metastases)
- It can detect **occult metastases** in 13–37%
- Laparoscopic ultrasound can detect **metastases in liver**
- It can identify adjacent **organ invasion**
- **Guided biopsies** are possible.
- Laparoscopy can help in doing a **peritoneal lavage and cytology**
- Laparoscopy can **eliminate the need for laparotomy.**

Q 24. What are the laparoscopic signs of inoperability?

Laparoscopic signs of inoperability

1. Positive cytology in peritoneal wash
2. Peritoneal deposits
3. Posterior fixation
4. Fixed celiac nodes
5. Para-aortic nodes
6. Liver metastases.

Q 25. What is the staging system for carcinoma stomach?

In the west, the AJCC TNM system based on the 7th edition is accepted. But the Japanese Investigators report their results based on the JRSGC (Japanese

Research Society for Gastric Cancer). The N_3 and N_4 nodes in the Japanese system correspond to extra-regional nodes in UICC system that is M_1 metastatic nodes.

AJCC 7th edition Staging

Tx: Primary cannot be assessed
T0: No evidence of primary tumor
Tis: Carcinoma in situ – intraepithelial tumor Without invasion of lamina propria
T1: Tumor invades lamina propria, muscularis mucosa or submucosa
T1a: Tumor invades lamina propria or muscularis mucosa
T1b: Tumor invades submucosa
T2: Invades muscularis or propria
T3: Tumor penetrates sub serosal connective tissue without invasion of visceral peritoneum or adjacent structures
T4: Tumor invades serosa (visceral peritoneum) or adjacent structures
T4a: Tumor invades serosa (visceral peritoneum)
T4b: Tumor invades adjacent structures
Nx: Regional node cannot be assessed
N0: No nodes
N1: Metastases in 1–2 regional nodes
N2: Metastases 3–6 regional nodes
N3: Metastases 7 or more regional nodes
N3a: 7–15 regional lymph nodes
N3b: Metastases in 16 or more regional lymph nodes
M0: No distant metastases
M1: Distant metastases (this includes peritoneum and distant lymph nodes)

Stage	0	Tis N0, M0
Stage	IA	T1 N0 M0
Stage	IB	T1 N1 M0/T2 N0 M0

Contd...

Contd...

Stage	IIA	T3 N0 M0 /T2 N1 M0/T1 N2 M0
Stage	IIB	T4A N0 M0 / T3 N1, M0 / T2 N2 M0 / T1 N0 M0
Stage	IIIA	T4a N1 M0/T3 N2 M0/T2 N3 M0
Stage T3	IIIB	T4b N0 M0/T4b N1 M0 / T4a N2 M0/ N3 M0
Stage IIIC	T4b	N2 M0 / T4b N3 M0 / T4a N3 M0
Stage	IV	Any T, any N, M1

Q 26. What are the nodal stations according to Japanese Research Society?

1. Right cardiac
2. Left cardiac
3. Lesser curvature
4. Greater curvature
5. Suprapyloric
6. Infrapyloric
7. Nodes along left gastric artery
8. Common hepatic artery
9. Celiac
10. Splenic hilar
11. Splenic artery
12. Hepatic pedicle
13. Retropancreatic
14. Mesenteric root
15. Middle colic artery
16. Para-aortic.

Lymph node stations

- 1–6 are considered **N_1 nodes (Perigastric nodes – along the curvatures)**
- 7 – 11 are considered **N_2 nodes** (**Along the named vessels)**
- 12 – 14 are considered **N_3 nodes** (**Intra-peritoneal nodes)**
- 15 – 16 are considered **N_4 nodes.**

Note:
- N1 and N2 nodes are regional nodes
- N3 nodes are metastatic node stations
- **Involvement of N3 node station is a contraindication for radical surgery.**

Q 27. What do you mean by D1 and D2 resection?
The extent of lymphadenectomy in the Japanese system is described using a D descriptor.

- **D0 lymphadenectomy** means all the JRSGC (Japanese Research Society for Gastric Cancer) N1 nodes have not been completely removed.
- **D1 lymphadenectomy** means all the N1 nodes have been removed but not all the N2 nodes.
- **D2 lymphadenectomy** means that all the N_1 and N_2 nodes have been removed but not all the N_3 nodes.

Thus, for example, a D2 lymphadenectomy for a tumor involving all 3 gastric areas would involve removal of lymph nodes at stations 1- 11.

The extent of lymphadenectomy before 1993 was classified by the **'R' descriptor**. Since 1993 in order to avoid confusion with the **UICC R descriptor** (which reflects an entirely different characteristics namely, the presence of known residual disease after surgical treatment), the extent of lymphadenectomy is denoted by **D-descriptor**.

Q 28. What are the bad prognostic factors for CA stomach?

1. Lymph node involvement is a poor prognostic factor—four or more lymph node involvement is a bad prognostic sign.
2. Serosal involvement is the single most important bad prognostic factor.
3. Free carcinoma cells in the peritoneum.
4. Intestinal type is having a better prognosis than diffuse (Lauren's).

Q 29. What are the poor prognostic variables that relate to surgery?

1. Positive resection margin
2. Inadequate lymphadenectomy
3. Need for splenectomy.

Q 30. What is Lauren's pathological classification?
DIO

- **D**iffuse
- **I**ntestinal
- **O**thers.

According to this classification, it is divided into **diffuse and intestinal type**. The **intestinal type** is having a better prognosis than the diffuse type. In intestinal gastric cancer, the tumor resembles a carcinoma elsewhere in the tubular GI tract and forms polypoid tumors or ulcers. It probably arises in areas of intestinal metaplasia.

In contrast, **diffuse gastric cancer** infiltrates deeply into the stomach without forming obvious mass lesions, but spreads widely in the gastric wall. A small proportion of gastric cancers are of mixed morphology.

- The diffuse type may be **localized or generalized**.
- The generalized type of diffused is called Linitis plastica (**leather bottle stomach**).

Q 31. What is Correa cycle?
Helicobacter seems to be principally associated with carcinoma of the body and distal stomach. **Helicobacter** is associated with **gastritis** leading on to gastric **atrophy**. Similarly exposure to nitroso compounds will lead on to nitrosamine leading to **gastritis** and **gastric atrophy** which in turn will produce intestinal **metaplasia** leading on to **dysplasia**, carcinoma in situ and finally **carcinoma.**

Q 32. What are the other risk factors for carcinoma stomach?

1. Pernicious anemia
2. Gastric atrophy

3. Gastric polyps
4. Heredity
5. Postgastrectomy patients—Post GJ, gastrectomy and post-pyloroplasty patients have approximately 4 times the average risk
6. Gastritis—Duodenogastric reflex and reflex gastritis are related to increased risk of malignancy
7. Diet—Smoked fish, excessive salt intake, chilly etc.
8. Smoking and dust ingestion
9. Deficiency of antioxidants
10. Exposure to N nitroso compounds.

Q 33. What is Borrmann classification of advanced gastric cancer?

Once there is involvement of the muscularis, it is called **advanced gastric cancer**. The macroscopic appearance is classified by Borrmann into 4 types: Type III and IV are commonly incurable.

Type I	–	Polypoidal
Type II	–	Ulcerative
Type III	–	Ulcerative and polypoidal
Type IV	–	Diffuse

Q 34. What is the most important epidemiological change in gastric cancer in recent cases?

1. The incidence of gastric cancer continues to fall at about 1% per year. This is specially seen in relation to carcinoma of the body and distal stomach. This may be because of the use of refrigerator widely for food preservation.
2. In contrast there appears to be an increased incidence of carcinoma of the proximal stomach. Particularly the GE junction.
3. The proximal and distal cancers are supposed to behave differently.

Q 35. What are the differences between proximal and distal gastric cancer?

Distal gastric cancer	*Proximal gastric cancer*
a. Diet related	Not diet related
b. Environmental	Not environmental
c. Epidemic variety	Endemic variety
d. Arise in the background of dysplastic mucosa	No such background
e. Intestinal histology	Diffuse type
f. Better prognosis	Bad prognosis (morbidity and mortality high)
g. Resectability is 30%	Resectability is 20%
h. Needs distal subtotal gastrectomy	Needs total gastrectomy

Q 36. What is the classification of esophagogastric junction tumors (OG junction tumors)?

Sievert classification of OG junction tumor
Type I – Esophageal cancer involving OG junction
Type II – Primary OG junction growth
Type III – Stomach lesion involving OG junction
Note: Type I needs esophageal resection with 10 cm clearance proximally.

Q 37. What are the modes of spread of carcinoma stomach?

Five modes of spread of carcinoma stomach

1. Horizontal spread along the stomach wall – **Submucosal spread**
2. Vertical – invasion of the stomach wall and to the **adjacent structures** like colon, pancreas, etc.
3. Lymphatic spread
4. Peritoneal dissemination
5. Bloodstream spread – to the liver.

Two types of horizontal extensions are met with.

a. Infiltrative growth
b. Expansive growth.

Q 38. What are the preoperative preparations in a patient with carcinoma stomach?

Preoperative preparations
a. Correction of anemia
b. Correction of nutritional status
c. Correction of fluid and electrolyte disturbance
d. Assessment of cardiac, respiratory and renal status
e. Arrange adequate blood
f. Preoperative stomach wash
g. Prophylactic antibiotic.

The stomach in normal individual is sterile because of the low pH. Patients with gastric cancer, however, often have an increased pH and colonization of the stomach. There is higher risk of wound complications in patients with high gastric pH and heavily colonized gastric secretions. The most common organism isolated from gastric juice are *Streptococcus faecalis, E.coli,* bacteroides, *S. albus,* etc. For this reason, a prophylactic antibiotic with a 3rd generation cephalosporin is advocated.

Q 39. What are the controversies regarding the surgical treatment of gastric adenocarcinoma?

The points of controversy are:

1. The extent of gastric resection
2. The extent of lymph node dissection.

Generally radical gastrectomies are performed for carcinoma stomach. A radical gastrectomy is one where the stomach along with the entire greater omentum, lesser omentum and lymph nodes are removed en-bloc.

1. *The extent of gastric resection*

   The distal division line is always placed at the duodenal bulb **at least 1 cm** from the tumor. As the diagnostic accuracy in infiltrative type is very low, the macroscopic proximal margin should be greater than **5 cm.**

   In the case of **Scirrhous carcinoma or Borrmann type IV**, the horizontal extension includes the whole stomach in the majority of cases and therefore **a total gastrectomy** is always indicated. In contrast, the diagnostic accuracy is high in **expansive growth type tumors** and also in early gastric cancer. A margin of **2 cm** is sufficient for these types and total or distal radical gastrectomy can be selected.

   Total versus subtotal radical gastrectomy

   The term radical is vague and lacks proper definition and may mean different operations to different surgeons.

   Surgical treatment is curative only in stage I and II diseases. A prospective randomized study by the French compared total versus subtotal gastrectomy and found that the morbidity and mortality were similar for both groups, but the five year survival was not improved. The morbidity and mortality appeared to be associated with distal pancreatectomy and splenectomy.

2. *The extent of lymph node dissection*

   The controversies regarding the extent of lymphadenectomy relate to D1 vs D2 resection. D_2 gastrectomy has 2 essential components.

   a. Adequate 5 cm clearance in the stomach
   b. Extensive lymphadenectomy—the omentum, superior leaf of mesocolon, and the pancreatic capsule are removed en-bloc, along with all N2 nodes (JRSGC) that is up to **station number 12.**

In order for a patient to have pathologically confirmed D2 lymphadenectomy more than **26 nodes** has to be identified in the specimen. Much of the mortality and morbidity in D2 resection is related to the distal pancreatectomy and splenectomy resulting in left subphrenic abscess.

So now a days, the D2 gastrectomy will **preserve spleen and pancreas**. Overall the oncological outcome may be better following D2 gastrectomy. The results of surgical treatment stage for stage in Japan are much better than commonly reported in the West and they attribute this to the staging and quality of surgery in Japan.

In general D1 resection involves the removal of perigastric nodes and D2 resection involves the clearance of the major arterial trunks.

Q 40. What is the ideal treatment for operable cancers of stomach ?

The ideal treatment consists of **D2 Gastrectomy and chemoradiation.**

Q 41. What is D2 gastrectomy?

Structures removed in D2 gastrectomy

- Removal of the stomach with the growth
- Omental bursa
- Entire greater omentum
- Lesser omentum
- Anterior layer of mesocolon
- Anterior pancreatitic capsule
- Lymphadenectomy up to D2 station.

Q 42. What are the divisions of the stomach from therapeutic point of view?

The most appropriate operation for a given patient with gastric cancer must take into account the location of the lesion and the known pattern of spread at that site. For this purpose the stomach can be divided into 3rds.

a. **The proximal 3**rd includes GE junction and the fundus.
b. **The middle 3**rd is the body of stomach and extends from the fundus to the incisura angularis of the lesser curvature.
c. **The distal 3**rd is the pyloric antrum and extends from the incisura angularis to the pylorus.

Q 43. What is the surgical treatment for middle third malignancy?

Lesions in this location are asymptomatic until they have become quite bulky with metastases to regional nodes. **Three procedures** are commonly performed in an attempt to encompass all gross and microscopic disease in the stomach and its lymphatic drainage network.

1. High radical subtotal gastrectomy
2. Radical total gastrectomy
3. Extended total gastrectomy with distal pancreatectomy and splenectomy.

As per the rules of the Japanese Research Society, tumors encroaching upon or crossing the line extending from the **bare area on the greater curvature** (between the portions of the stomach supplied by the gastroepiploic artery and the areas supplied by the short gastric) to a point 5 cm below **the cardioesophageal junction** on the lesser curvature required **total gastrectomy**. Pathoanatomic studies have demonstrated that carcinoma of the mid stomach metastasize to all regional lymph node basins of the stomach. There is, therefore, considerable theoretical basis for a radical total gastrectomy.

Q 44. How much stomach should be removed in a distal radical gastrectomy for a distal 3rd growth?

This involves resection of **approximately 75% of the stomach**, including **most of the lesser curvature**, where the margins of resection will often be the closest. At least **1 cm of the 1st part of the duodenum** is resected. **5 cm of normal stomach is removed proximal** to the tumor to assure adequate margin. Frozen section pathological evaluation of the surgical margin is performed before reconstruction. As with all gastric resections for carcinoma, greater and lesser omentectomy and regional lymph node resection is required in an attempt to remove all microscopic disease.

Q 45. What is the surgical treatment of proximal gastric cancer?

Esophagogastrectomy followed by reconstruction is the treatment of choice.

Q 46. What is the incision for a surgery for gastric malignancy?

For all types of gastric malignancy a bilateral subcostal incision (**Chevron**) is preferred.

Q 47. What is the management of inoperable lesions?

- Without complications and obstructions: **Chemotherapy**
- With complications: **Palliative surgery and chemotherapy**.

Q 48. What are the palliative surgical procedures?

Palliative procedures for carcinoma stomach

a. *Palliative gastrectomy* Is indicated for uncontrolled bleeding, obstruction and perforation
   A palliative resection is usually a palliative gastrectomy, which removes the tumor alone followed by reconstruction
b. *A palliative gastrojejunostomy*—this is a poor operation which does not allow proper emptying of the stomach but may produce additional problem of bile reflux
c. *Palliative esophagojejunostomy*
d. *Palliative intubation* for proximal growths
e. *Recanalization procedures.*

Q 49. What is combined resection?

The stomach is surrounded by pancreas, transverse colon, mesocolon, spleen, liver, diaphragm and omental bursa. All these structures can be surgically removed together with stomach if necessary. Combined resection shows survival benefits when there are no distant metastases.

Q 50. What is para-aortic dissection?

The fatty tissue is completely removed from around the abdominal aorta between the aortic hiatus and origin of the inferior mesenteric artery. The left adrenal gland is frequently removed to achieve complete dissection around the left renal artery. The overall incidence of metastases in this area is approximately 3%.

Q 51. What is the management of adjacent organ involvement?

- Liver involvement : Non anatomical resection
- Duodenum : 2 cm clearance
- Esophagus : 10 cm clearance
- Colon : Segmental resection
- Pancreas : Distal pancreatectomy

Note: Proximal pancreas is unresectable

Q 52. What is left upper abdominal evisceration?

It is one of the extended combined resections done in association with total gastrectomy. In addition to total gastrectomy, pancreatosplenectomy and transverse colectomy are minimum requirements. Sometimes it includes left hepatectomy, left nephrectomy, left adrenalectomy or resection of the diaphragm. The purpose is to achieve almost complete resection of the omental bursa which consists of the stomach, omentum, mesocolon, transverse colon, spleen and pancreas. The indications for the procedures are:

1. When the tumor is located in the upper or middle part of the stomach and the serosa is penetrated by cancer.
2. When the tumor mainly occupies the posterior wall of the stomach.

3. When there are no remote metastases
4. When there is no severe medical complication to prevent long aggressive intervention.

Q 53. What is the classification of early gastric cancer (EGC)?

The EGC is classified as:

- Type I Protruding
- Type II Superficial
- Type III Excavated.

Q 54. What are the minimally invasive procedures and function preserving procedures?

- These procedures are done for **early gastric cancer** limited to the **mucosa alone**.
- EGC affecting the **submucosa needs radical surgery**.

The procedures are:

1. Endoscopic mucosal resection
2. Laparoscopic wedge resection of the stomach
3. Pylorus preserving gastrectomy.

Q 55. What are the indications for endoscopic treatment of early gastric cancer (EGC)?

Absolute indications:

EGC small enough to be completely removed by single endoscopic treatment. They include:

1. Protruding cancers smaller than 1 cm
2. Ulcer-free depressed cancers smaller than 1 cm
3. Well-demarked cancers.

Relative indications:

1. Cancers associated with severe medical illness
2. Occurring in elderly patients
3. Occurring in patients who refuse surgery.

Q 56. What is pylorus preserving gastrectomy?

This is indicated in small cancers located in the **middle third of the stomach**. The purpose is to reduce dumping symptoms, gallbladder dysfunction and postoperative gallstone development. The hepatic and pyloric branches of vagal nerves are preserved.

Q 57. What is the prognosis of carcinoma stomach?

It rarely disseminates widely before it involves the lymph nodes and therefore there is an opportunity to cure the disease prior to dissemination. Distant metastases are uncommon in the absence of lymph node involvement.

a. The prognosis of **early gastric cancer is very good**. Early gastric cancer associated with lymph node involvement has **5 year survival rates in the region of 90%**.
b. In Japan, approximately 75% of the patients will have a curative resection and the **overall survival will be 50–70%**.
c. **In the West 25–50%** of patients will undergo curative resection and the **five year survival is 25–30%**.

Q 58. Is gastric cancer a different disease in Japan and West? What is the stage migration phenomenon (Will Roger's phenomenon)?

This proposition has no basis in evidence. A combination of differences in the staging and higher standard of surgery in Japan probably accounts for the difference. The more thorough staging, the higher the stage is likely to be and therefore stage for stage, the outcome seems better in patients adequately staged pathologically. This phenomenon is called **stage migration (Will Roger's phenomenon)**.

The pathologist will have considerable difficulty in orientating a fixed specimen and finding lymph node groups and therefore the surgeon should dissect the nodes from the specimen and send them separately to the pathologist—a practice commonly followed in Japan. Only by this method accurate staging can be achieved.

Q 59. Is there any role for chemoradiation?

- The standard adjuvant treatment is chemo-radiation.
- Chemotherapy is by 5-FU and Leucovorin.
- Three doses of bolus 5-FU during first and last weeks of radiotherapy.
- Radiotherapy: Dose is 4,500 Rads.
- Currently Epirubicin, Cisplatin and 5FU combination is favored

Q 60. Is there any role for neoadjuvant chemotherapy?

This is found to be beneficial to downstage cancer of the lower esophagus and occasionally stomach.

Q 61. What is the most common site for recurrence after surgery?

The most common site of recurrence is **stomach bed** followed by lymph nodes and anastomotic site.

Q 62. What is the treatment for recurrence?

- Self-expandable metal stents **(SEMS) is used for obstruction.**
- New chemotherapeutic regimens
  - Cisplatin based
  - Taxane based
  - Irinotecan based.

Q 63. What is the follow-up after surgery?

Follow-up after surgery for carcinoma stomach

- Clinical examination every three months × 2 years
- CT scan/chest X-ray every 6 months
- Endoscopy every year
- Laparoscopy - SOS.

FOR PG'S—WHAT IS NEW?

Current ICMR guidelines for gastric cancer surgery

- R0 Resection
- Resection of adjacent involved structures if resectable
- Minimum *15 lymph nodes* should be evaluated
- Splenectomy and pancreatectomy are not done routinely. If station 10 nodes are involved splenectomy is done If station 11 nodes are involved pancreatectomy may be done
- Staging is done by CT, endoscopic ultrasound and *staging laparoscopy.* PET scan also may be done
- If gross serosal disease is present there is no use of lymphadenectomy.

Case 8 Right Hypochondrial Lump Without Jaundice

Case Capsule

A 50-year-old male patient with history of **chronic alcoholism** and previous **jaundice,** now presents with **loss of appetite**, generalized weakness and **loss of weight** of **6 months** duration. On examination there is no jaundice but **pallor is present**. There are **no stigmata of liver disease**. On inspection of the abdomen, there is **right hypochondrial fullness.** The rest of the abdomen is normal and the abdomen moves with respiration. There are no dilated veins and no visible peristalsis. On palpation there is a **right hypochondrial mass** that is moving with respiration. It is about **6 × 10 cm** size and **hard in consistency**. The mass is seen to descend from below the right costal margin. One **cannot get above the mass** and **fingers cannot be insinuated** between the mass and costal margin. There is dullness on percussion over the swelling and the **dullness is continuous with liver dullness** that is dull up to the 8th rib in the midaxillary line. The **edge of the swelling is irregular and rounded** and the surface of the mass is irregular. On auscultation a **bruit is heard over the swelling.** There is no splenomegaly, there is no ascites. There is no evidence of encephalopathy (Fig. 8.1).

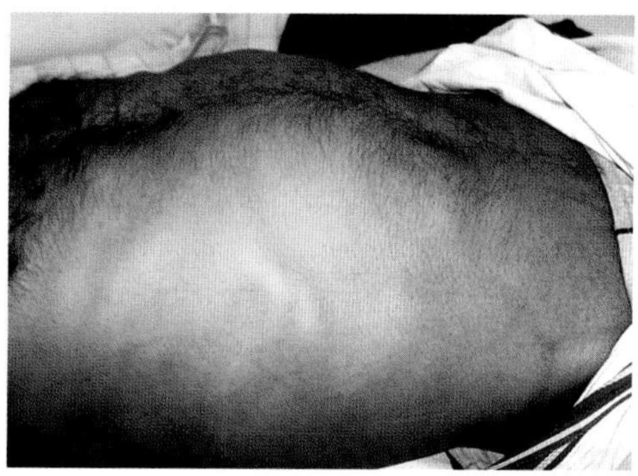

Liver swelling

Refer the checklist for examination in the previous chapter.

1. Look for **Jaundice**
2. Look for **stigmata of liver disease**—palmar erythema, spider nevi, testicular atrophy, absence of pubic and axillary hair, caput medusae, etc.
3. Rule out **Riedel's lobe**
4. Palpate for **spleen**
5. Rule out **ascites**
6. Look for **acquired umbilical hernia** in severe ascites.

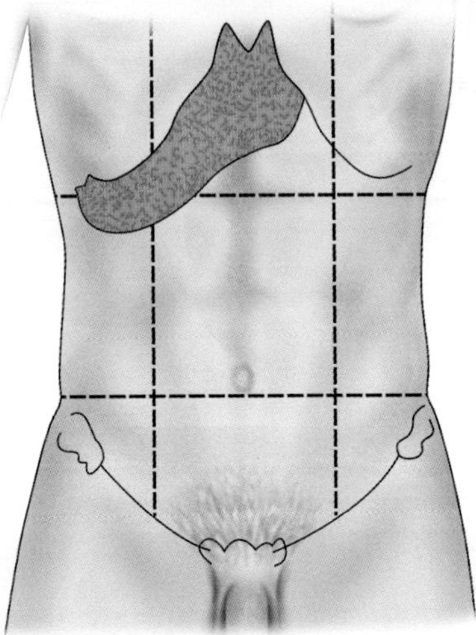

Fig. 8.1: Liver mass

Q 1. What is the probable anatomical diagnosis in this case?

It is a liver swelling.

Q 2. What are your points in favor of a liver swelling?

Clinical points in favor of liver swelling
a. Mass in the right hypochondrium moving with respiration
b. You cannot get above the swelling
c. Fingers cannot be insinuated between the swelling and the costal margin
d. It is dull on percussion and the dullness is continuous with liver dullness
e. The liver swelling will have an edge that may be sharp or round and a surface that will be smooth or irregular.

Q 3. What are the causes for a knobby generalized enlargement of liver without jaundice?

Causes for generalized knobby liver enlargement without jaundice
a. Secondary carcinoma (liver metastases)
b. Primary liver carcinoma
c. Polycystic disease
d. Macronodular cirrhosis.

Q 4. What are the causes for a knobby generalized enlargement of liver with jaundice?

a. Extensive secondary carcinoma
b. Cirrhosis of liver.

Q 5. What are the causes for localized swellings from liver?

Localized swelling from liver
a. Riedel's lobe
b. Secondary carcinoma
c. Liver abscess
d. Hydatid cysts
e. Primary liver carcinoma.

Q 6. What is Riedel's lobe?

This is an extension of the right lobe of the liver down below the costal margin along the anterior axillary line. It is often mistaken for a pathological enlargement of liver or gallbladder. It is a normal anatomical variation.

Q 7. What is the probable pathological diagnosis in this case?

A liver malignancy may be **primary** or **metastases.**

Q 8. What are the points in favor of a primary malignancy in this case?

a. Chronic alcoholism that can lead onto cirrhosis and a primary malignancy may arise in cirrhotic liver.

b. Previous history of jaundice—hepatitis B and hepatitis C lead on to primary malignancy.
c. Cirrhosis itself will predispose to primary malignancy.

Q 9. What are the points against metastases in the liver?

a. Usually multiple nodules are seen in metastases even though multifocal hepatocellular carcinoma is possible.
b. The classical sign of **umbilication** will be palpable in the liver nodule.
c. Other clinical swellings suggestive of a primary in another organ may or may not be palpable in the abdominal cavity.

Q 10. What is the most common malignant swelling in the liver?

Most common malignant swelling is **metastases** in the liver. Metastatic cancer is **20 times more** common than primary tumors in the liver. The cirrhotic liver, which often gives rise to primary hepatic tumors, is less susceptible than normal liver to implantation of metastases.

Q 11. What are the usual presentations of primary malignancy of the liver?

Clinical presentation of primary malignancy of the liver

a. Pain abdomen with or without hepatomegaly
b. Sudden deterioration of the condition of cirrhotic patient owing to the appearance of hepatic failure, bleeding varices or ascites
c. Sudden massive intraperitoneal hemorrhage
d. Acute illness with fever and abdominal pain
e. Distant metastases
f. No clinical finding

Q 12. Can there be associated metabolic or endocrine abnormalities in hepatocellular carcinoma (primary)? (PG)

Metabolic and endocrine abnormalities in hepatocellular carcinoma

a. Erythrocytosis
b. Hypercalcemia
c. Hypoglycemic attack
d. Cushing's syndrome
e. Virilization

Q 13. What are the complications of hepatocellular carcinoma? (PG)

a. Sudden intra-abdominal hemorrhage because of spontaneous bleeding
b. Obstruction of the portal vein resulting in portal hypertension
c. Obstruction of hepatic veins resulting in Budd-Chiari syndrome
d. Liver failure.

Q 14. What is the classification of liver tumors?

The broad classification is into benign and malignant.

Benign	*Malignant*
a. Hepatic adenoma (Hepatic adenoma, Cholangioadenoma or a combination)	A. *Primary* a. Hepatocellular carcinoma
b. Focal nodular hyperplasia	b. Cholangiocarcinoma
c. Hemangioma	c. Combination of hepato and cholangio-carcinomas
	d. Adenosquamous carcinoma

Contd...

Contd...

e. Squamous carcinoma of bile duct
f. Signet ring carcinoma
g. Undifferentiated carcinoma
h. Bile duct cystadeno-carcinoma

B. *Metastases*

Q 15. What is the classification of metastases?

Metastases may be classified as:

a. Carcinomatous, e.g. stomach, colon, pancreas, kidney, prostate, breast, etc.
b. Carcinoid metastases—Carcinoid syndrome will occur when the liver is metastasized and therefore 5HT cannot be metabolized to 5-hydroxyindoleacetic acid.
c. Melanomatous metastases—**beware of "missing toes and glass eyes"**
d. Sarcomatous metastases.
e. Lymphomatous deposits.

Q 16. What are the salient features of hepatic adenoma?

Salient features of hepatic adenoma
• Occur almost exclusively in women • Associated with the use of oral contraceptives • Well-circumscribed soft yellow tan tumors of 2–15 cm size • 2/3rd are solitary and remaining are multiple • Transition from adenoma to carcinoma may occur • Pain, intra-abdominal hemorrhage and shock may occur • Bleeding episode with menstruation is seen • Regression is possible when the size is less than 6 cm and when the oral contraceptive pill is withdrawn • Tumor should be followed-up periodically will ultrasound/CT • When in doubt remove the hepatic adenoma.

Q 17: What are the stigmata of liver disease?

Stigmata of liver disease
• Spider nevi (> 9 new crops indicate progressive disease) • Palmar erythema (thenar and hypothenar eminences) • Clubbing, leukonychia • Dupuytren's contracture • Body hair loss (axillary and pubic) • Fetor hepaticus • Gynecomastia • Testicular atrophy • Liver flap—flapping tremor • Encephalopathy—cog wheel limb rigidity.

Q 18. How to manage this patient with liver mass?

Management includes investigations and treatment. The investigations may be classified as:

1. Investigations for diagnosis
2. Investigations for staging
3. Investigations for surgical treatment.

*The most important investigations is **imaging.**

Q 19. What is the role of ultrasound for imaging liver?

- It is a screening test
- Can identify mass lesions
- Can identify bile duct dilatation
- Useful for guiding biopsy.

Note: But it is operator dependent.

Q 20. What is the role of CT in liver mass?

Triple phase, multislice spiral CT is the investigation of choice for liver mass.

- *A mass lesion up to 1 cm size can be identified*

Hepatocellular carcinoma in contrast enhanced CT shows:

- *Early arterial phase:* vascular enhancement.
- *The venous phase:* maps out portal vein and hepatic veins.

Q 21. What are the CT findings of various mass lesions?

Type of lesion	*Imaging finding*	*Mode of treatment*
Hemangioma	Hyperechoic in US Hypodense in CT without contrast Halo edge enhancement initially, then fills the center (**late, slow venous enhancement**)	No need for surgery
Hepatic adenoma	Well-circumscribed vascular solid tumor. Enlarged peripheral vessels in arteriography—needle biopsy will produce bleeding	Premalignant lesion. Resection is the treatment of choice. Withdrawal of oral contraceptives will produce regression
Focal nodular hyperplasia (FNH) focal over-growth of functioning liver with fibrous stroma	Central scarring in CT. Well-vascularized **Sulfur colloid liver scan** is the investigation of choice – the lesion includes both hepatocytes and Kupffer cells	No need for surgery
Metastases	**Nonenhancing** lesion after **IV contrast** in CT	Surgery for colorectal metastases
Hepatocellular carcinoma	Early arterial phase **enhancing** lesion with IV contrast	Liver resection/liver transplantation

Q 22. What is the gold standard investigation for the diagnosis of hepatocellular carcinoma?

Lipiodol enhanced CT scan is the goldstandard investigation. The practice is an injection of lipiodol into the hepatic artery during selective angiogram followed by CT after 2 weeks. The lipiodol will be taken up by the tumor.

Q 23. What is the role of magnetic resonance imaging (MRI)?

1. It is useful for patients with iodine sensitivity, who cannot undergo a lipiodol enhanced CT.
2. Imaging of the biliary tract (**MRCP**) is possible.
3. Hepatic artery and portal vein can be well-delineated.

Q 24. What is the role of needle biopsy / FNAC in mass lesions of liver?

Percutaneous biopsy of lesions in patients with potentially operable disease is **contraindicated** because of the high incidence of **needle track recurrence and high mortality** associated with this procedure (spontaneous bleeds).

Q 25. If so what is the indication for a needle biopsy?

1. Unresectable tumors
2. Diagnostic dilemma.

Q 26. What are the needles for liver biopsy?

1. Chiba needle (Chiba is the name of a University)
   - 20 cm long, 22 gauge, malleable needle with short bevel
2. Vim silverman needle
3. Menghini needle.

Q 27. What are the precautions to be taken before biopsy from liver?

- The coagulation profile should be checked and rectified (PT, aPTT and platelet count).

- In cases of jaundice (in coagulation failure also) **give vitamin K injections 10 mg IM/IV for 3 days.**

Note: The vitamin K1 (phytomenadione) only can be given IV. **Regular vitamin K is oily** and cannot be given intravenously.

Q 28. What are the macroscopic types of hepatocellular carcinoma? (PG)

Macroscopic types of hepatocellular carcinoma

a. *Unifocal*
   1. Expanding – Sharp demarcation between the tumor mass and compressed surrounding parenchyma
   2. Pedunculated - type 1—intrahepatic - type 2—extrahepatic (nourished by a branch of right hepatic artery) – not a true HCC
   3. Spreading (Engel's massive form)—lack of demarcation between tumor and normal liver—may involve the whole liver as nodules

b. *Multifocal*—synchronous swellings

c. *Indeterminate*—different features in different parts

d. *Diffuse*

Another macroscopic classification:

a. Pushing
b. Hanging
c. Infiltrative or diffuse

NCCN classification:

a. Nodular
b. Massive
c. Diffuse

Q 29. What are the pathological variants of HCC? (PG)

1. Fibrolamellar HCC—good prognosis
2. Mixed hepatocellular cholangiocellular—worse prognosis
3. Clear cell variant—better prognosis
4. Giant cell variant
5. Childhood HCC (bad prognosis)
6. Carcinosarcoma (sarcomatoid variant).

Q 30. What are the features of fibrolamellar carcinoma?

1. Younger age group (median 25 years)
2. Without history of cirrhosis
3. Well-circumscribed
4. Better resectability (50 – 75% in contrast to 25% in ordinary HCC)
5. Better prognosis
6. Left lobe is more commonly affected
7. Lymph node involvement is there
8. Does not produce AFP (α fetoprotein)
9. Neurotensin B and vitamin B12 binding proteins are the tumor marker
10. Equal sex incidence
11. CT finding—stellate scarring.

Q 31. What are the etiological factors for HCC?

1. Cirrhosis—Cirrhomimetic (develops in the background of cirrhosis) Noncirrhomimetic
2. HBV (hepatitis B virus)
3. HCV (hepatitis C virus)
4. Alcoholic liver disease
5. Hemochromatosis
6. Hereditary tyrosinemia
7. Mycotoxins (afla toxin B)
8. Hepatic helminthiasis – clonorchis sinensis for cholangiocarcinoma.

Q 32. What is the tumor marker for the HCC?

1. AFP (α fetoprotein)
2. PIVKA II (protein induced by vitamin K abnormality by antagonism) – it is positive in 80% HCC
3. Lens culinaris Agglutinin reactive AFP (isoform of alpha fetoprotein)

Q 33. What is small HCC? (PG)

A tumor that is < 2 cm as per Japanese General Rules. But a tumor < 3 – 5 cm may be considered small by some authorities. They are nodular and well-differentiated.

Q 34. What are the investigations for staging?

1. CT abdomen with oral and IV contrast
2. CT chest—to rule out metastases to lung
3. Bone scan—to rule out metastases
4. Laparoscopy.

Q 35. What is the role of Child-Pugh grading?

This is very important if one is planning for surgical resection. Resection should be contemplated in Child-Pugh A patients and occasionally in Child-Pugh B patients.

Child-Pugh classification of functional status of liver

	Class: A *Risk: Low* Score 1	*B* *Moderate* Score 2	*C* *High* Score 3
Ascites	Absent	Slight to moderate	Tense
Encephalopathy	None	Grades I – II	Grades III – IV
Serum albumin (g/dL)	> 3.5	2.8 – 3.5	< 2.8
Serum bilirubin (mg/dL)	< 2.0	2.0 – 3.0	> 3.0
Prothrombin time (seconds above control)	< 4.0	4.0 – 6.0	> 6.0

A – 5 to 6, B – 7 to 9, C – 10 to 15

Q 36. What are the surgical options available in HCC?

The two options are:

1. Resection
2. Liver transplantation.

Q 37. What are the investigations required for surgery?

- Liver function test
- Assessment of cardiac status
- Pulmonary status
- Renal status.

Q 38. What is the TNM staging? **(PG)**

Tx Primary tumor cannot be assessed
T0 No evidence of primary
T1 Solitary tumor without vascular invasion
T2 Solitary tumor with vascular invasion or multiple tumors none more than 5 cm
T3a Multiple tumors more than 5 cm
T3b Single tumor or multiple tumors of any size involving a major branch of portal vein or hepatic vein
T4 Tumor(s) with direct invasion of adjacent organs other than the gallbladder or with perforation of visceral peritoneum

Regional nodes:

Nx Regional node cannot be assessed
N0 No regional node metastasis
N1 Regional node metastasis

Metastasis

M0 No distal metastasis
M1 Distal metastasis

Q 39. What is MELD (Model for End-Stage Liver Disease) score? **(PG)**

The following factors are considered for MELD

- Creatinine
- Bilirubin
- INR.

Q 40. What are the bad prognostic factors? **(PG)**

In addition to MELD, alpha fetoprotein, fibrosis score and hepatitis serology

Q 41. What is Okuda staging? (PG)

Four factors are considered in this staging:

- Tumor size
- Ascites
- Albumin
- Bilirubin.

Q 42. What is CLIP (Cancer of Liver Italia Program) staging? (PG)

It consists of:

Child-Pugh and Alpha Fetoprotein and Portal vein thrombosis and Morphology

Q 43. What is CUPI (Chines University Prognostic Index)? (PG)

The following are considered in this:

TNM and ascites and Bilirubin and ALP and Symptoms

Q 44. What are the indications for resection in HCC? (PG)

Milan criteria:

1. Tumor less than 5 cm
2. Number less than 3 cm
3. Each less than 3 cm

University of California Sanfrancisco Criteria:

1. Single tumor less than 6.5 cm
2. Less than three tumors
3. Total diameter less than 8 cm
4. Largest less than 4.5 cm

Note: More than 30% of remnant liver must be kept. At least two contiguous liver segments must be retained and it should be a resection with tumor free negative margin.

Q 45. What are the contraindications for liver resection in HCC? (PG)

1. Extrahepatic disease
2. Lymph nodes
3. Peritoneal involvement
4. Distant metastases
5. 1 cm clear margin is not possible
6. Multifocal hepatoma (> 2 nodules)—Treatment is transplantation.

Q 46. How much liver should be left behind in case of liver resection? (PG)

Two segments of healthy liver must be left behind.

Q 47. What type of anesthesia is preferred for liver resection? (PG)

Low CVP anesthesia

- The inflow to the liver can be blocked by clamping the free edge of the lesser omentum
- Bleeding results from hepatic vein during resection
- If the CVP is decreased to zero, there will be little bleeding from hepatic veins
- As a result, there is no need for blood transfusion.

Q 48. What are the indications for transplantation? (PG)

Outlook is better for transplantation than resection provided:

- Tumor nodules are 3 cm or less in diameter
- Nodules are 3 or less in number.

Q 49. What are the nonsurgical ablative therapies available? (PG)

1. Radiofrequency ablation—complications are needle track recurrence, hemorrhage and liver failure.
2. Percutaneous alcohol injection—destruction of tumors up to 3 cm size is possible—ineffective in colorectal metastases.
3. **TACE** (Transartenal Chemo Embolization)—for small tumours only. A mixture of lipiodol and doxorubicin is injected directly into the hepatic artery. The complications are post embolization

syndrome, liver failure, and liver abscess. 50% reduction in tumor size is seen 50% of cases.

4. **TARE** (Transarterial Radioembolization).

Q 50. What is the role of chemotherapy in HCC? (PG)

The results of chemotherapy are disappointing. Therefore, there is no role for systemic chemotherapy. Subcutaneous **Octreotide** is being tried in advanced HCC.

Q 51. What is the prognosis of HCC?

- It is a tumor with poor prognosis
- Median survival is in the region of 1 year
- Symptomatic patients survive for 6 months
- Resected patients (if suitable) the 5 years survival is around 30%
- Transplantation gives better results
- **Life-expectancy is decided by the liver disease.**

Case

9 Right Iliac Fossa Mass (Suspected Ileocecal Tuberculosis)

Case Capsule

A 40-year-old female patient presents with **colicky abdominal pain** with **intermittent diarrhea** of 1 year duration. The pain is exacerbated by eating and relieved by vomiting. The **stool is watery**, small in amount and **mixed with blood**. She has got **flatulence and borborygmi** with frequent **distension** of abdomen. She also gives history of **loss of appetite and weight loss**. She gets **mild fever towards the evening**. There is a history of **exposure to tuberculosis** (her father-in-law had treatment for pulmonary tuberculosis). On general examination, she has **pallor** and she is **emaciated and malnourished**. The abdomen shows **visible peristalsis** and **distended small bowel loops**. The abdomen is found to have "**doughy**" feel on palpation and there is a **mass situated in the right iliac fossa** extending to the lumbar region of **12 × 8 cm** size which is firm in consistency. There is no intrinsic mobility for the mass. All the borders are well-defined except the lateral border. There is **no evidence of free fluid** in the abdomen. There are no other masses. No supraclavicular lymph nodes. There is **no evidence of pulmonary tuberculosis** on chest examination (Fig. 9.1).

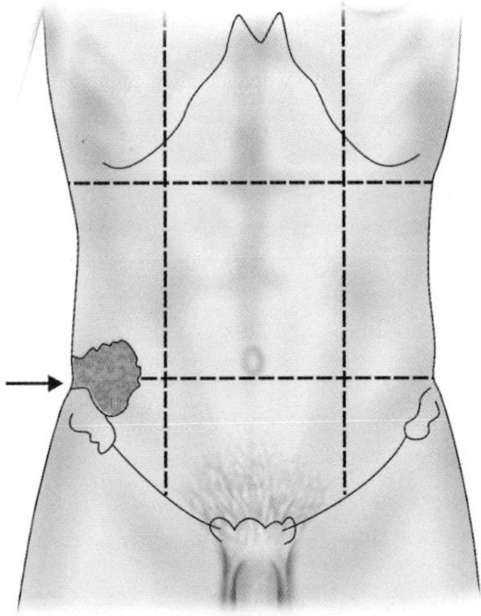

Fig. 9.1: Right iliac fossa mass

Refer the checklist for examination of abdominal lump.

Checklist for right iliac fossa mass

- Look for a primary growth in the **drainage area of inguinal and iliac nodes** (it may be a metastatic iliac group of nodes) including the genitalia, perineum, gluteal region and a per rectal examination

Contd...

Contd...

- Look for **edema of the right lower limb**—due to compression of iliac vein by a malignant lymph node mass
- *Examine the spine*—to rule out a gibbus as a result of tuberculosis (the mass may be an iliopsoas cold abscess)
- Rectal examination to rule out rectal shelf of Blummer and rectal growth
- Examination of **genitaliato rule out undescended testes**
- Examine for **left supraclavicular nodes**
- Look for **swelling below the inguinalligament,** if the right iliac fossa mass is soft. Look for cross fluctuation above and below the inguinal ligament. The psoas abscess will track down to the thigh behind the inguinal ligament
- In case of a soft swelling look for a **space between the swelling and ilium**. The space will be there in appendicular abscess and it will be absent in iliac abscess
- Examine the **sacroiliac joint**—tuberculous abscess from sacroiliac joint can present as right iliac fossa mass There are innumerable causes for mass in the right iliac fossa.

The important causes for mass right iliac fossa

- Appendicular mass
- Ileocecal tuberculosis
- Carcinoma cecum
- Right ovarian cyst/tumor
- Pelvic inflammatory disease
- Iliac lymphadenopathy
- Psoas abscess
- Tumor in undescended testis
- Unascended kidney
- Retroperitoneal tumors
- Chondrosarcoma of the ilium
- Crohn's disease
- Actinomycosis of the cecum
- Tubo-ovarian mass.

Q 1. What are the clinical characteristics of a swelling arising from the cecum?

Even though cecum has a complete peritoneal covering, it is relatively fixed and therefore the mass arising from the cecum will be **fixed.** There will be **no intrinsic mobility**. The mass will be **intraabdominal and intraperitoneal.** One can get above and below the swelling and there won't be any movement.

Q 2. What are the characteristic features of appendicular lump?

There will be typical history—the **Murphy's triad** – migratory pain (from umbilical region to the right iliac fossa), vomiting/nausea and fever. The right iliac fossa mass will be **tender**. The duration of the symptoms and the lump will be short. In late stages there will be **local rise of temperature** and reddening of the overlying skin. The patient may also have intermittent **fever** and tachycardia.

Q 3. What are the characteristic features of tuberculosis?

The patient often has central abdominal pain for months with general ill health, weight loss, and change in bowel habit. The mass is firm, the surface and edges are difficult to define. Ascites may or may not be there. The typical doughy feel may be there. The patient may have evening rise of temperature.

Q 4. What are the characteristic features of carcinoma cecum?

There won't be any history of acute pain. Some patients present with anemia, diarrhea, or intestinal obstruction. The right iliac fossa mass will be firm, or hard, distinct and fixed it is not tender, does not resolve with observation. The patient's temperature and pulse are normal.

Q 5. Comparison of the clinical features of three most important causes for right iliac fossa mass?

	Appendicular lump	*Ileocecal tuberculosis*	*Carcinoma cecum*
Age	Younger age group	Middle age	Above 50 years
Onset	Acute – 3 days after the initial symptoms	Subacute - recurrent attacks	Insidious/ asympto-matic
Symptoms	Murphy's triad • Migratory pain • Nausea/ vomiting • Fever	Recurrent attacks of abdominal pain, diarrhea, loss of weight, evening rise of temperature	Lump abdomen
Nature of mass Intrinsic move-ment	Irregular, firm and tender Fixed	Irregular, doughy Fixed	Hard Fixed
Response to antibiotic	Become smaller and then disappears	No response	No response
Radiological signs	No specific radiological signs	Pulled up cecum Fleischner sign, Sterlin sign, obtus eileocecal angle	Irregular filling defects in the cecum which is in the normal position

Q 6. What is the most probable diagnosis in this case?

May be a case of ileocecal tuberculosis, one should rule out carcinoma cecum.

Q 7. What are the points in favor of ileocecal tuberculosis?

- The long duration of symptoms
- Recurrent attacks of pain abdomen (central type)
- History of diarrhea
- Loss of weight
- Evening rise of temperature.

Q 8. How to confirm the diagnosis?

The investigations for confirming the diagnosis are:

1. *ESR*—will be raised in tuberculosis (complete Hemogram is done)
2. *Leukocyte count*—Leukopenia with lymphocytosis
3. *Hemoglobin*—Anemia may be present
4. *Mantoux test*
   - Mantoux is highly nonspecific
   - Mantoux can be negative in severely immuno-compromised individuals
   - It can be positive in BCG vaccinated individuals.
5. *X-ray chest*—May show pulmonary tuberculosis
6. *Plain X-ray abdomen*—May show calcified lymph nodes
   Evidence of intestinal dilatation
7. *Ultrasound abdomen*—May show mass lesion, fluid collection, enlargement of lymph nodes, etc. A tense tender tubular structure of more than 7 mm if identified is suggestive of appendicular mass, along with fluid collection
8. *Double contrast barium enema*—For visualizing the cecum barium enema is the investigation of choice. For visualizing the terminal ileum a barium meal follow through is the investigation of choice.

9. *CT scan* if required
10. *Peritoneal biopsy*
    a. Needle biopsy (not safe)—Abram's needle/Cope's needle.
    b. Laparoscopic biopsy (ideal)—Peritoneum loses its glistening and smooth appearance. Becomes dull, rough and irregular.
    c. Open biopsy (under local anesthesia).
11. *Ascitic fluid study*
    a. Adenosine De Aminase (ADA)—more than 32 units L—in ascitic fluid—indicates the degree of stimulation of lymphocytes (not significant in HIV patients and cirrhotic patients)
    b. Ascitic fluid total protein—more than 2.5 gm/L
    c. SAAG (Serum ascitic fluid albumin gradient)—more than 1.1
    d. Ascitic fluid blood glucose ratio of less than 0.96.
12. *PCR.*

Q 9. What are the radiological findings in favour of tuberculosis in barium meal follow through?

1. The cecum will be pulled up (normally it is seen in relation to the bone ilium)
2. Fleischner sign—Thickening of ileocecal valve and it is wide open
3. Sterlin sign—Fibrotic terminal ileum opening into a contracted cecum
4. Obtuse ileocecal angle.

Q 10. Which part of the intestine is commonly affected by tuberculosis?

It can affect any part of the GI tract. The commonly affected areas are ileum and proximal colon (57%).

Q 11. Why ileocecal region is more affected in tuberculosis?

a. More lymphatic follicles are seen in terminal ileum
b. Stasis in terminal ileum
c. Spread from adjacent fallopian tube (genital TB will spread via fallopian tube) in females.

Q 12. What are the other forms of abdominal tuberculosis?

Types of abdominal tuberculosis

a. Intestine
b. Peritoneum (38%)—6 types
    1. Chronic peritonitis
    2. Acute peritonitis
    3. Ascitic type
    4. Encysted type
    5. Fibrous type
    6. Purulent type
c. Mesentery
d. Lymph nodes (6%)
e. Omentum
f. Liver and spleen.

Q 13. What are the pathological types of intestinal tuberculosis?

Four pathological types of intestinal tuberculosis:

1. Ulcerative
2. Hypertrophic
3. Fibrotic
4. Ulcerofibrotic.

The first two account for majority of cases.

Q 14. What are the differences between ulcerative type and hypertrophic type of tuberculosis?

Ulcerative	*Hypertrophic*
1. Secondary to pulmonary tuberculosis by swallowing of tubercle bacilli	It is primary—due to ingestion of low virulent organisms by a person with high resistance
2. Patient is very ill	Not very ill
3. Multiple transverse ulcers in the ileum*	Thickening of intestinal wall and narrowing of the lumen
4. Clinical features—Diarrhea and bleeding, weight loss, night sweats, anorexia and evening rise of temperature	Mass right iliac fossa, intestinal obstruction, doughy feel, matted coils of intestine, anemia steatorrhea and weight loss
5. A primary will be there in the chest	No primary in the chest
6. Absence of filling of ileum, cecum and ascending colon	Filling defect in the terminal ileum, pulled up cecum, obtuse ileocecal angle
7. Presence of gross caseation	Absence of gross caseation
8. Obstruction not seen usually	Obstruction common

*Crohn's and typhoid are longitudinal ulcers

Q 15. What is the mechanism of involvement of peritoneum, mesenteric nodes and omentum?

They are involved by the following mechanisms:

a. Involvement during the bacteremic phase of pulmonary tuberculosis
b. From adjacent organ fallopian tube
c. From intestinal tuberculosis.

Note: When nodes and intestine nodes are involved, the node is considered primary because the earliest intestinal lesion is found to be submucosal.

Q 16. What are the complications of iliocecal tuberculosis?

1. Intestinal obstruction
2. Perforation.

Q 17. What is abdominal cocoon?

The plastic adhesions in abdominal tuberculosis, completely obliterate the peritoneal cavity forming a cocoon. Here the intestines are encased in a sheath.

Q 18. What is the importance of pelvic examination in abdominal tuberculosis?

1. To identify the associated genital TB in female
2. To take endometrial biopsy.

Q 19. What is the type of stricture in intestinal TB?
Napkin-ring stricture.

Q 20. What is the treatment for intestinal tuberculosis?

If the diagnosis is certain and in the absence of obstruction, antituberculous treatment alone is required.

Antituberculous Regime

Drug	*Adult dose*	*Bactericidal/Bacteriostatic*	*Important toxicity*
1. Rifampicin	450–600 mg/day (Before food) orally	Bactericidal	Hepatotoxicity (LFT monthly)
2. INH	300 mg OD orally	Bactericidal	Neuritis (Give pyridoxine 10 mg/day)
3. Ethambutol	800 mg OD after food	Bacteriostatic	Retrobulbar neuritis (Check vision)
4. Pyrazinamide (25 mg/kg/day)	750 mg BD after food	Bacteriocidal, acts on caseous materials, macrophages	Hepatotoxicity

Note: All four drugs are given for first two months. Next four months 1 and 2 are given.
Rifampicin can cause failure of oral contraception. It interferes with kinetics of the estrogen component.

Q 21. How will you classify antituberculous drugs?

Primary agents (Bactericidal)	*Secondary agents (Bacteriostatic)*	*Minor agents (Bacteriostatic)*
INH	Ethambutol	Kanamycin
Rifampicin	Ethionamide	Thiacetazone
Pyrazinamide	Cyclosporine	
Streptomycin	Viomycin	

Q 22. How will you classify *Mycobacterium tuberculosis*?

They are classified as:

- *Rapidly dividing*—Susceptible to bacteriocidal drugs
- *Intermittent metabolizers* (not more than a few hours)—Killed by **Rifampicin** because of the **rapidity of action**
- *Organismsin the acid environment of macrophages* - Killed by **Pyrazinamide**
- *Some are dormant* and not affected by drugs

Note: The INH will take one day for the action and therefore not effective for intermittent metabolizers.

Q 23. What are the drugs secreted in the milk?

- Rifampicin
- Pyrazinamide.

Note: Pyridoxine 2 mg for 100 mg of INH is given to mother and infant.

Q 24. What is the treatment of choice when there is obstruction?

a. Ileocecal resection in the form of a right **hemicolectomy**, when the disease involves ileum and cecum. When there is doubt regarding the nature of the mass, resection is recommended.
b. **Strictureplasty** when the lesion is confined to the ileum and the numbers of strictures are isolated and limited.

Q 25. If the investigations are found to be negative for tuberculosis, how one should proceed?

Carcinoma of the cecum should be ruled out by the following investigations:

1. Digital examination of the rectum
2. Rigid/fiberoptic sigmoidoscopy
3. Colonoscopy to rule out synchronous lesions
4. Carcinoembryonic antigen (CEA)—this will be elevated in cancer colon
5. Ultrasound abdomen to rule out liver metastases
6. CT of the abdomen to find out the extent of involvement of the surrounding structures
7. X-ray chest to rule out pulmonary metastases.

Case

10 Suspected Carcinoma of the Cecum

Case Capsule

A **male patient of 50 years** presents with abdominal **pain, anorexia and loss of weight** of eight months duration. It is a **dull ache in the right iliac fossa.** He also complaints of **melena.** There is no history of fever or vomiting. There is **no family history of any malignancy.** On examination the patient is **thin built and pale.** There is fullness of the abdomen in the right iliac fossa region. On palpation there is a **hard, irregular nontender mass** which is fixed, of the size of **16 × 12 cm** size extending to the lumbar region. All the borders are well-delineated except the lateral border. It is possible to get below the swelling. The mass is **dull to percussion.** The liver is not palpable. There is no other palpable mass. There is no evidence of free fluid. The bowel sounds are normal. The left supraclavicular lymph nodes are not enlarged. The rectal examination revealed **feces with blood staining.**

Checklist for examination:

- Take a thorough family history
- Digital rectal examination
- Left supraclavicular nodes
- Look for lumps in the breast
- Do vaginal examination to rule out endometrial and ovarian malignancies
- Look for sebaceous cyst
- Look for osteomas in skull, mandible and tibia
- Look for desmoid tumor in the abdomen
- Look for lipomas and fibromas
- Look for pigmented spots in retina.

Q 1. What are the diagnostic points in favor of carcinoma cecum?

1. Hard mass in the right iliac fossa
2. The mass is fixed
3. Appears to arise from the cecum (intra-abdominal)
4. Anemia
5. Melena.

Q 2. What is the importance of family history in carcinoma colon?

1. Familial adenomatous polyposis **(FAP)** is an inherited, autosomal, dominant condition affecting the **chromosome 5 p 21 (APC GENE)**– presenting as multiple adenomatous polyposis mainly involving **large bowel**, but it can also involve stomach duodenum and small intestine. It is clinically defined by the presence of more than 100 colorectal adenomas.
2. **HNPCC** (Hereditary nonpolyposis colorectal cancer) is also autosomal dominant problem where patient presents with colon cancers at an early age. It is also associated with cancers

of the endometrium, ovary, stomach and small intestine. The mutation is in the MLH1 and MSH2 genes. (It is also called Lynch Syndrome).

Q 3. What are the syndromes associated with polyps?

1. Gardner's syndrome—
   - FAP
   - Desmoid tumour of abdominal wall
   - Osteoma of skull, mandible, tibia
   - Epidermal cyst
   - Fibroma
   - Lipoma
   - Bone cyst
   - Impacted molars.
2. **Turcot's syndrome**—It is autosomal recessive
   - Polyposis
   - Childhood cerebellar medulloblastoma.

Q 4. What is the risk for malignancy in FAP?

1. All patients will develop **colorectal** carcinoma 10 to 20 years after the onset of polyp.
2. In addition there is a risk of **duodenal carcinoma, ampullary carcinoma**.

Q 5. What are the clinical features of FAP?

They may be **symptomatic or asymptomatic**

Symptoms:

- Loose stools
- Lower abdominal pain
- Weight loss
- Diarrhea
- Blood and mucus with stools.

Q 6. What are the investigations done to rule out FAP?

- Sigmoidoscopy
- Double contrast barium enema
- Colonoscopy and biopsy.

*More than 100 adenomas must be there to make a diagnosis of FAP.

Q 7. What is the screening policy for FAP? (PG)

1. The screening is by colonoscopy:
   - All members of the family (cousins, nephews, and nieces) are screened at the age of 10 to 12 years and thereafter once in 1–2 years. This should be continued upto the age of 20 years.
   - If no polyps till the age of 20, continue screening at 5 yearly intervals until 50 years.
   - At 50 years if there are no polyps—then no inherited gene is present.
2. Pigmented spots in retina (Congenital hypertrophy of retinal pigment epithelium > 4 in number on each eye).
3. DNA test for FAP (Genetic testing for at risk family members).

Q 8. Can you prevent carcinoma in FAP? (PG)

At present, the only means of prevention is by **prophylactic resection of the colon—total proctocolectomy** and **ileoanal pouch anastomosis.**

Q 9. Is there any role for upper GI endoscopy in FAP? (PG)

Yes. The patient can develop duodenal ampullary and stomach malignancies and therefore upper GI endoscopy is indicated.

Q 10. Is there any medical treatment for polyp? (PG)

Sulindac and Celecoxibare being tried.

Q 11. What are the features of HNPCC?

It is also an autosomal dominant condition affecting the chromosome **2P (short arm of 2) and** there are **2 syndromes** associated with this—

a. *Lynch I syndrome*—this produces multiple colonic cancers in the proximal colon at an early age **(hereditary site specific colon caner)**
b. *Lynch II syndrome*—here in addition to colon cancer **extracolonic adenocarcinomas** affecting (**Cancer family syndrome**)the following organs are seen:

- Breast, ovary, endometrium, pancreas, stomach, bile duct, ureter and renal pelvis, etc.

Q 12. What is Amsterdam criteria for HNPCC?(PG)

Amsterdam criteria 1 (Lynch 1)—at least 3 relatives must have histologically verified colorectal cancer.

1. One must be a 1st degree relative of the other two
2. At least two successive generations must be affected
3. At least one of the relatives with colorectal cancer must have received the diagnosis before the age of 50 years.

Amsterdam criteria 2 (Lynch 2)—at least 3 relatives must have a cancer associated with hereditary nonpolyposis colonic cancer namely colorectal, endometrial, ovarian, stomach, pancreas, hepatobiliary, etc.

1. One must be a 1st degree relative of the other two
2. At least two successive generations must be affected
3. At least one of the relatives with HNPCC associated cancer must have received the diagnosis before the age of 50 years.

Q 13. What is synchronous carcinoma?

In all cases of suspected colorectal cancer look for the presence of a second malignancy in another location in the colon. The development of simultaneous cancer is called synchronous carcinoma. If it is developing after the resection of one malignancy then it is called **metachronous** cancer. Therefore, even after identification of one malignancy the rest of the colon must be studied thoroughly by colonoscopy and double contrast barium enema to rule out a **second malignancy** (Synchronous).

Q 14. What are the macroscopical types of colorectal cancer?

There are 4 types:

- Type 1 – Annular
- Type 2 – Tubular
- Type 3 – Ulcerative
- Type 4 – Cauliflower—least malignant.

Q 15. Which type of lesion is seen on the right side of colon?

Ulcerative and polypoidal lesions are seen on the right side.

Q 16. What are the investigations for making a diagnosis in this case?

A. *Investigations for diagnosis:*
   1. Rigid sigmoidoscopy
   2. Flexible sigmoidoscopy (60 cm length)
   3. Colonoscopy—can visualize the growth and take biopsy.
      - Can demonstrate synchronous carcinoma (seen in 5%) and polyps
   4. Double contrast barium enema—
      - irregular filling defects
      - apple core appearance
      - shouldering
      - demonstrate polyps

B. *Investigations for staging:*
   1. Chest X-ray
   2. LFT
   3. Ultrasound
      - for liver metastases
      - for free fluid
      - for knowing the extent of the caecal mass
      - obstruction of ureter and subsequent hydronephrosis
   4. CECT (contrast enhanced)
      - for local invasion
      - for adjacent structure involvement

5. CEA

C. *Investigations for surgery:*
1. Cardiac status
2. Renal status
3. Hematological investigations.

Q 17. What is virtual colonoscopy?

High resolution 3D images of the colon can be made with a multislice CT scanner with improved software. It has a sensitivity and specificity of 94%. There is no need for sedation as in the case of colonoscopy.

Q 18. What are the methods of spread of carcinoma colon?

1. *Local spread*—may be **vertical**, **horizontal and radial.**
   Vertical is to the adjacent structures and horizontal is submucosal. Radial is circumferential.
   a. It will spread around—it takes one year for spreading 3/4th circumference and result in intestinal obstruction.
   b. Ulcerated type produce fistulization to urinary bladder
      Local perforation
      External fecal fistula.
2. Lymphatic spread
   Read the lymphatic drainage (below).
3. Bloodstream spread
   - Produce occult hepatic metastases
   - Responsible for late death
   - Metastases in lung, liver, bone, brain and skin.
4. Transperitoneal spread
   - Peritoneal metastases—Ascites
   - Carcinomatosis peritoneum
   - Rectal shelf of Blumer.
5. Intraluminal spread—This is responsible for anastomotic site recurrence.

Q 19. What are the predisposing causes for colorectal cancer?

Predisposing causes for colorectal cancer

- Ulcerative colitis—Inflammatory bowel disease of > 10 years
- Crohn's colitis
- Schistosomal colitis
- Exposure to radiation
- Ureterosigmoidostomy
- Breast carcinoma (small increased risk)
- Gallstone (postchole cystectomy-increased risk for right colonic malignancy)
- Diet—fiber diet protects, cooked meat—carcinogenic, bile acid—carcinogenic.

Q 20. What is the commonest site for colorectal cancer?

Incidence of colorectal cancer in various sites	
Maximum incidence in rectum	38%
Sigmoid	21%
Cecum 12%	
Transverse colon	5.5%
Ascending colon	5%
Descending colon	4%
Splenic flexure	3%
Hepatic flexure	2%

Q 21. What are the types of adenomatous polyps of colon?

There are 3 types
1. Tubular – 5% chance for malignancy
2. Tubulovillous – 22% chance for malignancy
3. Villous – 40% chance for malignancy

Q 22. What is the significance of adenomatous polyp and how will you manage polyp?

- Adenomas are premalignant
- They are usually multiple

- Synchronous cancer may occur
- Adenomas > 5 mm size should be removed because of malignant potential.

Q 23. What is the peculiarity of villous adenoma?

They are sessile frond-like spreading lesion. They produce mucus discharge, diarrhea and hypokalemia. Unlike other polyp, removal by colonoscopic snaring and diathermy obliteration with hot biopsy forceps are not possible in villous adenoma. Proctectomy may be required.

Q 24. What is adenoma-carcinoma sequence? (PG)

Fearon-Vogelstein Adenoma-carcinoma multi-step model of carcinogenesis

Normal epithelium
↓← 5q loss
Dysplasia
↓
Early adenoma
↓←12p activation K-ras
Intermediate adenoma
↓←18q loss
Late adenoma
↓←17p loss, p53
Carcinoma
↓
Metastases

Q 25. What is the staging for carcinoma colon?

Duke's classification originally described for rectum is used for colon with modification.

Duke's A: Tumor restricted, but not through the bowel wall
Duke's B: Indicating penetration through the bowel wall
Duke's C: Spread to local and regional nodes
- *C1:* Nodes in the immediate vicinity
- *C2:* Along the vessels

Duke's D: Distant metastases.

The staging system by Astler and Coller is a modification of Duke's.

TNM-AJCC 6th edition is the staging system followed now.

Q 26. What is the AJCC 7th Edition - TNM staging? (PG)

Tx	Primary tumor cannot be assessed
T0	No evidence of primary tumor
Tis	Carcinoma in situ, intraepithelial or invasion of lamina propria
T1	Tumor invades submucosa
T2	Tumor invades muscularis propria
T3	Tumor invades through the muscularis propria, into the subserosa or into non-peritonealized pericolic or perirectal tissues
T4a	Tumor penetrates to the surface of the visceral peritoneum
T4b	Tumor directly invades or is adherent to other organs or structures

Nx	Regional lymph nodes cannot be assessed
N0	No regional lymph node metastases
N1	Metastases in 1 to 3 nodes
N1a	Metastasis in 1 regional lymph node
N1b	Metastases in 2–3 regional lymph nodes
N1c	Tumor deposits in the subserosa, mesentery, or non-peritonealized pericolic or perirectal tissue without regional nodal metastases
N2	Metastases in 4 or more nodes
N2a	Metastases in 4 - 6 regional lymph nodes
N2b	Metastases in 7 or more regional lymph nodes
Mx	Distant metastases cannot be assessed
M0	No distant metastases
M1	Distant metastases
M1a	Metastases confined to 1 organ or site (e.g. liver, lung, ovary, non regional node)
M1b	Metastasis in more than 1 organ/site or the peritoneum

Q 27. Comparative chart showing TNM, Duke's and modified Astler-Coller staging? (PG)

Stage	*T*	*N*	*M*	*Dukes*	*MAC*
0	Tis	N0	M0		
I	T1	N0	M0	A	A
	T2	N0	M0	A	B1
IIA	T3	N0	M0	B	B2
IIB	T4a	N0	M0	B	B3
IIC	T4b	N0	M0		
IIIA	T1-T2	N1/N1c	M0	C	C1
	T1	N2a	M0		
IIIB	T3-T4a	N1/N1c	M0	C	C2/C3
	T2-T3	N2a	M0		
	T1-T2	N2b	M0		
IIIC	T4a	N2a	M0	C	C1/C2/C3
	T3-T4a	N2b	M0		
	T4b	N1-N2	M0		
IVA	Any T	Any N	M1a	D	D
IVB	Any T	Any N	M1b		

Q 28. What are the differences between right and left sided colonic malignancy?

Right sided	*Left sided*
1. Right side colonic diameter is large	Narrow
2. On right side the content is fluid (fecal)	Content is solid
3. Growth is ulcerated/ cauliflower like	Stenosing growth
4. Present with pallor	Present with intestinal obstruction
5. Ill defined pain	Colicky pain
6. Bowel symptom - Melena	Alternating constipation and diarrhea
7. Late diagnosis	Because of obstruction early diagnosis
8. For right colectomy only the branches of superior mesenteric are ligated	Flush ligation of inferior mesenteric artery done for left colectomy
9. Bad prognosis because of late diagnosis	Good prognosis because of early diagnosis

Contd...

Contd...

Q 29. What is the cause for alternating constipation and diarrhea in left sided colon cancer?

The left sided cancers are usually tubular or annular producing obstruction. As a result of obstruction there will be constipation. Subsequent to constipation there will be stasis of fecal matter proximal to the stenosis. This will produce stercoral enteritis which in turn will produce diarrhea—the so-called spurious diarrhea where the liquid fecal matter will escape through the narrow segment. Again the patient will go in for constipation. This is a vicious cycle.

Q 30. What is the site of perforation of the colon in cases of obstruction?

The perforation can occur in the following places.

a. At the site of the growth
b. Just proximal to the growth as a result of stercoral enteritis
c. At the cecum for any distal growth if the ileocecal valve is competent.

Q 31. What are the acute manifestations of colonic cancer?

- Intestinal obstruction
- Perforation
- Peritonitis
- Bleeding

Contd...

Contd...

- Fistulization with urinary bladder resulting in pneumaturia
- Gastrocolic fistula
- Acute appendicitis/appendicular abscess (obstructive appendicitis as a result of the growth in the cecum)
- Intussusceptions (always rule out a growth in all cases of adult intussusception. There is no role for hydrostatic reduction in adults).

Q 32. Having made the diagnosis of carcinoma cecum, how do you manage the patient?

After doing investigations in the form of X-ray chest to rule out metastases in the lungs, ultrasound abdomen to rule out metastases liver and free fluid, the patient is prepared for resection.

Q 33. What are the preparations for surgery?

- Make the patient fit for anesthesia (evaluate cardiac, respiratory status)
- Correction of anemia
- Correction of hypoproteinemia
- Dietary regulation
- Bowel preparation
- Prophylactic subcutaneous heparin
- Prophylactic antibiotics.

Q 34. What is the role of mechanical bowel preparation?

- Dietary restriction in the form of liquid diet for 24 hours before surgery.
- The role of mechanical bowel preparation for elective surgery is highly controversial. There is enough evidence in the literature for safe surgery without mechanical bowel preparation.
- Conventionally
  - Bowel washes
  - Laxatives in the form of sodium picosulphate
  - Cleansing agents like Polyethylene glycol (PEG) orally are given the day before.

Q 35. What is the role of antibiotic prophylaxis in colonic surgery?

The routine practice of Nichol's regime by giving 3 doses of antibiotics 18, 17 and 10 hours preoperatively with neomycin and erythromycin is no longer practised.

A single dose of ampicillin—sulbactam or quinolone and metronidazole or parenteral cefoxitin are recommended for antibiotic prophylaxis (1 hour before skin incision).

Q 36. How will you assess the operability? (PG)

a. After laparotomy look for metastases in peritoneum (small white seed-like), liver, pelvic deposits, Krukenberg's tumor (metastatic ovarian tumor) ascites and lymph nodes
b. Look for tumor mobility and adjacent structure involvement
c. Liver metastases if found are not biopsied—it will cause tumor dissemination
d. Hepatic metastases resection is done as a staged procedure later
e. Tumor dissemination is not a contraindication for resection of the primary.

Q 37. What is the surgical procedure of choice when there is a cecal growth?

Right hemicolectomy is the operation of choice, where a radical resection of the involved colon along with its lymphovascular drainage is done. Any devascularized segment should be removed in addition. Suspicious lymph nodes are taken for biopsy.

Q 38. How much is the clearance required in colonic resection?

The clearance of a minimum of 5–10 cm on either side is recommended.

Q 39. What are the vessels ligated for right hemicolectomy?

The ileocolic, right colic, and right branch of the middle colic vessels are ligated for right hemicolectomy.

Q 40. What are the technical precautions taken during surgery and how much ileum is removed? (PG)

- The cecum is mobilized by incising the lateral peritoneum which is carried around the hepatic flexure
- Take care not to injure the ureter, spermatic vessels (in males) and duodenum
- The mesentery of last 30 cm of ileum is removed
- The colon is divided as far as the proximal third of transverse colon
- The anastomosis is done between the rest of ileum and transverse colon in layers.

Q 41. What is non touch technique of Turnbull? (PG)

Its usefulness has been debated. Here early ligation of vascular pedicle and control of proposed resection edges is done before mobilization of the tumor bearing area. It aims to prevent the luminal, vascular and lymphatic pathways for tumor emboli or tumor cells while handling the lesion.

Q 42. What are the anatomical peculiarities of the colon from anastomotic point of view?

1. *The content* of the colon is fecal matter and therefore there is more chance for infection after resection and anastomosis
2. *The wall*—longitudinal muscle coat is thin and therefore there is more chance for anastomotic leak
3. *The arterial supply*—It is precarious and special (Fig. 10.1).

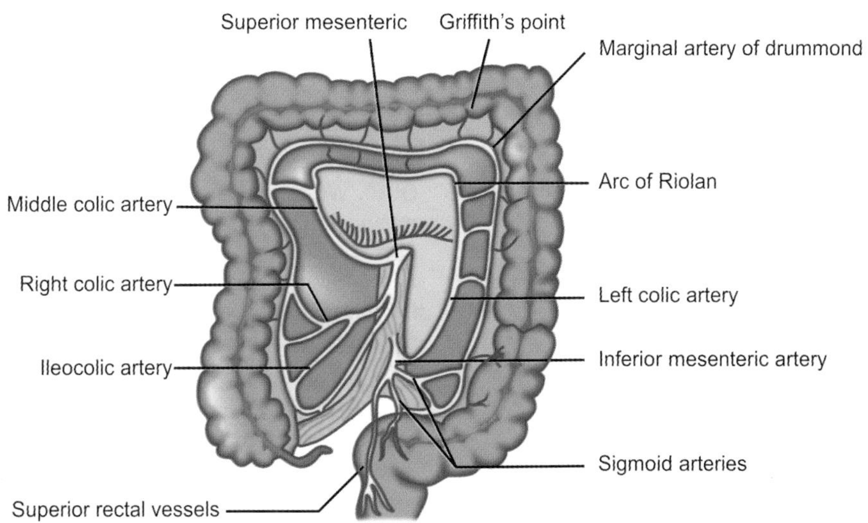

Fig. 10.1: Colonic blood supply

The colon is supplied by branches of the superior mesenteric artery namely the ileocolic artery, the right colic artery, and middle colic artery.

The inferior mesenteric artery arises from the aorta opposite L3 vertebrae and the branches are left colic artery and sigmoid arteries.

The marginal artery of drummond: It is present in almost all patients. It is a single arterial trunk along the concave part of large intestine from ileocecal junction to rectosigmoid junction forming a communicating channel between the superior and inferior mesenteric artery. It gives off vasa recta which run perpendicular to the colonic wall.

Meandering artery (Arc of Riolan): These are collateral branches connecting proximal middle colic artery to left colic artery. During colonic mobilization this artery should be protected.

Griffith's point: It is the weak point in the vascular anastomosis between middle and left colic arteries. Therefore it is important to avoid anastomosis at the splenic flexure.

Sudek's point: It is at the level of lowest sigmoid and superior rectal artery. There is a higher chance of avascularity if anastomosis is performed here.

Q 43. What is the lymphatic drainage of colon?
Lymph nodes are divided into four groups.

a. Epicolic—located on the bowel wall
b. Paracolic—located along the marginal artery
c. Intermediate—located along the colic vessels
d. Principal—located along SMA and IMA.

Q 44. What is white line of Toldt?
The ascending and descending colon has no peritoneal covering on their posterior aspects but has areolar tissue (fascia of Toldt), which represent the embryonic fusion of mesentery to posterior peritoneum. At the lateral parietal wall it reflects as the white line of Toldt. This line is used as the plane for avascular mobilization of the colon.

Q 45. Which part of the colon has the largest diameter?

- Cecum—7.5 cm
- Narrowest part is rectosigmoid—2.5 cm.

Q 46. Which are the mobile portions of the colon?
Transverse colon and sigmoid colon. (The rest of the colon is fixed).

Q 47. What are the ligaments attaching the hepatic flexure of colon (which is fixed)?

- Nephrocolic ligament
- Hepatocolic ligament
- Duodenocolic ligament.

Q 48. What is the attachment of splenic flexure?
Phrenicocolic ligament.

Q 49. What is the extent of descending colon?
It extends from the splenic flexure to the brim of the true pelvis.

Q 50. What is the attachment of transverse mesocolon?
The transverse mesocolon is attached to the descending part of duodenum, to the head and lower aspect of the body of the pancreas, and to the anterior surface of the left kidney—horizontally.

Q 51. What is the attachment of mesosigmoid?
It is inverted 'V' shaped, the apex of this peritoneal attachment is at the bifurcation of the left common iliac vessels over the left sacroiliac joint (at the left ureter). The right limb, comes down to the third piece of sacrum and the left limb traverses along the brim of the left side of pelvis (Fig. 10.2).

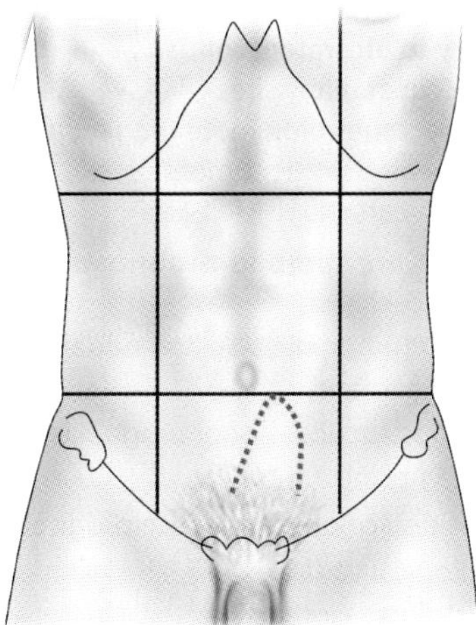

Fig. 10.2: Mesosigmoid attachment

Q 52. What is the management of carcinoma colon when there is obstruction? (PG)

a. If risk factors are present—Resection plus exteriorization of the bowel ends is preferred.
b. Healthy patients (no risk factors)—Resection plus primary anastomosis. If primary anastomosis is done always do a protective colostomy.
c. Unresectable cases—Ileo transverse anastomosis is done or ileostomy.

Note: Primary anastomosis is worrisome in left sided lesions because of increased anastomotic dehiscence seen in dilated and edematous unprepared bowel.

Q 53. What is the management of unresectable lesion with widespread metastases and severe comorbidity? (PG)

- Colonic stenting (SEMS).
- Complications of stenting are stent migration and restenosis.

Q 54. What is "On - Table - Lavage"?

This is done for unprepared bowel during emergency surgery. In left sided obstructed colonic growths presenting as emergency, a Foley catheter is introduced via terminal ileum to the cecum or directly to cecum through an appendectomy stump and the colon is irrigated. The colon is transected above the growth and the effluent is collected through a tubing (Boyle's apparatus tubing), until the colon is clean.

Q 55. What is the treatment of synchronous lesion? (PG)

- If lesions are in the same segment—segmental resection
- If they are widely separated—subtotal colectomy.

Q 56. What is CEA (Carcinoembryonic antigen)?

CEA (Carcinoembryonic antigen)
• It is a glycoprotein found in cell membrane of many tissues including colorectal cancer
• Some antigen enters the circulation and this is identified by radioimmunoassay
• It is present in other body fluids like urine and feces
• CEA is not specific for carcinoma of colorectum
• It is present in other GI cancers, nonalimentary cancers, and benign diseases
• It is high in 70% of carcinoma colon
• It is not useful as a screening investigation
• It is useful for detecting recurrence after a curative surgery if the serial CEA values are rising after 6–9 months
• CEA level of > 2.5 ng/mL is significant
• CEA level of > 5 ng/mL indicates poor prognosis
• If preoperative elevated CEA does not fall to normal within 2–3 weeks after resection, the resection is incomplete or there is occult metastases
• CEA values are highest in lung and liver metastases.

Q 57. What is left hemicolectomy?

This is done for tumors of descending colon and splenic flexure. Here resection of the colon from splenic flexure to rectosigmoid is done.

Q 58. What is the treatment for sigmoid cancer?

Sigmoidectomy.

Q 59. What are the indications for total colectomy/ subtotal colectomy?

- Multiple primary tumors
- Completely obstructing sigmoid cancers
- HNPCC
- Transverse colon carcinoma.

Q 60. What is extended right hemicolectomy?

This is done for proximal transverse colon growth.

Q 61. What is extended left hemicolectomy?

This is done for distal transverse colon growth.

Note: For transverse colon growth subtotal colectomy is another option.

Q 62. What are the surgical procedures of choice for growth in various regions of the colon?

Surgical procedures of choice for growth in various regions of the colon.

Site	*Surgical procedure*
Cecum, ascending colon, hepatic flexure	Right hemicolectomy
Proximal part of transverse colon	Extended right hemicolectomy
Distal transverse colon	Extended left hemicolectomy
Descending colon and splenic flexure	Left hemicolectomy
Sigmoid colon	Sigmoidectomy
Transverse colon, sigmoid colon, multiple tumors, HNPCC	Subtotal colectomy

Q 63. What are the peculiarities of cancer secondary to ulcerative colitis?

- May occur at many sites
- May affect the colon more than rectum
- They are high grade tumors
- After 20 years the risk is 12%.

Q 64. What are the bad prognostic factors in colonic cancer? (PG)

1. Depth of tumor invasion and nodal metastases (most important)
2. Bowel obstruction—poor prognosis
3. CEA > 5 ng/mL
4. Right sided colon carry worse prognosis
5. Pathological variables
   - Histological grade
   - Signet ring type-poor prognosis
   - Small cell carcinoma
   - Lymphovascular invasion.

Q 65. What is the indication for adjuvant therapy in colorectal cancer? (PG)

- In stage I lesion no further adjuvant therapy
- In stage II and III – adjuvant therapy has most important impact
- In Stage II – 5FU and Leucoverin (folenic acid)
  - Folenic acid is a potentiator of 5 FU
  - (immunomodulator levamisole with 5 FU is used less nowadays)
  - Histopathologically positive lymph nodes is an indication for chemotherapy.
- In Stage III – FOLFOX 4 regimen
  - (Oxaliplatin and 5FU - 2 times a month for 12 cycles)

    OR
  - FOLFIRI regimen (folic acid, and 5FU and Irinotecan).

Q 66. What is the most effective single chemotherapeutic agent for adenocarcinoma?

5-Fluorouracil.

Q 67. What is the follow-up for carcinoma colon?

Clinical examination once in six months.

Annual examination of the following:

- CEA
- Chest X-ray
- Colonoscopy
- LFT
- CBC.

Q 68. What is fast track surgery?

It is a multimodal rehabilitation regimen for elective colonic surgery for enhanced recovery consisting of—

Fast track surgery

- Preoperative counseling and optimization
- Epidural catheter for pain control
- General anesthesia using propofol (no nitrous oxide)
- No bowel preparation
- Transverse abdominal incision instead of vertical
- Continuous epidural analgesia for two days
- Oral feeding with protein drink (60–80 gm protein/day) from the day of surgery
- Early mobilization
- Laxative and prokinetics for bowel function from the day of surgery
- POP day 1 remove urinary catheter
- POP day 2 remove epidural catheter
- POP day 3 discharge after lunch.

FOR PG'S—WHAT IS NEW?

- Cancer of the descending colon with obstruction current treatment choice is endoscopic stenting followed by elective surgery after two weeks or Hartmann's procedure or colostomy
- All carcinomas arise from adenomas
- All adenomas need not produce carcinoma
- NSAIDs will reduce the number and size of polyps but will not prevent carcinoma
- Full colonoscopy is a must for all colonic carcinoma
- CEA – Indian patients are non secretors
- For metastatic disease FOLFOX 4 cycles followed by surgery followed by 4 cycles of FOLFOX
- Adjuvant—usually 8 cycles
- Cheaper OP Regimen—Cape OX Regimen – Oxaliplatin and Capecitabine orally for 15 days
- New agent for colonic cancer is Cetuximab—agent against Kras
- For synchronous metastasis in liver two approaches are there (a) Surgery of liver along with primary (b) Surgery of liver later (majority of surgeons favor the second approach).

Case 11 Appendicular Mass

Case Capsule

A 25-year-old female patient presents with history of abdominal pain of 4 days duration. Initially the pain started as a vague central abdominal pain in the early morning hours. This pain was preceded by loss of appetite. The patient was constipated for a few days. She felt nauseated and vomited once on the first day of pain. Later the pain shifted to the right iliac fossa. Her pain is aggravated by moving and coughing. The patient is married and has two children. Her menstrual cycles are regular having normal blood flow. Her last menstrual period was 6 days back. There is no history of discharge from vagina. On examination the patient looks pale. There is mild pyrexia. The tongue is furred and there is fetor oris (halitosis). Her pulse rate is 90 per minute. Abdominal examination revealed a tender mass of 16 × 9 cm size in the right iliac fossa with overlying muscle guard and rigidity confined to the right iliac fossa. There is no intrinsic movement for the mass and all the borders are well made out except the lateral border. The mass is intra-abdominal and intraperitoneal. There is no extension of the mass below the inguinal region. The rest of the abdomen is soft and nontender. There is no free fluid demonstrated. The bowel sounds are normally heard. On digital rectal examination, the patient complained of pain deep in the pelvis and the mass is palpable per rectum. On vaginal examination movement of the cervix did not cause pain. Other systems are normal.

Read the checklist of previous case

Checklist with special reference to this case

- A careful gynecological history is taken in all women
- Last menstrual period—to find out whether it is a mid-menstrual pain (mittelschmerz) and to rule out pregnancy
- History of vaginal discharge—pelvic inflammatory disease
- History of dysmenorrhea
- Pelvic examination to rule out adnexal and cervical tenderness
- High vaginal swab to rule out *Chlamydia trachomatis*
- Urine for pregnancy test
- Ultrasound abdomen.

Q 1. What is the most probable diagnosis in this case?

Appendicular mass.

Q 2. What are the differential diagnoses?

- Read the differential diagnosis of right iliac fossa mass

- The patient being a female, in addition to those conditions consider the following:
  - Torsion of ovarian cyst/tumor
  - Tubo-ovarian mass
  - Ectopic pregnancy
  - Pelvic inflammatory disease
  - Uterine swellings.

Q 3. What are the diagnostic points in favor of appendicular mass?

1. History of Murphy's triad of symptoms—migratory pain, vomiting/anorexia, and fever
2. Short duration
3. Patient—ill looking and febrile
4. Tender mass in the right iliac fossa
5. The tender mass is indistinct, dull to percussion and fixed to the right iliac fossa (unlike ovarian).

Q 4. What are the clinical point in favor of an ovarian cyst?

Clinical points in favor of ovarian cyst

- Smooth, spherical with distinct edges
- You cannot get below the swelling (arises from the pelvis)
- It may be mobile from side to side (horizontally) No up and down mobility
- It is dull to percussion
- The lower part of the swelling may be palpable during pelvic examination
- The movement of the cyst per abdominally will be transmitted to the examining finger in the pelvis.

Q 5. What are the clinical points in favor of fibroid uterus?

- Fibroids can grow to enormous size and fill the whole abdomen
- It arises out of the pelvis and so lower edge is not palpable
- It is firm or hard
- Bosselated or knobby
- It is dull to percussion
- Slight transverse mobility will be present.

Q 6. What is appendicular mass?

It is a complication of acute appendicitis. As a result of small perforation in the appendix, the policeman of the abdomen, i.e. omentum will come and try to seal the perforation, as a protective mechanism leading to mass formation. The mass is a palpable conglomerate consisting of the inflamed appendix (usually perforated), adjacent viscera namely cecum and ileum and greater omentum. This is also called phlegmon.

Q 7. What is appendicular abscess?

One should suspect appendicular abscess during the course of conservative treatment of appendicular mass. The clinical criteria for the diagnosis of appendicular abscess are:

1. A rising pulse rate
2. Increasing or spreading abdominal pain
3. Increasing size of mass
4. Patient looking ill.

Q 8. What are the differences between appendicular mass and abscess?

Appendicular mass	*Appendicular abscess*
1. Mass forms around the 3rd day	Abscess around 5 – 10 days
2. Fever absent	Fever present
3. Local signs subside with antibiotics	Local signs aggravate with antibiotics
4. Leukocytosis will return to normal	Rising leukocyte count
5. Imaging—absence of fluid inside	Imaging—presence of fluid inside
6. Clinically patient is not sick	Patient is very sick

Q 9. What is initial management of appendicular mass?

When a mass is diagnosed, the patient is not operated but treated conservatively. It is a contraindication for appendicectomy. The classical treatment is the so-called Ochsner-Sherren regimen (conservative treatment). This consists of:

1. Bed rest (preferably hospitalized)
2. Fluid intake output chart
3. Mark out the limits of mass on the abdominal wall (using a skin pencil)
4. Pulse, temperature and respiration chart (4th hourly)
5. Initiate antibiotic therapy
6. Patient is given fluid diet only initially (if required IV fluids may be given—if patient cannot tolerate oral fluids)
7. Contrast enhanced CT is done to rule out abscess inside.

Q 10. Why appendicectomy is contraindicated in appendicular mass?

1. Immediate appendicectomy is technically more difficult
2. Fear of disturbing the natural barrier present in the mass
3. The mass will resolve without surgery (90% will resolve with conservative treatment)
4. Operation can always be resorted to, should the initial conservative trial fail.

Q 11. What is the indication for stopping the conservative treatment and proceed to surgery?

1. Clinical deterioration
   - rising pulse rate
   - Febrile
2. Failure of the mass to resolve
3. Peritonitis.

Q 12. What is the management of appendicular abscess?

- Traditionally appendicular abscess used to be treated with surgery in the form of extraperitoneal drainage of the abscess.
- But now sono-guided percutaneous catheter drainage is the option.

Q 13. What are the indications for CT scan in appendicitis?

Indications for CT scan in appendicitis

1. Equivocal clinical findings
2. Diagnostic dilemma
3. Appendicular mass/abscess
4. Older patients in whom, acute diverticulitis, neoplasms are differential diagnoses.

Q 14. What are the CT finding in appendicitis? What are the advantages and problems of CT?

- A distended appendix of more than 6 mm size with intramural gas or with stranding of the periappendiceal fat is indicative of inflammation.
- CT scan has been demonstrated to have a sensitivity ranging from 96–100% for the appendix.
- Utilization of CT has been associated with decrease in the negative appendicectomy rate [use of ultrasound is recommended for evaluation of pelvic organs in women of child-bearing age].

Note: A wholesale move to the routine use of spiral CT for the diagnosis of appendicitis will emasculate the clinical skills of the next generation of the surgeons.

It is important not to substitute clinical uncertainty for radiological ambivalence.

Q 15. What is the CT classification of appendicular abscess?

Group I – Comprises phlegmons and abscesses with maximum diameter smaller than 3 cm

Group II – Larger but well-localized abscesses

Group III – Includes extensive periappendicular abscesses involving multiple intra or extraperitoneal compartments.

Q 16. What is the management for each of these CT groups?

Group I patients—antibiotic alone (identification of pus collection alone is not an indication for drain)
Group II patients—percutaneous catheter drainage
Group III patients—surgical drainage.

Q 17. What are the complications of appendicular abscess?

Complications of appendicular abscess

- Obscure subacute intestinal obstruction
- Formation of granulation tissue leading to frozen pelvis
- Stricture of the rectum subsequent to frozen pelvis
- Pelvic abscess.

Q 18. What is the role of laparoscopy in appendicular mass/abscess?

Appendicular abscess is considered a relative contraindication for laparoscopy because of the following reasons:

1. Spread of sepsis
2. Risk of injury to the bowel and mesentery
3. Periappendiceal adhesions.

Q 19. What is the sonological finding in acute appendicitis?

Tense, tender, noncompressible tubular structure of more than 6 mm size in the right iliac fossa.

Q 20. What is interval appendicectomy?

- After treating an appendicular mass conservatively by Ochsner-Sherren regimen, conventionally the patient is advised to undergo appendicectomy after 6–12 weeks of waiting period. This is nowadays shortened to the time required for complete resolution of the mass.
- However, now, many have questioned the practice of interval appendicectomy, since the recurrence rate of acute appendicitis after management of the mass is only 10% (3–15%).
- Routine interval appendicectomy is unnecessary in the majority of patients.
- An argument can be made in favor of interval appendicectomy in patients who in the future, may not have easy access to modern surgical facilities.

Q 21. How to tackle the issue of missing or missed diagnosis of a malignancy in cases of appendicular mass?

It is recommended that patients over the age of 40 years undergo a barium enema examination (double contrast) or a colonoscopy after successful conservative treatment of appendicular mass.

Q 22. What is Alvarado score?

It is a clinical and laboratory based scoring system devised to assist the diagnosis of acute appendicitis. A score of 7 or more is strongly predictive of acute appendicitis. A score of 5–6 is considered equivocal and needs contrast enhanced CT examination to reduce the rate of negative appendicectomy. In Alvarado score, points are given for 3 symptoms, 3 signs, 2 laboratory findings. The mnemonic for Alvarado score is—MANTRELS—migratory pain, anorexia, nausea/vomiting, tenderness, rebound tenderness, elevated temperature, leukocytosis, shift to the left.

Alvarado score	Score
Symptoms	
• Migratory RIF pain	1
• Anorexia	1
• Nausea and vomiting	1
Signs	
• Tenderness (RIF)	2
• Rebound tenderness	1
• Elevated temperature	1
Laboratory	
• Leukocytosis	2
• Shift to left (increase in the number of immature neutrophils) or banded forms	1
	Total score 10

Q 23. What is the acceptable negative appendicectomy rate?

- It should ideally be less than 20% (with the introduction of CT for the diagnosis of acute appendicitis the negative appendicectomy rate should be less than 5%)
- If the rate is more it means we are over doing it
- If the rate is very less it means we are too much waiting, so that perforation will occur.

Q 24. In the course of an operation for presumed acute appendicitis, the appendix is found to be engulfed in a mass of uncertain etiology. How to proceed?

The safe approach is a segmental intestinal resection with primary ileocolonic anastomosis. Whether a limited resection through the same incision or to have a formal right colectomy depends on the likelihood of malignancy.

Q 25. What are the differential diagnoses of right iliac fossa pain of acute onset? (Fig. 11.1)

The Attic (the nasopharynx and thorax)

- Tonsillitis in children (swallowed exudate causes tonsil tummy)
- Lobar pneumonia and pleurisy.

Upper storey (diaphragm to the level of the umbilicus):

- Perforated peptic ulcer (the visceral content passing along the paracolic gutter to the right iliac fossa)
- Acute pancreatitis
- Acute cholecystitis
- Leaking aortic aneurysm
- Cyclical vomiting in children
- Ruptured liver abscess.

The ground floor (umbilicus to the brim of pelvis):

- Nonspecific mesenteric lymphadenitis
- Meckel's diverticulitis
- Gastroenteritis
- Enterocolitis
- Intestinal obstruction
- Intussusception
- Carcinoma of the cecum
- Diverticulitis
- Torsion of appendix epiploicae
- Mesenteric infarction
- Leaking aortic aneurysm
- Regional ileitis
- Diverticulum of cecum (solitary)
- Rectus sheath hematoma.

The basement (the pelvis):

- Pelvic inflammatory disease
- Salpingitis
- Ectopic gestation
- Ruptured ovarian follicle (mittelschmerz)

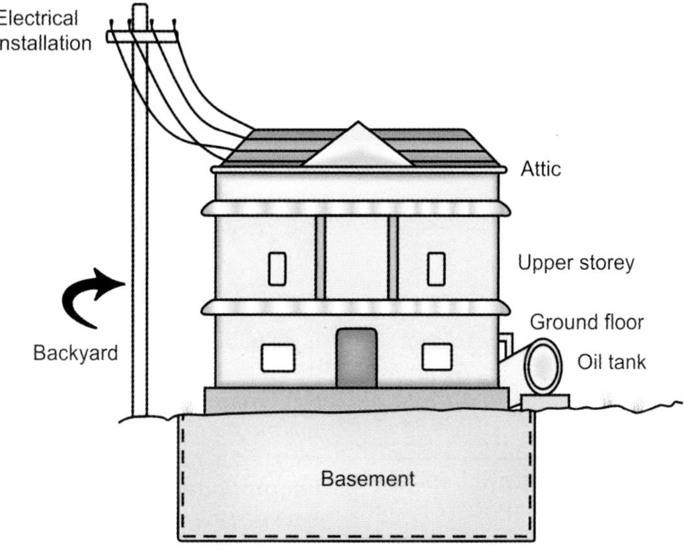

Fig. 11.1: Appendicitis building

- Twisted right ovarian cyst
- Endometriosis.

The backyard (the retroperitoneal structures):
- Right ureteric colic
- Right sided acute pyelonephritis.

The electrical installation ***(****central nervous system****)***
- Preherpetic pain of the right tenth and eleventh dorsal nerves
- Tabetic crisis
- Spinal conditions
  - Pott's disease of the spine,
  - Secondary carcinomatous deposits
  - Senile osteoporosis
  - Multiple myeloma.

Fuel supply (blood)
- Henoch-Schönlein purpura
- Blood dyscrasias
- Use of anticoagulants.

Other conditions:
- Abdominal crisis of porphyria
- Diabetic abdomen
- Leukemic ileocecal syndrome
- Clostridial septicemia.

Case

12 Obstructive Jaundice

"Jaundice is the disease that your friends diagnose"

Sir William Osler (1849–1919)

Case Capsule

A **68-year-old male patient** presents with **epigastric discomfort, anorexia and weight loss** of 6 months duration. Initially these complaints were dismissed by his doctor. Later he noticed **yellow discoloration** of **urine and conjunctiva** for the last two months. The jaundice is **painless and progressive**. There is no history of **waxing and waning of symptoms**. At present he complaints of **generalized itching** for the last 1 month. He passes **clay-colored stools** for the last two months. He is a **recently detected diabetic**. He is a **heavy smoker** for the last 50 years. On examination he is ill **built and cachexic**. The **sclera is yellow orange** in color (deeply jaundiced). **Scratch marks are seen** in the abdomen and chest. Abdominal examination revealed a **globular mass** below the costal margin in the midclavicular line impinging upon the examining hand on inspiration of about **10 × 4 cm** size. The **mass is visible** and moving up and down with respiration. This mass is **better seen than felt** and better **palpated by superficial palpation** than deep palpation. The **liver is palpable** about 4 cm below the costal margin. It is firm in consistency, the edges are sharp and the surface is smooth. There is no other palpable mass in the abdomen. There is no free fluid. Digital rectal examination is normal. There is a **hard mobile lymph node in the left supraclavicular area** between the two heads of sternomastoid muscle.

Read the checklist for abdominal examination

Checklist for history

- *Family history of jaundice*: Gilbert's familial nonhemolytic hyperbilirubinemia, Crigler-Najjar's familial nonhemolytic jaundice, Dubin-Johnson's familial conjugated hyperbilirubinemia
- History of *cigarette smoking:* Carcinoma pancreas
- History of *alcoholism*: Acute alcoholic jaundice
- High dietary *consumption of meat*: Carcinoma pancreas
- History of *transfusion*: Hepatitis B
- History of *omphalitis*: Infection of umbilicus → incomplete obliteration of umbilical vein → jaundice
- *History of drugs*: Chlorpromazine, Methyl testosterone, etc.
- History of *injections*, drug abuse, tattoos (hepatitis B)
- Past history of *biliary surgery* (postoperative stricture)

Contd...

Contd...

- Family history of jaundice with anemia (*hemolysis*) – Hereditary spherocytosis
- *Back pain*: 25% of patients with carcinoma pancreas (relief of pain in sitting position)
- Whitish *clay-colored stools*: Suggestive of obstructive jaundice
- *Melena*: Periampullary carcinoma (silver paint stool)
- *Waxing and waning* of jaundice: Suggestive of CBD stone and periampullary carcinoma
- *Diabetes mellitus*: Early manifestation of 25% of carcinoma pancreas
- *Charcot's triad*: Intermittent jaundice, pain and intermittent fever.

Checklist for examination of a case of obstructive jaundice

- *Examination in daylight* for yellow discoloration—sclera, skin, nails bed, posterior part of the hard palate, under surface of the tongue
- Look for *presence of scratch mark* in the lower limbs, chest and abdomen—accumulation of bile salt
- Look for *migratory thrombophlebitis* (Trousseau's sign seen in carcinoma pancreas
- Look for *spleen* (hereditary spherocytosis)
- Look for *stigmata of liver disease*—liver palms, spider angioma, ascites, collateral veins on the abdomen and splenomegaly
- Look for a *distended gallbladder* → Courvoisier's law
- Gallbladder is *better seen than felt*. Better palpated by superficial palpation than by deep palpation
- Look for *ascites*
- Look for *leg ulcers*—Hereditary spherocytosis, sickle cell disease
- Look for left *supraclavicular nodes*
- Rectal examination—*rectal shelf* of Blumer, presence of primary growth, color of stool, and blood stained finger stall.

Q 1. What are the physical findings of an enlarged gallbladder?

Physical findings of an enlarged gallbladder

- It is better seen than felt
- It is better felt by superficial palpation than deep palpation
- It appears from beneath the tip of the ninth rib on the right side
- It is ovoid and smooth and moves with respiration
- It is dull to percussion
- You cannot feel a space between the lump and the edge of the liver.

Q 2. What are your points in favor of obstructive jaundice?

- It is a painless progressive jaundice
- Presence of itching and scratch marks
- Presence of palpable gallbladder
- Loss of weight.

Q 3. What is the definition of jaundice?

Jaundice is yellow staining of body tissues produced by an excess of circulating bilirubin. Normal serum concentration is **5–19 mmol/L** (**0.2–1.2 mg/dL**) Jaundice is detected clinically when the level rises above **40 mmol/L** (**2.5 mg/dL**).

Q 4. How bilirubin is formed and how is bile pigments metabolized?

Bilirubin is formed from *hem,* a compound of iron and protoporphyrin and about 85% of that produced daily comes from the breakdown of hem from mature RBC's in the reticuloendothelial system. 15% is derived from heme compounds in liver and bone marrow. This bilirubin is **unconjugated** (which is **insoluble** in water) and transported attached to the plasma proteins to the liver cells. In liver, conjugation occurs and the conjugated bilirubin is called **bilirubin glucuronide** (which is *water-soluble)* and transported to the bile ducts. Disturbance to the flow of bile leads to stagnation and retention of conjugated bilirubin. Therefore, in hemolytic anemia, liver is overloaded with unconjugated bilirubin produced from excessive breakdown of hem; hence the **rise in indirect bilirubin** in **prehepatic and hepatic jaundice**. In obstructive jaundice, the conjugated bilirubin is raised (*direct*). Bacterial deconjugation of bilirubin occurs in the colon to form **stercobilinogen**. Part of this stercobilinogen is absorbed into the circulation and re-excreted by the liver and kidneys (**urobilinogen**). This stercobilinogen is partly converted to **stercobilin** and excreted in the feces (Fig. 12.1).

Q 5. What are the types of jaundice?

Jaundice is classified as:

A.
- Prehepatic (hemolytic)
- Hepatic
- Posthepatic (obstructive).

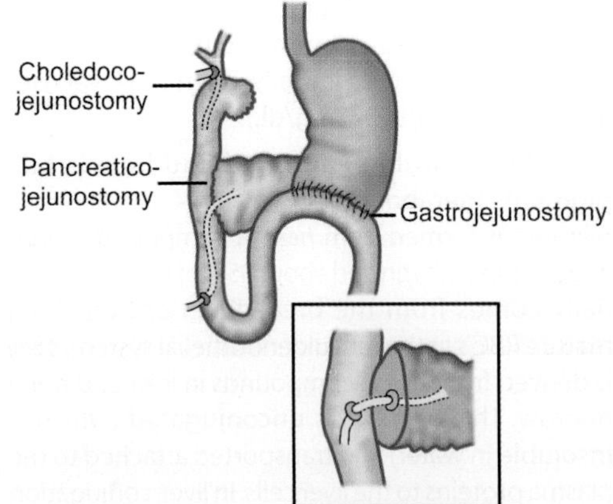

Fig. 12.1: Bile pigment metabolism

B.
- Intermittent
- Continuous
- Progressive.

C.
- Painful jaundice
- Painless jaundice.

Q 6. Can you differentiate the types clinically by the color of jaundice?

Lemon yellow – Hemolytic jaundice
Orange – Hepatocellular jaundice
Deep and greenish – Obstructive jaundice

Q 7. Clinically what are the other differentiating features of various jaundice?

Clinical features of various types of jaundice

Disease	*Symptoms*	*Pain*	*Jaundice*
Hemolytic	General malaise, loss of weight	No pain	Slow onset and jaundice persists
Infective hepatitis	Loss of appetite, nausea, malaise	Dull ache	Gradual onset and disappearance
Gallstone	Episodes of flatulent dyspepsia	Intermittent severe pain	Sudden onset, fades slowly in days
Carcinoma head of pancreas	Loss of weight, loss of appetite, itching	Backache	Progressive jaundice

Q 8. What are the causes for each type of jaundice?

Causes for prehepatic, hepatic and posthepatic jaundice		
Prehepatic (hemolytic)	*Hepatic*	*Posthepatic (obstructive)*
• Hereditary spherocytosis • Hereditary nonspherocytic anemia • Sickle cell disease • Thalassemia • Acquired hemolytic anemia • Hypersplenism • Crigler-Najjar syndrome* • Gilbert's disease*	*Hepatocellular*—Acute viral hepatitis, alcoholic cirrhosis Dubin Johnson syndrome** *Cholestatic*—Toxic drugs, cholestatic jaundice of pregnancy, postoperative cholestatic jaundice, biliary cirrhosis	*In the lumen*— • Gallstone • Parasites (hydatid, liver fluke roundworms) • Foreign body—broken T tube • Hemobilia • Benign stricture • Malignant stricture *In the wall*— • Congenital atresia • Traumatic strictures • Choledochal cyst • Caroli's disease • Tumors of bile duct • Klatskin's tumor • Sclerosing cholangitis *Outside the wall*— • Carcinoma head of pancreas • Periampullary carcinoma • Porta hepatis metastasis • Pancreatitis • Chronic duodenal diverticulum • Pseudocyst of pancreas • Metastatic carcinoma

***Crigler-Najjar and Gilbert's** disease are due to defective uptake and conjugation of bilirubin and therefore the hyperbilirubinemia is of the **unconjugated type.** They are differential diagnoses for hemolytic jaundice.

****Dubin Johnson's familial conjugated hyperbilirubinemia** is a condition where the hepatic excretion of conjugated bilirubin into the biliary system is impaired and therefore a differential diagnosis for obstructive jaundice (Fig. 12.2).

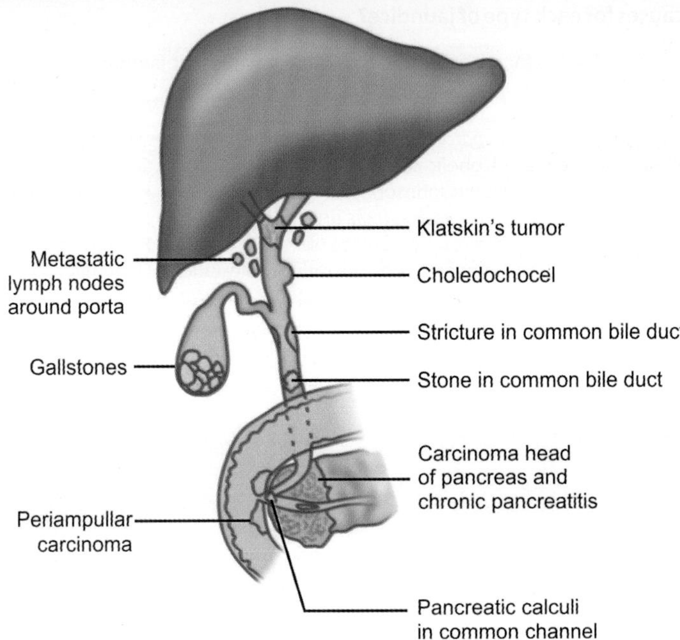

Fig. 12.2: Common causes of obstructive jaundice

Q 9. What is the problem of this classification?

Obstruction can occur without any evidence of a lesion requiring surgical correction, e.g. intrahepatic cholestasis due to drugs and early primary biliary cirrhosis. A patient with viral hepatitis may have considerable cholestasis suggesting obstruction. A patient with obstructive jaundice may go on to develop a degree of hepatocyte insufficiency too. **Hence, the classification has considerable overlapping.**

Q 10. How to differentiate the types of jaundice biochemically?

There are two types of bilirubin—**conjugated** (direct) and **unconjugated** (indirect).

The direct bilirubin is increased in obstructive jaundice whereas the indirect bilirubin is increased in hemolytic jaundice. **In obstructive jaundice** conjugated bilirubin from the hepatocytes and biliary radicles overflow into the bloodstream, whereas in **hemolytic jaundice**, unconjugated bilirubin overloads the liver and is detected as elevated in blood.

- The serum bilirubin level rarely exceeds 4–5 mg/dL in hemolytic jaundice.
- The bilirubin exceed to **10–20 mg/dL in obstruction due to neoplasm.**
- In obstruction due to stones usually it ranges **up to 5 mg,** rarely does it exceed 15 mg.

Q 11. What is the role of liver enzymes in the diagnosis of jaundice?

The two most important enzymes are ALT, AST and alkaline phosphatase (ALP).

- ALT above 1000 is suggestive of viral hepatitis
- In alcoholic liver disease AST is raised (AST : ALT is >2)
- Alkaline phosphatase is raised in **obstructive jaundice and infiltrative liver diseases like tumor or granuloma.**

Note: Normal values: ALT: 5 – 35 U/L
AST: 5 – 40 U/L

Q 12. What are the sources of alkaline phosphatase and what are the conditions in which the enzyme is increased?

There are three sources for alkaline phosphatase

1. Liver } Equal contribution
2. Bone }
3. Intestine—Small contribution
   - In the liver, it is a product of epithelial cells of the cholangioles
   - **It is expressed in Bodansky units (previously KA units)**

Note: Normal value: 30 – 115 U/L.

Clinical conditions in which alkaline phosphatase is increased
• Intrahepatic cholestasis • Cholangitis • Extrahepatic obstruction • Focal hepatic lesions without jaundice • Solitary metastases • Pyogenic abscess • Granulomas • Bone tumors (primary and secondary).

Q 13. How to rule out alkaline phosphatase rise because of bone pathology? (PG)

- Serum calcium and phosphorus (which will be abnormal in bony pathology)
- **5′nucleotidase** and **γ-glutamyl transpeptidase** which are specific for obstructive jaundice.

Q 14. What is acholuric jaundice?

It is nothing but the result of **hereditary spherocytosis.** It is called acholuric because there is no excretion of bilirubin in the urine. In this condition, because of the hemolysis as a result of spherocytosis, the bilirubin produced is insoluble (unconjugated). This is not filtered by glomerulus. There will be **family history of jaundice.** In addition you get—

- Pigmented stones in gallbladder
- Enlarged spleen
- Leg ulcers.

It produces *hemolytic crisis*—

- Pyrexia
- Abdominal pain
- Nausea and vomiting
- Extreme pallor.

The fragility of the RBC's will be increased because of the biconvex nature of the RBC in contrast to the normal biconcave.

Q 15. What are the investigations for hemolytic jaundice?

Investigations for hemolytic jaundice
1. Peripheral smear for spherocytosis 2. Osmotic fragility test for red cells (which will be increased). 3. Reticulocyte count which will be increased (compensatory hemopoesis) 4. Positive *Coombs' test.*

Q 16. What is surgical jaundice?

Surgical jaundice is a condition where the jaundice can be corrected by surgery. The posthepatic jaundice is mainly included in this category. Hemolytic conditions like hereditary spherocytosis require splenectomy as part of the treatment, but are not referred to commonly as surgical jaundice.

Q 17. Any other classification for surgical jaundice?

- Complete jaundice – Carcinoma head of pancreas
- Intermittent jaundice – Periampullary carcinoma
- Chronic and incomplete – Biliary stricture
- Segmental – Traumatic

Q 18. What is Courvoisier's law?

Courvoisier first drew attention to the association of an enlarged gallbladder and a pancreatic tumor in 1890 and this law states.

"When the gallbladder is palpable and the patient is jaundiced, the obstruction of bile duct causing the jaundice is unlikely to be a stone because previous inflammation will have made the gallbladder thick and nondistensible."

- But he never said when the gallbladder is not palpable, it is due to stones (that is, the converse – jaundice without palpable gallbladder certainly does not implicate stones).
- Gallbladder is palpable only in 30% of cases of carcinoma head of the pancreas.
- **There are exceptions to Courvoisier's law**

Exceptions to Courvoisier's law

1. Stones, simultaneously occluding the cystic duct and the distal CBD (Double impaction)
2. Pancreatic calculus obstructing the ampulla

Contd...

Contd...

3. Oriental cholangiohepatitis because of Clonorchis sinensis (Ductal stones formed secondary to the liver fluke infestation)
4. Mucocele/empyema of gallbladder
5. Carcinoma of the gallbladder with or without jaundice—it's although rare it can also cause a palpable gallbladder (In 1 to 4 the gallbladder is palpable in a jaundiced patient with stones)
6. Nodes in porta hepatis
7. Carcinoma gallbladder with multiple metastases in liver.

Q 19. What is oriental cholangiohepatitis?

It is because of Clonorchis sinensis (**Chinese liver fluke**) and in this condition, stones are formed primarily in the bile ducts and therefore the **gallbladder is often palpable**.

Q 20. What is choledochal cyst?

It is a dilation or diverticula of all or a portion of the common bile duct. Women are more affected than men and Asians are more affected than Western people. The incidence is very high in Japan. Various causes are postulated:

- Infectious agents
- Reflux of pancreatic enzymes via long common channel
- Genetic
- Autonomic dysfunction.

Q 21. What are the types of choledochal cysts? (PG)

Types of choledochal cyst

Type 1 –	Fusiform (85%)
Type 2 –	Saccular
Type 3 –	Choledochocele (wide mouth dilatation of the common bile duct at its confluence with duodenum)
Type 4 –	Cystic dilatation of both intra and extra-hepatic bile duct
Type 5 –	Lakes of multiple intrahepatic cysts (Type 5 along with hepatic fibrosis is called Caroli's disease).

Alonso-Lej/Todani classification of choledochal cyst	
Type I	Classic cyst type characterized by cystic dilatation of CBD. Most common (50–85%) IA (Cystic); IB (Fusiform); IC (Saccular)
Type II	Simple diverticulum of extrahepatic biliary tree; located proximal to the duodenum (5%)
Type III	Cystic dilatation of the intraduodinal portion of the extrahepatic CBD also known as choledochocele (5%)
Type IV	Involve multiple cysts of intrahepatic and extrahepatic biliary tree
Type IV A	Both intrahepatic and extrahepatic cysts (30–40%)
Type IV B	Multiple extrahepatic cysts without intrahepatic involvement
Type V	Isolated intrahepatic biliary cystic disease (Caroli's disease) associated with periportal fibrosis or cirrhosis; can be multilobar or confined to a single lobe.

Q 22. What is the treatment of choledochal cyst? (PG)

There is increased chance for malignancy, if part of cyst is left behind. Therefore, **complete excision followed by hepaticojejunostomy** is the treatment of choice.

Q 23. What is Caroli's disease? (PG)

It is a congenital cystic disease having saccular intra-hepatic dilatation of the ducts. It may be isolated or associated with:

- **Congenital hepatic fibrosis**
- **Medullary sponge kidney**

It may manifest as cholangitis or obstructive jaundice.

Q 24. What is hemobilia? (PG)

It is a complication of hepatic **trauma** as a result of bleeding from intrahepatic branch of the hepatic artery into a duct. The **triad of hemobilia** (**Sandblom's** triad) consists of

- Biliary colic
- Obstructive jaundice
- Occult/gross intestinal bleeding.

Causes for hemobilia

- Trauma
- Oriental cholangiohepatitis
- Hepatic neoplasm
- Rupture of hepatic artery aneurysm
- Hepatic abscess
- Choledocholithiasis.

The diagnosis is by Technicum 99m labeled RBC scan and arteriogram.

Q 25. What is the treatment of hemobilia? (PG)

Therapeutic embolization using:

- Stainless steel coils
- Gel foam
- Autologous blood clot.

Q 26. What are the causes for intermittent jaundice?

1. CBD stones
2. Periampullary carcinoma
3. Repeated hemolytic episode
4. Parasite
5. Hemobilia
6. Duodenal diverticula.

Q 27. What are the symptoms of a patient with carcinoma head of pancreas?

- **Progressive jaundice 75%** (it is possible to get carcinoma head of the pancreas without obstructive jaundice).
- **Pain**: Pain is frequent even though classical description is painless.
- **Hematemesis and melena** in late cases.
- **Chills and fever** when there is cholangitis.
- **Diabetes mellitus:** Carcinoma pancreas induces glucose intolerance resulting in diabetes mellitus (25% of patients).
- **Courvoisier sign**: Palpable gallbladder noted only in 25% of patients with resectable lesions.

Q 28. How will you proceed to investigate the given case of jaundice?

A. *Investigations for diagnosis and staging are* (Flow chart 12.1):
   1. *Ultrasound* examination—look for intrahepatic biliary radicle dilatation
      - Size of the CBD normally should be less than 8 mm sonologically
      - Dilatation of pancreatic duct (dilatation of CBD and pancreatic duct is suggestive of carcinoma head of the pancreas)
      - For biliary stones
      - For free fluid
      - For mass lesions (difficult to identify pancreatic head malignancy in ultrasound because of the gas in intestines in front of the organ)
      - For liver metastases.
   2. *Contrast enhanced helical CT*
      - Can identify the tumor in the head of pancreas (**Central zone of decreased**

Flow chart 12.1: Management of pancreatic cancer

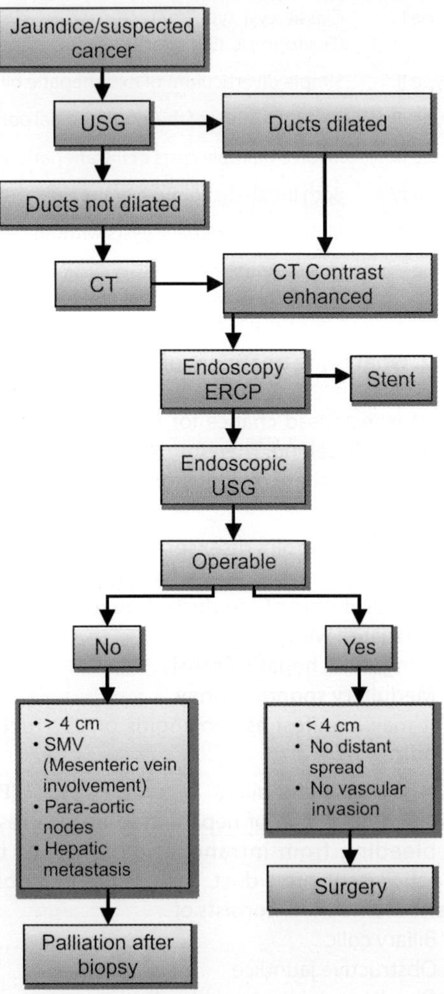

attenuation will be present). Pancreatic duct and bile duct dilatations are strong evidence of pancreatic carcinoma
   - Note the size of the tumor
   - Infiltration to the adjacent structures like portal vein
   - Nodal involvement.
3. *Endoscopy/ERCP (Endoscopic retrograde cholangiopancreatography)—useful for non dilated ducts*—in the absence of mass in the CT, ERCP is indicated. It is the most sensitive test for such situations.
   - The periampullary carcinoma can be visualized
   - Biopsy can be taken from the periampullary lesion
   - The lower limit of the growth can be identified by ERCP
   - Stenting can be done to relieve the jaundice
   - Sphincterotomy can be done to remove the bile duct stone.
4. *Endoscopic ultrasound*
   - To assess the operability
   - Size of the tumor
   - To know the involvement of mesenteric lymph nodes, para-aorticnodes and superior mesenteric vein
   - Hepatic metastases.
5. *Percutaneous transhepatic cholangiography (PTC)—useful for dilated ductal system.*
   - The coagulation profile is checked and antibiotic coverage is given. In this procedure a pliable needle is inserted under local anesthetic and sonological guidance into the dilated biliary duct. Should **decompression of the biliary tree** be desired preoperatively, then a fine bore catheter may be left in the ducts to allow continuous drainage of bile.
   - It is also possible to insert an endoprosthesis to relieve the obstruction for unresectable lesions.
   - The PTC is ideal for demonstrating the anatomy above an extrahepatic obstruction and the **upper limit of the obstructing lesion** can be identified by injecting dye.
6. *Upper GI series*—to decide whether a gastrojejunostomy is indicated or not. The classical findings are (largely replaced by Helical CT).
   - Widening of the C-loop of the duodenum in carcinoma head of the pancreas.
   - Reverse 3 sign in periampullary carcinoma.

B. *Biochemical investigations*
   - **Total bilirubin**, direct and indirect (direct is increased obstructive and indirect is increased in hemolytic jaundice (total and direct bilirubin raised in hepatic).
   - **Alkaline phosphatase**—(over 100 international unit is indicative of cholestasis if bone disease is absent).
   - **Total protein, albumin and globulin** (albumin and globulin levels are reversed in chronic hepatocellular damage). Globulin level will be very high in biliary cirrhosis. In biliary obstruction *per se* there won't be any change in the values.
   - **Serum transaminase** levels are above normal in viral hepatitis.

C. *Coagulation profile—Prothrombin Time*—normal in hemolytic jaundice. Prolonged but correctable with vitamin K in cholestatic jaundice (provided their remains some functioning liver tissue). This will be prolonged and not correctable in advanced hepatocellular disease.

- **Platelet count, bleeding time and clotting time.**

D. *Urine examination*

1. **Absent urobilinogen** indicates obstruction to the common bile ducts.
2. **Excess urobilinogen** occurs in hemolytic jaundice and sometimes in liver damage.
3. **Absent bilirubin** indicates hemolytic jaundice (Bilirubin predominantly unconjugated).
4. **Excess bilirubin** is present in obstructive jaundice.

E. *Stool examination*

1. Absence of bile pigment indicates biliary obstruction (**Clay-colored stool**).
2. Positive occult blood indicates ampullary carcinoma, bleeding esophageal varices and alimentary carcinoma.

Q 29. What is the dose of vitamin K and how is it given?

The dose of vitamin K is 10 mg and it is given IM for 3 days.

The vitamin K_1 (phytomenadione) is given intravenously—10 mg daily for 3 days.

Q 30. What are the preoperative preparations if you are planning for surgery?

1. Hydration
2. Nutrition
3. Correction of coagulation deficiency—vitamin K, FFP, platelet transfusion, etc.
4. Correction of anemia.

Q 31. What are the indications for preoperative biliary decompression? (PG)

Indications for preoperative biliary decompression

- Bilirubin > 12 mg
- Sepsis
- Hepatorenal failure
- Severe cardiopulmonary disease
- Severe malnutrition.

NB: Routine drainage is not recommended.

Q 32. What is the other simple option for drainage?

Simple cholecystostomy, if other options are not available.

Q 33. What are the causes for fever in jaundice?

Causes for fever in jaundice	
1. Cholangitis	2. Hemolysis
3. Septicemia	4. Hepatic abscess

Q 34. What are the 3 important special risks in obstructive jaundice? (PG)

1. Hypocoagulability
2. Renal failure—may be because of increased bile pigment load on the tubules, increased postoperative distal tubular reabsorption of water and failure of liver to trap enteric nephrotoxins
3. Sepsis of bile with or without calculi.

Q 35. What are the signs of unresectability in carcinoma head of the pancreas?

1. Hepatic metastases
2. Distant metastases (Distant lymph nodes from pancreatic head)
3. Ascites (Peritoneal metastases)
4. Encasement of superior mesenteric, hepatic or celiac artery by tumor.

Note: Nowadays the superior mesenteric artery is approached from behind as the first step before contemplating Wipple's resection and if the artery is involved resection is abandoned.

Q 36. Should portal vein involvement preclude a resection? (PG)

Involvement of a short segment (< *1.5 cm*) of portal vein is not a contraindication to a curative resection.

Q 37. What is the treatment of itching because of obstructive jaundice? (PG)

a. Cholestyramine—It is an ion exchange resin, usually provides relief by binding bile salts in the intestinal lumen, thus, inhibiting their reabsorption into blood.

b. Opiates.

Q 38. What is the role of percutaneous biopsy (Aspiration) of pancreatic tumor? (PG)

- It is done under ultrasound/CT guidance
- It is contraindicated in candidates for surgery—risk of spreading
- Done in patients with radiographic evidence of unresectability
- It is also done preoperatively in operable cases
- Biopsy may miss the lesion because a variable area of pancreatitis surround the tumor, leading to sampling error.

Q 39. What are the complications of needle biopsy of pancreatic tumor? (PG)

- Pancreatitis
- Fistula
- Hemorrhage
- Infection.

Q 40. What is the tumor marker for pancreatic malignancy? (PG)

- CA 19-9 (**Carbohydrate antigen**)—It is useful in following the results of the treatment
- CEA (**Carcinoembryonic antigen**).

Q 41. Perioperatively can you differentiate chronic pancreatitis from carcinoma? (PG)

- It is very difficult.
- A hard noncystic mass in the head and obstructive jaundice and dilatation of CBD is more in favor of carcinoma.
- A hard noncystic mass in the retroampullary part and no jaundice and no dilatation is in favor of chronic pancreatitis.

Q 42. What are the signs of inoperability in carcinoma head of pancreas?

Signs of inoperability in carcinoma head of pancreas

Clinically

- Supraclavicular nodes
- Ascites
- Rectal shelf of Blumer
- Liver metastases, etc.

Preoperatively

- Ascites
- Liver metastases
- Peritoneal metastases
- Rectal shelf of Blumer
- Involvement of the portal vein and superior mesenteric vessels (preoperatively assess the resectability after Kocherizing the duodenum and passing the surgeon's finger between the pancreas and the portal vein) – *"Tunnel of love"*.

Q 43. What are the surgical options for the operable carcinoma head of the pancreas?

1. The classical **Whipple's** procedure (pancreaticoduodenectomy followed by pancreaticojejunostomy/gastrostomy, choledochojejunostomy and gastrojejunostomy) (Fig. 12.3).

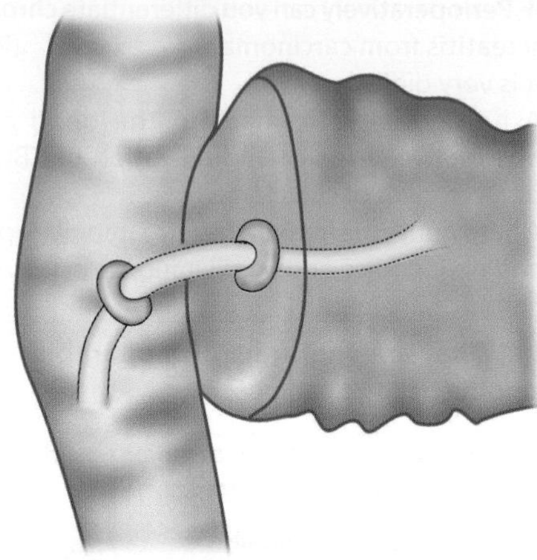

Fig. 12.3: View of pancreaticojejunostomy

2. Pylorus preserving pancreaticoduodenectomy (*PPPD*).

The second procedure is favored nowadays.

Note: Currently the pancreatic head is accessed from behind to see invasion of mesenteric artery as the first step and if it is found to be involved, it is considered inoperable.

Q 44. What is the morbidity and mortality of this procedure? (PG)

Mortality is 3 – 5% in high volume center

Morbidity is around—40%—**pancreatic leak**—*10%*—infection.

Q 45. What are the surgical options for inoperable cases?

To relieve jaundice

1. After ruling out a **low insertion of cystic duct**, a cholecystojejunostomy is done to relieve the jaundice. This may be combined with a jejunojejunostomy.
2. If there is low insertion of cystic duct, a choledochojejunostomy is done to relieve the obstruction.

Relieve duodenal obstruction

1. If duodenal obstruction (15% of cases) is suspected in addition, a **gastrojejunostomy** is done.
2. **Self-expanding metal stent** placed endoscopically, is an alternative to gastrojejunostomy.

Q 46. What is the management of pain in inoperable cases?

Transthoracic splanchnicectomy (dividing the splanchnic nerve transthoracically preferably through thoracoscope).

Q 47. What percentage of pancreatic head malignancy is resectable?

At the time of presentation 90% are unsuitable for resection because of local spread to the superior mesenteric vein, para-aortic and mesenteric nodes and liver metastases.

Q 48. What is the role of chemotherapy in pancreatic cancer?

Chemotherapeutic agent of choice is 5 fluorouracil (5FU)

- A new drug **Gemcitabine** produces remission in 15 – 25% of patients.

Q 49. What is the prognosis of carcinoma head of the pancreas?

- The overall median survival is only 20 weeks
- Less than 3% of patients survive for 5 years
- In carcinoma of the ampulla of Vater, the 5 years survival after resection is 40%.

OBSTRUCTIVE JAUNDICE DUE TO STONES

Q 50. What are the manifestations of CBD stones?

The classical presentation is **Charcot's triad** consisting of:

- Intermittent pain
- Intermittent fever
- Intermittent jaundice.

Q 51. What is cholangitis?

Obstruction of bile duct will lead on to bacterial infection of the bile duct. Obstruction is synonymous with infection. The obstruction may be partial or complete. **The causes for cholangitis are—**

- Choledocholithiasis
- Biliary stricture
- Neoplasms (15%)
- Ampullary stenosis (less common)
- Chronic pancreatitis
- Pseudocyst
- Duodenal diverticulum
- Parasitic.

Q 52. What is the pathology of cholangitis ? (PG)

- The ductal pressure increases when there is obstruction
- Bacteria escape to the systemic circulation via hepatic sinusoids
- Organism will reach the blood and blood culture will positive.

Q 53. What are the common organisms for cholangitis ? (PG)

Organisms causing cholangitis
• *E. Coli*
• *Klebsiella*
• *Pseudomonas*
• Enterococci
• *Proteus*
• Bacteroides.

Q 54. What is Reynold's pentad?

It is a manifestation of **acute toxic cholangitis** as a result of obstruction of the bile duct (It is also called **suppurative cholangitis**). It is a life-threatening condition and should be managed as emergency. The Pentad consists of:

- Pain
- Fever
- Jaundice
- Mental confusion
- Shock.

Q 55. What is the management of acute toxic cholangitis? (PG)

It is an emergency. The antibiotic of choice is aminoglycoside and clindamycin/metronidazole. The ductal system is decompressed by **emergency sphincterotomy** or by transhepatic drainage. The associated gallbladder pathology may be tackled as an elective procedure later by laparoscopic cholecystectomy.

Q 56. What is the management of obstructive jaundice due to CBD stone?

The investigations and preparations are the same as for obstructive jaundice. (which is given above). There are 3 surgical options:

1. **Endoscopic sphincterotomy** initially, followed by **laparoscopic cholecystectomy** preferably in the same admission. (currently favored where laparoscopic expertise is not available).
2. **Laparoscopic cholecystectomy** and **laparoscopic CBD exploration** (if expertise is available); the CBD exploration may be done through the cystic duct or if the duct is more than 1.5 cm through a choledochotomy.
3. **Open**—Laparotomy, cholecystectomy and CBD exploration and stone removal.

Q 57. What are the contraindications for sphincterotomy?

- Stone size more than 2 cm.
- Stenosis of bile duct proximal to the sphincter.

Q 58. What is the management of bile duct tumor? (PG)

The bile duct tumors may be benign or malignant. The benign tumors are rare and far less common. The malignant tumors are called cholangiocarcinomas. **Cholangiocarcinoma is a term now applied to malignant intrahepatic, perihilar and distal extra hepatic tumors of the bile ducts.** The incidence of this condition is rising. The management may be **palliative stenting** or **surgery**. Most patients will receive only palliative surgery. **The consensus of surgical opinion is that the surgical treatment is difficult and should be reserved for the fittest patients** getting 5 mm clearance, node and liver resection if required. In all cases, reconstruction is made using **hepaticojejunostomy** (Roux–en–Y). On the right side an extended right **hepatic lobectomy** is done because of anatomical reasons. The length of right hepatic duct is smaller in contrast to the left which has got significant length of extrahepatic duct.

Q 59. What are the risk factors for cholangiocarcinoma? (PG)

These include:

Risk factors for cholangiocarcinoma

- Sclerosing cholangitis
- Chronic intrahepatic gallstones
- Caroli's disease
- Choledochal cyst
- Ulcerative colitis
- Liver flukes.

Possible association:

- INH (Inhibitor)
- Methyldopa
- Oral contraceptives
- Asbestos.

Q 60. What is Klatskin tumor? (PG)

The perihilar cholangiocarcinoma is called Klatskin tumor. About 50% of all cholangiocarcinomas are Klatskin tumor. Of the reminder, half are intrahepatic and half are related to extrahepatic bile ducts.

Q 61. Is there any role for fine needle aspiration cytology? (PG)

Percutaneous fine needle aspiration cytology is absolutely contraindicated in patients who may be operable.

Q 62. What is the Bismuth classification of cholangiocarcinoma? (PG)

Type I – involving the **common hepatic duct.**

Type II – the growth involving the **proximal common hepatic** duct that **extends to the bifurcation**, but both hepatic ducts are free.

Type III – growth involving one **hepatic duct.**

Type IV – is the **hilar** involving both hepatic and proximal common hepatic ducts.

Q 63. What are the contraindications for surgery? (PG)

- Lymph node involvement
- Encasement of hepatic hilar vessels.

Q 64. What is Taj Mahal resection? (PG)

The technique of central liver resection for cholangiocarcinoma is called Taj Mahal resection owing to the shape of the defect in the liver. This involves removal of segments **1, 4 and 5** and the **relevant bile ducts.**

Q 65. What is the palliative surgical treatment? (PG)

Palliative surgical drainage is done by anastomosing a Roux loop to the segment III duct.

Q 66. Is there any role for surgery in hereditary spherocytosis?

- Splenectomy is done
- Gallbladder stones, if present are managed by cholecystectomy.

Q 67. What type of gallstone you get in hereditary spherocytosis?

Pigment stone.

FOR PG'S—WHAT IS NEW?

- The imaging modality of choice for pancreatic malignancy is MDCT (Multi Detector Computed Tomography) and angiography, MRI and MRCP
- Tumor marker CA 19-9 is measured routinely in pancreatic carcinomas and levels greater than 1000 units/mL have been found to be linked to unresectable disease
- PTC—is an investigation done for proximal biliary obstruction and not routine
- There is no role for mannitol in the preoperative preparation of obstructive jaundice patient. In fact, it will worsen the renal function
- Uncinate—First approach for pancreaticoduodenectomy—this approach is suitable for infiltration of the superior mesenteric vein or portal vein. It is also suitable for infiltration of the arterial axis
- SMA—First approach for pancreaticoduodenectomy—It comprises early dissection of superior mesenteric artery after kocherization of the duodenum along with the posterior pancreatic capsule. The advantage of this technique is that the tumor infiltration of SMV, portal vein, or tumor proximity to SMA can be handled at the initial stage or resection can be abandoned. This will reduce the chances of margin positive pancreatic head resection. It will also help improved lymph node yield
- The indications for preoperative biliary drainage are:- 1. Acute cholangitis (systemic sepsis of biliary origin is called cholangitis), 2. Obstructive jaundice with secondary renal impairment, 3. Comorbidities delaying the surgery
- Classic Whipple's operation is reserved for duodenal cancers
- Removal of lymph nodes of the right side of the hepatoduodenal ligament, posterior pancreaticoduodenal nodes, nodes to the right side of the superior mesenteric artery from the origin to the inferior pancreaticoduodenal artery are important
- Neoadjuvant chemotherapy is beneficial
- For pancreatic leak irradiation of pancreas is useful
- R1 cases needs postoperative radiotherapy
- Multimodality treatment is now recommended for pancreatic carcinoma
- Chemotherapeutic agents are 5FU, Cisplatin and alpha interferon
- Gemcitabine alone or in combination with other drugs.

Case

13 Varicose Veins

Case Capsule

Middle-aged **multiparous female** patient presents with **dilated tortuous veins on both lower limbs of 10 years duration**. She complains of **dull ache felt in the calves** and lower leg that **get worse through the day** especially during standing. It is relieved **by lying down** for 30 minutes. She also complaints of **mild swelling of the ankle** by the end of the day. She does not give history of previous accidents, major operations or prolonged illness. Her mother and elder sister had similar complaints.

On inspection, large tortuous visible veins are noted in the **distribution of long saphenous vein.** Skin of the **lower third of the medial side of the right leg shows brown pigmentation** and there is an **ulcer situated just above the medial malleolus** of the size of **7.5 × 5 cm.** On palpation there is **pitting edema of the right ankle region.** The **skin and subcutaneous tissue are thickened** over the area. Palpation along the course of the long saphenous vein behind the medial border of the tibia revealed **three defects in the deep fascia 5, 10 and 15 cm** above the medial malleolus. There is a palpable **cough impulse in the groin** at the saphenous opening region. The veins collapse when the patient lies down and the limb is elevated. **Trendelenburg test I and II are positive** on the right side and test I positive on left side. **Modified Perthes test is negative** on both sides. Multiple tourniquet test shows **perforator incompetence** in the right leg corresponding to the fascial defects mentioned above. Schwartz test is positive **on right** side. There is no bruit heard over the veins.

The ulcer is of the size of **7.5 × 5 cm** with a **sloping edge** and the surrounding skin is purple blue in color. The floor of the ulcer is covered with pink granulation tissue. The base of the ulcer is fixed to the deeper tissues. There is **serous discharge** from the ulcer. **Equinus deformity** is present at the ankle joint. Regional lymph nodes are enlarged, firm in consistency and mobile (the **vertical group of inguinal nodes on right side**). On abdominal examination there is no vein seen crossing the abdomen and there is **no mass lesions.** Per rectal and per vaginal examination shows no pelvic cause for the dilated tortuous veins. Examination of the **peripheral vascular system is normal.**

Checklist for history

History of

- Major surgery
- Major illness necessitating prolonged recumbency
- Recent long air travel (economy class syndrome)—deep vein thrombosis
- Sudden undue strain
- Drug intake—hormone containing pills (like contraceptives)
- Computer professionals requiring long hours in a sitting posture—E thrombosis
- Occupation demanding prolonged standing
- Family history of varicose veins.

Checklist for examination of varicose veins

- Examine the patient in standing position
- Expose the patient from umbilicus to the toes
- Examine the front and back of the limb
- Examine the limbs for inequality of circumference
- Know the anatomy of long saphenous and short saphenous veins with its named tributaries
- Identify the anatomical distribution of the varicose veins
- Feel the veins—tender/fibrous /thrombosed
- Examine the ankle—congestion, prominent veins, pigmentation, eczema, ulcer
- Pelvic examination to rule out secondary causes of varicose veins—intrapelvic neoplasms (uterus, ovary and rectum)
- Examine the abdomen for dilated veins that will be secondary to obstruction of inferior vena cava (commonest cause—intra-abdominal malignant disease)
- Always do abdominal examination—for intrapelvic tumor such as ovarian cysts, fibroid, cancer cervix, abdominal lymphadenopathy
- Look for large suprapubic veins and abdominal varices which are present in cases of patients with chronic iliac vein occlusion

Contd...

Contd...

- Digital rectal examination
- Auscultate the veins to rule out continuous murmur (for AV fistula)
- Always examine the peripheral pulses—venous and arterial disease often coexist.

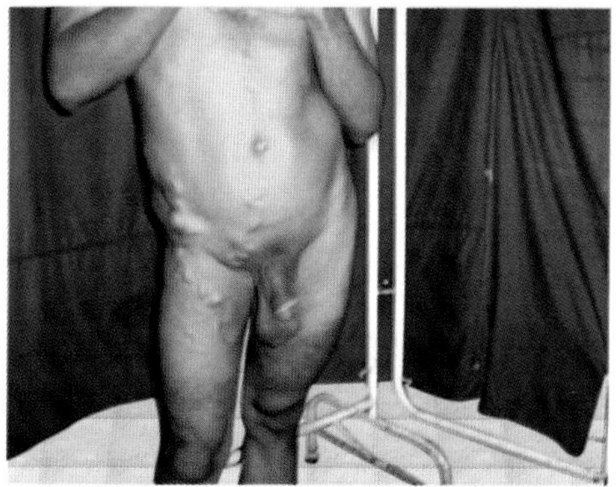

Abdominal varices in iliac vein occlusion

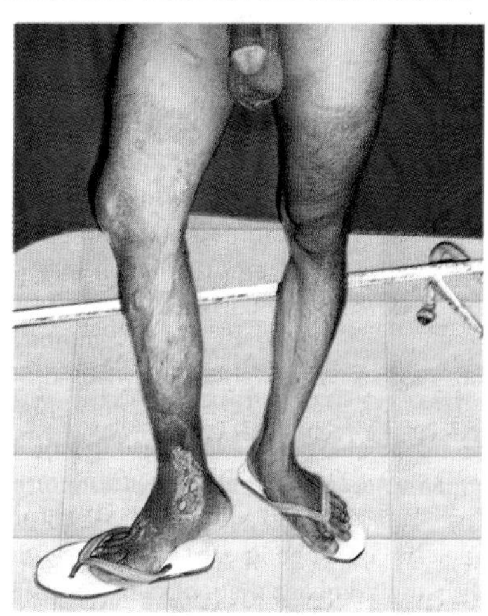

Venous ulcer

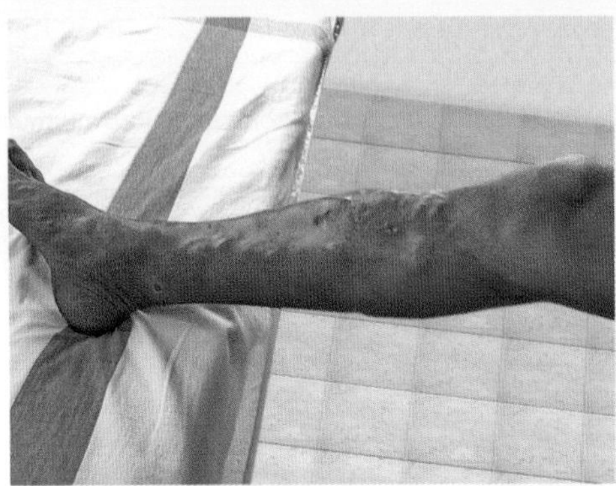

Varicosity of the long saphenous system with lipodermatosclerosis

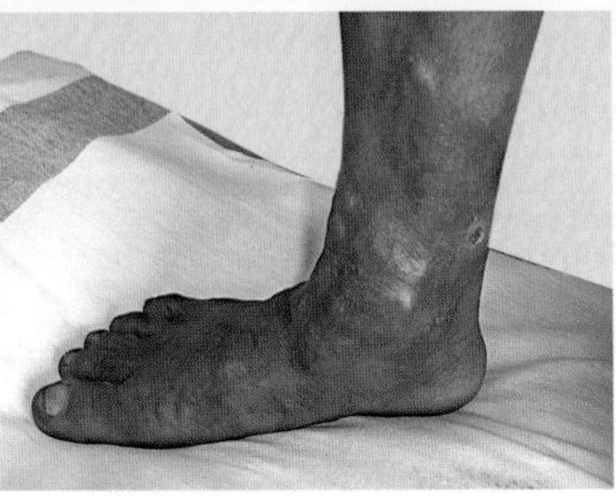

Varicosity of the long saphenous system with lipodermatosclerosis

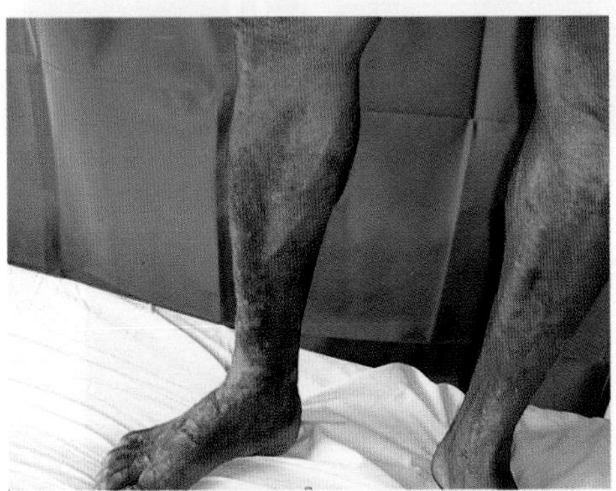

Pigmentation in gaiter area

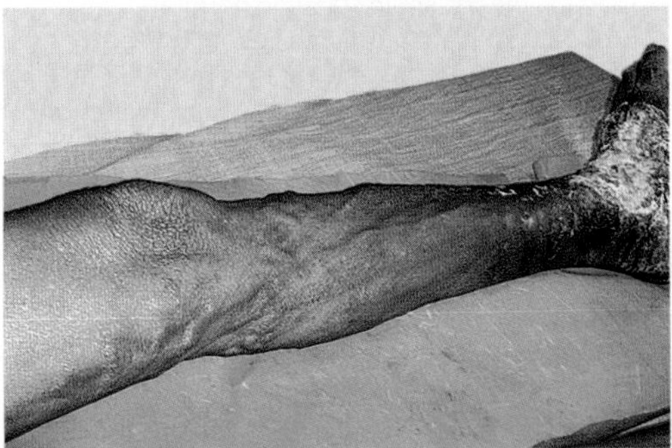

Venous ulcer with Marjolin's

Q 1. What are varicose veins?

By definition varicose veins are thin-walled, tortuous, dilated, and lengthened veins with incompetence of the contained valves. This excludes the normal prominent and dilated veins on healthy muscular legs in nonobese people. Physiologically varicose vein is one that permits reversal of flow through its faulty valves.

Q 2. What are the causes for varicose veins?

- *Congenital*—rare (congenital absence of valves)
- Primary varicose veins (cause not known, often familial)—wall theory (weakness of walls) and valve theory
- *Secondary varicose veins*:
  - Post-thrombotic (destruction of valves)
  - Post-traumatic

- Pregnancy
- Fibroids and ovarian cysts
- Abdominal lymphadenopathy
- Pelvic tumors
- Retroperitoneal fibrosis
- Ascites
- Iliac vein thrombosis
- High flow and pressure states, e.g. AV fistula.

Q 3. How can you distinguish primary varicose veins associated with a normal deep venous system from varicose veins secondary to a diseased deep venous system (the postphlebitic syndrome)?

Primary varicose veins	*Secondary varicose veins*
Seen in early adolescence	Older age group
Positive family history	No family history
Saphenous distribution alone is involved	In addition to the saphenous, the perforators and the deep veins are involved
Positive Trendelenburg—1— test	Trendelenburg—1 and 2 positive
No stasis sequelae (dermatitis and ulceration)	Stasis sequelae present
No morning ankle edema	Ankle edema present
Patent deep veins in doppler and duplex	Deep veins and perforators are abnormal in Doppler and duplex
History of varicose veins of long duration without any previous acute event like edema	The limb is normal until swelling begins as a sudden event. Varicose veins develop later

Note: Primary varicose veins can ultimately lead to stasis sequelae, even ulceration because with time, retrograde flow down the superficial system and back into the deep system can produce sustained venous hypertension. At this end-stage the appearance may be indistinguishable from postphlebitic syndrome, but the history is very different.

Q 4. What is the incidence of varicose vein?

About 20% of the population suffer varicose veins.

Q 5. How much blood is there in the venous system?

About 70% of the body's blood is in the venous system at any one time and there are at least 3 times as many veins as arteries in the limbs.

Q 6. What percentage venous blood is carried by the superficial system?

10%.

Q 7. What is the anatomy of veins in the lower limb?

The venous system in the lower limb has three portions.

Superficial: Long saphenous system and short saphenous system with their tributaries (they terminate at the saphenofemoral and saphenopopl junctions respectively.

Deep veins: Three pairs below the knee each with its associated artery—anterior tibial, posterior tibial, and peroneal. In the upper third of calf they join to form the popliteal vein which proximally becomes the superficial femoral vein.

Perforating veins: In the case of long saphenous vein four sets:

- Dodd's perforator in relation to the subsartorial canal.
- Boyd's perforator in relation to the calf muscles just below the knee.
- Cockett's perforators just above the ankle –5, 10, and 15 cm above the malleolus.
- Ankle perforators of May or Kuster.

In the case of short saphenous vein:

- Bassi's perforator—5 cm above the calcaneum
- Soleus point perforator
- Gastrocnemius point perforator.

Q 8. What is the anatomy of long saphenous system?

This is the biggest vein in the body, arises in front of the medial malleolus. It ascends behind the medial femoral condyle along the medial aspect of the thigh and terminates in the common femoral vein through the saphenous opening in the groin. The important tributaries are:

- The posterior arch vein (Leonardo's vein) (Fig 13.1)—starts behind the medial malleolus and runs upwards to the long saphenous vein joining it at the knee level. This vein is important because it has 3–4 constant perforators—(the cockett's perforators) joining it at the posterior border of the tibia linking the superficial with the posterior tibial vein of the deep system. This vein has a tendency to become varicose rather than the long saphenous vein.
- Anterior superficial tibial vein—ascend along the shin and joins the long saphenous system again at knee level (Fig. 13.2).
- The medial and lateral accessory saphenous vein (posteromedial and anterolateral) in the thigh joining of the long saphenous vein at variable levels near to the saphenofemoral junction.
- The saphenofemoral junction tributaries—superficial inferior epigastric, superficial circumflex iliac and superficial external pudendal (Fig. 13.2).

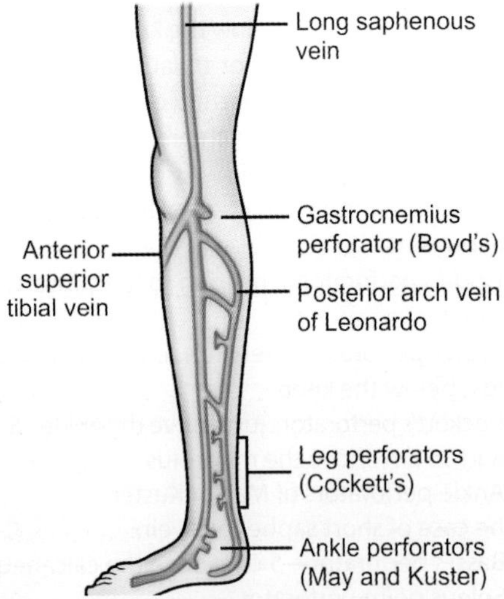

Fig. 13.1: Posterior arch vein

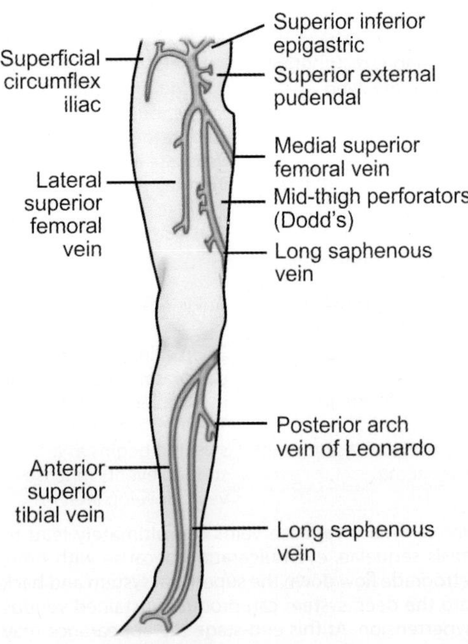

Fig. 13.2: Long saphenous

Q 9. What is the anatomy of the short saphenous system?

The vein starts behind the lateral malleolus and ascends superficially through the posterior aspect of the calf to terminate in the popliteal vein after piercing the deep fascia. In about 50% of individuals the short saphenous vein terminates above the popliteal fossa (Fig. 13.3).

Q 10. What is 'Blow out syndrome'? (PG)

This was described by Cockett. When the valves of the perforating veins become incompetent, contraction of the muscle will result in retrograde flow of venous blood from the deep to the superficial veins. The resultant high pressure reflux is called venous hypertension (described by Cockett as blow out syndrome).

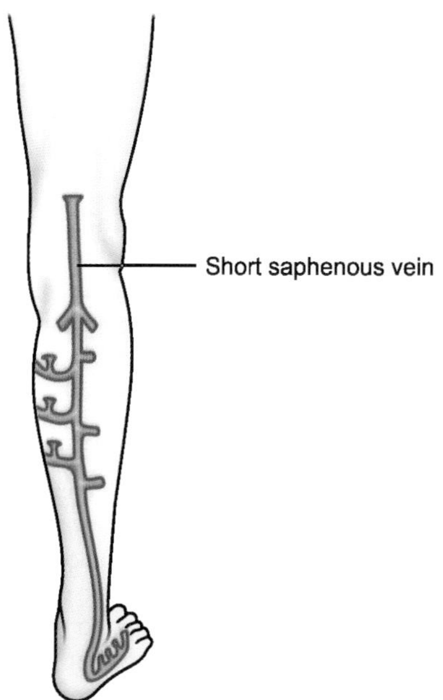

Fig. 13.3: Short saphenous vein

Q 11. What are the functions of veins?

There are three principal functions.

- Return of blood to the heart
- Blood storage
- Thermoregulation.

Q 12. What is the normal hemodynamics of venous system in the lower limb? What is ambulatory venous hypertension?

Normally the venous blood flow is from the superficial to the deep system through the perforators if the valves are competent. On standing the venous pressure in the foot vein is equivalent to the height of the column of blood extending from the heart to the foot. Normally the pressure in the superficial veins of the foot and ankle is around 80–100 mm of Hg. The venous blood is pumped to the heart from the limb by the series of muscle pumps in the calf and thigh. They are called peripheral hearts. In addition there is a foot pump that ejects blood from the plantar veins during walking (there are three pumps altogether— the foot pump, the calf pump and thigh pump). During walking the pressure within the calf compartment rises to 200–300 mm of Hg and the blood is pushed up from the deep system. During the relaxation of the calf muscle the pressure within the calf falls to a low level and the blood from the superficial veins flows through the perforators to the deep veins. The pressure in the superficial system will then automatically fall to about 20 mm of Hg. When the perforators are incompetent, the pressure in the superficial system will not fall and eczema, skin damage and leg ulceration develops. The failure of superficial venous pressure to fall during exercise is called ambulatory venous hypertension and is the main cause of venous leg ulceration. Incompetence of the deep veins has a more severe effect on the venous physiology than superficial venous incompetence because the deep veins are much larger than the superficial veins. Persistently raised venous pressure tracks back to the microcirculation of the skin and causes skin damage, resulting in venous ulceration.

Q 13. What are the causes for venous ulcer?

Venous ulcers occur in the following situations:

1. In patients with deep vein thrombosis (DVT)—post-thrombotic limb
2. Ankle perforator incompetence
3. Sometimes long-standing superficial varicose veins.

Q 14. What is the pathophysiology of venous ulcer?

1. The fibrin-cuff theory of Browse:

Persistently raised venous pressure
↓
Capillary proliferation and inflammation in the skin and subcutaneous tissue (Like a glomerulus) ↓
increased capillary leakage
↓
Perivascular cuff of fibrin, collagen type IV and fibronectin around the capillaries
↓
Fibrotic process affecting the skin and subcutaneous fat (lipodermatosclerosis)
↓
Barrier to diffusion preventing nutrient exchange ↓
Ulcer

Note: This theory is no more accepted because it has been found that there is no physical barrier to the diffusion.

2. White cell trapping theory (Dormandy)—presently accepted theory:

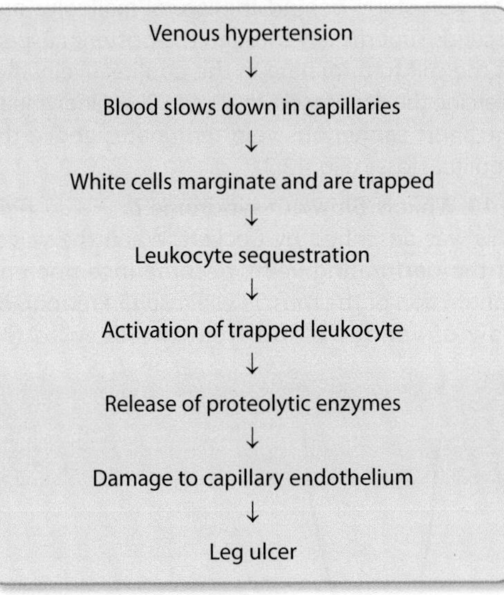

Q 15. What is venous claudication?

After deep vein thrombosis recanalization will usually occur. When recanalization fails to occur after iliofemoral venous thrombosis, venous collaterals develop to bypass the obstruction to the venous outflow. These collaterals usually suffice while the patient is at rest. However, any leg exercise induces increased arterial inflow to the lower extremities along with a commensurate increase in venous outflow requirements. This may exceed the capacity of the venous collateral bed resulting in venous hypertension. The pressure built up is manifested as tight or bursting pain. Relief is obtained with rest but not as prompt as in arterial claudication. This pain is seen after walking and towards the evening.

Q 16. What are thread veins (dermal flares)?

They are smaller veins of 0.5 mm diameter seen in the skin in varicosity. They are `usually purple or red in color. These tiny veins are associated with superficial venous incompetence in 30% of cases.

Q 17. What are reticular veins?

Reticular veins are small vessels of 1—3 mm in diameter lying immediately beneath the skin. They may present as small varices. These tiny varices are associated with superficial venous incompetence in about 30% of cases.

Q 18. What are the symptoms of varicose veins?

Symptoms of venous insufficiency
1. Asymptomatic
2. Cosmetic problems
3. Aching
4. Heaviness and cramps
5. Itching—especially on standing (the whole lower leg may itch)
6. Venous claudication
7. Ankle swelling - towards the end of the day
8. Pigmentation on the medial aspect of lower leg
9. Eczema
10. Ulcer—on the medial aspect of lower leg (gaiter area)

Note:

1. Aching, swelling, cramps, heaviness, itching are absent in the morning and become evident and aggravates as the day goes by
2. The severity of the symptoms is unrelated to the size of the veins and is often more severe during the early stages of the development of varices.

Based on symptoms patients may be classified into three groups:

Group I (Cosmetic only)	*Group II (Symptomatic)*	*Group III (Complications)*
• Venous telangiectasia • Thread veins (0.5 mm) • Reticular varices (1–3 mm) • Visible varicose veins	• Ache/ cramps/ tenderness • Heaviness/ swelling • Champagne bottle leg • Itch/restless legs/ paresthesia	• Bleeding from trauma • Superficial phlebitis • Ankle venous flare/ edema • Atrophie blanche • Venous eczema • Lipodermatosclerosis • Venous ulcers

Q 19. What is the cause for ankle edema?

Ankle edema is a feature of persistent venous obstruction. In some patients veins remain permanently blocked following a deep vein thrombosis. This causes symptoms which are worse than venous valvular incompetence. The passage of time will allow recanalization and the ankle edema may become less. The recanalized veins are likely to be incompetent and the features of venous hypertension may then predominate.

Q 20. From the location of varicose veins can you identify the system affected?

1. Varicosities of the medial calf and thigh → originate from great saphenous vein.
2. Varicosities on the posterior and lateral calf and popliteal fossa → short saphenous system.
3. Varicosities in the groin and along the anterior abdominal wall → iliac vein obstruction.

Q 21. What is Klippel-Trenaunay syndrome?

In this condition you get prominent veins along the lateral aspect of thigh mostly present from very young age, with dysplastic deep veins. The classical clinical triad consists of:

a. Hemangiomas
b. Hypertrophy of soft tissue and over growth of extremity
c. Varicose vein.

Q 22. What is postphlebitic syndrome?

It includes a chronically swollen limb with hyperpigmentation, lipodermatosclerosis and nonhealing ulcers with or without varicose veins around the ankle. One of the common presentations is a patient with chronic ulcer around the ankle. A definite history of DVT may not be present in most of these patients. Almost all of them will have destroyed deep veins due to the previous DVT.

Q 23. What are the clinical tests to be done in a patient suspected with varicose veins?

Tests for varicose veins
1. Morrissey's cough impulse test
2. Brodie-Trendelenburg test—1 and 2
3. Modified Perthes' test
4. Multiple tourniquet test
5. Schwartz's test—(tap sign)
6. Pratt's test
7. Fegan's test
8. Assessment of the short saphenous vein.

Q 24. What is Raju's test? **(PG)**

This is a useful test for venous obstruction. With patient lying supine, pressure is measured in the veins of hand and foot. Normally the foot pressure is equal to or slightly higher (by 5 mm of Hg) than the hand pressure. In venous obstruction this difference is more (10–15 mm of Hg).

Note: The venous pressure is measured by inserting a cannula to the dorsal vein of foot and measuring the pressure by a saline manometer with the help of a three way.

Q 25. What is Morrissey's cough impulse test?

In this test the patient is recumbent. The lower limb is elevated and the veins are emptied. The limb is elevated to about 30° and then the patient is asked to cough. If there is saphenofemoral incompetence expansile impulse is seen and felt at the saphenous opening. One can also see retrograde filling of the proximal part of the long saphenous vein.

Q 26. What is Brodie-Trendelenburg test?

The patient lies down on a couch and the limb is raised to allow the blood to drain out of the veins. The saphenous vein at the upper 3rd of the thigh is then compressed with a tourniquet (the saphenofemoral junction may be occluded with the thumb). The patient is then asked to stand up. The varices are observed for 30 seconds. Normally the venous filling occurs from the periphery slowly when the patient gets up and takes more than 20 seconds. When the tourniquet is released if the veins fill rapidly from above, it indicates valvular incompetence of the saphenofemoral junction. This is a positive Trendelenburg-1 test.

If the veins fill rapidly from below despite the applied tourniquet this indicates incompetence of the perforating veins (here the tourniquet is not released). This is a positive Trendelenburg-2 test.

Note: Test 1 is done first that is followed by the 2nd test.

Q 27. How is the assessment for sapheno- popliteal incompetence done? (short saphenous system).

This can be done in the same manner applying a tourniquet around the calf below the popliteal fossa.

The long saphenous vein should simultaneously be occluded at the upper thigh for accurate interpretation.

Q 28. What is modified Perthes' test?

This is a test for assessing the patency of the deep veins. In this test, with the patient standing, a rubber tourniquet is applied around the upper 3rd of thigh tight enough to occlude the long saphenous vein but not the deep veins (note—here the veins are not emptied before the test). Now the patient is asked to walk quickly for 5 minutes. If the patient complains of bursting pain in the lower leg, it is proof that the deep veins are occluded. The additional evidence is that the superficial varicosities, if present, will become more prominent as their exit is blocked by the tourniquet.

In original Perthes' test the affected limb is wrapped with elastic bandage and then allowed to walk.

Q 29. Is there any alternative test for assessing the patency of deep veins ?

Apply a tourniquet at the upper third of the calf with the patient in standing position. The patient is asked to perform 10 repeated tip toe movements. The patient will experience bursting pain.

Q 30. How is multiple tourniquet test done and what is the purpose?

This is done for seeking the sites of perforators.

The patient is in the supine position. Elevate the affected lower limb and empty the veins. The first tourniquet is tied at the ankle, second one below the knee, third one above the knee and the fourth one below the saphenous opening. The purpose of fourth tourniquet is to prevent retrograde filling from above into the long saphenous vein.

Make the patient stand up, and ask the patient to stand on toes. The resultant pumping action will throw the blood from the deep system through the perforators to the superficial. Now the tourniquets are sequentially released from below upwards. Look for varicosities at the ankle after releasing the tourniquet at the ankle. Next release the tourniquet at the calf below the knee. If the veins are prominent here perforators in this region are incompetent. Lastly release the tourniquet above the knee and look for varicosities.

Q 31. What is Schwartz's test? (Tap sign)

In standing position a tap is made on the long saphenous varicose vein with the right middle finger in the lower part of the leg after placing the fingers of the left hand just below the saphenous opening at the groin. A thrill (impulse) will be felt in the left hand, if it is a varicosity of the long saphenous system.

Q 32. What is Pratt's test?

In this test Esmarch bandage is applied to the leg from below upwards followed by tourniquet below the saphenofemoral junction. Now the bandage is released slowly keeping the tourniquet in position to see the **blow outs**.

Q 33. What is Fegan's test?

This is done for seeking the sites of perforators. In the standing position mark the excessive bulges within the varicosities. Now the patient lies down. The affected limb is elevated to empty the varicose veins, resting the heel against the examiners upper chest. The examiner palpates along the line of the marked varicosities carefully to find out gaps or circular defects with sharp edges in the deep fascia which transmit the incompetent perforators. They are marked with an 'X'.

Tests for varicose veins

Sl. No	*Test for varicose vein*	*Purpose of the test*
1.	Trendelenburg-1	To identify saphenofemoral incompetence
2.	Trendelenburg-2	To identify perforator incompetence
3.	Morrissey's cough impulse test	To identify saphenofemoral incompetence
4.	Modified Perthes' test	For noting the patency of the deep veins and ruling out deep vein thrombosis—Clinically identified as bursting pain during walking and increase in the prominence of varicosities
5.	Multiple tourniquet test	Done to identify the segment of perforator incompetence when Trendelenburg test 2 is found positive
6.	Schwartz's test	Demonstrates incompetent saphenofemoral junction by tapping below just above the ankle region
7.	Pratt's test	To demonstrate "blow outs" at the site of perforators
8.	Fegan's test	Demonstrate deep fascial defects at the site of incompetent perforators

Q 34. What is CEAP (American Venous Forum 1994) classification? (PG)

This acronym CEAP stands for:

- C—Clinical classification
- E—Etiological classification
- A—Anatomic classification
- P—Pathophysiological classification

C—Clinical classification—7 clinical grades have been identified

Class 0—No visible or palpable sign of venous disease
Class 1—Telangiectasis or reticular veins
Class 2—Varicose veins
Class 3—Edema
Class 4—Skin changes (pigmentation, eczema or lipodermatosclerosis)
Class 5—Skin changes defined above with healed ulceration
Class 6—Skin changes defined above with active ulceration

E—Etiological classification—3 etiologies
Ec—Congenital
Ep—Primary (undetermined cause)
Es—Secondary (post-thrombotic, post-traumatic, other causes)

A—Anatomic classification—18 anatomic segments have been described in 3 anatomic regions
As—Superficial veins
Ad—Deep veins
Ap—Perforating veins

P—Pathophysiological classification—3 pathologic mechanisms
Pr—Reflux
Po—Obstruction
Pro—Reflux and obstruction

Q 35. What is gaiter area?

This is an area immediately above the medial malleolus and less commonly above the lateral malleolus where the changes of chronic venous hypertension (venous stasis) are seen in the form of lipodermatosclerosis, dermatitis, eczema, pigmentation and ulceration.

Gaiter is a type of protective clothing for a person's ankles and legs below the knees. Gaiter area is the area of lower extremity over which a gaiter fits roughly from ankle to the proximal calf.

Q 36. What is champagne bottle leg (inverted beer bottle appearance)?

The lipodermatosclerosis will present as palpable induration in the gaiter area. Contraction of the skin and subcutaneous tissue in this region will result in narrowing of the ankle area. The combination of a narrow ankle and prominent calf is referred to as the champagne bottle.

Q 37. What is atrophie blanche?

In this condition the superficial veins are lost from the skin and white patches develop. This is called atrophie blanche. This indicate that the skin has been severely damaged by the venous valvular incompetence. Venous ulceration may develop in these areas.

Q 39. What are the investigations for diagnosis?

Investigations for varicose veins

- Duplex ultrasound imaging
- Doppler ultrasound
- Photoplethysmography
- Venography (phlebography)—invasive
- Ambulatory venous pressure studies
- Raju's test—arm foot venous pressure study
- Ultrasound of the abdomen.

1. *Duplex ultrasound imaging*—The examination is performed with the patient in standing position. The examiner steadily work his way from the groin to the ankle. This is the most important noninvasive investigation for practically all venous disorders. It produces high quality pictures using a combination of B mode imaging and Doppler ultrasound. Anatomical, physiological and functional details can be obtained. Venous lumen, flow, direction and reflux of blood can be visualized. The site of perforator incompetence can be located with accuracy. **It has replaced the venography**. All patients with recurrent varices, history of previous DVT and patients with skin changes should be fully investigated by using duplex ultrasonography or venography.
2. *Doppler ultrasound*—This investigation is also done in the standing position. A bidirectional flow probe will identify venous reflux. The Doppler probe is first placed over the sapheno-femoral junction. With one hand the examiner squeezes the calf to produce an acceleration of blood flow in the veins. This is heard as a 'whoosh' from the speaker of the Doppler machine. The calf compression is released and look for any reverse flow in the veins. This procedure is repeated over the saphenopopliteal junction and over other areas. The saphenopopliteal junction is inconstant. It can be identified and marked with Doppler. Doppler assessment is the minimum investigation required before treating a patient with venous disease. The arterial disease can also be excluded.

- Four characteristics descriptions are **patent, augmented, spontaneous and phasic.**

Patent	–	Flow is heard at the anatomical level of the vein
	–	Rarely does the flow completely disappear with DVT

	–	DVT is associated with continuous, high pitched signal
Augmented	–	Firm, gentle compression of the limb for a few seconds distal to the vein should result in augmentation of the flow
	–	Proximal compression followed by release should also result in augmentation
	–	Augmentation produced by proximal compression before release or distal compression after release indicates valvular incompetence
Spontaneous	–	DVT results in loss of spontaneous flow
	–	Anything causing vasoconstriction also causes loss of spontaneity
Phasic	–	Variation with respiration is called phasicity
	–	A Valsalva maneuver should decrease the signal and a deep breath should augment the signal with normal venous physiology
	–	This is lost in DVT.

3. *Venography (Phlebography)*—invasive- not done now-a-days. For identifying incompetence of the valves a descending phlebography is done where the dye is injected into the femoral vein with the patient standing.
   For ruling out deep vein thrombosis an ascending phlebography is done by injecting the dye to the foot vein after occluding the superficial veins above the ankle by a tourniquet.
4. *Ambulatory venous pressure study*—is not done routinely. It is considered by many to be the gold standard venous function test (the significance of the pressure is described earlier).
5. *Raju's test*—arm foot venous pressure study—(described earlier).

Ultrasound of the abdomen—to rule out abdominal pathology in suspected cases of secondary varicose veins.

Q 39. What are goals of treatment?

- Alleviation of pain
- Reduction of edema
- Healing of ulcers if present
- Prevention of recurrence.

Compression remains the cornerstone of treatment.

Q 40. What is the contraindication for surgery?

Deep venous thrombosis. Superficial varices developing after a venous thrombosis may be the only route of venous drainage in the lower limb and should not be removed until the patency of the deep veins of the limb has been shown.

Q 41. What are the treatment options available? (Flow chart 13.1).

Treatment options for varicose veins

- Reassurance
- Elastic compression stockings
- Injection sclerotherapy—foam sclerotherapy, echo-sclerotherapy and microsclerotherapy
- Surgical treatment
- Laser therapy.

Q 43. What are the indications for treatment?

Better results are obtained with early treatment before continuous reflux:

- Varicose veins that cause discomfort

Flow chart 13.1: Management of varicose veins

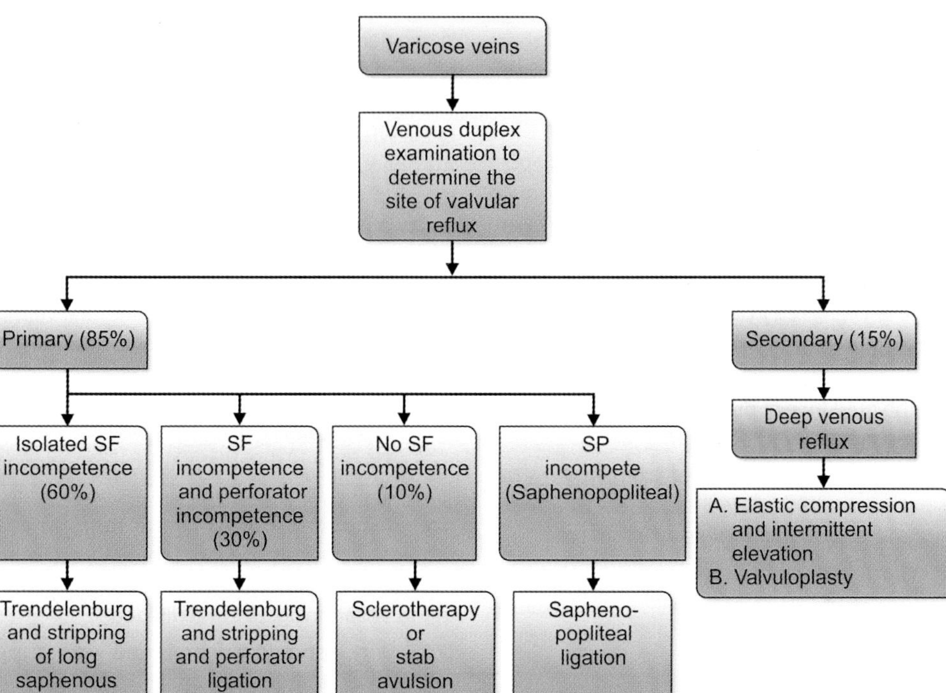

- Cosmetic embarrassment
- Complications like venous ulcers.

Q 43. What is the role of compression stockings?

The symptoms of varicose veins may be relieved by the use of compression stockings. Which are available in 3 grades—Class 1, 2 and 3.

Q 44. What are the agents used for injection sclerotherapy?

- STD—Sodium Tetradecyl Sulphate (3%)
- Polidocanol
- Ethanolamine oleate.

Q 45. What is the indication for sclerotherapy?

1. This is used to treat varicose veins in the absence of junctional incompetence and major perforating veins.
2. Used for smaller veins < 3 mm in size.

Q 46. What is the technique of injection sclerotherapy?

The sclerosant is injected into an empty vein and the vein is compressed. The endothelial lining is destroyed. If the vein is not compressed it will produce thrombosis which will later get recanalized producing recurrence.

Q 47. What is foam sclerotherapy (by Tessari)?
In this technique the STD is drawn into one syringe and air is taken in another syringe. Using a three way, rapid too and fro movements of the piston of the syringe, the foam is produced. This foam is then injected into the long saphenous vein after cannulation. The air is absorbed, the vein collapses and the endothelial lining is destroyed. A much larger volume can be injected into the vein with a small quantity of sclerosant so that it will fill the superficial varicosities. The patient is lying supine with the leg elevated instead.

Q 48. What is echosclerotherapy? (PG)
When the procedure of foam sclerotherapy is done under the guidance of duplex ultrasound imaging it is called echosclerotherapy.

Q 49. What is the advantage of sclerotherapy?
The patients can undergo repeated treatment sessions to ensure that all veins are removed.

Q 50. What are the complications of sclerotherapy?

Complications of sclerotherapy
• Skin pigmentation • Injury to the skin and ulceration • Allergic reaction • Thrombophlebitis • Deep vein thrombosis.

Q 51. What is microsclerotherapy? (PG)
The thread veins and reticular varices are injected by inserting a 30 G needle. The solutions used are STD and polidocanol. After the injection compression bandage is given for a period of 1–5 days.

Q 52. What is the surgical treatment of saphenofemoral incompetence?
Trendelenburg's operation and stripping of the long saphenous vein.

Q 53. What is the contraindication for Trendelenburg's operation?
When **deep vein thrombosis** is destroying the main axial limb vein and the patient will depend on the superficial veins for venous drainage.

Q 54. What is Trendelenburg's operation?
An oblique incision is made in the groin and the long saphenous vein is exposed. The procedure has got two portions:

a. Saphenofemoral flush ligation
b. Ligation of the proximal five tributaries:
    1. The superficial external pudendal vein
    2. The superficial inferior epigastric vein
    3. The superficial circumflex iliac vein
    4. The posteromedial vein (medial accessory saphenous vein)
    5. The anterolateral (lateral accessory saphenous vein).

Note: It is important that the femoral vein is inspected carefully at least 1cm above and below the saphenofemoral junction (SFJ) and all tributaries in this situation ligated and divided.

Q 55. Why it should be combined with stripping of the long saphenous vein?
The main principle of the surgical treatment is to ligate the source of venous reflux and to remove the incompetent saphenous trunk. The Trendelenburg procedure alone is associated with high rate of recurrence. To ensure elimination of as much reflux as possible it is necessary to remove the long saphenous vein. Similarly in case of saphenopopliteal incompetence the part of the short saphenous vein must be removed.

Q 56. What type of stripping is recommended for saphenous vein?
To avoid injury to the saphenous nerve the long saphenous vein should not be removed below the

midcalf level. The conventional way of removing the long saphenous vein is with a stripper (Babcock). Here the stripper wire is passed down the long saphenous vein. The end is identified in the upper calf and a 2 mm incision is made to retrieve the stripper. An olive of about 8 mm diameter is attached to the upper end and the saphenous vein is removed by firm traction on the wire in the calf.

Q 57. What is invaginating stripping (inverting)? (PG)

The aim of this type of stripping is to reduce the damage to the tissues around the vein. There will be less pain and less bleeding in this operation. A rigid metal pin stripper (Oesch) has been developed and this is passed down the inside of the saphenous vein which is recovered from the upper calf. A strong suture is attached to the stripper and firmly ligated to the proximal end of the vein. During pulling of the stripper the long saphenous vein will invert and can be delivered through a 2 mm incision in the midcalf region. Here no olive is used.

Q 58. What are the nerves at risk during venous surgery?

1. Saphenous nerve—this is likely to be injured during stripping of the long saphenous vein
2. Sural nerve—this is likely to be injured during stripping of the short saphenous vein.

Q 59. What is the peculiarity of the sapheno-popliteal junction?

The saphenopopliteal junction is not constant. The termination may lie from 2 cm below the knee to 15 cm above the knee. It is very important to identify the termination sonologically and mark it on the skin before surgery.

Q 60. What is hook phlebectomy? (PG)

After stripping, the residual veins and tributaries are left behind. These veins conventionally used to be managed by incisions long enough to insert artery forceps for ligating the veins. Now these veins can be tackled by means of small hooks that may be inserted through incisions of 1–2 mm size. The closure of these small incisions is achieved using adhesive strips. This gives excellent cosmetic outcome.

Q 61. What is the postoperative management?

1. Compression bandaging is applied to the limb at the end of the operation to prevent bruising.
2. Some surgeons apply compression to the limb before stripping.
3. After two days the bandage may be replaced with thigh length high compression stockings (class 2).

Q 62. What is VNUS closure? (PG)

This is intraluminal destruction of the long and short saphenous vein using ablation catheter under ultrasound guidance.

Q 63. What are the complications of varicose vein surgery? (PG)

Complications of varicose vein surgery
1. Pain, discomfort and bruising 2. Nerve injury—Saphenous for long saphenous surgery—Sural for short saphenous surgery 3. Venous thrombosis in residual varices 4. Deep vein thrombosis—1/1000 operations (give prophylactic heparin when there is history of previous DVT).

Q 64. What are the complications of varicose veins?

Complications of varicose veins
• Hemorrhage • Superficial thrombophlebitis

Contd...

Contd...

- Eczema
- Pigmentation
- Lipodermatosclerosis
- Deep vein thrombosis (rarely)
- Venous ulcer
- Marjolin's ulcer
- Calcification
- Periostitis
- Talipes equinus.

Q 65. What are the causes for superficial thrombophlebitis ?

Causes for superficial thrombophlebitis

- TAO (Buerger's disease)
- Occult carcinoma (visceral malignancy)
- Varicose veins
- Polycythemia
- Iatrogenic—IV Injection.

Q 66. What is the classical location for venous ulcer?

Just proximal to the medial and lateral malleolus (gaiter area).

Q 67. What are the differences between venous ulcer and varicose ulcer?

When the ulcer is secondary to deep venous pathology or perforator incompetence producing chronic venous hypertension, it is called **venous ulcer**. When the ulcer is due to superficial insufficiency alone, it is called **varicose ulcer**. It is better to use the term venous ulcer because the ulcer is not caused by the varicose veins but by the disordered pattern of the venous blood flow.

Differences between varicose ulcer and venous ulcer

Varicose ulcer (40–50%)	*Venous ulcer*
Due to pure superficial venous insufficiency (long standing SFJ incompetence)	Due to incompetence of the perforators and deep venous incompetence. It may be post-thrombotic venous damage
History of long standing superficial varicosity	History suggestive of deep vein thrombosis followed by lower limb edema
Ankle edema may not be there	Ankle edema, calf muscle increase and narrow ankle suggestive of deep vein problem
Painless	Painful
Does not penetrate deep fascia	Penetrate deep fascia
Respond to surgical treatment of the superficial varicosity	Does not respond to treatment

Q. 68. What are the most important causes for leg ulceration?

Causes of leg ulcers

- Peripheral arterial disease
- Venous disease of the lower limb
- Diabetes
- Neuropathy
- Infective ulcers
- Traumatic ulcers
- Malignant ulcers
- Rheumatoid disease
- Autoimmune disease—systemic sclerosis, SLE.

Q 69. What are the characteristic features of venous ulcer?

Features of venous ulcer

1. Seen at the gaiter area (usually on the medial side)—lower 3rd of the leg (never found above the junction of middle and upper third of leg)
2. The surrounding tissues show signs of chronic venous hypertension—pigmentation, eczema and lipodermatosclerosis
3. Presence of obvious varicose veins (may not be visible sometimes)
4. The ulcer can take any shape
5. The edge will be sloping
6. The floor will be covered with granulation tissue/slough/white fibrous tissue
7. The tendons and bone may be sometimes exposed
8. The base of the ulcer is fixed to the deeper tissues
9. The movements of the ankle joint may be limited by the scarring of the ulcer—equinus deformity.

Q 70. What are the investigations in venous ulcer?

1. Examine the peripheral pulses to rule out arterial problem
2. Examine the sensation to rule out neuropathy
3. Doppler ankle blood pressure
4. Duplex ultrasonography of the veins and arteries
5. Blood examination to rule out SLE, rheumatoid disease
6. Biopsy of the ulcer.

Q 71. What is the management of venous leg ulcers?

This consists of :

1. Management of the ulcer
2. Surgery for the superficial venous incompetence
3. In patients with deep venous insufficiency surgery may not be effective.

Q 72. Is it necessary to delay surgery until the ulcer has healed? (PG)

It is not necessary and surgery may be carried out before the ulcer has healed. It is found that the ulcer healing is rapid in this situation.

Q 73. What is the management of ulcer?

The standard old regimen is called **Bisgaard regime** consisting of:

- Elevation of the limb
- Elastocrepe bandage (compression stocking)
- Exercise
- Education.

Note: Do culture and sensitivity and give appropriate antibiotics.

Biopsy of the ulcer if nonhealing

Blood examination—Blood sugar
ESR
Rheumatoid factor, etc.

Q 74. What is Marjolin's ulcer?

Malignant change may occur in long standing venous ulcers. This should be suspected, when there is evidence of raised or rolled out edge. They are nothing but squamous cell carcinoma.

Q 75. Is there any role for topical applications and topical antibiotics?

- No
- Topical applications will not speed up healing
- It will produce allergy and skin sensitization
- Topical antibiotics are ineffective
- If eczematous reaction is there around the ulcer, topical steroid may be useful.

Q 76. What is the role of compression?

- A pressure of 30–45 mm of Hg applied to the ulcer is found to be effective for healing of the ulcer.

- Class III stockings exert about 30 mms of Hg compression
- The compression is applied to the ulcer region alone (**below knee stockings**)
- Those who cannot use compression stockings use multilayer bandaging regimes (4 layer bandage developed by Charing Cross Hospital, London). This bandage is changed once or twice weekly.

Q 77. What is the principle of compression?

The exact mechanism by which compression is of benefit is not known but the following physiological alterations occur.

1. Relieves the leg edema
2. Controls the chronic venous insufficiency
3. Reduction in ambulatory venous pressure
4. Improvement in skin microcirculation
5. Increase in subcutaneous pressure preventing transcapillary fluid leakage.

Q 78. What is the drug treatment for venous ulcer?

Drugs are inferior to compression bandaging. The following drugs are used:

- Aspirin
- Prostaglandin E Analog
- Diosmin
- Pentoxifylline
- Calcium Dobesilate
- Flavonoids

Q 79. What is the role of systemic antibiotics in venous ulcer?

- Antibiotics have no effect on ulcer healing
- Evidence of infection in the form of cellulitis and fever, are indications for antibiotics.

Q 80. What is the treatment of deep venous insufficiency? (PG)

The surgical treatment is difficult and being done only in a few centers. The surgical options are:

a. Direct vein valve repair by valvuloplasty (Kistner)
b. Vein valve transposition
c. Transplantation of a segment of axillary vein.

Q 81. What is the indication for deep venous surgery? (PG)

Those who have persisting swelling of the lower limb after a previous venous thrombosis.

Q 82. What is the surgical treatment for deep venous obstruction? (PG)

1. *Palma operation:* This involves mobilizing the long saphenous vein in the opposite leg, tunnelling the distal end of the LSV across suprapubically and inserting it into the femoral vein of the affected side below the obstruction.
2. *May-Husni procedure:* This is done for the obstruction of the superficial femoral vein. The long saphenous vein is connected to the popliteal vein in the same limb allowing blood to flow along the superficial vein.

Q 83. What is the treatment of perforator incompetence?

1. Subfascial endoscopic perforator surgery (SEPS)
2. Foam sclerotherapy
3. Open subfascial ligation—Linton flap and Dodd and cocket procedure
4. Multiple perforator ligation.

Q 84. What are the new alternatives of treatment?

1. *Radiofrequency ablation*—a catheter is passed up the saphenous vein from the lower leg and withdrawn under ultrasound guidance while radio frequency waves are used to destroy the endothelial lining through a series of metal prongs.
2. *Endovenous laser ablation (EVLA)*—A laser probe is passed up inside a catheter inserted into the lower part of the saphenous vein

under sono-guidance. Large amounts of crystalloid fluid containing local anesthesia are placed around the vein to separate the skin from the laser probe to avoid cutaneous burns. The laser probe is kept just below the saphenofemoral junction and a set number of joules are given to the endothelial lining. Flush occlusion is not possible with radio-frequency ablation and laser.

Poem on Varicose Veins

"Varicose vein disease is sometimes diagnosed with ease,
But of the best attempts will meet with sad and sorrowful defeat

So let us give you good advice
Examine once, Examine twice:
Examine from head to toes,
Before you dare to diagnose
More harm is done because you do not look
Than from not knowing what is in the book
Above all do not try to spot
Because you think you know a lot
Spot diagnosis you should hate
Until you are a surgeon great!
By then of course you will have learnt
Some lessons bitter and you daren't"

Case 14 Peripheral Occlusive Vascular Disease

Case Capsule

A **60-year-old male patient** presents with **left calf muscle, thigh muscle and gluteal pain** of 18 months duration. He gets a **cramp-like pain** only **while he walks** and the pain disappears when he stops walking. **At the beginning** of the walk he gets **numbness, pins and needles and paresthesia** in the skin of the foot. Initially the **claudication distance** was about 200 meters. The walking distance gradually shortened over a few months. There is **no history of chest pain, fainting, blurred vision or weakness or paresthesia** of the upper limbs. For the last 3 weeks he gets **continuous severe pain aching in nature** which is present at rest **throughout the day and night**, mostly in the foot and leg. After a few days he noticed **black color of the left big toe** and **ulcer in the left heel region**. The maximum pain he gets is at the **junction of black area of the big toe** and the **remaining normal foot**. He prefers to **sleep sitting in a chair**, if at all in the bed, **he hangs his leg over the side of the bed**. The patient is **requesting for amputation** of the leg.

On examination, the patient is found to be **hypertensive.** The patient **sits with the left knee bent, holding the left foot still**. He is **unwilling to lie flat**. When the limb is kept horizontal the **foot is pale**. The **capillary filling is retarded**. The **pulps of the toes show wasting**. The **veins of the limb are empty and guttered**. The entire **left big toe is gangrenous**. A **line of demarcation** is seen between the gangrenous area and the normal foot. There is an **ulcer of 4 × 3 cm** size situated **in the left heel** region. The **floor of the ulcer is covered with slough** and the **edge is punched out**. The surrounding area of the ulcer is very tender. The **skin temperature from midcalf** downwards **is cold**. The femoral, popliteal, dorsalis pedis and posterior tibial **pulses are absent on the left side**. On the right side all the pulses are present except dorsalis pedis and posterior tibial. There is **wasting of left leg muscles**. There is an **audible bruit over the right femoral artery**. Cardiovascular system and neurological examination are normal.

Checklist for history

- Character of the pain, severity aggravating and relieving factors
- Claudication distance
- History of sudden onset or gradual onset
- History of smoking
- History of diabetes mellitus
- History of cardiac illness

Contd...

Contd...

- History of cerebrovascular accidents/TIA
- History of dyslipidemias
- History of superficial phlebitis
- History of fainting, blurred vision, abdominal pain
- History of impotence
- Family history of atherosclerosis.

Checklist for examination

- Always examine the heart because vascular diseases are part of the cardiovascular system
- Listen for aortic, renal, celiac and iliac bruits
- Look for signs of congestive cardiac failure—raised JVP, edema, basal creps, pleural effusion, ascites
- Take blood pressure in both arms
- Look for palpable thrill over the vessels
- Examine all peripheral pulses including both lower limbs and upper limbs, common carotid arteries and their bifurcation, facial and superficial temporal vessels
- Assess the mental status and speech abnormalities
- Look for visual defects
- Examine for evidence of motor and sensory disorders—(hemiplegia of the contralateral leg, arm and face)
- Look for speech problems—aphasia
- Ipsilateral temporary visual loss (Atheromatous fragments in retinal vessels)
- Look for nutritional changes (trophic changes) of the toes, foot, fingertips and hands—thin and atrophic skin, loss of pulp, brittle and deformed nails, with loss of hair, wasting of muscles. Painful cracks appear across the heel

Contd...

Contd...

- Look for ulceration in the pressure points and bony prominences—the heel, malleoli, tips of toes, 5th metatarsal head region, and ball of the foot.

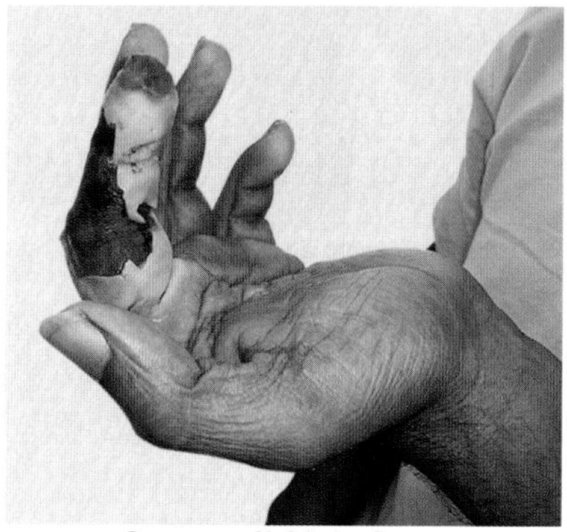

Gangrene of left index finger

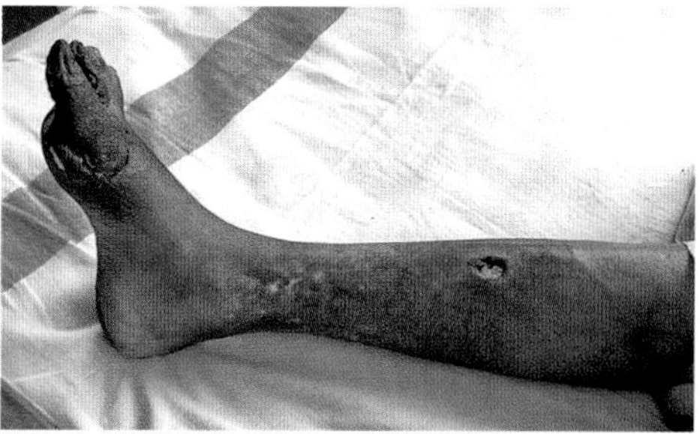

Gangrene of right big toe and second toe with a patch

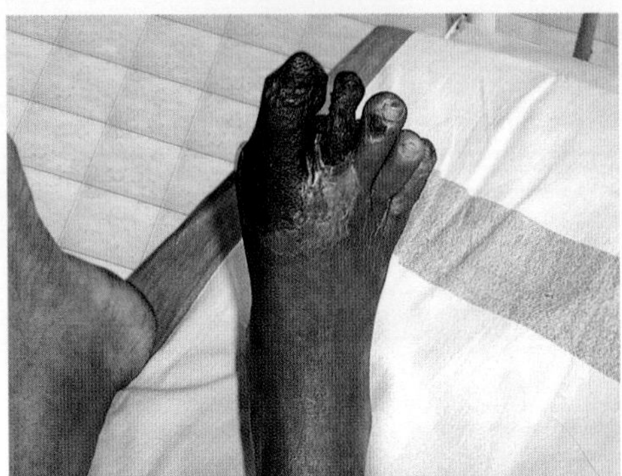

Gangrene of right big toe and second toe

Q 1. What is the most probable diagnosis in this case?

- Peripheral occlusive arterial disease
- Probably atherosclerotic obstruction
- Level of obstruction being aortoiliac
- With gangrene of the left big toe
- Ischemic ulcer of left heel.

In all cases of peripheral occlusive vascular disease ask the following questions

- Find out the level of occlusion clinically and include it in the diagnosis?
- Look for bruit in all arterial diseases over the vessels even if they are palpable—carotids, subclavian, aorta, renal, celiac axis, and femoral
- Find out the nature of obstruction? Thrombosis/embolism
- Decide whether patient needs invasive investigations?
- Invasive investigations are done only if patient is suitable for surgery?
- Assess the comorbid conditions?

Q 2. What are diagnostic points in favor of your diagnosis?

- Intermittent claudication
- Ischemic rest pain
- Absent popliteal, dorsalis pedis and posterior tibial pulsations with audible bruit over the left femoral
- Ischemic ulcer (nonhealing heel ulcer)
- Pallor of foot on elevation and pink color on dependency
- Gangrene of left big toe
- Low ankle brachial index.

Q 3. Why this is a case of atherosclerosis rather than TAO (Buerger's)?

The difference between atherosclerosis and Buerger's disease are given below: In the given circumstances the diagnosis is atherosclerosis.

Differences between ASO and Buerger's disease

Feature	*Atherosclerosis*	*Buerger's*
Age of onset	Above 40 years	20–40 years
Sex	Male > female	Rare in women
Smoking	Can occur without smoking	Seen only in smokers
Progression of disease	Proximal to distal	Distal to proximal
Venous involvement	Not seen	Common
Thrombophlebitis	Not seen	Common
Inflammatory reaction	Not seen	Common
Layer of vessel affected	Affects the intima	Affects all layers—panarteritis, periarteritis, and panphlebitis

Contd...

Contd...

Site of lesion	Large and medium sized arteries (aorta, iliac, femoral and popliteal)	Small arteries
Arteriography	Proximal lesion	Distal lesion
Collateral in arteriography	Extensive collaterals (tree root appearance)	Poor collaterals (cork screw appearance)
Distal run off in arteriogram	Usually present	Usually absent
Bypass surgery	Possible	Not possible

Note: Atherosclerotic obstructionn (ASO)

Q 4. What is claudication?

Claudication means limping (Claudio = **I limp**). The term is now used to describe the cramp-like muscle pain which appears following exercise as a result of inadequate arterial blood flow. **The three criteria for claudication are:**

1. It is a cramp-like muscle pain (usually calf)
2. Pain develops only when the muscle is exercised—(not present on taking the first step in contrast to osteoarthritis)
3. The pain disappears when the exercise stops (contrast lumbar intervertebral disk nerve compression).

Q 5. What are the types of claudication?

There are **three types of claudication**

1. Arterial claudication
2. Venous claudication
3. Neurogenic claudication.

Q 6. What is the cause for paresthesia in the skin of the foot?

The patient notices numbness, pins and needles and other paresthesia in the skin of the foot at the when muscle pain begins. This is as a result of shunting of blood from the skin to the muscle.

Q 7. What is the cause for claudication pain?

The cause of the pain can be explained as a response to the accumulation of acidic, anaerobic metabolite (**P** - substance) due to inadequate blood and oxygen supplies to meet the requirements of the increased activity. On stopping the activity the blood supply is replenished, the anoxia is abolished and the painful metabolites are washed away.

Q 8. What is claudication distance?

The distance a patient can walk on normal ground and at a normal speed without pain and having to stop.

Q 9. What are the sites of claudication pain?

Depending on the level of occlusion, the site of claudication pain will differ. The following chart shows the claudication sites for each level of occlusion.

Levels of occlusion with clinical features

Level of occlusion	*Site of claudication and other clinical findings*
1. Absent ankle pulses	Claudication of calf and foot
2. Femoropopliteal obstruction (*femoral pulse present and popliteal pulse absent*)	Unilateral claudication in calf
3. Iliac vessel obstruction (*the femoral and distal pulses absent*)	*Unilateral claudication* in thigh and calf and some times buttock. *Bruit* over iliac or femoral vessel
4. Aortoiliac obstruction (*all pulsations from femoral down absent on both sides*)	*Bilateral claudication* of both buttocks, thighs and calves. Presence of *bruit* over both femoral *Impotence*-common

Q. 10. What is Leriche's syndrome?

It occurs in men as a result of aortoiliac disease and consists of:

- Claudication of the hip, thigh and buttock muscles (Gluteal claudication)
- Atrophy of the leg muscles
- Sexual impotence
- Diminished/absent femoral pulses
- Transient numbness of the extremity accompanies the pain and fatigue of claudication.

Q 11. What is the cause for impotence in Leriche's syndrome?

It is due to the lack of blood supply to the penis. The penis is getting blood supply through the internal iliac vessels which is occluded in this conditions.

Q 12. What is rest pain? What is the site of rest pain?

- It is the continuous pain caused by severe ischemia. This pain is present at rest throughout the day and night. The pain is relieved by **putting the leg below the level of the heart** (the patient hangs his legs over the side of the bed and prefers to **sleep sitting in a chair**. In the bed he often sits with the knee bent holding the foot still to try and relieve the pain).
- The rest pain usually occurs in the **most distal part of the limb.** The toes and the fore foot. If there is associated gangrene the patient feels the pain at the junction of the living and dead tissue.

Q 13. What is Boyd's grading of claudication?

	Boyd's grading of claudication
Grade I	Patient experiences pain after walking some distance. Pain disappears and patient continues to walk
Grade II	Pain persists and still the patient continues to walk
Grade III	Pain compels the patient to take rest.

Q 14. What is Fontaine classification for the severity of chronic ischemia?

Fontaine classification of limb ischemia	
Stage I	Asymptomatic
Stage II	Intermittent claudication limiting lifestyle • IIa—Well compensated (> 200 meters) more than 1 block • IIb—Poorly compensated < 200 meters
Stage III	Rest pain due to ischemia
Stage IV	Ulceration or gangrene due to ischemia.

Q 15. What is ischemic ulcer? What are the features of ischemic ulcer?

Ischemic ulcer is an ulcer caused by inadequate blood supply

The features of ischemic ulcers

- They are usually found at the tips of toes/fingers and over the pressure areas
- The ulcer and surrounding tissues are very tender
- The surrounding tissues are very cold
- The edge of ischemic ulcer is punched out (because there is no attempt at healing)
- Skin at the edge of the ulcer is usually blue grey in color
- The floor may contain slough
- Ischemic ulcers are very deep and penetrate down to the bone and joints
- The base of ulcer may be bone, ligaments or tendons.

Q 16. What are the causes for ischemic ulcerations?

Causes for ischemic ulcers

- Large artery occlusion—Atherosclerosis
  - Embolism
- Small artery occlusion
  - Buerger's disease
  - Diabetes
  - Embolism

Contd...

Contd...

- – Trauma
- – Scleroderma
- – Raynaud's disease
- – Physical agents—radiation, electric burns
- Systemic diseases affecting the vessels.

Q 17. How will you assess the skin temperature?

The skin temperature can be assessed reliably only when both limbs are exposed to the same ambient temperature for a full **five** minutes. Do not examine immediately after pulling back the sheets. The temperature assessment is done by **back of the fingers of the clinician** because the palmar surface of the hand is usually warm and moist and is not a good temperature sensor as the **cool dry** back of the fingers.

Q 18. What are the clinical tests to be carried out?

Clinical tests in a vascular case

- Assess the skin temperature of the affected limb
- Buerger's vascular angle
- Capillary filling time
- Venous filling
- Capillary refilling
- Feel the peripheral pulsations
- Crossed leg test of Fuchsig
- Reactive hyperemia test

Test for upper limb

- Adson's test
- Allen's test
- Elevated arm stress test.

Note:

- Auscultate for bruit in all cases
- Measure blood pressure in all cases.

Q 19. What is Buerger's vascular angle?

It is the angle to which the leg must be raised before it becomes white (**pallor**). In a normal person the straightened limb can be raised by 90° and the toes and foot will remain pink. In an ischemic leg elevation to 15–30° may cause pallor. The angle is directly proportional to the pressure in the small vessels of the foot. The height in cm, between the **sternum and heel** at the elevation when it becomes pale is equal to the **pressure in the foot** vessel in mm of Hg. **A vascular angle < 20° indicates severe ischemia.**

Q 20. What is capillary filling time?

After determining the vascular angle by **elevating the limb**, ask the patient to sit up and **hang his legs down** over the side of the couch. A normal leg will remain pink in color. The ischemic leg will slowly turn from white to pink which is caused by the blood filling the dilated skin capillaries. **The time taken for the foot to become pink** is the capillary filling time. More than **20–30 seconds** indicates severe ischemia.

Q 21. What is venous filling?

The limb should be **elevated for 30 seconds** and then laid flat on the bed. The veins collapse when the legs are raised above the level of the heart. But if the circulation is normal they do not empty completely. Normal venous filling occurs within 5 seconds. When there is ischemia, the **veins collapse** and become **guttered at 10–15°** elevation. Normally at room temperature, the veins are relaxed and full of blood when the patient is lying horizontal. In ischemia the veins will be collapsed and some times look like **blue gutters**.

Q 22. What is capillary refilling?

Press the tip of **nail or the pulp** of a toe or a finger for **2 seconds**. Then observe the time taken for the blanched area to turn pink after releasing the pressure. This gives a crude indication of the rate of blood flow in the capillaries.

Q 23. What are the peripheral pulsations to be examined?

The arteries are palpated **against a bone** (where it is crossing the bone). Diminution of a pulse can be appreciated by comparing it with the pulse in the other limb. The following arterial pulsations are looked for against the areas mentioned below.

Pulsations	*Area to be examined*
Dorsalis pedis artery	Proximal intermetatarsal space on the dorsum of the foot, lateral to the tendon of extensor hallucis longus The pulse is felt against the navicular bone and base of 1st metatarsal. Absent in 10% of populations
Posterior tibial artery	Pulsation is felt against the medial aspect of the calcaneum, or against the back of the medial malleolus
Peroneal artery	1cm medial to the lateral malleolus
Anterior tibial artery	Midway between the malleoli against the lower end of the tibia just above the level of ankle at the head of the talus
Popliteal artery (an easily palpable popliteal artery may be aneurysm)	*Three methods:* 1. Flex the knee to 135° with the heel resting on the couch. The thumb of the examiner is on the tibial tuberosity and the fingers over the lower part of the popliteal fossa. Press the neurovascular bundle against the posterior surface of the tibia (in the upper part of popliteal fossa it is difficult to palpate the artery because it is deep between the condyles of the femur) 2. The most reliable method is perhaps the most inconvenient. Here the patient is examined in the prone position. Flex the knee to relax the popliteal fossa and feel the artery with fingertips of both hands in the lower part of the fossa over the posterior surface of the upper end of tibia (medial tibial condyle) 3. With the leg straight, place one hand of the examiner around the knee with the fingertips on the midline of popliteal fossa and hyperextend the knee against this hand and the couch with the other hand
Femoral artery	At the groin mid way between the symphysis pubis and the anterior superior iliac spine against the neck of femur
Radial artery	Is felt at the wrist in front of the lower end of the radius laterally, lateral to the flexor carpi radialis tendon
Ulnar artery	Is felt at the wrist against the lower end of the front of ulna, lateral to the flexor carpi ulnaris tendon
Brachial artery	Is felt against the lower part of humerus, medial to the biceps brachii tendon
Axillary artery	Felt in the apex of the axilla against the neck of the humerus
Subclavian artery	Felt against the first rib in the middle of supraclavicular fossa
Common carotid artery	Felt medial to the sternomastoid muscle at the level of the thyroid cartilage against the carotid tubercle (Chassaigne tubercle) of the 6th cervical vertebra
Facial artery	Felt against the body of the mandible where the masseter is attached
Superficial temporal artery	Felt in front of the tragus of the ear against the temporal bone.

Q 24. What is disappearing pulse?

In arterial occlusion with well-developed collateral circulations, the distal pulses will be normal to palpation. The patient is exercised to the point of claudication, which may unmask the effect of an arterial obstruction by disappearance of the pulse. The pulse will reappear after a minute or two after rest. The exercise produces vasodilatation below the obstructing lesion and the arterial inflow cannot keep pace with the increasing vascular space and the pulse disappears.

Q 25. What is crossed leg test of Fuchsig?

This test is done for the assessment of the **patency of the popliteal artery**. The patient sits with legs crossed in a chair. Oscillatory movements of the foot occur synchronously with the pulsation of the popliteal artery, if the artery is patent. Attention of the patient is distracted from the legs.

Q 26. What is Adson's test (for cervical rib/scalenus anticus syndrome)?

The patient will be sitting in a chair and the radial pulse of the patient is felt. Patient is asked to turn the face to the same side where the pulse is being felt. Now ask the patient to take a deep breath to narrow the cervicoaxillary channel. If the radial pulse disappears or becomes feeble it is suggestive of a **cervical rib** or a **scalenus anticus syndrome**. The purpose of taking deep breath is for allowing the rib cage to move upwards so that it will narrow the cervicoaxillary channel. The purpose of turning the face to the same side is to contract the scalenus anterior muscle.

Q 27. What is Allen's test (to look for completeness of the palmar arch formed by radial and ulnar artery)?

This test is done for assessing the patency of radial and ulnar arteries and digital arteries. The patient is asked to clench his fist tightly and then the clinician will compress the radial and ulnar arteries at the wrist. The patient opens and closes the fist several times for venous return. After 1 minute ask the patient to open his fist. The palm will be white. Now release the compression on the radial artery and watch the blood flow to the hand. Normally the hand will become pink immediately, whereas if there is obstruction to the artery or one of the digital arteries the concerned area will remain pale. Slow flow into one finger caused by digital artery occlusion will be apparent from the rate at which that finger turns pink. Now repeat the procedure by releasing the pressure on the ulnar artery first.

Q 28. What is elevated arm stress test (for thoracic outlet syndrome)?

This is a test for thoracic outlet syndrome. In this test the patient is asked to keep both arms in abducted position at 90°. The patient is then asked to make fist and release it repeatedly on both sides for 5 minutes. The patient will continue to do the manoeuvre in the normal side. On the effected side patient will get pain and paresthesia with difficulty to continue the manuever.

Q 29. What is reactive hyperemia test?

This gives an indication of severity of the arterial ischemia. Inflate sphygmomanometer cuff around the limb to 250 mm of Hg for five minutes and then measure the interval between releasing the cuff and appearance of red flush in the skin. In the normal limb it appears within 1–2 seconds. In a severely ischemic leg it may never appear.

Q 30. What is bruit?

It is the sound produced by the turbulent blood flow through a stenotic arterial segment which is **transmitted distally along the course of artery.** When a bruit is heard over the peripheral vessel, stenosis is present **at or proximal to that level**. It is heard loudest during systole and with greater stenosis it may extend into the diastole. The pitch of the bruit rises as the stenosis become more marked. When the vessel become completely occluded, the bruit may disappear. **Absence of bruit does not indicate absence of occlusion.** You need a **bell on your stethoscope** to listen along the line of an artery. Do not press too hard over a superficial artery.

Q 31. What are the common sites to listen for bruits?

Common sites to listen for bruit

Name of artery	*Where to look for*
Subclavian artery	Supraclavicular fossa
Carotid	Behind the angle of mandible
Renal artery	Posteriorly below the 12th rib
Celiac axis	Epigastrium
Femoral artery	In the groin—half way between the anterior superior iliac spine and the symphysis pubis and over the adductor canal (a hand's breadth above the knee).

Note: The systolic bruits are conducted distally. A bruit at the level of angle of mandible without any supraclavicular bruit means a carotid artery stenosis. When a bruit is heard over supra clavicular fossa and angle of mandible, the origin may be more proximal i.e. aortic valve, aortic arch, brachiocephalic or subclavian arteries.

Q 32. What are the investigations for diagnosis?

1. Doppler ultrasound
2. Ankle brachial pressure index (ABPI) - (Cornerstone of diagnosis)
3. Duplex imaging
4. Arteriography—if intervention is planned
5. DSA (if required)
6. Magnetic resonance angiogram (MRA)
7. Plethysmography
8. Photoplethysmography Not routinely done
9. Transcutaneous oximetry.

Q 33. What is Doppler ultrasound?

The **Doppler signal indicates moving blood**. It does not indicate that the blood flow detected is sufficient to prevent limb loss. A continuous wave of ultrasound signal is transmitted from the probe at an artery. The reflected beam is picked up by a receiver within the probe itself in a case of **hand held Doppler**. The Doppler ultrasound equipment can be used as a sensitive stethoscope in conjunction with sphygmomanometer to assess the systolic pressure in small vessels. This is possible even at sites where the arterial pulse can not be palpated. It can be used to assess the difference in arterial blood pressure between segments of the limb and hence can identify the site of stenosis. In the leg the cuff is commonly placed above the ankle, mid calf, and mid thigh to provide segmental pressure.

Note: **Christian Johann Doppler enunciated Doppler** principle in 1842.

Q 34. What is ankle brachial pressure index (ABPI)?

The ABPI is a quick screening test and is the **cornerstone of diagnosis** in arterial occlusion. A blood pressure cuff is applied above the ankle and the systolic pressure is determined using a Doppler probe at the dorsalis pedis or posterior tibial artery region. Similarly systolic pressure is recorded in the brachial artery using Doppler probe. The higher systolic BP at the ankle is divided by the brachial pressure to give the ABPI. Normally it is **more than 1 or about 1 (100%)**. Vascular disease is confirmed if it is **less than 0.9.** The test may be **repeated after exercise**. Normally ABPI will rise after exercise. In occlusive arterial disease it will fall.

Q 35. What is the relationship between ABPI and vascular symptoms?

ABPI	*Symptoms*
> 0.9	None
0.5 to 0.8	Claudication
0.3 to 0.5	Rest pain
< 0.3	Gangrene

Q 36. What is the fallacy of ABPI?

In **elderly** patients or **diabetics** the tibial artery may be calcified. An elevated pressure is recorded even though the intraluminal pressure is low, since such a vessel cannot be compressed leading to **false-negative** examination. **Wall calcification** should be suspected when ABPI is **more than 1.2** or when the value is out of proportion to the patients clinical status.

Q 37. What are the indications for Doppler and ABPI? **(PG)**

1. For confirming the diagnosis.
2. Objective estimation of the degree of ischemia.
3. Follow-up of patients on conservative treatment.
4. Follow-up of patients after surgery (graft surveillance). A successful bypass must demonstrate a significant increase in ABPI, even if the distal pulse is not palpable.
5. For the diagnosis of diabetic vascular disease.
6. Prediction of healing of ischemic ulcers.
7. Deciding the level of amputation.
8. For intraoperative assessment of the Doppler signal over the graft.

Q 38. What is Duplex imaging?

The duplex imaging is a combination of B mode ultrasound and Doppler. The B mode ultrasound will image the vessels. The Doppler is then used to insonate the imaged vessels and the Doppler shift obtained is analyzed by a computer which will give knowledge about the **blood flow and turbulence.** The new machines are capable of color coding indicating the direction of flow. High flow in a segment suggest stenosis. The duplex imaging is as accurate as arteriography.

Q 39. Do you recommend arteriography in all cases?

No. **Arteriogram is undertaken only after deciding intervention**. This is because arteriography is *invasive* and it is associated with risk (especially so in the case of carotid arteries having the risk of stroke).

Q 40. What are the techniques available for arteriography?

1. Trans lumbar method for aortography (not done now-a-days)
2. The Seldinger technique.

Q 41. What is Seldinger technique?

It is a **retrograde percutaneous catheter method** usually done through the **femoral artery**. It can also be done through **brachial and axillary vessels**. The catheter can be pushed up into the aorta and its various branches depending on the requirement. When vessels like superior mesenteric or inferior mesenteric vessels are selectively cannulated and dye is injected, it is called **selective arteriography.** Through the radial artery or brachial artery the coronary arteries can be cannulated and angiograms obtained to search for coronary artery blocks.

Q 42. What are the complications of arteriogram? **(PG)**

1. Allergic
2. Anaphylactic reactions
3. Thrombosis of the vessel
4. Hematoma formation
5. Arterial dissection
6. Neurological dysfunction
7. Renal dysfunction.

Q 43. What are the dyes used for arteriography?

1. Meglumine diatrozoate
2. Ionohexal
3. Carbon dioxide
4. Gadolinium.

Q 44. What are the angiographic informations to be looked for?

1. Site of the occlusion
2. Extent of the occlusion
3. Nature of occlusion
4. **Run in**—patency of the vessel proximal to the occlusion
5. **Distal run off**—patency of the vessel distal to the occlusion
6. State of collateral circulation.

Q 45. What is distal run-off?

It is the patency of the artery distal to the obstruction demonstrated by arteriography. Arterial bypass surgery is feasible only if a named distal artery is open beyond the block where the anastomosis can be done.

Q 46. What is run-in?

It is the state of arteries proximal to the stenosis (whether it is normal or not). If the proximal artery also is occluded the patient will not benefit from a bypass. In a planned femeropopliteal bypass, it will not function if the ipsilateral iliac artery has got a significant stenosis.

Q 47. Is it possible to do arterial revascularization in Buerger's disease?

It is not usually possible because it is a disease of the small arteries and distal run-off is absent.

Q 48. What is Digital substraction angiography (DSA)?

A computer system is used to digitize the angiographic images. This allows precontrast injection images to be substracted from the contrast image, removing the extraneous background and providing clarity. This can be carried out by injecting the contrast intra-arterially or intravenously. Intravenous injection of the contrast avoids arterial puncture but the only problem is that large volumes of contrast agent is required for the investigation.

Q 49. What is magnetic resonance angiography (MRA)?

It is a **multiplanar imaging** without arterial puncture, catheters, or ionizing radiation. The principle is **rearrangements of hydrogen atoms** in a strong magnetic field. We can image the vascular tree and the soft tissue surrounding the vessel. The dye used is called **gadolinium** (non-iodine containing). This dye is not nephrotoxic and therefore can be used in patients with compromised renal function.

Q 50. What is plethysmography? (PG)

It is a device to measure the volume of an organ or extremity. The pulse volume recording, i.e. the change in the volume of an extremity between systole and diastole is a reflection of the pulsatile blood flow. **It is not routinely done**.

Q 51. What is photoplethysmography? (PG)

It is a measurement of the blood in the cutaneous microcirculation by detecting the reflection of infra-red light.

Q 52. What is transcutaneous oximetry? (PG)

It is the measurement of intracutaneous oxygen tension (PO_2) by placing the probe over the skin surface. Normally it is **40–70 mm of Hg.** When the $TCPO_2$ is less than 30 mm of Hg, the part will go in for gangrene.

Q 53. What is gangrene? (See definitions)

Macroscopic death of tissue with putrefaction is called gangrene.

Q 54. How will you classify gangrene according to etiology?

Causes for gangrene

1. *Secondary to arterial obstruction*
   - Atherosclerosis
   - Buerger's disease
   - Embolism
   - Diabetic arteriopathy
   - Raynaud's disease
   - Iatrogenic—intra-arterial injection like thiopentone
2. *Infective gangrene*
   - Carbuncle
   - Gas gangrene
   - Fournier's gangrene (gangrene of scrotum)
3. *Traumatic*
   - Direct arterial injury—Crush injury, pressure sores
   - Indirect arterial injury—Injury to vessels at some distance from the site of gangrene, e.g. Injury to popliteal artery by fractured lower end of femur
   - Physical agents—burns, scalds, frost bite, electrical, irradiation, etc.
   - Chemical
4. *Venous gangrene.*

Note: **Mnemonic** for the secondary causes of **gangrene is BREASTED.**

B – Buerger's disease
R – Raynaud's disease
E – Ergot intake
A – Arterial injection (Thiopentone)
S – Senile (Atherosclerosis)
T – Thrombosis
E – Embolism
D – Diabetes

Q 55. What is the clinical appearance of gangrene?
Gangrenous part **lacks** the following:

- Arterial pulsation
- Venous return
- Capillary response to pressure
- Sensation
- Warmth
- Function.

The color of the part varies from pallor, mottled grey, dark brown, greenish black, and finally black.

Q 56. What is the cause for black appearance?
It is due to the formation of **iron sulphide** as a result of disintegration of hemoglobin.

Q 57. What are the clinical types of gangrene?

a. Dry gangrene—slow arterial occlusion alone —the affected part becomes **dry and wrinkled.**
b. Wet gangrene (moist gangrene)—arterial and venous obstruction is present. **Infection** is always present. The affected part is **swollen and discolored.** The epidermis may be raised as **blebs. Crepitus** may be palpated (gas forming organisms).

Q 58. What is the line of demarcation?

It is zone of demarcation between the truly viable and dead or dying tissues indicated on the surface by a band of **hyperemia and hyperesthesia.** The separation of the dead and living tissue is achieved by the development of a layer of **granulation tissue** which will advance into the dead tissue until it can get nourishment.This is followed by ulceration and final line of the demarcation.

In **dry gangrene** the separation is by **aseptic ulceration** (final line of demarcation in a few days).

In **moist gangrene** the separation is by **septic ulceration** (here there is more infection and suppuration reaching the neighbouring living tissues and the separation takes long time and will be more proximal than dry gangrene). The moist gangrene should be converted to dry gangrene.

Q 59. What is skip lesion?

Appearance of black patches on the other side of the foot or proximally in the calf is suggestive of spreading of gangrene due to arterial occlusion and a proximal amputation may be required.

Q 60. What is pre-gangrene?

The term pre-gangrene is used by clinicians to describe the changes in tissues indicating that the blood supply to the part is precarious and it will soon be inadequate to keep the tissues alive. The principle symptom is rest pain and the **signs** are:

1. Pallor on elevation
2. Congestion when dependent
3. Coldness
4. Tenderness.

Q 61. What is the treatment of gangrene?

- Exposure of gangrenous area for desiccation
- Protection of local pressure areas (the skin of heel and malleoli)
- Removal of the hard desiccated skin for release of pus in other areas
- The gangrenous part must be removed
- A limb saving attitude is required
- The poor blood supply proximal to the gangrene in the given case can be improved by surgery or percutaneous angioplasty.
- General measures—control of diabetes
  - Control of pain
  - Treatment of cardiac failure
  - Correction of anemia
  - Improve tissue oxygenation.

Q 62. What is the difference between Raynaud's disease and Raynaud's syndrome?

Raynaud's disease is an idiopathic condition occurring in young women due to **abnormal sensitivity of the arterioles to cold** affecting upper limbs more than the lower limbs.

Raynaud's syndrome is a **secondary phenomenon**, secondary to underlying systemic disorder often one of the collagen diseases. The clinical features are much more aggressive. It is seen in diseases like:

- Collagen diseases

Peripheral arterial manifestations of the diseases like:

- Systemic lupus erythematosus (SLE)
- Rheumatoid arthritis (RA) manifestations of the disease
- Vibration white finger (seen in those who are using vibrating tools like pneumatic drills, chain saws, etc.).

Q 63. What are the manifestations of Raynaud's disease?

Characteristically it is **painful and paroxysmal** and the sequences are:

- *Blanching*—constriction of arterioles
- *Dusky cyanosis*—capillaries then dilate and fill with deoxygenated blood
- *Red engorgement*—the arterioles relax and oxygenated blood returns to the capillaries Gangrene is usually uncommon.

Q 64. What is the treatment of Raynaud's disease?

1. Protection from cold—Electrically heated gloves in winter
2. Avoidance of pulp and nail bed infection
3. Calcium antagonists—Nifedipine
4. Sympathectomy.

Q 65. What is the treatment of Raynaud's syndrome?

1. Treatment of the primary condition
2. Gangrene will occur in secondary and may require multiple amputations
3. Nifedipine
4. Steroids
5. Sympathectomy is ineffective.

Q 66. What is acrocyanosis?

It is painless and not paroxysmal affecting the young females producing cyanosis of fingers and legs accompanied by paresthesia. Sympathectomy may be useful.

Q 67. How will you classify limb ischemia?

Can be classified as—

- Acute limb ischemia
- Chronic limb ischemia
- Acute on chronic limb ischemia.

Q 68. What is the basic difference between acute and chronic limb ischemia? (PG)

Acute occlusion leads to gangrene unless revascularization is done. **Chronic occlusive disease** allows time for collateral arterial formation. In chronic, mild ischemia gives rise to intermittent claudication. But when the residual vessels are unable to provide enough blood to support the resting metabolic needs a state of **critical ischemia** is reached accompanied by the symptoms of rest pain and gangrene.

Q 69. What is critical limb ischemia? (PG)

Two criteria:

1. Recurring **rest pain that persists for more than 2 weeks,** requiring regular analgesics with ankle systolic pressure of < **50 mm of Hg** or toe systolic pressure < **30 mm of Hg** and ABPI < 0.5.
2. **Ulceration or gangrene** of the foot or toes with similar hemodynamic parameters.

Q 70. What are the causes for chronic arterial occlusion?

Common causes:

1. Atherosclerosis
2. Buerger's disease
3. Arteritis—Takayasu's disease, SLE
4. Post-traumatic—direct injury, radiation.

Rare causes:

1. External – Thoracic outlet syndrome compression
   – Popliteal entrapment
2. Developmental – Coarctation anomalies
3. Arterial wall disorders – Fibromuscular dysplasia
   – Cystic medial necrosis.

Q 71. What is the management of the given case?

General measures

- Stop smoking (vascular bypass will get occluded earlier in smokers)
- Keep walking (exercise is to be encouraged, walking within the limit of disability)
- Care of the foot – well fitting footwear
  – heel raise—the claudication distance can be improved by 1cm heel raise
- Diet—weight reduction in obese patients
- Control of diabetes and hypertension.

Pharmacological therapy

- Analgesics—opioid should be avoided
- Antiplatelet agents—aspirin – 75–300 mg daily—Clopidogrel
- Pentoxifylline 400–800 mg tablet 3 times daily alters the blood viscosity (useful in intermittent claudication)
- Naftidrofuryl oxalate (Praxilene)—May alter the tissue metabolism and increase the claudication distance
- Prostaglandin E1 (Alpostin)—Useful in critical limb ischemia in doses of 100 mg daily (over 10 hrs) for five days monthly × 6 months.

Surgical procedures

The given case needs **above knee amputation** because of the nonhealing ischemic ulcer in the heel with aortoiliac occlusion. His general condition and comorbid factors makes him unsuitable for aorto femoral revascularization. If patient's general condition is good and there is no ischemic ulcer of the heel the following surgical procedures are recommended for him.

- Ray amputation of big toe
- Aortofemoral bypass graft or if the contralateral femoral is normal a femoro-femoral cross over graft or an axillofemoral bypass graft may be tried for revascularization of the limb.

Q 72. What is the role of surgery in peripheral vascular disease?

Can be divided into **3 broad groups**.

1. **Direct arterial surgery**
   - Percutaneous transluminal angioplasty and stenting
   - Endarterectomy
   - Bypass graft.
2. **Lumbar sympathectomy**
3. **Amputations.**

Q 73. What are the indications for direct arterial surgery? (PG)

1. Critical limb ischemia
2. Severe intermittent claudication which is incapacitating
3. To lower the level of the amputation.

Q 74. What is percutaneous transluminal angioplasty and where it is used?

It involves a femoral angiogram during which a guide wire is inserted and a balloon catheter is then inserted over the guide wire and positioned within the stenosis. Now the balloon is inflated for 1 minute and then deflated. In cases where the vessels fail to stay adequately dilated it may be possible to hold the lumen using metal stent. The catheter is removed. Now self-expanding stents are available. It is used in the following situations.

- Coronary artery (widely used)
- Iliac vessels
- Vessels of the lower limb
- Vessels of the upper limb
- Renal arteries
- Mesenteric vessels.

Q 75. What is endarterectomy?

The occluded intima and a part of the media are removed by coring them out through an artificial plane created in the media. This is usually done for large arteries like aorta. Nowadays it is rarely done.

Q 76. What is bypass graft? (PG)

A native vein (usually *saphenous vein*) or a *prosthetic material* is used for bypassing the obstruction in the vessel. The bypass procedures can be classified as—

- Anatomic, e.g. femoropopliteal bypass
- Extra anatomic—femoro-femoral crossover graft.
  - iliofemoral crossover graft
  - Axillobifemoral.

Q 77. What are the materials used for bypass graft?

- Reversed long saphenous vein (**the most useful and successful conduit**)—if the long saphenous vein is not available short saphenous vein or arm vein may be used.
- PTFE (Poly Tetra Fluro Ethylene)
- Dacron - two types—Woven and Knitted (Knitted prosthesis are sealed with gelatin or collagen)
- Human umbilical vein (Glutaraldehyde—tanned, Dacron supported).

Q 78. How will you choose the prosthetic material? (PG)

It depends on the site of disease and the type of operation.

The patients own saphenous vein gives the best results when used either as a reversed conduit or as **in situ** after valve disruption.

Q 79. What are the bypass operations done for peripheral vascular disease?

Bypass operations depending on the level of occlusion	
Site of disease	*Type of operation*
1. Aortoiliac occlusion	Aortobifemoral bypass surgery.
2. Unilateral Iliac occlusion alone	Percutaneous transluminal angioplastyalone (PTA) with or without stent or endarterectomy In patients unable to withstand abdominal surgery femorofemoral or iliofemoral crossover bypass graft (8 mm PTFE or dacron graft tunnelled subcutaneously above the pubis)
3. Bilateral iliac occlusion with pregangrenous limb on one side	Axillofemoral graft to the affected side with 8 mm PTFE
4. Superficial femoral with profunda femoris occlusion	Femoropopliteal graft artery using autogenoussaphenous vein or human umbilical vein

Note:

- For long distance claudication conservative treatment is wise.
- Salvage operations should not be performed for intermittent claudication alone. Gangrene and loss of limb may occur if the operation fails.
- Any vein used for anastomosis requires a diameter of at least 3 mm.
- The size of suture material used for anastomosis from groin down is 4/0–5/0 polypropylene.
- Femoro-distal bypasses are usually carried out using long saphenous vein preferably in situ.

Q 80. What is in situ bypass graft? (PG)

This is done for femoropopliteal bypass graft. The long saphenous vein is not removed and reversed in this operation. Instead it is left in place (in situ) and the valves disrupted with a valvulotome. The vein is then anastomosed to the femoral artery proximally and to the popliteal vessel distally.

Q 81. What is profundaplasty? (PG)

The common femoral artery and its branches are exposed. After giving heparin IV and clamping the vessel an incision is made into the common femoral artery and carried down into the profunda dividing the stenotic profunda origin. The arteriotomy is then closed with a patch of vein to widen the narrowed segment.

Q 82. What is the role of lumbar sympathectomy?

This should only be done if there is no chance for direct arterial surgery or angioplasty**. It has no role in the treatment of intermittent claudication.** The indications are:

- Nonhealing ischemic ulcers
- Ischemic rest pain
- Vasospastic conditions
- Hyperhidrosis
- Causalgia.

Q 83. What is lumbar sympathectomy?

In lumbar sympathectomy the **second, third and fourth** lumbar sympathetic **ganglia** are removed. The removal of bilateral first lumbar ganglia will result in retrograde ejaculation. The operation can be done either by **open or laparoscopic** method. The open method is done by extra-peritoneal approach using a loin incision. The sympathetic trunk lies on the side of the bodies of the lumbar vertebrae on the right side overlapped by IVC. **Care is taken** not to mistake and remove small lymph nodes and tendinous strip of psoas minor. It is also important to avoid the genitofemoral nerve.

Q 84. What is chemical sympathectomy?

Under **radiographic fluoroscopic control** with the patient in the lateral position after giving local anesthesia a **long spinal needle** is inserted to seek the side of vertebral body to reach the lumbar sympathetic chain. **5 mL of phenol in water** (1:16) is injected after confirming the needle position by injecting contrast agent. It is carried out in two sites beside the bodies of second to fourth lumbar vertebrae. It is important to avoid aorta, IVC and ureters. It is contraindicated in patients taking anticoagulants.

Q 85. What is the role of amputation?

Amputation is inevitable when the arterial surgery and conservative treatment fail. The commonly performed amputations are:

1. Ray amputations for gangrene of toes
2. Transmetatarsal for fore foot gangrene
3. Below knee (BK) amputation—if the gangrene is limited to foot
4. AK (above knee) amputation—if the gangrene is approaching to the leg.

Note: The BK amputation is functionally far superior to AK amputation provided the popliteal is patent.

Discussion on Acute Lower Limb Ischemia

Q 1. What are the causes for acute limb ischemia?

The causes may **traumatic or non-traumatic.**

Non-traumatic

Common causes:

1. **Embolism** (commonest in developing countries)
2. **Thrombosis of a native artery**—at sites of arterial stenosis due to disorders like atherosclerosis, Buerger's disease, etc. Thrombosis of an artery can occur in hypercoagulable states like malignancy, protein C, protein S, and antithrombin III deficiency.
3. Thrombosis of a **bypass graft** (commonest in developed countries).

Rare causes:

1. Thrombosed popliteal artery aneurysm
2. Aortic dissection
3. Popliteal artery entrapment syndrome.

Q 2. What are the clinical features of acute embolism?

Six Ps

- Pain
- Pallor
- Pulseless ness
- Paresthesia
- Paralysis
- Poikilothermia (cold limb).

Clinically important features are:

- Sudden loss of previously palpable pulse
- Coldness of the limb
- Severe continuous pain
- Sensory disturbances like tingling, numbness and complete loss of sensation
- Paralysis of the limb—which is usually a late feature.

Q 3. What is the critical period for revascularization. (PG)

Ischemia of the tissues distal to the site of occlusion begins from the moment of occlusion. The extent of damage to various tissues depends on the cell type and their metabolic rate. In the limb the **peripheral nerves** are most sensitive to ischemia followed **by muscles, subcutaneous tissue and skin.** Reversible ischemia will occur after **6 hours.** Histological changes can develop by **4 hours** of warm ischemia. Pre-existing collaterals may delay this event. By **12 hours** ischemic muscles undergo irreversible changes. Muscle rigidity will occur over the next **12–24 hours.**

Q 4. What are the clinical differences between acute thrombosis and embolism?

Differences between thrombosis and embolism

Feature	*Thrombosis*	*Embolism*
Onset	Gradual	Sudden
History of claudication	Common	None
Contralateral pulse	Often absent	Normal
Source of embolus	None	Usually heart showing either valvular disease or fibrillation
Temperature changes	Less marked	More marked
Loss of function	Slow - because collaterals are there	Rapid loss of function (4–6 hrs)
Angiography	Diffuse disease	Minimal disease
"	Tapered and irregular cut off	Sharp cut off
"	Collaterals well-developed	Few collaterals

Q. 5. What are the causes for peripheral arterial embolism?

It is classified as cardiac, noncardiac and cryptogenic.

Cardiac—(80–90%)

- Atrial fibrillation
- Myocardial infarction
- Cardiac valvular prosthesis
- Rare causes like atrial myxoma.

Noncardiac

- Atherosclerotic disease (plaques in proximal arteries)
- Aneurysm in proximal arteries
- Noncardiac tumors
- Foreign bodies—broken cannula.

Cryptogenic—Unknown inspite of investigation (5–10% of cases).

Q 6. What is the classification for severity of acute limb ischemia? (PG)

Class 1 (viable)
- No persisting pain
- No motor and sensory deficits
- Doppler signals audible

Class 2a (marginally threatened)
- Numbness/paresthesia
- Digital sensory loss
- No audible Doppler signals

Class 2b (immediately threatened)
- Above and persistent ischemic pain
- Sensory and motor deficit

Class 3 (irreversible)
- Profound anesthesia and paralysis may be early and late.

Q 7. What is the management of acute limb ischemia? (PG)

Once the diagnosis is made patient should be heparinized.

Contrast angiography is still considered the gold standard investigation of choice.

C-arm facility and peroperative angiograms are necessary.

The site of entry for angiogram should be preferably the contralateral limb.

In case of bilateral lower limb problem the brachial artery should be the entry point.

Immediate revascularization is required either by **surgical** (**embolectomy by Fogarty or open thrombectomy with or without bypass procedures**) **or endovascular procedures.**

Class 1 and 2	– Angiography and thrombolysis
Class 2b and 3 early	– Emergency surgery
Class 3 late	– Delayed amputation

For distal embolism thrombolytic therapy is preferred.

Q 8. What is embolectomy?

- The femoral artery is exposed under general anesthesia or local anesthesia.
- Longitudinal arteriotomy is made after placing vascular clamps.
- A Fogarty catheter of appropriate size is passed proximally, the bulb inflated, and catheter gently pulled down to extract the blood clot. This is repeated until a good antegrade flow is obtained.
- The same procedure is repeated in the distal artery until good back flow is obtained.
- Heparin is given IV. (5000 units) and anti-coagulation is continued postoperatively.
- Arteriotomy is closed by continuous suture with 5/0 or 6/0 polypropelene.
- Fasciotomy of the distal muscle is recommended if the ischemic time has exceeded 6 hours.

Q 9. What is thrombolytic therapy? (PG)

This will bring about lysis of fibrin by stimulating the plasmin system. **It cannot be done in a limb threatened with gangrene.** It may take upto 48 hours to lyse the thrombus. Old clots cannot be lysed by thrombolytic therapy. Duration of the procedure is lengthy. The commonly used agents are:

- Streptokinase (A bacterial enzyme)—Cheap but antigenic—Anaphylaxis is a problem.
- Urokinase (Extracted from renal parenchymal cells).
- Tissue plasminogen activator (TPA-Synthetic).

Q 10. What are the contraindications for Thrombolytic therapy? (PG)

- Recent stroke
- Recent surgery
- History of GI hemorrhage
- Pregnancy
- Uncontrolled hypertension
- Allergy to the agent.

Case

15 Lymphoma

Case Capsule

A 20-year-old male patient presents with **weight loss, malaise, pyrexia of unknown origin and drenching night sweats that require change of cloths** for the last 9 months. There is neither history of pruritus, nor alcohol intolerance. There is no abdominal pain after drinking alcohol. He also complains of bilateral supraclavicular swellings for the last 7 months which is painless. There is no history of bone pain.

On examination the patient is **febrile and pale**. There is a **10 × 6 cm** size swelling in the right supraclavicular region and **12 × 8 cm** size swelling in the left supraclavicular region. On palpation, there is neither local rise of temperature nor tenderness over the swelling. It appears to be a **group of lymph nodes** on either side. It **is possible to define individual nodes** and they are **ovoid, smooth and discrete**. The nodes are having **rubbery consistency**. These nodes can be **moved from side to side**. There is no fixity of the nodes. The abdominal examination revealed **enlargement of the liver**, about 4 cm below the costal margin, firm in consistency and the surface is smooth and edge is sharp. The **spleen is also enlarged.** No palpable abdominal nodes detected. There is no free fluid in the abdominal cavity. Examination of other lymph node areas like axillary and inguinal is normal. There is **no evidence of collaterals veins across the chest wall** suggestive of mediastinal mass. There is **no venous congestion of the neck**. Examination of the genitalia is normal.

Read the checklist for examination of abdomen.

Checklist for lymph node examination in section on short cases

Mnemonics for lymph node examination –'PALS' (short case section)

P – Primary (examine the drainage area of the lymph node for a primary lesion)

A – Another node (always look for another node when one group is palpable)

L – Liver (always examine the abdomen for enlargement of liver)

S – Spleen

Remember the 3 lymphatic water sheds of the skin (on each side):

A vertical line through the sagittal plane of the body divides the lymphatic drainage of the skin into 3 areas on each side. There is some communications across the midline. The 3 areas on each side of the body are demarcated from each other by two **horizontal lines one at the level of the clavicle**, the other **at the level of the umbilicus.** These lines are the lymphatic water sheds and the skin lymph flows in a direction away from them. Each line also represents the meeting place of adjacent territories, so that the cancer situated in one of these lines may spread by two routes along the lymphatics running away from the water shed, e.g. **cancer situated at the umbilicus may spread in four directions. Viz: towards both axillae and both groins**, as lymphatics draining to these glands come into communication at the umbilicus. Similarly a cancer situated anywhere in the **midline of the surface of the body** may spread in at least two directions because of the lymphatic communication **across the midline.** Thus, we get 3 groups of lymph nodes draining the three areas.

1. Cervical lymph nodes
2. Axillary lymph nodes
3. Inguinal lymph nodes
    - The lymphatic above the clavicle will drain to the cervical nodes.
    - The lymphatics below the clavicle up to the level of umbilicus will drain to the axilla (both front and back).
    - The lymphatics below the level of umbilicus will drain to the inguinal nodes.
    - If axillary node is enlarged, examine the following drainage areas—breast, front of the chest and upper abdomen up to the umbilicus, back of the chest down up to the level of umbilicus, and the entire upper limb.
    - If the **inguinal lymph node is enlarged**, examine the following drainage areas—the lower abdomen from the level of umbilicus, the corresponding area in the back, the gluteal region, natal cleft, perineum, genitalia, the lower part of the anal canal and the entire lower limb. **The lower limb lymphatics will drain to the vertical group of nodes.** The remaining areas will drain to the **horizontal group** of inguinal nodes. **A digital rectal examination** must be done in all cases of horizontal inguinal lymph node enlargement.
    - When the cervical lymph node is enlarged the drainage areas to be examined will start from the scalp down to the level of the clavicle, including examination of the oral cavity, pharynx (oral and nasal) nasal sinuses and the hidden areas.

Checklist for history

- H/o weight loss (> 10% loss of weight in 6 months)
- H/o fever occurring in a periodic fashion (Pel-Ebstein fever)
- H/o pruritus
- Alcohol-induced nodal pain
- Bone pain (lymphomatous infiltration)
- Pallor
- Family history of leukemias and similar illness.

Checklist for examination

- Look for other groups of lymph nodes
- Look for liver and spleen
- Look for anemia
- Look for jaundice
- Look for venous congestion of the neck and upper chest—superior venacaval obstruction produced by mediastinal masses
- Look for edema of both legs—abdominal masses obstruct the inferior vena cava
- Examine the skin for scaly elevated reddened patches of skin—mycosis fungoides (dermatological manifestations of lymphoma).

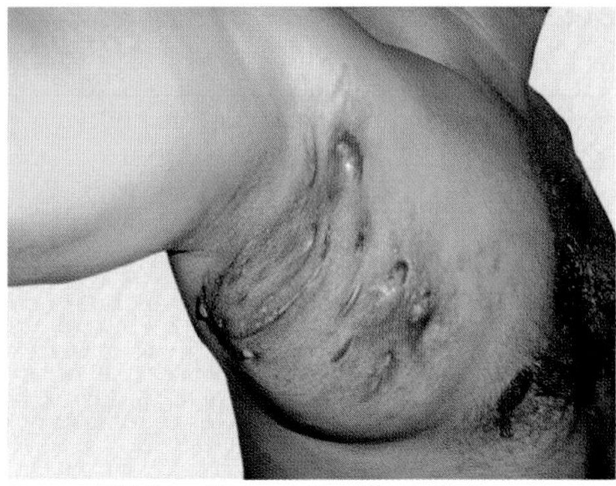

Right axillary node with multiple sinuses-lymphoma

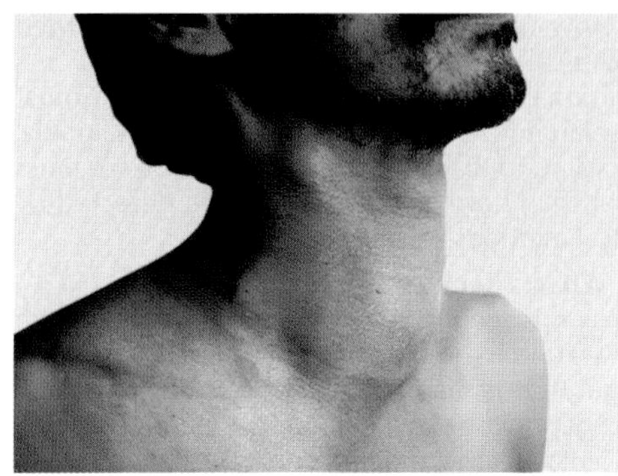

Hodgkin's lymphoma of right cervical node

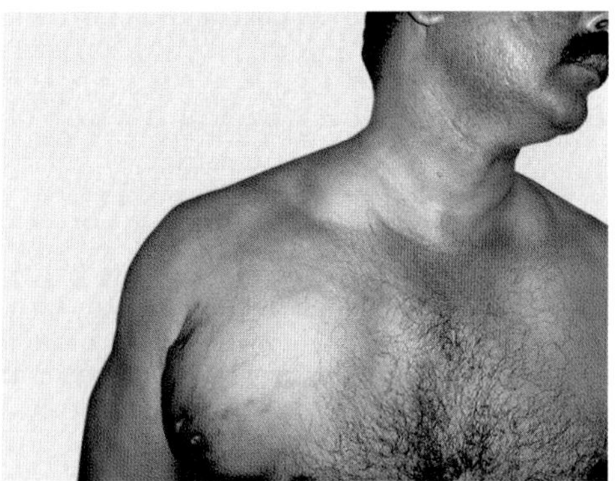

Non-Hodgkin's lymphoma with axillary and right supraclavicular nodes

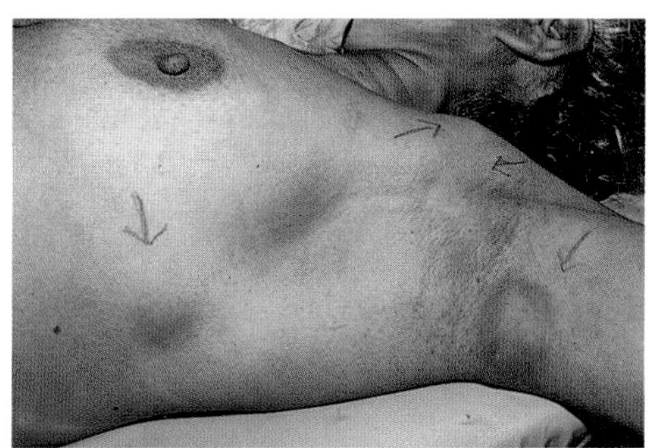

Multiple swellings of Non-Hodgkin's lymphoma

Q 1. What are the physical signs of an enlarged spleen?

Physical signs of enlarged spleen

- It appears from below the tip of the 10th rib
- It enlarges along the line of the rib towards the umbilicus

Contd...

Contd...

- Definite notch will be felt (splenic notch)
- One cannot get above it
- Moves with respiration
- It is dull to percussion
- It is not bimanually palpable.

Q 2. How many times the spleen must be enlarged for clinical palpation?

Traditionally it was taught that the spleen must be enlarged *2–3 times* before it become palpable. According to Blackburn, spleen must be *1½ times* larger than normal, before it can be detected by clinical methods.

Q 3. What is Kenawy's sign?

This sign is seen in splenomegaly associated with **bilharzial cirrhosis** of liver **(Egyptian splenomegaly).** It is also seen in portal hypertension secondary to the above condition. The stethoscope is applied beneath the xiphoid process. This will reveal a venous hum which is louder on inspiration. This is because of the engorgement of the splenic vein and the hum is louder during inspiration because the spleen is compressed during inspiration.

Q 4. What are the causes for splenomegaly?

The causes for splenomegaly can be classified as follows:

Splenomegaly	
Cause	*Conditions*
Neoplastic	• **Benign** conditions like hemangioma (commonest)· • **Malignant** - Hodgkin's lymphoma - Non-Hodgkin's lymphoma (NHL) - Myelofibrosis (abnormal proliferation of mesenchymal elements in the bone marrow, spleen, liver and lymph nodes) - Metastatic disease
Hematologic malignancies	• **Acute leukemia** • **Chronic leukemia**
Hemolyticnemias	• Hereditary spherocytosis • Autoimmune hemolyticnemia • Thalassemia (cooley's anemia, Mediterranean anemia) • Sickle cell disease
Other blood diseases	• Idiopathic thrombocytopenic purpura • Pernicious anemia • Polycythemia vera • Erythroblastosis fetalis
Tropical splenomegaly	• Malaria • Kala-azar • Schistosomiasis • Tropical splenomegaly • Trypanosomiasis
Infective	• **Bacterial** - Typhoid, paratyphoid, tuberculosis, splenic abscess and septicemia • **Viral** - Infectious mononucleosis, HIV related, psittacosis. • **Spirochaetales** - Weil's disease, syphilis • **Parasitic**—Hydatid cyst
Metabolic	• Porphyria (hereditary error of hemoglobin catabolism in which porphyrinurea occurs— the orange colored urine turns to a port-wine color after exposure to the air) • Gaucher's disease (Lipid storage disease) • Amyloid
Collagen disease	• Felty syndrome • Still's disease
Nonparasitic cysts	• True cyst—(lined by flattened epithelium) dermoid and mesenchymal inclusion cyst • False cyst—(pseudocyst)
Circulatory disease	• Portal hypertension • Segmental portal hypertension of pancreatic carcinoma

Q 5. What is hypersplenism?

Hypersplenism is an indefinite clinical syndrome characterized by splenic enlargement, any combination of anemia, leukopenia or thrombocytopenia, compensatory bone marrow hyperplasia and improvement of the condition after splenectomy.

Q 6. What are the clinical characteristics of lymph nodes in lymphoma?

- They cause lymphadenopathy in the posterior triangle
- The nodes are ovoid, smooth and discrete
- Possible to define individual nodes even when they are large (in contrast to tuberculosis)
- The nodes are solid and rubbery
- The nodes can be moved from side-to-side and are rarely fixed to the surrounding structures.

Q 7. What is lymphoma?

It is a primary malignant neoplasm originating from lymphoid tissue of the lymphatic system. There are two types:

1. Hodgkin's disease
2. Non-Hodgkin's disease (NHL).

Q 8. What is lymphoid neoplasm?

Lymphoid neoplasm consists of the following:

- Hodgkin's
- Non-Hodgkin's lymphoma (NHL)
- Lymphatic leukemia
- Plasmacytoma.

Q 9. Why this new nomenclature of lymphoid neoplasm is preferred over lymphoma?

Traditionally, neoplasms that typically present with an **obvious tumor or mass** of lymph nodes or extra nodal sites are **called lymphomas** and neoplasms that typically **involve the bone marrow and peripheral blood** without tumor mass are called **leukemias**.

However, we now know that many B and T/NK – cell neoplasms may have both tissue masses and circulating cells, either in the same patient or from one patient to another. Thus, it is artificial to call them different diseases, when in fact, they are just **different stages or phases of the same disease**.

- Neoplasms that typically produce tumor masses are called **lymphomas**.
- Neoplasms that typically have only circulating cells are called leukemias.
- Those that have both solid and circulating phases are designated lymphoma/leukemia.
- Plasma cell neoplasms including multiple myelomas and plasmacytoma have their origin from B cell are also now included under lymphoid neoplasms.

B cell chronic lymphocytic leukemia and B cell small lymphocytic lymphoma are simply different manifestations of the same neoplasm. (Similarly, lymphoblastic lymphoma and acute lymphoblastic leukemia are different manifestations of the same neoplasm).

Q 10. What is the classic cell of Hodgkin's disease?

The Hodgkin's lymphoma is defined by the histological finding of **Reed-Sternberg** cells. They are binucleate cells. The binucleate cell is having vesicular nuclei and prominent eosinophilic neucleoli (**pennie on plate** appearance or owl eye appearance). The subtype is decided by the pattern of lymphocyte infiltrate.

Q 11. What are the clinical features of mediastinal lymph nodes?

When the nodes are large in the mediastinum, they occlude the superior vena cava, causing venous congestion in the neck and the development of collateral veins across the chest wall. This is called **superior vena cava syndrome**. It may also produce dysphagia or hoarseness of voice. This is one of the classic presentations for **nodular sclerosis** in Hodgkin's.

Q 12. What is the clinical feature of intra-abdominal lymph node mass?

Large nodal masses in the abdomen can obstruct the inferior vena cava and iliac veins producing edema of both lower limbs.

Q 13. Can you differentiate Hodgkin's lymphoma from non-Hodgkin's lymphoma (NHL) clinically? What are the differences between Hodgkin's and NHL?

Clinically it is difficult to differentiate these conditions. The differences are given in Table 15.1.

Q 14. What is the probable diagnosis in this case?

Hodgkin's disease.

Q 15. What are the points in favor of Hodgkin's disease?

- Cervical and axillary lymph node enlargement with hepatosplenomegaly
- Clinical nature of the lymph nodes as mentioned earlier
- The age group of patient (younger age is in favor of Hodgkin's rather than NHL).

Q 16. What are the differential diagnoses?

- NHL
- Leukemias
- Myeloproliferative disorders.

Q 17. Why cannot this be tuberculosis?

- Tuberculosis will produce usually matting of lymph nodes.
- It will not produce hepatosplenomegaly.

Q 18. What are the causes for matting of lymph nodes?

1. Acute lymphadenitis
2. Tuberculosis (Read tuberculosis of lymph nodes)
3. Late stages of lymphoma
4. Late stages of metastasis.

Q 19. What is the WHO Classification of lymphoma (REAL classification)?

Revised European-American classification of Lymphoid neoplasms).

It is a list of distinct disease entities, which are defined by combination of **morphology, immunophenotype** and **genetic features** and which have distinct clinical features. The classification includes all lymphoid neoplasms: Hodgkin's lymphoma, non-Hodgkin's lymphoma, lymphoid leukemias and plasma cell neoplasms.

B Cell Neoplasms

Precursor B-cell Neoplasm

- Precursor B-lymphoblastic leukemia/lymphoma (precursor B-cell acute lymphoblastic leukemia).

Mature (peripheral) B-cell neoplasms

- B-cell chronic lymphocytic leukemia/small lymphocytic lymphoma
- B-cell pro lymphocytic leukemia
- Lymphoplasmacytic lymphoma
- Splenic marginal zone B-cell lymphoma (with or without villous lymphocytes)
- Hairy cell leukemia
- Plasma cell myeloma/plasmacytoma
- Extra nodal marginal zone B-cell lymphoma of MALT type
- Nodal marginal zone B-cell lymphoma (with or without monocytoid B cells)
- Follicular lymphoma
- Mantle cell lymphoma
- Diffuse large B-cell lymphoma
- Burkitt lymphoma/Burkitt cell leukemia.

T Cell and NK Cell Neoplasms

Precursor T-Cell Neoplasm

- Precursor T-lymphoblastic lymphoma/leukemia (precursor T-cell acute lymphoblastic leukemia).

Mature (peripheral) T/NK-cell neoplasms

- T-cell pro lymphocytic leukemia
- T-cell granular lymphocytic leukemia
- Aggressive NK-cell leukemia
- Adult T-cell lymphoma/leukemia (HTLVI +)
- Extra nodal NK/T cell lymphoma, nasal type
- Enteropathy—type T-cell lymphoma
- Hepatosplenic T-cell lymphoma
- Subcutaneous panniculitis-like T- cell lymphoma
- Mycosis fungoides/Sezary syndrome
- Anaplastic large cell lymphoma, T/null cell, primary cutaneous type
- Peripheral T-cell lymphoma, not otherwise characterized
- Angioimmunoblastic T-cell lymphoma
- Anaplastic large cell lymphoma, T/null cell, primary systemic type.

Q 20. What is the staging of Hodgkin's lymphoma?

Ann-Arbor staging

Stage	*Description*
Stage I	Involvement of a single lymph node region (*I*) or localized involvement of a single extra lymphatic organ or site in the absence of any lymph node involvement **(1E) (rare in Hodgkin's lymphoma)**
Stage II	Involvement of **two or more lymph node regions on the same side of the diaphragm (II)**; or localized involvement of a single extralymphatic organ or site in association with regional lymph node involvement with or without involvement of other lymph node regions on the same side of the diaphragm **(IIE)**. The number of regions involved may be indicated by a subscript, as in, for example, $\mathbf{II_3}$
Stage III	Involvement of **lymph node regions on both sides of the diaphragm (III)** which also may be accompanied by extra lymphatic extension in association with adjacent lymph node involvement **(IIIE)** or by involvement of the spleen **(IIIS)** or both **(III E, S)**
Stage IV	**Diffuse or disseminated** involvement of one or more extralymphatic organs, with or without associated lymph node involvement or isolated extralymphatic organ involvement in the absence of adjacent regional lymph node involvement, but in conjunction with disease in distant site (s). **Any involvement of the liver or bone marrow or nodular involvement of the lung (s)**. The location of stage IV disease is defined further by specifying the site according to the notation.

Note: All stages are having A/B stages depending on the absence or presence of B symptoms.

Q 21. What are B symptoms?

The B symptoms are:

- Weight loss—unexplained weight loss of > 10% of the usual body weight in 6 months prior to diagnosis

- Fever—unexplained fever with temperature > 38°C
- Drenching night sweats—that require change of bedclothes.

Note: Pruritus alone does not qualify for B classification nor does alcohol intolerance, fatigue or a short febrile illness associated with suspected infection.

Q 22. What are the pathological types of Hodgkin's disease?

Major categories of Hodgkin's lymphoma are:

- Nodular lymphocyte predominance Hodgkin's lymphoma (NLPHL)
- Classic Hodgkin's lymphoma (CHL)—further divisions given below:

Classic Hodgkin's Lymphoma

Sub type	*Characteristics*
1. Lymphocyte rich classic Hodgkin's lymphoma (*LRCHL*)	*Uncommon-6%*. Few Reed-Sternberg cells Diffuse lymphocytes – *excellent prognosis*
2. Lymphocyte depletion Hodgkin's lymphoma (*LDHL*) *Older males* affected *Aggressive*	*Rare-2%* Abundant Reed-Sternberg cells Paucity of lymphocyte
3. Mixed cellularity Hodgkin's lymphoma *(MCHL)*	*Common 20 – 25%* often presents with disseminated disease
4. Nodular sclerosis Hodgkin's lymphoma *(NSHL)*	*Commonest – 70%* Fibrosis present, Reed-Sternberg cells and lymphocytes seen. *Young women* affected Cervical and Mediastinal disease

Q 23. What are the features of the lymphocyte predominant Hodgkin's lymphoma?

- Considered to be an indolent B-cell lymphoma
- More common in young men and old ages
- Infradiaphragmatic disease common than Hodgkin's disease
- Bulky disease and splenic involvement uncommon
- Natural history like low grade NHL
- Can have delayed relapses
- Can progress to large B-cell lymphomas.

Q 24. What is nodal/extra nodal disease?

For the purpose of coding and staging, **lymph nodes, Waldeyer's ring, and spleen are considered nodalor lymphatic sites.**

Extra nodal or extra lymphatic sites include the following:

- Bone marrow
- Gastrointestinal tract
- Skin
- Bone
- Central nervous system
- Lung
- Gonads
- Ocular adnexa
- Liver
- Kidneys and uterus.

Note:

- Hodgkin's lymphoma rarely presents in extra-nodal site
- About 25% of NHL is extra nodal at presentation
- Mycosis fungoides (a type of NHL affecting the skin) and MALT lymphomas are virtually always extra nodal.

Q 25. What is the 'E Lesion' for Hodgkin's lymphoma?

- The Ann-Arbor system defined E as extra lymphatic.
- Disease in sites such as Waldeyer's ring, the thymus, and the spleen although extra nodal is not extra lymphatic and therefore not considered to be 'E Lesion'.

According to the revised AJCC system the E Lesion is defined as disease that involves extra lymphatic sites (s) adjacent to site (s) of lymphatic involvement but in which direct extension is not necessarily demonstrable. **Examples of E lesions include extension into**:

- Pulmonary parenchyma from adjacent pulmonary hilar/mediastinal nodes
- Extension into the anterior chest wall and into the pericardium from mediastinal mass
- Involvement of iliac bone from adjacent lymph node
- Involvement of lumbar vertebral body from para-aortic nodes
- Involvement of pleura from internal mammary nodes
- Involvement of thyroid from adjacent cervical lymph nodes.

Note 1: It is proposed that for *NHL, the E designation should indicate the presentation of lymphoma in extra nodal sites* and the lack of an E designation should indicate lymphoma presenting in lymph nodes.
Note 2: Liver is designated as H; bone marrow designated as M and spleen is designated as S.

Q 26. In which core nodal region, the infraclavicular nodes are included (Read core nodal regions in NHL section)?

It is considered as part of the axilla.

Q 27. What are the other lymphatic structures other than lymph nodes?

The lymphatic structures in the body:

- Lymph nodes
- Spleen
- Appendix
- Peyer's patches
- Waldeyer's ring
- Thymus.

Q 28. What is splenic involvement in Hodgkin's disease?

- Evidence of one or more nodules in the spleen of any size on imaging evaluation
- Histologic involvement documented by biopsy or splenectomy.

Note: Splenic enlargement alone is insufficient to support a diagnosis of splenic involvement.

Q 29. What is hepatic involvement in Hodgkin's?

- One or more nodules in the liver of any size on imaging
- Histological involvement documented by biopsy.

Note: Hepatic enlargement alone is insufficient.

Q 30. What is bone marrow involvement?

Bone marrow involvement must be documented by biopsy from a clinically/radiographically uninvolved area of bone. Bone marrow involvement is designated by the letter M. **Bone marrow involvement is always considered as diffuse extra lymphatic disease (stage IV).**

Q 31. What are the unfavorable types of Hodgkin's disease?

1. The presence of B symptoms
2. Unfavorable histology—**mixed cellularity and lymphocyte depleted**.

Q 32. What is the most important confirmatory investigation for this case?

Lymph node biopsy.

Q 33. Is there any role for FNAC of the lymph node?

For the diagnosis of lymphoma a **node biopsy is a must** in order to study the histological background and architecture of the lymph node. FNAC can be done as a screening investigation if more than one node is palpable. The needle aspiration will produce anomalies in the node and it will be difficult for the histopathologist to interpret this node, if it is taken for biopsy later.

Q 34. Which lymph node is taken for biopsy and what are the precautions for lymph node biopsy?

- The largest and most central node in a group is most likely to be diagnostic.
- The inguinal nodes are avoided because they often show changes of chronic infection (if other enlarged nodes are available).
- A cervical node is preferred to the axillary or inguinal group.
- Always take an intact node for biopsy.
- Biopsied node should be handled gently.
- Imprint of freshly cut node may be done if this is available (imprint cytology).
- Avoid nodes which are aspirated for biopsy.
- For imprint cytology purpose the node should be send in a bottle containing saline.

Q 35. What is the staging work up?

Clinical staging includes:

- Careful recording of medical history
- Physical examination
- Imaging of chest, abdomen and pelvis
- Complete blood count
- Blood chemistry
- Bone marrow biopsy

Recommendations for the diagnostic evaluation of patients with lymphoma.

A. Mandatory procedure

1. Biopsy, with interpretation by a qualified pathologist
2. History, with special attention to the presence and duration of fever, night sweats, and unexplained loss of 10% or more of body weight in the previous 6 months
3. Physical examination
4. Laboratory tests
   a. Complete blood cell count and platelet count
   b. Erythrocyte sedimentation rate
   c. Liver function tests
5. Radiographic examination
   a. Chest X-ray
   b. CT of chest, abdomen and pelvis
   c. Gallium scan
6. Bone marrow biopsy.

B. Ancillary procedures

1. Laparotomy and splenectomy if decisions regarding management are likely to be influenced
2. Liver biopsy (needle), if there is a strong clinical indication of hepatic involvement
3. Radioisotopic bone scans, in selected patients with bone pain
4. CT of head and neck in extra nodal or nodal presentation to define disease extent
5. Gastroscopy and/or GI series in patients with GI presentations
6. MRI of spine in patients with suspected spinal involvement
7. CSF cytology in patients with Stage IV disease and bone marrow involvement, testis involvement, or parameningeal involvement.

Q 36. What are the indications for bone marrow biopsy?

- B symptoms
- Anemia

- Leukopenia
- Thrombocytopenia.

Q 37. What is the role of staging laparotomy? (PG)

Staging laparotomy is **not done nowadays** after CT has become part of the staging work up where by most of the nodal status and disease process can be ascertained. 40% of the patients require chemotherapy because of the reasons mentioned below and therefore, a staging laparotomy is omitted.

- It has got significant morbidity in 10% of patients.
- It is considered when the results are likely to alter the treatment strategy (chemotherapy vs radiation). If the chemotherapy will be used regardless of the finding on laparotomy, there is no need for staging laparotomy. Hodgkin's disease that is localized may be curable by radiation therapy if all involved nodes are included in the treatment field. Non-Hodgkin's lymphomas are usually treated with chemotherapy because of wide-spread nodal and extra-nodal involvement especially of the bone marrow. Therefore, laparotomy is unnecessary in NHL.
- Considered only in special situations of stage IIa or less in which mantle radiation is planned.
- In children, splenectomy will produce overwhelming postsplenectomy sepsis (OPSI)—0.1%/year
- In 20% of the cases, the stage is upstaged by staging laparotomy and therefore, will require chemotherapy
- About 20% of the patients will develop relapse requiring chemotherapy.

Q 38. What are the important steps in staging laparotomy? (PG)

In staging laparotomy the following procedures are done:

- Splenectomy
- Wedge biopsy of liver
- Biopsy—nodes of the paraaortic, splenic hilar, hepatic, portal, and iliac nodes—the suspicious nodes are clipped
- Oophoropexy in women (childbearing age) which will allow radiation therapy to be given to the inverted 'Y' field which covers the iliac and inguinal nodes without radiation damage to the ovaries.

Q 39. Which are the nodal regions affected by Hodgkin's disease?

Mediastinal	– 60%
Pure infradiaphragmatic	– 3%
Extra nodal	– 5 – 10%
Splenomegaly	– 10%

Q 40. What are the etiological factors for Hodgkin's disease? (PG)

1. Siblings with Hodgkin's disease
2. HLA antigens
3. Patients who have undergone tonsillectomy
4. Immunodeficiency states
5. Autoimmune disorders
6. Oncogenic viruses
7. Epstein-Barr virus (EBV)—Nuclear protein in 40% of Hodgkin's
8. Lymphotropic viruses.

Q 41. What is the antigen in Hodgkin's disease? (PG)

It is *CD 30* positive, which is a surface antigen seen in Reed-Sternberg cells.

Other CD markers:

- NK cell—CD 54
- Leukocyte antigen—CD 45
- Stem cells—CD 34
- T cells—CD 3, 4, 5, 15 and 30
- B cells—CD 19, 20, 21, 22

Rituximab is a Monoclonal antibody against CD 20.

Q 42. What is the stage of the disease in the given case?

Stage III because of the infradiaphragmatic involvement.

Q 43. What is early stage disease?

- Stage IA and IIA
- Nonbulky disease.

Q 44. What is bulky disease? (PG)

- 10 cm diameter mass or more
- Mediastinal disease with transverse diameter exceeding 1/3rd of the transverse thoracic diameter is defined as bulky disease.

Q 45. What is the treatment of Hodgkin's disease?

The treatment is classified as:

- Radiotherapy—curative radiation therapy is given to 3 major fields known as:
  - Mantle
  - Para-aortic
  - Pelvic (inverted Y fields)
- The lungs, heart, larynx, kidneys, gonads and iliac crest are protected by shields
- The dose of radiotherapy is approximately 40-45 grey delivered at the rate of 10 Gy/week
- When used with chemotherapy the dose of radiation is reduced.

Chemotherapy

Combined modality—Radiation and Chemotherapy

Q 46. What is the indication for radiotherapy?

Localized disease—I A and II A.

Q 47. What is the indication for chemotherapy?

Stages III and IV are generally treated with combination chemotherapy.

Q 48. What is the management of B symptoms of I and II?

Even if the disease seems to be localized, **B symptoms and unfavorable** histology (mixed cellularity and lymphocyte depletion), usually calls for the use of **chemotherapy with or without radiation**. The relapse rates are high after radiation therapy alone.

Q 49. What is Mantle radiation?

Irradiation of -

- Cervical
- Axillary
- Mediastinal
- Hilar lymph nodes.

Q 50. What is Subtotal Lymphoid Irradiation (STLI)? (PG)

Irradiation of Mantle area and upper abdominal and para-aortic and splenic bed nodes.

Q 51. What is Total Lymphoid Irradiation (TLI)? (PG)

Irradiation of the pelvic field in addition to STLI is given.

Q 52. What is the indication for chemotherapy for early stage Hodgkin's disease? (PG)

Chemotherapy is given to eradicate subclinical disease outside the radiotherapy ports.

The ABVD regimen is used because of the better toxicity profile and effectiveness.

Q 53. What is combined modality therapy? (PG)

This is done to prevent relapse, where radiation is combined with chemotherapy. The indications are:

- Unfavorable disease (Stage III and IV)

- Unfavorable histology (mixed cellularity and lymphocyte depletion type)
- Extensive splenic involvement
- Children who cannot tolerate full dose of radiotherapy.

Q 54. What is the chemotherapeutic regime for Hodgkin's disease (HD)?

There are two regimes:

- ABVD regime
- MOPP regime.

Q 54. What is ABVD regime?

(6 – 8 cycles)

It is a widely used regimen for Hodgkin's disease. The drugs used are:

- **A**driamycin
- **B**leomycin
- **V**inblastin
- **D**acarbazine.

Q 56. Why ABVD is preferred over MOPP?

- Better disease free survival and over all survival
- Better toxicity profile.

Q 57. What is MOPP regime?

The drugs used in this regime for the treatment of Hodgkin's disease are:

- Nitrogen mustard
- Vincristine (Oncovin)
- Procarbazine
- Prednisolone.

Q 58. What is high dose chemotherapy? (PG)

Chemotherapeutic drugs are given in high doses with stem cell transplant (Bone marrow transplant).

Q 59. What are the problems of chemotherapy?

- Infertility
- Second cancers—leukemia, solid tumors like breast and thyroid
- Cardiopulmonary complications.

Q 60. What is radioimmunotherapy? (PG)

- This is usually given for relapse for which ^{131}I labeled anti CD30 Monoclonal antibodies are used
- Dendritic cell vaccines against EB virus
- Antibodies against CD3, CD28, CD25 are also available.

Q 61. What are the bad prognostic factors?

Bulky disease
Anemia
High ESR
Inflammatory signs
Inguinal node involvement
Tissue eosinophilia
High serum LDH
Pathological grade
Sex: Male
Age > 45
WBC > 15000/cumm
Serum albumin < 4 gm
Stage 4 disease
Lymphocyte count < 600/cumm

NON-HODGKIN'S LYMPHOMA

Q 62. What is the definition of NHL?

It is a heterogenous group of B and T cell malignancies having diversity in — cellular origin, morphology, cytogenetic abnormalities, response to treatment and prognosis.

Q 63. What are the features of NHL?

These are neoplasms of the immune system usually presenting as disseminated and extra-nodal disease of the old age. The peculiarities are:

1. Multicentricity
2. Wide spreading
3. Showing malignant cell in the blood
4. Leukemic transformation may occur in 10–15% of patients.

Q 64. What are the clinical features of NHL?

1. Asymptomatic
2. B symptoms
3. Enlarged lymph nodes
4. Abdominal mass
5. GI symptoms—pain, vomiting, bleeding
6. Loss of weight.

Q 65. What are the predisposing factors? (PG)

The following predisposing factors are attributed:

1. Immunosuppression
2. Autoimmune diseases
   - Hashimoto's disease
   - Sjogren's syndrome.
3. Infective agents
   - EB virus – African Burkitt's
   - AIDS related
   - Nasopharyngeal lymphoma
   - Transplant lymphoma
   - Lymphoma after infectious mononucleosis
   - HTLV-I infection – (**H**uman **T** cell **L**ympho-tropic **V**irus)
   - HTLV -II – T cell lymphoma and Leukemia
   - *H. pylori* – Gastric lymphoma
   - Hepatitis C virus – 8 and 6
   - Human herpes virus
4. Prior chemotherapy
5. Prior radiotherapy.

Q 66. What are the congenital disorders having increased incidence of NHL? (PG)

- Ataxia telangiectasia
- Wiskott-Aldrich syndrome
- Celiac disease.

Q 67. What are the core nodal regions?

They are as follows:

- Right cervical (including cervical, supraclavicular, occipital and preauricular lymph nodes)
- Left cervical nodes
- Right axillary
- Left axillary
- Right infraclavicular
- Left infraclavicular
- Mediastinal lymph nodes
- Hilar lymph nodes
- Para-aortic lymph nodes
- Mesenteric lymph nodes
- Right pelvic lymph nodes
- Left pelvic lymph nodes
- Right inguinofemoral lymph nodes
- Left inguinofemoral lymph nodes.

Q 68. Can NHL involve any other nodes other than the core nodal regions?

Yes. NHL may involve the following nodes in addition:

- Epitrochlear lymph nodes
- Popliteal lymph nodes
- Internal mammary lymph nodes
- Occipital lymph nodes
- Submental lymph nodes
- Preauricular lymph nodes
- Many other small nodal areas.

Q 69. What is the E designation for NHL?

For NHL the **E designation** should indicate the presentation of lymphoma in extra nodal site and the lack of E designation should indicate lymphomas presenting in lymph nodes. For example, **lymphoma presenting in thyroid gland** with cervical lymph node involvement should be staged as **IIE**. Lymphoma presenting only in cervical node is Stage I.

Q 70. What are the extra nodal sites?

Extra nodal sites
• Paranasal sinuses • Thyroid • GI tract • Liver • Testicles • Skin • Bone marrow • Bone • CNS • Lung • Gonads • Kidneys • Uterus • Ocular adnexa.

Q 71. What are the classifications for NHL?

1. Rappaport
2. Working classification
   - Low grade: B cell lymphomas
   - Intermediate grade: B cell or T cell (lymphoblastic group)
   - High grade.
3. *REAL* (**R**evised **E**uropean - **A**merican **L**ymphoma)/ WHO classification
   - B cell — precursor B cell cancers —peripheral B cell neoplasms – *Burkitt's*
   - T cell and natural killer cells (NK)
     - Precursor T-cell neoplasm
     - Peripheral T-cell and NK cell neoplasm – **Mycosis fungoides**
     - Intestinal T-cell lymphoma.
4. Functional classification (for treatment purposes).
   - Indolent—smaller cells, differentiated cells
     - Low grade, very difficult to cure
     - **Progress to more aggressive type**
   - Aggressive—larger cells, less differentiated — Better chance for cure
   - Highly aggressive.

Q 72. Since low grade lymphomas can progress to aggressive type, what are the criterion for suspecting a disease transformation? (PG)

1. Increased LDH
2. Rapid enlargement of the nodes
3. Constitutional symptoms
4. Extra nodal disease.

Q 73. What is Burkitt's lymphoma?

It is a B-cell tumor.

Q 74. What is Mycosis fungoides?

It has a T cell and NK cell origin and will manifest as skin lesion. Skin is followed by lungs and lymph node involvement (**Cezary syndrome**—circulating T and NK cells).

Q 75. What is the staging of NHL?

The Ann-Arbor classification is used for staging (see Hodgkin's disease).

Q 76. What is stage IV disease?

By convention, any involvement of the following calls for classification as stage IV disease.

Stage IV disease
• Bone marrow • Liver • Pleura • CSF.

Q 77. What are the investigations required for diagnostic evaluation of NHL?

Read the chart for Hodgkin's lymphoma.

Q 78. What is the treatment of NHL?

Chemotherapy is the primary modality of treatment in NHL, because NHL spreads widely and there is early hematogenous spread. For localized disease radiotherapy may be useful.

Indolent lymphoma—treatment

a. Localized—Radiotherapy
   Disseminated—rarely curative
b. Palliation—watch and wait until they progress to more aggressive type.
   The quality of life is better here.

Aggressive

- Stage I and II—Radiation alone
- Stage III and IV—CHOP regimen
- High dose chemotherapy—with autologous marrow transplantation.

Q 79. What is the chemotherapeutic regime for NHL?

NHL is generally treated with *CHOP* regimen, which is combination chemotherapy of the following drugs.

- Cyclophosphamide
- Adriamycin (is designated H – Hydroxy-daunorubicin or Doxorubicin)
- Oncovin
- Prednisolone.

Q 80. What is CD - 20? (PG)

It is a **cell surface protein** involved in the development and differentiation of natural **B cells.**

Q 81. What is Rituximab? (PG)

It is a monoclonal antibody that binds to the B cell surface antigen CD-20. The dose is 375 mg/m^2 slow IV infusion once weekly for 4 doses.

Q 82. What is the chemotherapeutic agent for CNS lymphoma? (PG)

The CHOP therapy has poor penetration to the blood brain barrier (BBB) and therefore it is ineffective. It can be treated with **whole brain irradiation. Methotrexate** is effective and it may be given systemically or intrathecally.

Q 83. What is international prognostic index (IPI) for NHL?

Five pretreatment characteristics were found to be independent statistically significant factors for prognosis.

International Prognostic Index

- Age > 60 years
- Ann-Arbor stage III or IV
- Increased LDH
- Reduced performance status (ECOG > 2)
- Extra nodal site-one or more.

Q 84. What are the extra nodal sites which are more aggressive?

1. GIT
2. Nasopharynx
3. Testis.

Q 85. What are the lymphomas having predilection for CNS metastasis? (PG)

- Testis
- Paranasal sinuses
- AIDS related.

Note: Prophylactic intrathecal methotrexate is given in such situations.

Q 86. What is the role of surgery in NHL?

1. For establishing the diagnosis
2. For resection of extra nodal GI lesions.

Q 87. What is the treatment of NHL of stomach and small bowel?

It is controversial, whether to treat it with chemotherapy or surgery. **Resection** is recommended because of the following reasons:

- Risk of perforation
- Risk of fatal bleeding (with chemotherapy)

Stage 1 and 2 non bulky—*H. pylori* eradication – if it disappears surveillance for three years.

Stage 1 and 2 bulky—Chemotherapy and surveillance for three years.

Stage 3 and 4—Chemotherapy

Q 88. What is paraneoplastic syndrome? (PG)

Many tumors develop the ability to elaborate **hormones or cytokines** that can have deleterious consequences for the host. The effects may be affecting a single organ system or systemic. The common cancer sequelae like hypercoagulation, cachexia, fever and anemia of chronic disease are due to this syndrome.

Case

16 Renal Swelling

Case Capsule

A **55-year-old male patient** presents with **fever, hematuria, flank pain and mass abdomen of 8 months duration**. He also complains of **loss of weight**. He noticed recently that his left side of the **scrotum and testes are hanging too low** than what it used to be. He is found to be hypertensive recently.

On examination his **blood pressure is 166/110** mm of Hg. He is **febrile** and there is **pitting edema of both lower limbs**. On examination of the abdomen, **distended subcutaneous veins** are seen in the anterior abdominal wall. The shape of the abdomen is normal and it moves with respiration. On palpation there is no local rise of temperature and tenderness. There is a **mass in the left lumbar region** of about **15 × 12 cm size** which moves with respiration (Fig. 16.1). The mass is firm in consistency and the surface is smooth. All the borders of the mass are well-delineated. One **can get above the swelling**. The mass is **ballotable and bimanually palpable**. Percussion over the mass revealed that it is **resonant**. There is no mass lesion on the right side. The supraclavicular lymph nodes are not enlarged. Examination of the genitalia revealed **left sided varicocele**. On examination of the spine, there is **no scoliosis**. The **left renal angle is full and it is dull to percussion.** There is **no bruit** at the lumbar area adjacent to the lumbar spine. Examination of the chest is normal. There is no evidence of bony metastasis. (The mass is intra-abdominal and retroperitoneal).

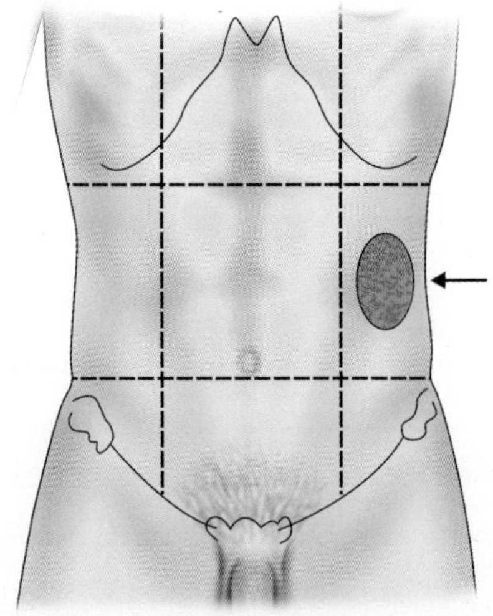

Fig. 16.1: Left lumbar mass

Read the checklist for abdomen.

Checklist for examination of suspected renal swelling

1. Always check the blood pressure reading—hypertension can be a cause or consequence of renal disease (renal artery stenosis)—patient may present with headache
2. Remember the triad of renal cell carcinoma—flank pain, hematuria, and flank mass
3. Examine the genitalia for varicocele—tumor thrombus in the renal vein
4. Examine for lower limb edema—tumor thrombus in the inferior vena cava
5. Gross distension of the abdominal veins as a result of venacaval obstruction Examine the contralateral flank for bilateral renal swellings
6. Examine the renal angle—for fullness, tenderness and dullness
7. Look for scoliosis—inflammatory conditions will produce scoliosis with concavity towards the side of the lesion
8. Auscultation for a bruit at the lumbar areas adjacent to the lumbar spine at the level of L2 (renal artery stenosis)
9. Always examine the chest for pulmonary metastasis
10. Always examine the bones for pain and pathological fractures.

Q 1. What are the physical signs of an enlarged kidney?

Physical signs of an enlarged kidney

1. It moves with respiration
2. It is resonant on percussion (because it is covered by colon in front)
3. Fingers can be insinuated between the mass and costal margin
4. Bimanual palpable
5. Ballotable.

Q 2. Why the kidney is moving up and down with respiration?

Upper posterior aspect of the kidney is related to the diaphragm (diaphragmatic area) and therefore it will move up and down with respiration.

Q 3. What is Ballottement?

This sign is useful for the diagnosis of the following conditions.

a. This is a sign used for the confirmation of pregnancy of more than 3 months standing
b. For ballottement of kidneys
c. It is also used for mobile intraperitoneal fluid filled swellings like ovarian cyst
d. Ballottement of swellings rising out of the pelvis where one hand is laid over the hypogastrium and the other inserted to vagina or rectum.

Q 4. What is renal ballottement?

The patient is supine and one hand of the examiner is laid flat upon the abdomen, so that the greater part of the flexor surfaces of the fingers overlies the swelling. This hand is called the **watching hand**. The slightly flexed fingers of the other hand are insinuated behind the loin so that they contact the area lateral to the sacrospinalis muscle. This hand is the **displacing hand**. Short, quick, forward thrusts are made by the displacing hand (posterior). If these movements impart a bouncing sensation to the anteriorly placed watching hands, the sign is positive.

Q 5. What is the significance of a bimanually palpable swelling?

It is a palpation done by both hands, right hand placed anteriorly and the left hand placed posteriorly. All the big abdominal masses in the loin are bimanually palpable. Therefore, it is important to decide with **which hand the mass is better felt**. If it is better felt with the anterior hand, it is likely to be arising from colon or one of the viscera. If it is better felt with the posterior hand, it is likely to be kidney.

Q 6. What is the significance of scoliosis of lumbar spine in a renal mass?

Scoliosis of lumbar spine with **concavity towards the affected side** is a constant sign in inflammatory conditions of the kidney like perinephric abscess. Bending the trunk away from the side of lesion is likely to cause more pain in such conditions.

Q 7. What is renal angle? What is the significance of examination of renal angle?

It is the angle formed by the lateral border of the sacrospinalis muscle and the last rib. The renal angle is **normally resonant** to percussion because of the colonic flexure in front of the kidneys. The renal angle is dull, when there is enlargement of the kidney.

The renal angle is checked for:

Fullness—when there is mass lesion/enlargement.

Tenderness—in inflammatory pathology.

Dullness—when there is mass lesion/enlargement.

Q 8. What is Murphy's kidney punch? (The renal angle test)

The patient sits up and folds his arms in front of him. The thumb is then placed under the 12th rib to the lateral side of the sacrospinalis muscle. Sharp and jabbing movements are made with the thumb. Initially the movements are very gentle and if the patient is not experiencing pain, the strength is increased. This test is useful for demonstration of deep-seated tenderness.

Q 9. What is renal pain?

It is a persistent fixed ache situated mainly in the costovertebral angle. If there is significant renal enlargement, stretching of the peritoneum may localize the pain more anteriorly to the upper and outer quadrants of the abdomen. The pain is not strictly lumbar.

Q 10. What is the triad of renal cell carcinoma (RCC)?

Triad of renal cell carcinoma
Hematuria—40%
Flank pain—30%
Palpable flank mass—20%

Note: Only 10% of patients have all these symptoms.

Q 11. What is the most probable diagnosis in this case?

The first diagnosis will be a **renal tumor**.

Q 12. What are the differential diagnoses?

Clinically **carcinoma of the descending colon** can have a clinical presentation like this.

The points against colon are:

- Ballottement is positive that is in favor of kidney
- Renal angle is obliterated and dull
- There are no bowel symptoms
- In colon, the swelling will be better felt with the anterior hand in bimanual palpation and ballottement will be negative.

The other differential diagnoses of a renal mass are:

Differential diagnoses of renal mass other than colon

1. Hydronephrosis
2. Adult polycystic kidney disease
3. Tuberculosis
4. Adrenal tumors
5. Retroperitoneal tumors
6. Angiomyolipoma
7. Benign renal tumors
8. Xanthogranulomatous pyelonephrosis
9. Solitary cyst of the kidney
10. Abscess (Perinephric).

Q 13. What is the definition of hydronephrosis?
Aseptic dilatation of pelvicalyceal system because of **partial or intermittent** obstruction.

Q 14. What are the causes for unilateral hydronephrosis?

Causes for unilateral hydronephrosis
1. Pelviureteric obstruction— a. *Congenital pelvi-ureteric junction stenosis* b. Stones in the renal pelvis c. Tumors in the renal pelvis d. Pressure from aberrant arteries 2. Ureteric obstruction a. Stones b. Tumor infiltration of the ureter—carcinoma colon, rectum, cervix and prostate c. Tumors of the ureter d. Bladder tumors e. Ureterocele.

Q 15. What are the causes for bilateral hydronephrosis?

Causes for bilateral hydronephrosis
• Prostatic enlargement—benign or malignant • Urethral strictures and valves • Carcinoma of the bladder • Retroperitoneal fibrosis • Phimosis

Q 16. What is the most common tumor in this age group?
Renal cell carcinoma (RCC) is the correct terminology. The older names are:

- Grawitz's tumor
- Hypernephroma
- Adenocarcinoma
- Clear cell tumor

The most common of the neoplasm of the kidney is RCC.

Q 17. Why is it called hypernephroma?
Hypernephroma means above the kidney. Grawitz initially thought that they arose from adrenal rests within the kidneys. Later on, Lubarsch stated that these tumors are definitely adrenal in origin leading to the term hypernephroma.

The tumors usually occupy the poles most commonly the upper pole. The tumors of the hilum are less common.

Q 18. Why is it called the 'golden tumor' and what is the cut section appearance?
The tumor is **yellowish** because of the abundance of lipids including cholesterol. It is also rich in glycogen and exhibits areas of necrosis and hemorrhage.
Cut section appearance:
The tumors are irregular in shape with central hemorrhage and necrosis. It is semitransparent. The tumor is often divided into lobules by fibrous septa, some of which are cystic.

Q 19. What is the histology of RCC?
Histologically it is an adenocarcinoma containing clear, granular and spindle cells in varying proportions.

Q 20. What are the pathological types of RCC?

- Clear cell
- Granular cell
- Spindle cell
- Sarcomatoid
- Papillary
- Chromophilic.

Q 21. What are the methods of spread of RCC?

1. Local
2. Lymphatic spread—lymph nodes of hilum and later on to the para-aortic nodes.
3. Tumor thrombus into the veins—renal vein, inferior vena cava and then up to the *right heart*—

pieces of growth may end up in the lungs where they grow to form cannon ball secondary deposits.
4. Metastases to bone—they are highly vascular and may pulsate (pulsatile bony metastasis DD follicular carcinoma thyroid metastasis).

Q 22. What is the cause for hypertension in renal tumors?

The renal cell carcinoma produces renin and thus causes hypertension.

Q 23. What is the cause for erythrocytosis in renal cell carcinoma (RCC)?

About 60% of the tumors will produce raised level of erythropoietin. This will result in erythrocytosis (not polycythemia).

Q 24. What is paraneoplastic syndrome?

Nonendocrine tumor producing ectopic hormone inappropriate for the tissue of origin.

Q 25. What are the paraneoplastic syndromes produced by renal cell carcinoma (RCC)? (PG)

1. Hypertension
2. Parathyroid hormone like substances—Hypercalcemia
3. Adrenocorticotropic hormone—Cushing
4. Human chorionotropic hormone
5. Kinin substances—*fever* (renal tumors may present as pyrexia of unknown origin). Persistence of fever after nephrectomy suggests the presence of metastasis
6. Thrombocytosis
7. Anemia
8. Erythrocytosis
9. Coagulopathy
10. Vasculopathy
11. Amyloidosis
12. Nephrotic syndrome
13. Stauffer's syndrome (Hepatopathy)
14. Polymyalgia rheumatica
15. Cachexia
16. Skin rash.

Q 26. What is Stauffer's syndrome? (PG)

It is a nonmetastatic liver dysfunction seen in cases of hypernephroma.

Q 27. What is the importance of genitalia examination in cases of renal tumors?

Renal carcinoma has a predilection for producing **occlusive thrombi in the renal vein** and the inferior vena cava. When the left renal vein is occluded it will produce acute **Varicocele** on the left side.

Q 28. Why varicocele is seen only on left side in case of renal tumors?

The left renal vein is the vein of three paired organs namely—the kidneys, the adrenal and the testis. The right testicular vein joins the inferior vena cava directly instead of the renal vein. On the left side the left testicular vein joins the renal vein at right angles. When there is tumor thrombus in the left renal vein, the resultant pressure is transmitted to the left testicular vein resulting in varicocele.

Q 29. What is the cause for lower limb edema in renal tumors?

As mentioned earlier tumor **thrombus will occlude the inferior vena cava** and manifest as lower limb edema.

Q 30. What are the ectopic hormones produced by RCC? (PG)

1. Parathyroid hormone like substances
2. Adrenocorticotropic hormone
3. Human chorionotropic hormone
4. Kinin substances.

Q 31. What are the causes for hematuria?

Causes for hematuria

Site	*Cause*
Urethra	Trauma

Contd...

Contd...

	Urethritis
	Stricture
	Stone
	Carcinoma of the urothelium
Prostate	Benign prostatic hyperplasia (BPH
	Carcinoma of the prostate
	Prostatitis
Bladder	Cystitis
	Carcinoma
	Stone
	Trauma
	Schistosomiasis
Ureteric	Stone
	Carcinoma of the urothelium
Renal	Carcinoma of the kidney
	Stone
	Polycystic kidney
	Tuberculosis
	Carcinoma of the renal pelvis
	Trauma
	Glomerulonephritis

Note: Frank hematuria indicates a urological malignancy until proven otherwise.

Q 32. What is clot colic?

When the patient is having hematuria, the clot will obstruct the ureter and will present with clinical features of ureteric colic.

Q 33. What are the investigations for this patient?

Investigations can be classified as:

- Investigations for diagnosis
- General investigations
- Staging investigations.

General Investigations

1. Urine analysis—may reveal hematuria
2. ESR – may be increased but nonspecific
3. Hematocrit—elevated in RCC
4. Hb—anemia is present in RCC—with or without hematuria (anemia unrelated to blood loss occur in 20-40% of patients
5. Serum calcium—elevated in RCC
6. Alkaline phosphatase—increased.

Investigations for Diagnosis and Staging

1. *X-ray chest*—reveal '**cannon balls**'—It is the metastatic lesions in the lungs from RCC.
2. *Plain X-ray abdomen*—Reveal **calcified renal mass** and distortion of renal outline—only 20% contain demonstrable calcification (20% of the masses with **peripheral calcification** are malignant and 80% with **central calcification** are malignant).
3. *IVU*—(**Initial technique for workup of hematuria**) the calyces may be stretched and distorted. The typical '**spider leg**' deformity occupying the upper or lower pole (splaying of calyceal system) is seen. It is important to know the **function of the contralateral kidney**.
4. *Ultrasonography*—Can define solid and cystic lesions. The ultrasound will reveal **solid mass** within the renal parenchyma in RCC. It can also identify **venacaval tumor thrombus**.
5. *CT scan and CT urography* (contrast enhanced)—**It is the diagnostic procedure of choice** when a solid renal mass is identified in ultrasound (delineates RCC in 95% of cases) RCC will show heterogeneous **enhancing lesion** (in 80%).

In addition to diagnosis, CT is also useful for:

- Local staging
- Involvement of perinephric fat
- Hilar lymph nodes
- Tumor thrombus in renal vein and IVC.

6. MRI — It is the investigation of choice for renal vein and venacaval thrombi. MR angiography is useful for mapping the blood supply of the tumor and the relationship of the tumor to adjacent structures.
7. *Isotope bone scanning*—It is indicated in patients with bone pain, elevated alkaline phosphatase and known metastasis cases.
8. *Renal angiography*—It is not done nowadays after the CT became available. The practice of preoperative embolization has also waned.

Q 34. What are the risk factors for RCC? (PG)

- Cigarette smoking
- Coffee drinking
- Cadmium exposure
- Von Hippel-Lindau disease (Cerebellar hemangioblastoma, retinal angiomatosis, bilateral renal cell carcinoma)
- Adult polycystic kidney disease
- Acquired renal cystic disease in end stage renal disease.

Q 35. What is the tumor suppressor gene in Von Hippel-Lindau renal cancer? (PG)

Suppressor gene on *3p*

Q 36. What is Robson's staging?

Stage 1 Tumor confined within the renal parenchyma

Stage 2 Extracapsular extensions into the perinephric fat or the adrenal but within Gerota's fascia

Stage 3 Spread to the **regional nodes** and lymphatics within the Gerota's layer and or tumor thrombus invasion of the wall of the **renal vein or IVC**

Stage 4 Adjoining **organ invasion**—Colon, posterior muscle wall or distant metastasis.

Q 37. What is the TNM Staging as per AJCC 7th edition? (PG)

Primary Tumor (T)

TX Primary tumor cannot be assessed

T0 No evidence of primary tumor

T1 Tumor 7 cm or less in greatest dimension, limited to the kidney

T1a Tumor 4 cm or less in greatest dimension, limited to the kidney

T1b Tumor more than 4 cm but not more than 7 cm in greatest dimension limited to the kidney

T2 Tumor more than 7 cm in greatest dimension, limited to the kidney

T2a Tumor more than 7 cm but less than or equal to 10cm in greatest dimension, limited to the kidney

T2b Tumor more than 10 cm, limited to the kidney

T3 Tumor extends into major veins or perinephric tissues but not into the ipsilateral adrenal glands and not beyond Gerota's fascia

T3a Tumor grossly extends into the renal vein or its segmental (muscle containing) branches, or tumor invades perirenal and/or renal sinus fat but not beyond Gerota's fascia

T3b Tumor grossly extends into the vena cava below the diaphragm

T3c Tumor grossly extends into the vena cava above the diaphragm or invades the wall of the vena cava

T4 Tumor invades beyond Gerota's fascia (including contiguous extension into the ipsilateral adrenal gland).

Regional Lymph Node (N)

NX Regional lymph nodes cannot be assessed

N0 No regional lymph node metastasis

N1 Metastasis in regional lymph node (s)

Distant Metastasis (M)

M0 No distant metastasis

M1 Distant metastasis

Anatomic stage/prognostic groups Renal cell carcinoma			
Stage	T	N	M
I	T1	N0	M0
II	T2	N0	M0
III	T1 or T2	N1	M0
	T3	N0 or N1	M0
IV	T4	Any N	M0
	Any T	Any N	M1

Q 38. This patient is having stage II RCC. What is the management?

Stage I, II and IIIA are best treated by radical nephrectomy.

Q 39. What is radical nephrectomy?

This is an en-block removal of the following structures.

- Kidney
- Surrounding Gerota's fascia (including the ipsilateral adrenal)
- Renal hilar lymph nodes
- Proximal half of the ureter.

Q 40. What are the approaches for nephrectomy? (PG)

The kidney may be approached by the following routes:

1. *Loin incisions (Retroperitoneal)*
   - **Transcostal** starts from the angle of 12th rib and goes for 8–15 cm beyond the tip of the 12th rib
   - **Subcostal** – from the renal angle downwards and forwards between the12th rib and iliac crest and stops 4–5 cm above the anterior superior iliac spine
   - **Supracostal** – between the 11th and 12th rib
   - **Lumbotomy** – the incision starts from the upper border of the 12th rib vertically downwards along the lateral border of the erector spinae and then forwards to the iliac crest for 10 cm
   - **Nagamatsu** is used for better renal artery control—this incision starts at the angle of 11th rib down to the 12th rib angle and then along the 12th rib to the umbilicus. This is an extrapleural retroperitoneal approach.
2. *Abdominal (Transperitoneal)* — this approach has as the advantage that the renal pedicle and inferior vena cava can be widely exposed.
   - Midline
   - Paramedian
   - Transverse abdominal (for bilateral renal tumors).
3. *Thoracoabdominal*

   For lesions of the upper pole, and lesions invading the inferior vena cava.

Q 41. What are the precautions to be taken in radical nephrectomy? (PG)

- The vascular pedicle should ligated before the kidney is mobilized (malignant cells will be released into the circulation)
- Initially the renal artery is ligated in continuity (massive bleeding during mobilization is less likely)
- Palpate the renal vein gently to rule out tumor thrombus (renal vein extension may embolize to the pulmonary circulation during nephrectomy). If it is empty, it is divided between ligatures

- The renal artery is then divided and the kidney mobilized
- The ureter is then traced downwards and divided and ligated at appropriate level.

Q 42. If the renal vein or inferior vena cava is invaded what is the procedure? (PG)

- The surgeon must obtain control of the cava above and below
- Cardiac bypass may be required, if there is extension into the thorax (Get the cardiac team) and the tumor thrombus may be removed from the right side of the heart.

Q 43. Is there any role for partial nephrectomy (nephrone sparing surgery)?

Yes. Partial nephrectomy is recommended in the following situations:

- Patients with tumors in solitary kidney
- Those with diabetes mellitus
- Patients with renal insufficiency
- Tumors under 4 cm size (Even with normal opposite kidney)

(In patients with negative surgical margins the prognosis will be the same as that of the radical nephrectomy).

Q 44. What is the role of laparoscopic nephrectomy?

It is becoming the gold standard in institutions with appropriate expertise. Laparoscopic radical or partial nephrectomy has been advocated as a method equal to the open approach with the following advantages:

- Less blood loss
- Shorter hospitalization
- Less pain
- Earlier return to normal activity.

Q 45. What is the treatment for a patient with solitary pulmonary metastasis? (PG)

Joint surgical removal of both the primary lesion and metastatic lesion is recommended.

Q 46. Is there any role for preoperative arterial embolization? (PG)

This will not improve survival rate. It is recommended as a single treatment in symptomatic patients with nonresectable primary lesions.

Q 47. What is the role of radiotherapy?

It is useful only for the treatment of symptomatic bone metastases.

Q 48. What are the chemotherapeutic agents used in RCC? (PG)

Vinblastine

Medroxy progesterone—for metastatic RCC.

Q 49. What is the role of immunotherapy? (PG)

- Interferon alpha—15 – 20% response rate
- IL-2 (interleukin)
- Combination of interferon alpha and IL-2.

Q 50. What is the prognosis of RCC? (PG)

Removal of even the largest neoplasm may cure the patient. In operable cases, 70% are well after 3 years and 60% after 5 years.

Q 51. What are the bad prognostic factors? (PG)

- Tumor invasion beyond the capsule
- Macroscopic involvement of renal vein and IVC
- Lymph node involvement.

Q 52. What is congenital polycystic kidney disease?

It is a hereditary condition transmitted by autosomal dominant trait affecting both kidneys (one kidney may contain larger cysts than the contralateral). The disease manifests in 2nd or 3rd decade of life and usually does not manifest before the age of 30 years. The etiology is uncertain. In 18% of cases, there is associated congenital cystic liver disease. The pancreas and lungs are occasionally affected. The disease is more common in women. The most important theory is failure of fusion between the secretory part and collecting system during the development (the secretory part is developed from the meta-nephrogenic tissue cap, and collecting part from the ureteric bud).

Q 53. What is the genetic abnormality in polycystic kidney disease? (PG)

There are two types:

1. *Autosomal recessive polycystic kidney disease (ARPKD)*—Previously called infantile. In this condition small cysts arise from collecting ducts resulting in bilateral symmetrical enlargement. Occurs in 1/14000 births and may be detected in utero. Infants usually die of respiratory failure.
2. *Autosomal dominant polycystic kidney disease (ADPKD)*—The gene located on chromosome 16p. Another gene responsible is PKD 2gene located in chromosome 4q 21-23. ADPKD occurs in 1/1000 individuals.

Q 54. What is the median age for end stage renal disease?

In PKD1—54 years
In PKD2—74 years

Q 55. What are the manifestations of polycystic disease?

Manifestations of polycystic disease of kidney

- Upper abdominal mass (bilateral knobby enlargement)
- Hypertension—present in 75% of patients above 20 years
- Loin pain—becuase of the weight of the organ or stretching of the capsule
- Uremia—large volumes of urine of low specific gravity (10:10 or less)—chronic renal failure (headache, drowsiness, vomiting and anorexia)
- Infection—pyelonephritis
- Hematuria—rupture of cyst into the renal pelvis.

Q 56. What is the gross appearance of polycystic disease?

The gross appearance is that of a collection of bubbles beneath the renal capsule. The renal parenchyma is riddled with cysts of varying sizes containing clear fluid, thick brown material or blood.

Q 57. What are the investigations for polycystic disease of the kidney?

- IVU—Enlarged kidneys with marked elongation of the calyces which are compressed by the cysts. The spider leg deformity or bell-like appearance
- Ultrasound multiple cysts in both kidneys, some times in liver and other organs
- CT.

Q 58. What are the treatment options for polycystic disease of the kidney?

- Medical—Low protein diet, treatment of infection, anemia and renal failure
- Dialysis
- Renal transplantation is the ideal treatment
- Rovsing's operation—(deroofing the cysts)—This is a palliative procedure for relieving the pressure on the parenchyma, and for reducing the pain. The open operation is not done nowaday. If required, it can be done laparoscopically.

Q 59. What is Dietl's crisis?

This is seen in intermittent hydronephrosis. After an attack of acute renal pain, swelling appears in the loin. After a few hours following the passage of a large volume of urine, the pain is relieved and the swelling disappears. This is called Dietl's crisis.

Causes for disappearing mass:

1. Dietl's crisis
2. Intussusception
3. Choledochal cyst

4. Communicating pseudocyst
5. Worm mass
6. Fecal impaction.

Q 60. What are the clinical features of hydronephrosis due to idiopathic pelviureteric junction obstruction?

- Renal colic
- Renal mass
- Intermittent hydronephrosis.

Q 61. What is the IVU finding in hydronephrosis?

- The minor calyces lose their normal cupping
- They become flattened
- Finally the classical clubbing is seen
- In very advanced cases the thin rim of poorly functioning renal parenchyma may give a faint nephrogram around the dilated calyces—the soap bubble appearance.

Q 62. What is the most helpful test to establish the dilatation because of obstruction?

Isotope renography using DTPA (Diethylene Triamine Penta Acetic acid) ^{99}Tc – DTPA is used for this investigation.

Q 63. What is the principle behind ^{99}Tc - DTPA?

The DTPA is injected intravenously, which is filtered by the glomeruli and not absorbed. When the DTPA is labeled with ^{99}Tc it will emit gamma rays. The passage of this technetium labeled DTPA through the kidneys can be tracked using a gamma camera. When the ureter is obstructed, the marker is trapped in the renal pelvis and will not be washed out, even if the flow of urine is increased by administering frusemide.

Q 64. What is Whitaker test?

A percutaneous puncture of the kidney is made through the loin and fluid is infused at a constant rate with monitoring of intrapelvic pressure. An abnormal rise in pressure confirms obstruction. This test is done occasionally.

Q 65. What is RGP (Retrograde pyelogram)?

After cystoscopy, the affected ureter is cannulated and dye is injected, which will reveal the anatomy of obstruction. This is done when the kidneys are not functioning in IVU in order to get an idea about the site of obstruction before surgery.

Q 66. What are the indications for surgery in idiopathic pelviureteric junction obstruction (PUJ)?

- Increasing hydronephrosis
- Bouts of renal pain
- Parenchymal damage
- Infection.

Q 67. What are the operations available for PUJ?

The operations are classified into dismembered Pyeloplasty and nondismembered pyeloplasty. The example of nondismembered is Foley's VY – Pyeloplasty.

Anderson-Hynes is dismembered pyeloplasty, is the most commonly performed operation (it can be done laparoscopically or by open method).

Endoscopic pyelolysis—The disruption of the pelviureteric junction is done by specially designed balloon passed up the ureter under radiographic control.

Q 68. What is the indication for nephrectomy in hydronephrosis?

Conservation of renal parenchyma is the aim. Nephrectomy is considered only when the renal parenchyma has been largely destroyed. If renal function is adequate (> 10% of total renal function surgical repair of the stenosis is done.

Case 17 Pseudocyst of Pancreas

Case Capsule

A 45-year-old male patient presents with history of **upper abdominal pain, epigastric fullness, nausea and occasional vomiting of 6 weeks duration**. He is a **chronic alcoholic** and gives history of hospital admission for acute abdominal pain two months back. For the last one week he gives history of **severe pain** over the epigastric region with **mild fever and rigors**. There is no history of trauma.

On general examination, there is **mild icterus and pallor**. On abdominal examination the **upper abdomen shows fullness**. The abdomen moves with respiration and the umbilicus is normal. There are no dilated veins seen in the abdominal wall. On palpation of the abdomen there is a **firm, tender mass of 20 × 16 cm size (20 cm horizontal and 16 cm vertical)** in the epigastrium extending to both hypochondriums. The **lower border of the swelling is indistinct**. The **upper limit is not palpable**. On both sides the mass goes beneath the costal margin. It **does not move with respiration** and there is **no intrinsic mobility**. The surface of the swelling is smooth. The mass is **resonant to percussion**. The plane of the swelling is **intra-abdominal and retroperitoneal**. The rest of the abdomen is normal. There is no free fluid demonstrated and normal bowel sounds are heard. Digital rectal examination revealed no abnormality. The hernial orifices and genitalia are normal. The left supraclavicular nodes are not enlarged. The renal angles are normal.

Read the checklist for abdominal examination

Checklist for history in the case of pseudocyst examination

- History of acute abdominal pain suggestive of acute pancreatitis
- History of trauma
- History of chronic abdominal pain
- History of alcoholism
- History of jaundice—because of pressure from pseudocyst.

Q 1. What are the physical features of pseudocyst of pancreas?

Physical features of pseudocyst of pancreas

1. Epigastric mass with indistinct lower edge
2. The upper limit may or may not be palpable
3. It is **resonant to percussion** (because of the overlying stomach)
4. There is **no movement with respiration** (minimal movement may be there)
5. The mass will be firm or soft but it is not possible to elicit fluctuation or fluid thrill
6. The mass may be tender.

Q 2. What is pseudocyst?

This is a collection of pancreatic juice enclosed in a wall of fibrous or granulation tissue that arises following an attack of acute pancreatitis (old definition is collection of fluid in the lesser sac).

Q 3. Why it is called pseudocyst?

It denotes absence of an epithelial lining. The true cyst is lined by epithelium.

Q 4. What is the time gap between the attack of acute pancreatitis and pseudocyst?

Usually it is four weeks.

Q 5. What are the types of pseudocyst?

The pseudocysts may be:

Acute pseudocyst or Chronic pseudocyst.

Another classification is

- *Postnecrotic*: Following an attack of necrotizing pancreatitis (Confined to the lesser sac or into the retroperitoneal space or to the mesentery of small or large bowel)
- *Peripancreatic*: Associated with chronic pancreatitis
- *Intrapancreatic cyst*: In advanced chronic pancreatitis (majority in the head of the pancreas).

Q 6. What is acute pseudocyst?

It is a fluid collection arising in association with an episode of acute pancreatitis of > 4 weeks duration and surrounded by well-defined wall of granulation or fibrous tissue.

Q 7. What constitutes the fibrous tissue in the wall of the cyst?

It is constituted by the inflammatory fibrosis of the following:

- Peritoneum
- Mesentery
- Serous membrane.

Q 8. What are the locations of the pseudocyst?

- Lesser sac
- Neck
- Mediastinum
- Pelvis

Q 9. What is the incidence of acute pseudocyst?

It develops in about 2% of cases of acute pancreatitis.

Q 10. Can you get multiple pseudocysts?

Yes. The cysts are single in 85% cases and multiple in the remainder.

Q 11. What is chronic pseudocyst?

Chronic pseudocyst is a collection with a well-defined wall that arises in a patient with chronic pancreatitis, without antecedent episode of acute pancreatitis. It may also occur in trauma victims (after a blow) and alcoholics. The mechanism consists of ductal obstruction and formation of a retention cyst that loses its epithelial lining as it goes beyond the confines of the gland. It may also occur sometimes as iatrogenic after splenectomy.

Q 12. What is pancreatic abscess?

It is a circumscribed peripancreatic collection of pus occurring late (**more than 4 weeks**) after the onset of acute pancreatitis. Infected collections identified earlier are classified as either infected acute fluid collection or infected pancreatic necrosis.

Q 13. What is the difference between pseudocyst and acute fluid collection?

The acute fluid collection occurs early in the course of acute pancreatitis (less than 4 weeks) and is lacking a wall of fibrous or granulation tissue and is located in or near the pancreas (in pseudocyst there is a wall of fibrous or granulation tissue).

Q 14. What is the nature of fluid in acute pseudocyst?

It is a collection enzyme rich pancreatic juice and may contain small amounts of necrotic debris.

Q 15. What are the investigations for the diagnosis of pseudocyst?

- Serum amylase—elevated (if the serum amylase remains elevated for 3 weeks, about half will have pseudocyst).
- Leukocytosis—(about 50% of patients).
- Bilirubin—elevated (suggestive of biliary obstruction).
- CT scan is the diagnostic study of choice (the size, shape of the cyst and its relationship to other viscera can be seen).

Acute cysts are irregular in shape, chronic cysts are circular.

An enlarged pancreatic duct may be demonstrated in chronic pancreatitis.

A dilated CBD would suggest biliary obstruction either from the cyst or as a result of pancreatitis.

- *Ultrasound*—to follow changes in size of acute pseudocyst and to study the gallbladder
- *ERCP*—not done routinely (If CT shows ductal abnormalities and if LFT is abnormal)
- *Upper GI series*—to look for site of gastric or duodenal obstruction. The cyst will push the stomach wall anteriorly (the retrogastric space will be increased).

Q 16. What is the role of ERCP in pseudocyst?

The ERCP will reveal the communication of the cyst to the pancreatic duct. Based on this, the pseudocysts are classified as—

- Communicating—communicating to the pancreatic duct
- Noncommunicating.

Q 18. What are the differential diagnoses in pseudocyst?

Differential diagnoses of pseudocyst of pancreas:

- Pancreatic abscess
- Pancreatic carcinoma (if gallbladder is palpable)
- Neoplastic cyst—cystadenoma or cystadenocarcinoma (about 5% of all cases of cystic pancreatic masses)
- Other epigastric masses.

Q 18. What are the complications of pseudocyst?

The complications are—

1. Pancreatic pseudocyst hemorrhage—resulting from autodigestion of the pancreas leading to erosion of splenic, gastroduodenal, or pancreaticoduodenal artery. This will result in false aneurysm of the artery in the cyst wall. **The clinical presentations of hemorrhage in the cyst are:**
   - Increasing epigastric pain
   - Increase in the size of abdominal mass
   - Shock
2. Hematemesis and melena—cyst eroding into the stomach
3. Rupture of the cyst into the peritoneal cavity—peritonitis and shock—emergency surgery with irrigation of the peritoneal cavity and drainage for the pseudocyst.
4. Infection—high fever, chills and leukocytosis (percutaneous drainage or internal drainage is the treatment).

Q 19. What are the indications for intervention in pseudocyst?

Indications for intervention in pseudocyst

- Persisting pain
- Pressure effects caused by increasing size
- Cysts of > 6 cm size
- Cysts of > 6 weeks duration.

Q 20. Why the procedure is done after 6 weeks?

The cyst wall is mature enough only after 6 weeks to hold sutures for anastomosis of the gut.

Q 21. Why 6 cm size is taken as cut off for treatment?

The chance for spontaneous resolution is there in 40% of cases if the cysts are smaller and therefore expectant management is recommended in smaller cyst.

Q 22. What is the cause for jaundice in a patient with pseudocyst?

It is usually caused by pressure from the cyst on the bile duct—*Wadsworth syndrome*.

Q 23. What are the therapeutic options for the management of pseudocyst?

See the algorithm for the management of pseudocyst (Flow chart 17.1).

Q 24. What are the internal drainage procedures available for pseudocyst?

The internal drainage may be:

- Endoscopic—endoscopic cystogastrostomy or cystojejunostomy
- Laparoscopic
- Open.

Q 25. What are the viscera to which internal drainage procedures are carried out?

- Cystogastrostomy—technically simpler (Recurrence and GI hemorrhage occur after this procedure)
- Cystojejunostomy (Roux-en-Y)—is the most versatile
- Cystoduodenostomy—risk of biliary injury.

Q 26. What is the prerequisite for the internal drainage?

Cyst wall should be sufficiently mature for anastomosis (usually 4–6 weeks).

Q 27. What is external drainage?

The external drainage is done when the wall surrounding the fluid collection is too fragile for internal drainage. It can be done under sonological guidance. This is also called percutaneous catheter drainage.

Q 28. What is the incidence of recurrence of pseudocyst after catheter drainage? (PG)

The recurrence is 4 times greater after external drainage than after internal drainage.

Q 29. What are indications for external drainage (nonsurgical drainage)? (PG)

- Critically ill patients
- Infected pseudocyst
- Uncomplicated pseudocyst
- To shrink a huge pseudocyst occupying half of the abdominal cavity.

Q 30. What is the complication of external drainage? (PG)

Pancreaticocutaneous fistula in 20–30% of patients.

Q 31. Is there any other method of external drainage? (PG)

A percutaneous drainage where a catheter is passed through the anterior abdominal wall, the anterior wall of the stomach and through the posterior stomach into the cyst. After several weeks the catheter is removed.

Q 32. What are the essential steps of cystogastrostomy?

- Upper midline incision
- Anterior gastrotomy (longitudinal incision in the anterior wall of stomach)
- Identify an area where the cyst wall is maximum bulging to the lumen of the stomach
- A 4 cm longitudinal window is created in the posterior wall along with the cyst wall (evacuate the contents of the cyst)
- A full thickness mattress suture is used to suture the edge of the posterior gastrotomy and cyst wall together

Flow chart 17.1: Management of pseudocyst of pancreas

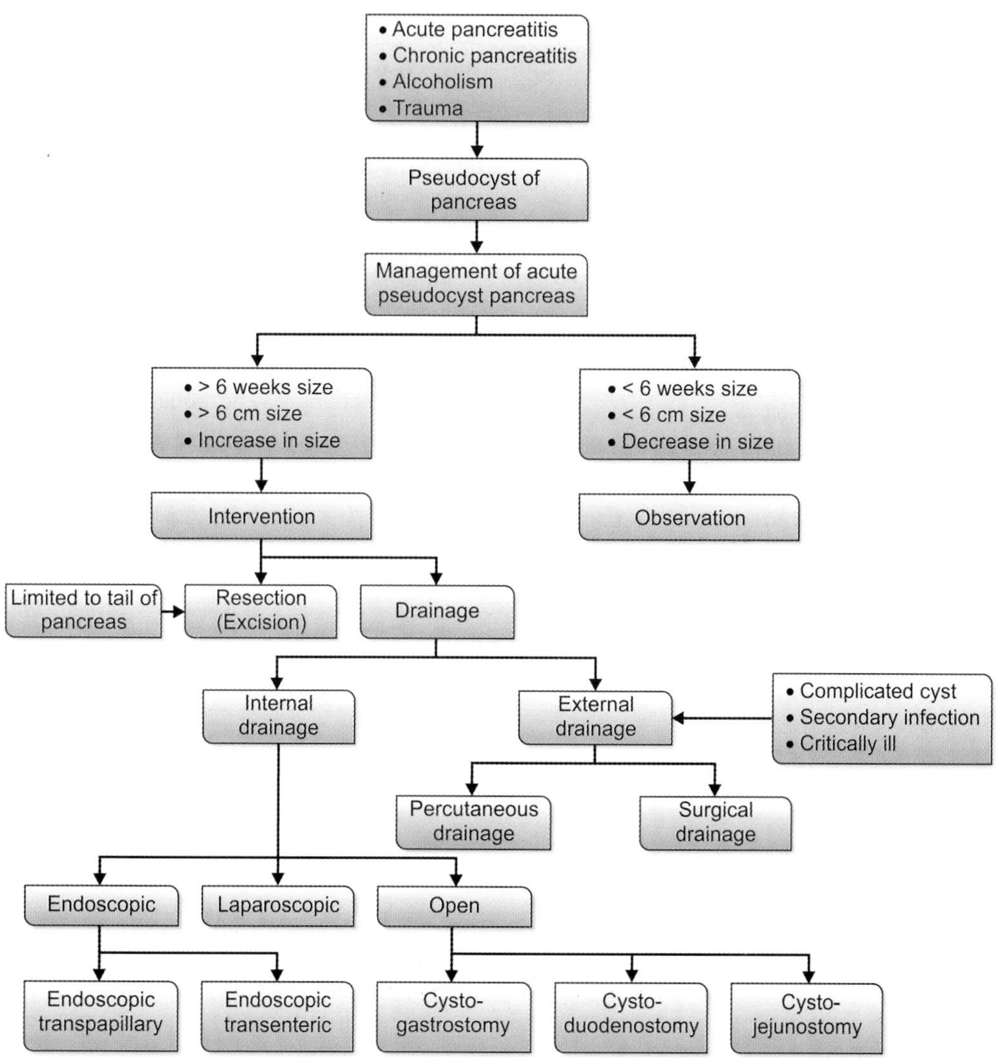

- The anterior gastrotomy is closed
- The abdomen is closed.

Q 33. What are the important things to be done with the pseudocyst during surgery? (PG)

Aspirate the cyst fluid and send for culture and sensitivity.

Send the cyst fluid for CEA (> 400 ng/mL suggestive of mucinous neoplasm) and amylase estimation.

Take biopsy from the cyst wall (this will rule out a cystic tumor).

Q 34. What will happen to the passage of food after cystogastrostomy? (PG)

Surprisingly the food will not go to the cyst cavity and the cystogastrostomy will get obliterated within a few weeks and heal in due course of time.

Q 35. What is the recurrence rate for pancreatic pseudocyst? (PG)

Its 10% (Recurrence is more frequent after external drainage).

Q 36. What is the postoperative complication of cystogastrostomy? (PG)

Hemorrhage occurs rarely.

Q 37. What is excision for pseudocyst? (PG)

This is the most definitive treatment. Usually this is done for chronic pseudocysts in the tail of gland. This is usually recommended for cysts following trauma.

Q 38. What is the treatment of pseudocyst hemorrhage? (PG)

- Angiographic embolization
- Subsequent elective treatment of the pseudocysts (after several weeks)
- Emergency laparotomy and ligation of the bleeding vessel after opening the cyst, and drainage of pseudocyst
- For lesions in the pancreatic head, pancreatico-duodenectomy may be required.

Q 39. What is Degidio and Schein classification? (PG)

	Type I	*Type II*	*Type III*
Occurrence	Acute	Acute in chronic	Chronic
Pancreatic duct	Normal	Diseased but no stricture	Stricture present
Communication with duct	No	No	With communication

Case

18 Retroperitoneal Tumor

Case Capsule

A 55-year-old male patient presents with **backache and pain radiating down the left lower limb of 6 months duration**. He in addition complains of **anorexia and loss of weight**. For the last 3 months he complains of **distension of abdomen**. There is **no history of therapeutic irradiation**. There is no family history of swelling all over the abdomen.

On examination, the patient is **afebrile; the blood pressure is 140/86 mm of Hg**. There is **pitting edema of the left lower limb**. On examination of the abdomen, there is **distension of abdomen which is more towards the left half**. A **big bosselated mass of 25 × 15 cm** (25 cm vertically and 15 cm horizontally) is felt in the left half of the abdomen occupying the **left lumbar region, left hypochondrium and left iliac fossa**. The mass is **firm in consistency** and **does not move with respiration**. All the borders except the lateral border are well-defined. **Medially it is not crossing the midline**. It is bimanually palpable, but **not ballotable.** It is intra-abdominal as demonstrated by the cough test. The mass is not falling forwards as demonstrated by examination in the knee elbow position and therefore **retroperitoneal**. There is **no intrinsic mobility** for the mass. On percussion there is **resonance over the mass.** The rest of the abdomen is normal. There is no free fluid in the abdomen and there is no organomegaly. Normal bowel sounds are heard on auscultation. There is **no evidence of varicocele**. The hernial orifices are normal. The left **lower limb pulsations are normal** and there is **no neurological deficit** in the left lower limb. Chest examination is normal.

Read the checklist for abdominal examination.

Checklist for history

- History of therapeutic radiation
- History of exposure to vinyl chloride family
- History of Gardner's syndrome
- Family history of Gardner's
- Familial retinoblastoma
- Risk factors such as Neurofibromatosis, Li-Fraumeni syndrome
- History of hypertension—because of catecholamine production
- History of back pain and leg pain
- History of hypoglycemia—liposarcoma produces insulin
- History of precocious puberty
- History of myoclonus in children.

Checklist for examination

- Take the temperature—RP tumors produce fever
- Take the blood pressure—tumors produce catecholamines
- Check the plane and remember the clinical points for retroperitoneal tumors given below:
- Look for dilated abdominal veins—because of the pressure on vena cava
- Look for lower limb edema
- Look for varicocele
- Look for ascites (nonmalignant ascites of RP tumor)
- Look for features of Costello syndrome.

Q 1. What is the most probable diagnosis in this case?

Retroperitoneal tumor.

Q 2. What are the clinical points in favor of retroperitoneal tumor?

Clinical points in favor of retroperitoneal tumor

- The mass is intra-abdominal as demonstrated by head raising test (Carnet's test)
- The mass is not falling forwards in the knee elbow position (suggesting the plane to be retroperitoneal)
- There is no movement with respiration (retroperitoneal swelling will not move)
- The mass is fixed (no intrinsic movement)
- The mass is resonant on percussion because of the intestinal loops in front
- The mass is not crossing the midline (retroperitoneal swellings usually will not cross the midline).

Q 3. What is the most probable diagnosis in this case?

Malignant retroperitoneal tumor, most probably liposarcoma.

Q 4. Why liposarcoma?

It is the most common retroperitoneal sarcoma in adults.

Q 5. What is the age group affected in liposarcoma?

Usually 40–70 years and they are asymptomatic in early stages.

Q 6. What is the cause for left lower limb edema and pain in this patient?

These are symptoms of **compression on the iliac veins.** The backache and lower limb pain in this case is due to stretching of the **lumbar and pelvic nerves.**

Q 7. What are the symptoms and signs of liposarcoma?

Symptoms and signs of liposarcoma

- Mass abdomen (91%)
- Mass pelvis (21%)—DD ovarian malignancy
- Abdominal pain and discomfort (71%)
- Anorexia, vomiting, fatigue
- Weight loss
- Caval compression—limb edema, varicocele, ascites (nonmalignant), dilated abdominal veins
- Back pain and leg pain—compression and stretching of lumbar and pelvic nerves
- Fever.

Q 8. What is retroperitoneum?

According to Ackerman retroperitoneum is defined as:

A region of the trunk covered—

- Anteriorly by the parietal peritoneum
- Superiorly by the 12th rib and diaphragm
- Inferiorly by the pelvic diaphragm and fascia of the levator ani and coccygeus
- Posteriorly by the fascia of the muscles of the anterior abdominal wall.

Q 9. Is it a real space?
It is an actual or potential space.

Q 10. What are the contents?
The contents are structures of mesodermal and endodermal origin with their embryonic remnants. This consists of **loose connective tissue, fat, nerves, lymphatics and lymph nodes.**

Q 11. What about the retroperitoneal organs?
Tumors of the **retroperitoneal organs are not included** in the retroperitoneal tumors traditionally (like kidneys, adrenals, pancreas and ureters).

Q 12. What is the incidence of retroperitoneal tumors?
They are uncommon heterogeneous group of tumors arising either primarily in the retroperitoneum or metastasis from elsewhere. The incidence is 0.3 to 3%.

Q 13. What is the classification?

Classification

Retroperitoneal tumors — Cystic, Solid

Retroperitoneal tumors — Benign, Malignant

- Cystic swelling is usually benign
- Majority are accidentally discovered
- Majority of the solid tumors are malignant (75–95%)

Q 14. What are the benign swellings?

Classification of benign tumors

- Lipomas
- Neurofibromas, neurilemmomas
- Leiomyomas
- Extra-adrenal chromaffinomas (pheochromaftinomas may be malignant)
- Mucinous cystadenomas
- Hemangiopericytomas
- Paragangliomas.

Q 15. What is Costello syndrome? (PG)
It is a syndrome consisting of mental retardation and benign tumors usually papillomata. Children with Costello syndrome develop **embryonal rhabdomyosarcoma.**

Q 16. What is Paraganglioma? (PG)

Features of paraganglioma

- They are tumors of embryonal origin from the neural crest
- May arise from any location along the aorta or the sympathetic chain
- They may be functioning or nonfunctioning (secrete norepinephrine)
- 20% are catecholamine secreting
- May be multiple
- Malignant paragangliomas can occur
- 0.1 – 0.5% cases produce hypertension
- May produce syndrome similar to pheochromocytoma
- May be familial (hereditary paragangliomas)
- Associated with von Hippel-Lindau disease and RET proto-oncogene.

Q 17. What is the pathology in paraganglioma? (PG)
The paraganglioma may arise from **type I or type II** cells.
Type I cells are chromogranin A positive (NSE positive).
Type II cells are S 100 positive (with good prognosis).

Q 18. What are the features of retroperitoneal neurilemmomas? (PG)
They are well-demarcated round or oval mass in CT with heterogeneous contrast enhancement. Nonenhancement of the lesion may be due to cyst formation or tumor calcification.

Q 19. What is mucinous cyst adenoma? (PG)
Mucinous cyst adenoma and cyst adenocarcinoma are similar to ovarian mucinous tumors.

Q 20. What is hemangiopericytoma? (PG)

They are vascular benign tumors derived from pericytes. They are very bulky and silent tumors. Treatment is excision.

Q 21. What are the malignant retroperitoneal tumors?

They may be Primary or Secondary.

Primary	*Secondary (metastatic)*
Sarcomas	Adenocarcinoma
Lymphomas	Endometrium
Malignant variety of germ cell tumors (common in children and are benign)	Prostate
Teratocarcinoma	Pancreas
Endodermal sinus tumor	Lung
Tumors of embryonal origin	GIT
Urogenital ridge tumors	Squamous cell carcinoma (SCC) cervix, vagina and lung
Chordoma	

Q 22. What is the origin of malignant retroperitoneal tumors?

They may originate from mesodermal, neurectodermal or embryonic remnant

- 75% mesodermal in origin
- 24% neurectodermal
- 1% embryonic remnant

The most common malignancy is sarcoma.

Q 23. What is the most common retroperitoneal malignancy?

Sarcoma.

Q 24. What is the most common sarcoma?

Liposarcoma is the most common sarcoma in adults.

- Liposarcoma – 50%
- Leiomyosarcoma – 29%
- Malignant fibrous histiocytoma (MFH).

[**In children** the most common sarcoma is *Rhabdomyosarcoma*:

- 18% present with neurological deficit
- 37% with distant metastasis.

Q 25. What are the etiological factors for retroperitoneal sarcoma? (PG)

Etiological factors for retroperitoneal sarcoma

- Idiopathic
- History of therapeutic radiation
- Exposure to vinyl chloride
- Thorium dioxide
- Familial disorders
- Gardner's syndrome
- Familial retinoblastoma
- Neurofibromatosis
- Li-Fraumeni syndrome
- Germ line mutations of p53 (chapter 17)

Q 26. What is the origin of liposarcoma?

About 1/3rd of the liposarcoma originate from **perinephric fat.**

Q 27. What is the cause of death in liposarcoma?

- Local treatment failure is the cause of death
- Distant metastasis is rare (30% of cases)—liver and lungs.

Q 28. What is the pathology of liposarcoma?

They may be well-differentiated or highly aggressive and undifferentiated. The tumor grows along the fascial planes and **envelops** rather than directly invading the nearby organs. Histologically they exhibit **meningothelial like whorls. Metaplastic bone** is seen in these whorls. **Myofibroblastic or osteoblastic** differentiation may occur.

Q 29. What are the sarcomas which will spread to the lymph nodes?

Lymph node spread is rare (< 5%). The following sarcomas spread to the lymph nodes.

Sarcoma with lymph node metastasis

- Rhabdomyosarcoma
- Lymphangiosarcoma
- Epitheliod sarcoma.

Q 30. What are the paraneoplastic syndromes of the retroperitoneal tumors? (PG)

1. Liposarcoma/Lipoma – *Intermittent hypoglycemia* (Insulin like substance production or rapid use of glucose by metabolically active sarcoma)
2. Paragangliomas – *Catecholamine excess*
3. Germ cell tumors – *Precocious puberty*
4. Neuroblastoma – *Myoclonus in children*

Q 31. How will you proceed to investigate?

Investigations in a case of retroperitoneal tumor

- Helical CT with contrast enhancement
- MRI
- CT scan of the chest/X-ray chest—to rule out metastasis
- PET scan
- Retroperitoneal core needle biopsy under CT/USG guidance
- IVU
- Retroperitoneoscopy
- Laboratory investigations –
  Alpha - fetoprotein
  HCG
  Liver function tests
  Renal function tests
- Role of FNAC – Recurrence
  Metastasis
  Lymph node involvement.

Q 32. What are the advantages of MRI over CT? (PG)

- Greater accuracy than CT (100% vs 80%)
- Extent of recurrence can be identified
- Points out areas of desmoplastic reaction.

Q 33. What are the MRI findings in various sarcomas? (PG)

Liposarcoma—decrease in signal in T_1 W increase in signal in T_2 W

MFH – Heterogeneous signal pattern

Hemangiopericytoma is multiloculated, cystic mass with areas of solid tissue.

Q 34. What is the role of retroperitoneoscopy? (PG)

It is not established for routine use. The sensitivity of this investigation for lymphoma is 84%, for Hodgkin's is 94%, for metastasis 95% and for retroperitoneal tumors 100%. In future this may replace CT guided biopsy.

Q 35. What is the metastatic evaluation for RP sarcoma?

CT scan of the chest.

Q 36. Why CT scan of the chest is preferred over X-ray chest? (PG)

The X-ray chest may not show metastasis because sarcoma metastasizes to the periphery of the lung which may be missed in X-ray chest.

Q 37. What is the TNM staging (AJCC 7th edition)? (PG)

TNM Staging

Primary Tumor (T)

Tx – Primary tumor cannot be assessed
T0 – No evidence of primary tumor
T1 – Tumor 5 cm or less greatest dimension
T1a – Superficial tumor
T1b – Deep tumor
T2 – Tumor more than 5 cm in greatest dimension
T2a – Superficial tumor
T2b – Deep tumor

Regional Lymph Node (N)

Nx—Regional lymph nodes cannot be assessed
N0—No regional lymph node metastasis
N1—Regional lymph node metastasis

Distant Metastasis (M)
M0 – No distant metastasis
M1 – Distant metastasis
Gx – Grade cannot be assessed
G1 – Grade 1
G2 – Grade 2
G3 – Grade 3

Q 38. What is the staging as per AJCC 7th edition? (PG)

AJCC Staging

Stage of the disease	*T stage*	*N stage*	*M stage*	*Grade of tumor*
Stage IA	T1a	N0	M0	G1, GX
	T1b	N0	M0	G1, GX
Stage IB	T2a	N0	M0	G1, GX
	T2b	N0	M0	G1, GX
Stage IIA	T1a	N0	M0	G2, G3
	T1b	N0	M0	G2, G3
Stage IIB	T2a	N0	M0	G2
	T2b	N0	M0	G2
Stage III	T2a, T2b	N0	M0	G2
	Any T	N1	M0	Any G
Stage IV	Any T	Any N	M1	Any G

Q 39. What is the grading as per AJCC 7th edition? (PG)

The AJCC 7th edition incorporates a three tiered grading system determine by three parameters—mitotic activity, extent of necrosis and differentiation. Each parameter is scored: differentiation (1–3), mitotic activity (1–3) and necrosis (0–2). The scores are summed to designate grade.

Grade 1	2 or 3
Grade 2	4 or 5
Grade 3	6 to 8

Q 40. What is the significance of nodal involvement?

Nodal involvement has very poor prognosis. Outcome of the N1 is similar to M1 disease.

Q 41. What is the treatment of retroperitoneal liposarcoma?

Complete en-block surgical excision at first laparotomy is the treatment of choice. This is possible only in 30% of cases.

Q 42. What are the preoperative preparations and precautions?

- Bowel preparation
- Consent for removal of whole or part of the adjacent organs
- Consent for fecal or urinary diversion
- Arrange adequate blood
- Operation is undertaken at a tertiary referral center.

Q 43. What anesthesia is used for surgery? (PG)

Hypotensive anesthesia.

Q 44. What are the incisions recommended?

Midline incision for pelvic level tumors and thoracoabdominal for upper level tumors.

Q 45. What is the clearance required for en-block excision?

Best results are seen in which a surgical margin of 3 cm or more can be obtained beyond the tumor.

Q 46. What is the most difficult area for clearance? (PG)

If a plane of dissection is there posteriorly, the clearance will be adequate. Decide whether the tumor has traversed along a spinal nerve root into the spinal canal and its cord.

Q 47. What is the role of radiotherapy?

Radiotherapy has a definite role in lowering the incidence of local recurrence. The dose recommended is 5500 cGy. Radiotherapy will delay the progression of the disease but does not improve the survival.

Q 48. What is the role of IORT (Intraoperative radiotherapy)? (PG)

The IORT reduces local recurrence and reduces radiation enteritis.

Q 49. What is the chemotherapeutic agent of choice for RP sarcoma? (PG)

Adriamycin—as a single agent—15–35% response. This may be combined with granulocyte macrophage colony stimulating factor (GM-CSF). There are three important regimes.

1. AIM—Adriamycin, Iphosphamide, Mesna
2. AD—Adriamycin and Dacarbazine
3. MAID—Mesna, Adriamycin, Ifosfamide and Dacarbazine.

Q 50. What are the important prognostic factors? (PG)

The two most important factors are:

- Histological grade
- Completeness of surgical excision (R0).

Q 51. What is the prognosis of RP sarcoma? (PG)

A 5-year-survival of 62–92% for well-differentiated tumor after radical excision. 16–48% in undifferentiated tumors.

Q 52. What is the local recurrence rate? (PG)

About 40–82% with median time of 15 months to 44 months.

Q 53. What is the follow-up? (PG)

- Physical examination every 2–3 months
- If symptoms occur do CT/MRI
- Asymptomatic patients—CT/MRI to be done at every 6 months for first 3 years.

Retroperitoneal Cystic Lesions

Q 54. What are the cystic lesions of the retroperitoneum?

Cystic lesions of the retroperitoneum

- Cystic lesions from the developmental remnants (Wolffian) of urogenital tract situated near the kidney
- Retroperitoneal mesenteric cyst
- Teratomatous and dermoid cysts
- Abdominal cystic lymphangioma (lymphogenous cyst)
- Parasitic cysts.

Q 55. What are the clinical features of the abdominal cystic lymphangioma?

This is usually seen in infants and children (3 months to 5 years). The most common presentation is abdominal pain. 30% of the children present with mass abdomen. 90% of the cysts are intraperitoneal. 10% are retroperitoneal. Children may present with complications like intestinal obstruction.

Q 56. What is the diagnostic investigation?

USG abdomen.

Q 57. What is the treatment of the abdominal cystic lymphangioma?

Surgical excision.

Q 58. Can you get abdominal cystic lymphangioma in adults?

Yes. There will be a history of long duration. Acute presentations are rare in adults.

Case

19 Testicular Malignancy

Case Capsule

A 40-year-old male patient presents with **lower abdominal pain, loss of appetite and loss of weight of 6 months duration**. The **right testis was absent from the scrotum** from childhood. He developed a **swelling in the right inguinal region** at the age of 15 years which was operated, the nature of surgery is not known. He gives history of **infertility since 10 years.** There is no history of chest pain, dyspnea or hemoptysis.

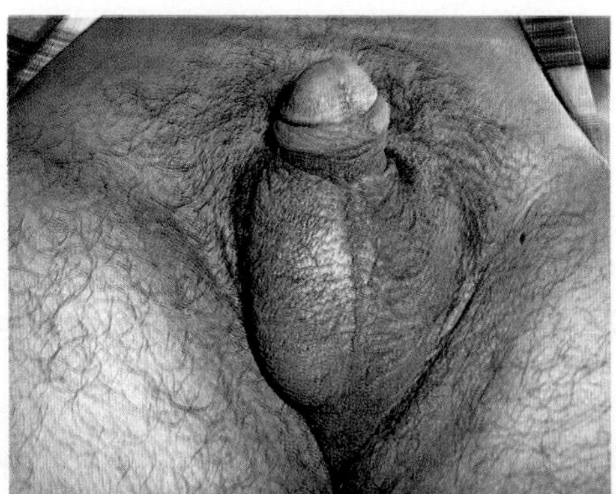

Left undescended testis with agenesis of left scrotum

On examination there is **pallor.** There is no jaundice and no generalized lymphadenopathy. Abdominal examination revealed fullness **in the right side of the hypogastrium and right iliac fossa-region.** On palpation, there is a firm **mass of 18 × 12 cm (18 cm horizontal and 12 cm vertical)** occupying the right side of the hypogastrium and right iliac fossa. All the borders of the mass except the lower border are well defined. One **cannot get below the mass.** The **mass is fixed** and the **surface is nodular.** The rest of the abdomen is normal. Liver is not palpable. There is no free fluid in the abdomen. The supraclavicular lymph nodes are not enlarged.

On examination of the genitalia, the **right scrotal sac is found to be empty** with **absence of rugae.** The **left testis is small and atrophic.** The **left vas is normally** palpated. Pubic hair and other secondary sexual characteristics are normal. There is no gynecomastia (Fig. 19.1).

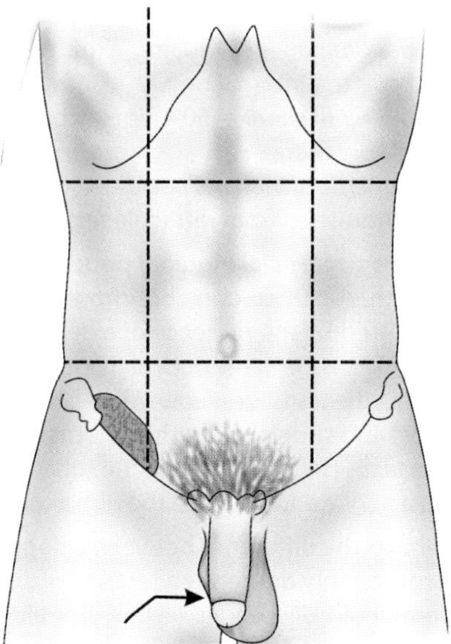

Fig. 19.1: Hypogastric mass (undescended right testis)

Read the checklist for abdominal examination.

Checklist for history
• History of trauma • Undescended testis • Scrotal surgery • Nausea and vomiting—retroduodenal metastasis • Cough and dyspnea—pulmonary metastasis • Backache—retroperitoneal metastasis • Bone pain—skeletal metastasis.

Checklist for examination
• Look for empty hemiscrotum with absent rugae • Look for lower limb edema (unilateral or bilateral)—Pressure from the retroperitoneal nodes • Gynecomastia—seen in 5% of cases

Contd...

Contd...

• Supraclavicular lymph nodes, iliac lymph nodes • Look for secondary hydrocele • Palpate the abdomen in the supraumbilical region for retroperitoneal nodes • Rule out liver metastasis • Examine the chest to rule out pulmonary metastasis • Look for pallor (in advanced cases).

Q 1. What is the most probable diagnosis in this case?

Malignant tumor arising from the undescended testis. Most probably **seminoma**.

Q 2. Why seminoma?

That is the most common tumor in the undescended testis.

Age group is also in favor of seminoma.

Q 3. What is the clinical sign for undescended testis?

Empty hemiscrotum with absent rugae is suggestive of undescended testis.

Q 4. What is "sign of the vas"?

In testicular neoplasm the vas deferens is normal, whereas it is thickened in inflammatory lesions of the testis and epididymis. In order to differentiate tumor from inflammation, this clinical sign is used.

Q 5. What will happen to the undescended testis?

Degenerative changes will occur in the seminiferous tubules. The lining cells become progressively atrophic and hyalinized with peritubal fibrosis. Degenerative changes begin to occur at 2 years of age. If not corrected all bilaterally, cryptorchidism in adult males becomes sterile.

Q 6. What is the chronology of descent of testis?

The testis is formed in front of the kidneys from the genital fold medial to the mesonephros

(Wolffian body) in early fetal life. They lie in the retroperitoneum below the developing kidneys. The primitive testis is attached to the posterior abdominal wall by the mesorchium. Its descent is a complicated process, which depends on the gubernaculum testis, steroid hormones and maternal gonadotropins. The testis is intra-abdominal up to 7 months of intrauterine life. Shortly before birth the testis reaches the bottom of the scrotum being invaginated into a tube of peritoneum—the processus vaginalis. The chronology of descent is as follows:

Chronology of descent of testis	
3rd month of intrauterine life	– from loin to iliac fossa
4–7 months of intrauterine life	– rest at the site of internal ring
7th month of intrauterine life	– it is travelling through the inguinal canal
8th month of intrauterine life	– lies at the external ring
9th month of intrauterine life	– it enters the scrotum, reaching its base at or after birth

Note: The descent may continue after birth, 50% reaching the scrotum during the first month of life.

Q 7. What are the complications of undescended testis?

Mnemonic—MAT SHOP

M – Malignancy
A – Atrophy – because of recurrent minor trauma
T – Torsion
S – Sterility – in bilateral cases
H – Hernia – in 95% there is patent processus vaginalis and 25% develop clinical hernia
O – Orchitis (epididymo – orchitis)
P – Pain – because of trauma.

Q 8. What are the positions of undescended testis?

1. *Intra-abdominal*—(33%) lying extra peritoneal just above the internal ring
2. *In the inguinal canal*—(50%) it may or may not be palpable there
3. *In the superficial inguinal pouch*—(50%) it must be distinguished from retractile testis.

Q 9. What is superficial inguinal pouch?

Failure of the testis to descend into the scrotum may be caused by the presence of a dense layer of subcutaneous tissue at the neck of the scrotum. As a result of this, the testis turns upwards to lie in a **pouch just above and superficial to the external inguinal ring.** The testis is therefore felt in the subcutaneous tissue just above and lateral to the pubic tubercle.

Q 10. What is the difference between ectopic testis and incompletely descended testis?

An incompletely descended testis will lie along the line of the normal descent at the neck of scrotum, over the external ring to the canal and on the posterior abdominal wall. In this situation, the testis is **palpable only when it is at or outside the external ring. The ectopic testis is always palpable** in contrast to incompletely descended testis and it is not in line of the normal descent.

Q 11. What are the common positions of ectopic testis?

Common positions of ectopic testis

1. Femoral triangle—confused with lymph node
2. Base of the penis
3. Perineum
4. Superficial inguinal pouch.

Q 12. What is the timing of surgery for undescended testis?

It is usually done between **6 months to 1 year** of age (the degenerative changes will start at the age of 2 years).

Q 13. What is the fertility after orchidopexy?

- Unilateral orchidopexy—fertility rate is 80%
- Bilateral orchidopexy—fertility rate is 50%.

Q 14. What is retractile testis?

During childhood the testis are mobile. In children < 3 years with **very active cremasteric reflex** due to the **small size of testis** the gonad will retract into the external ring or within the canal. It can be manipulated back into the mid or lower scrotum. No treatment is required in this condition.

Q 15. What is 'vanishing' testis?

It is a condition where the testis develops but disappears before birth. The most likely cause is **prenatal torsion**.

Q 16. What is true agenesis?

It is very rare. **Laparoscopy** is useful in distinguishing true agenesis from cryptorchidism with intra-abdominal testis.

Q 17. What are the anomalies associated with cryptorchidism?

This is seen in 15% of cryptorchidism. The following are the associated anomalies:

Anomalies associated with cryptorchidism
• Klinefelter's syndrome
• Hypogonadotropic, hypogonadism
• Prune belly syndrome
• Horse shoe kidney
• Renal agenesis or hypoplasia
• Exstrophy of the bladder
• Ureteral reflux
• Gastroschisis
• Cloacal exstrophy.

Q 18. What is the incidence of undescended testis?

- 4% of full-term infants
- 30% in premature babies.

Q 19. Can the unilateral cryptorchid develop malignancy in the normally descended contralateral testis?

Yes. 10% of patients with history of cryptorchidism develop malignancy in contralateral testis.

Q 20. What is the risk of malignancy according to the position of the testis in undescended testis?

The relative risk for malignancy in:

Intra-abdominal testis – 1 in 20

Inguinal testis – 1 in 80.

Q 21. What is the most common pathological type of malignancy seen in undescended testis?

Seminoma

Embryonal carcinoma—It is seen nowadays in patients in whom the testis has been brought down.

Q 22. Will orchidopexy change the malignant potential of the cryptorchid testis?

No. It facilitates examination and tumor detection.

Q 23. What are the factors responsible for the malignant change in cryptorchidism?

Factors responsible for malignant change in cryptorchidism
1. Abnormal germ cell morphology
2. Gonadal dysgenesis
3. Elevated temperature
4. Interference of blood supply
5. Endocrine dysfunction.

Q 24. What are the differential diagnoses of a solid swelling in the testis?

Differential diagnoses of solid swelling in the testis
1. Testicular tumor
2. Acute and chronic epididymo-orchitis
3. Hematocele
4. Gumma
5. Orchitis (mumps).

Q 25. What is 'billiard ball' testis?

Syphilis in adults will cause interstitial inflammation turning the testis into a round, hard and insensitive mass, which is called 'billiard ball testis'.

Q 26. What is Gumma of the testis?

Gumma of the testis is due to syphilis. The testis is painless and therefore presents as a lump on the surface of the testis or enlargement of the whole organ. The testicular sensation is lost early. H/o exposure will be there. A search is made for stigmata of syphilis like **Clutton's joint**, **interstitial keratitis**, etc. It is indistinguishable from tumor. If untreated it will breakdown to form **Gummatous ulcer**.

Q 27. What is the relationship of testicular tumor and trauma?

Many patients attribute the symptoms of the swelling to trauma. But this is to be ignored. **We do not know whether the lump is due to the hump or the hump is due to the lump!!**

Q 28. What is the most common starting point of the tumor in the testis?

Lower pole of the body of the testis, later they occupy the whole of the testis.

Q 29. What is the classification for testicular tumors?

Various classifications are there:

- Dixon and Moore
- WHO
- British tumor panel
- Histopathological classification.

The testis is composed of actively dividing germ cells, the supporting cells and connective tissue stroma. The tumors of the testis arise from the actively dividing germ cells. Comprising 90 – 95% and the rest contributed by nongerminal neoplasms. The histopathological classification is given below:

Histopathological Classification

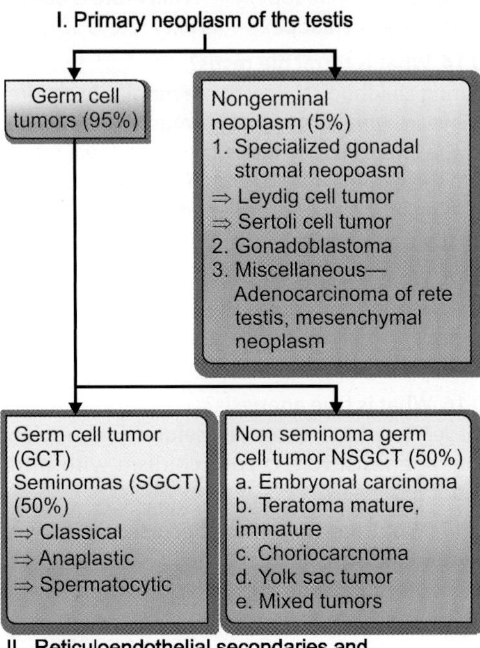

II. Reticuloendothelial secondaries and metastasis

III. Paratesticular neoplasms
   a. Adenomatoid
   b. Cystadenoma of epididymis
   c. Mesenchymal of epididymis
   d. Mesothelioma
   e. Metastasis.

Q 30. What is teratoma? What is the classification of teratoma?

Teratoma arises from totipotent cells in the rete testis and contains a variety of cell types with predominance of one or more cells. The usual variety is yellowish in color with cystic spaces containing gelatinous fluid. Cartilaginous areas are often present. The tumor may be as small as a peanut or as large as a coconut.

Testicular Panel Classification of Teratoma

- Teratoma differentiated (TD)—Uncommon.
- Even though there is no histologically recognizable malignant component, it cannot be considered benign. It may contain cartilage, muscle and glandular tissue.
- Malignant teratoma intermediate or Teratocarcinoma (MTI) (most common) (A and B Type). Contains definitely malignant and incompletely differentiated components.
- Malignant teratoma anaplastic or Embryonal carcinoma (MTA). The cells are presumed to be derived from yolk sac and are responsible for elevation of AFP.
- Malignant teratoma trophoblastic (MTT)—Uncommon

It contains syncytial cell mass with malignant villous or papillary cytotrophoblast (choriocarcinoma). It produces chorionic gonadotropin (hCG). It is one of the most malignant tumors having spread by bloodstream and lymphatics early.

Q 31. What are the differences between seminoma and teratoma?

No.	*Seminoma*	*Teratoma*
1.	*Age group:* 35 – 45 (older age group)	20 – 35 (younger age group)
2.	*Cut surface* is homogeneous and pinkish in color	Yellowish in color with cystic spaces containing gelatinous fluid. Cartilages are often present
3.	*Origin:* histologically arising from seminiferous tubules	Originate from totipotent cells in the rete testis containing variety of cell types
4.	*Cell type:* Oval cells with clear cytoplasm and prominent acidophilic neucleoli	Cell type depends on the type of teratoma – TD, MTI, MTA, MTT
5.	*Main spread* by lymphatics	Spread by *bloodstream*
6.	Sensitive to *radiotherapy*	Not sensitive to *radiotherapy*

Note: The non seminomatous tumors are classified into three groups – Good risk, Intermediate risk and bad risk

- The HCG value will be > 50,000 for bad risk and < 50,000 for good risk. The intermediate risk values are in between.

Q 32. What is Leydig cell tumor?

It is an interstitial cell tumor arising from Leydig cells, which **masculinizes**. They are prepubertal tumors causing sexual precocity and extreme muscular development. The regression of the symptoms is incomplete after orchidectomy because of the hypertrophy of the contralateral testis.

Q 33. What is Sertoli cell tumor?

They are interstitial cell tumor arising from Sertoli cells, which produces **feminizing** hormones. This will produce **gynecomastia, loss of libido and aspermia.** These tumors are benign and orchidectomy is curative.

Q 34. What are the testicular tumors producing gynecomastia?

- Teratoma
- Feminizing tumors (Sertoli).

Q 35. What is the cause for gynecomastia in testicular tumor?

Raised β-hCG is responsible for gynecomastia.

Q 36. What are the etiological factors for testicular tumors?

Etiological factors for testicular tumors

- Congenital—Cryptorchidism (3–14 times greater incidence than normal)
- Acquired
- Trauma
- Viral—Mumps (Atrophy of testis)—atrophic testis is more prone for malignancy
- AIDS
- Hormones—Estrogen administration results in Leydig cell tumor—Testicular tumor in children of mother's treated with diethyl stilbestrol
- Ethnic factors
- Environmental factors
- Klinefelter's syndrome.

Q 37. What are the modes of spread of testicular tumor?

1. Local – Local involvement to epididymis and cord is hindered by tunica albuginea
2. Lymphatic
3. Hematogenous.

Q 38. What is the lymphatic drainage of testis?

From the testis several lymphatic vessels emerge from the mediastinum testis and accompany the gonadal vessels in the spermatic cord. Where the spermatic vessels cross ventral to the ureter, some of these lymphatics diverge medially and drain into the retroperitoneal lymph nodes, while others follow the spermatic vessels to their origin and reach the para-aortic nodes.

Lymphatics from the medial side of the testis may run with the artery to the vas and drain into a node at the bifurcation of the common iliac artery (common iliac nodes).

The **inguinal lymph nodes** are affected when the **scrotal skin is involved**.

Q 39. What you mean by landing zones for lymphatics?

The primary landing zones for right testicular tumor lies in the interaortocaval nodes immediately below the renal vessels. (At the level of L2 lumbar vertebrae). The ipsilateral lymphatics will also go to paracaval, preaortic and right common iliac and external iliac nodes.

For the left testicular tumor it lies in the true para-aortic nodes just below the left renal vessels. (Left renal hilum). The ipsilateral distribution also includes para-aortic, preaortic and left common iliac nodes.

The metastasis reach the common iliac, external iliac and inguinal nodes usually secondary to retrograde spread because of large volume disease.

Q 40. Clinically what is the level of retroperitoneal nodes?

Above the umbilicus in the abdomen.

Q 41. What is the spread beyond the regional nodes?

The retroperitoneal lymphatics empty into the cisterna chyli via the right and left lumbar trunks. From here, it will reach the left supraclavicular nodes.

From the para-aortic nodes, the lymphatics will reach the retrocrural nodes and from there it will reach the mediastinal nodes (posterior mediastinum). Involvement of the anterior mediastinum is rare.

Q 42. What is the method of contralateral spread? (PG)

The contralateral spread is usually seen with right sided tumors especially in large volume tumors (rare with left sided tumors). If the patient has undergone herniorrhaphy, vasectomy or other trans scrotal procedures unrelated to the tumor, pelvic and inguinal nodes may get enlarged.

Q 43. What is the mechanism of inguinal node metastasis?

This will occur only if the tunica albuginea has been invaded by the tumor or as a result of previous surgical procedures like orchidopexy or herniorrhaphy.

Q 44. What are the sites of extranodal metastasis?

Sites of extranodal metastasis in order of decreasing frequency are:

Lung
Liver
Brain
Bone
Kidney
Adrenal
GI tract
Spleen.

Q 45. Can testicular tumor occur bilaterally? (PG)

Yes. About 2–3% of testicular tumors are bilateral. They may occur simultaneously or successively. Primary bilateral tumors occur synchronously or asynchronously.

Q 46. What is the most common cause for bilateral testicular tumor? (PG)

- Testicular lymphoma
- Seminoma is the most common bilateral primary tumor.

Q 47. How will you size the testis? (PG)

They can be sized according to Prader orchidometer.

Q 48. When examining the testes, which side is examined first?

The normal side is examined first.

Q 49. What is the incidence of testicular tumor? (PG)

- They make up 1–2% of the male cancers
- The life time probability of developing a tumor of the testis is 0.2%
- The highest incidence is seen in Scandinavia
- Lowest incidence is in Africa and Asia
- Higher socioeconomic class has higher incidence
- Incidence is 4 times in whites compared to black.

Q 50. Why testicular tumor is more common on the right side?

There is increased incidence of cryptorchidism on the right side and therefore tumor is more common on the right side.

Q 51. What are the clinical features of testicular tumor?

Painless enlargement of the testis 90% (Dull ache, sensation of heaviness in the lower abdomen, anal area or scrotum) acute testicular pain due to infarction or intratesticular hemorrhage is seen in about 10% of cases.

Extra testicular manifestations

- Cough and dyspnea—pulmonary metastasis
- Anorexia, nausea, vomiting (retroduodenal metastasis)
- Supraclavicular lymph node metastasis
- Back pain—retroperitoneal metastasis
- Lower extremities swelling—venacaval obstruction (unilateral or bilateral limb)
- Metastatic para-aortic lymph nodes (present behind and above the umbilicus)
- Gynecomastia (5% of cases)
- Bone pain (skeletal metastasis)
- CNS involvement (spinal cord/root involvement)
- Asymptomatic (10%)—identified incidentally.

Q 52. What is the incidence of secondary hydrocele in testicular tumors?

Its *10%*. The secondary hydrocele is usually lax.

Q 53. What is the cause for thickening of the spermatic cord? (PG)

This is a late feature and it is because of the **cremasteric hypertrophy** and the enlargement of the testicular vessels.

Q 54. What is the importance of testicular sensation in tumors?

The testicular sensation is lost completely in the early stage of the tumor. This **sign is better not demonstrated because of the fear of dissemination**. Palpation of the tumor also should be avoided to the minimum.

Q 55. What is "hurricane tumor"?

It is a ferocious type of malignancy that kills the patients in a matter of weeks because of the rapid spread of the tumor.

Q 56. Can you feel the epididymis separately in testicular tumor?

Epididymis is normal during initial stages. But it becomes more difficult to feel as it is flattened and **incorporated in the growth in later stages**.

Q 57. What are the tumor markers?

Tumor markers for testicular tumors

1. α - Fetoprotein (AFP)
2. β - Human chorionic gonadotropin (β-hCG)
3. Lactate dehydrogenase (LDH).

Q 58. What is the significance of serum tumor markers? (PG)

In 85% of patients at least 1 marker is raised.

Markers are used for assessment of tumor regression and recurrence.

Remember !!Tumor is possible without elevation of the tumor marker.

Q 59. What is the significance of LDH? (PG)

It is increased in 60% of nonseminomatous GCT and 80% of patients with advanced seminoma.

It has independent prognostic significance in patients with advanced germ cell tumor.

Increase in the serum concentration is a reflection of tumor burden, growth rate and proliferation.

Q 60. What is the significance of AFP? (PG)

- AFP is elevated in 70% of nonseminomas (not in pure seminomas)—restricted to embryonal cell carcinoma and endodermal sinus tumor (yolk sac tumor).
- If AFP is elevated in seminoma, suspect non-seminoma elements in either the primary or metastasis.
- The normal adult concentration is usually < 15 ng/mL.
- The physiological half-life is 5–7 days.

Q 61: What is the significance of β-hCG? (PG)

- It is a glycoprotein produced by 65% of non-seminomas and 10% of seminomas (all patients with choriocarcinoma and 40% patients with embryonal carcinoma).
- It is produced by syncytiotrophoblasts.
- Half-life of β-hCG is 24–48 hours

Q 62. What are the investigations in a patient with suspected testicular tumor?

Investigations in testicular tumor

1. *Blood*—radioimmunoassay of tumor markers
2. *Chest*—radiograph – for pulmonary metastasis
3. *Ultrasound*—of the affected testis and abdomen—abdomen for lymph nodes and liver metastasis
4. *CT/MRI*—for intra-abdominal and intrathoracic secondaries
5. *IVU*—deviated or obstructed ureters as a result of the retroperitoneal nodes will be demonstrated
6. *High orchidectomy.*

Q 63. What is the sonological finding in testicular tumor? (PG)

Sonologically the tumor will appear as **hypoechoic lesion.** It may also reveal secondary hydrocele.

Q 64. Why high orchidectomy is included along with investigations?

Orchidectomy is considered as the basic investigation in testicular tumors. It is essential to remove the primary tumor to obtain the histological type of malignancy. The pathological knowledge is important for the **AJCC** staging because the tumor status in this staging is always PT0, PT1, etc.

Q 65. What is the incision for high orchidectomy?

Transinguinal incision.

Q 66. Why not transscrotal incision?

If a transscrotal incision is made in testicular tumor, the tumor will spread to the lymphatic territory of the inguinal nodes (testis will normally drain to para-aortic nodes). Therefore, if transscrotal incision is made, the inguinal nodes also must be tackled by radiotherapy. This must be avoided. There are three things to be avoided in testicular tumors:

Three Nos in testicular tumors

- No transscrotal incision
- No transscrotal aspiration
- No transscrotal biopsy.

Q 67. What is high orchidectomy (inguinal orchidectomy)? (PG)

Through a transinguinal incision the spermatic cord is displayed by dividing the external oblique aponeurosis. A soft clamp is placed across the cord as the initial step to prevent dissemination of malignant cells as the testis is mobilized into the wound. The cord is then doubly ligated at the level of the deep inguinal ring and divided, so that the testis can be removed.

Q 68. What is Chevassu maneuver? (PG)

During the above procedure when the testis is brought to the inguinal wound, if there is doubt regarding the diagnosis, the testis should be bisected along its anterior convexity so that its internal structure can be examined by frozen section. If a tumor is ruled out the bisected testis can be closed and returned to the normal position.

Q 69. If the patient is explored by transscrotal route already what is the course of action? (PG)

Hemiscrotectomy and radiation of inguinal nodes is recommended.

Q 70. What is the clinical staging?

Clinical staging of testicular tumors

Stage 1—Tumor confined to the testis
Stage 2—Nodes below the level of the diaphragm—spread to regional lymph nodes—retroperitoneal, para-aortic
Stage 3—Nodes above the level of the diaphragm—spread beyond the retroperitoneal nodes, to the mediastinum or extra lymphatic metastasis
Stage 4—Pulmonary or hepatic metastasis

Q 71. What is the TNM staging (AJCC 7th Edition)? (PG)

T stage

*The extent of primary tumor is usually classified after radical orchiectomy and for this reason; a Pathological Stage is assigned using the prefix *P*

*pTX Primary tumor cannot be assessed

pTO No evidence of primary tumor (e.g. histologic scar in testis)

pTis Intratubular germ cell neoplasia (carcinoma *in situ*)

pT1 Tumor limited to the testis and epididymis without vascular/lymphatic invasion, tumor may invade into the tunica albuginea but not the tunica vaginalis

pT2 Tumor limited to the testis and epididymis with vascular/lymphatic invasion, or tumor extending through the tunica albuginea with involvement of the tunica vaginalis

PT3 Tumor invades the spermatic cord with or without vascular/lymphatic invasion

pT4 Tumor invades the scrotum with or without vascular/lymphatic invasion

Note: Except for pTis and pT4, extent of primary tumor is classified by radical orchiectomy. TX may be used for other categories in the absence of radical orchiectomy.

N Stage (Clinical)

NX Regional lymph nodes cannot be assessed

N0 No regional lymph node metastasis

N1 Metastasis with a lymph node mass 2 cm or less in greatest dimension; or multiple lymph nodes, not more than 2 cm in greatest dimension

N2 Metastasis with a lymph node mass more than 2 cm, but not more than 5 cm in greatest dimension; or multiple lymph nodes, any one mass greater than 2 cm but not more than 5 cm in greatest dimension

N3 Metastasis with a lymph node mass more than 5 cm in greatest dimension.

Pathological N Stage (pN)

pNX Regional lymph nodes cannot be assessed

pN0 No regional lymph node metastasis

pN1 Metastasis with a lymph node mass 2 cm or less in greatest dimension and less than or equal to 5 nodes positive, not more than 2 cm in greatest dimension

pN2 Metastasis with a lymph node mass more than 2 cm but not more than 5 cm in greatest dimension; or more than 5 nodes positive, not more than 5 cm; or evidence of extranodal extension of tumor

pN3 Metastasis with a lymph node mass more than 5 cm in greatest dimension

M stage

MX Distant metastasis cannot be assessed

M0 No distant metastasis

M1 Distant metastasis

M1a Non regional nodal or pulmonary metastasis

M1b Distant metastasis other than to non- regional lymph nodes and lungs

Serum Tumor Markers (S)

SX Marker studies not available or not performed

S0 Marker study levels within normal limits

S1 LDH < 1.5 X N* and hCG (mIU/mL) < 5000 and AFP (ng/ml) < 1000

S2 LDH 1.5 – 10 X N or hCG (mIU/mL) 5000 – 50,000 or AFP (ng/mL) 1000 – 10,000

S3 LDH > 10 X N or hCG (mIU/mL) > 50,000 or AFP (ng/mL) > 10,000

*N indicates upper limit of normal for the LDH assay.

Q 72. What is the management of testicular tumors?

The management of seminomas and non-seminomatous germinal cell tumors is different.

Q 73. What is the management of seminoma?

After high orchidectomy seminoma is treated with radiotherapy (because seminoma is a radio sensitive tumor) for stage 1 and nonbulky for stage 2.

- Over a 3-week-period administer 2500 cGy hockey stick field including the following nodes
- Para-aortic, paracaval, bilateral common iliac and external iliac nodal regions

- Recently the radiation is confined to the para-aortic area alone
- With history of herniorrhaphy and orchidopexy include the contralateral inguinal region shielding the contralateral testis
- Mediastinal radiation is currently avoided (chemotherapy is more effective).

Q 74. Is there any role for semen banking? (PG)

If the function of the contralateral testis is in question, this should be considered. The semen of the patient may be collected and preserved if the patient is desirous of having children.

Q 75. What are the indications for chemotherapy in seminoma? (PG)

- Bulky abdominal disease
- Metastasis.

Q 76. What is the chemotherapeutic regimen? (PG)

It is treated with four cycles of chemotherapy with **BEP regimen**

- Bleomycin
- Etoposide
- Cisplatin.

Q 77. What is the treatment of residual abdominal mass after chemotherapy? (PG)

Residual tumor of more than 3 cm is treated by surgery.

Q 78. What is the management of non-seminomatous germ cell tumor?

After high orchidectomy, patients are treated with Retroperitoneal Lymph Node Dissection (RPLND) except bulky disease or distant metastasis.

Q 79. What are the approaches for RPLND? (PG)

- Transabdominal
- Thoracoabdominal.

Q 80. What is bulky disease? (PG)

All patients with retroperitoneal mass > 5 cm (high burden disease).

Q 81. What is the most important problem of RPLND? (PG)

Retrograde ejaculation.

Q 82. What is the extent of RPLND? (PG)

The standard RPLND is a bilateral dissection from renal vessel down to aortic bifurcation, along the external iliac artery to the deep inguinal ring on the affected side. The following lymph nodes are removed on both sides.

Lymph nodes removed in RPLND

Paracaval
Interaortocaval
Para-aortic
Preaortic
Common iliac nodes.

Q 83. What is the contraindication for RPLND? (PG)

Choriocarcinoma. Here the disease is systemic and the treatment is multi agent chemotherapy.

Q 84. What are the indications for withholding RPLND? (PG)

- Normal serum markers
- No nodes in abdominal CT
- No distant metastasis.

The rationale behind this policy is that only 20% of such patients will develop disease and in such a situation patient should be ready for regular follow-up.

Q 85. What is the follow-up of such a patient? (PG)

- Physical examination
- CT abdomen 3 monthly for first two years, 6 monthly thereafter
- Tumor markers.

They are done monthly for the first year, every 2 monthly for the second year and 3–6 months thereafter.

Q 86. What is modified RPLND (Nerve sparing RPLND)? (PG)

This involves bilateral dissection above the origin of the inferior mesenteric artery and unilateral dissection confined to the side of the tumor below the origin of the inferior mesenteric artery. This preserves the important sympathetic fibers from the contralateral side thus, maintaining ejaculation.

Q 87. What is the treatment of extensive retroperitoneal nodes with chest metastasis? (PG)

High orchidectomy and multi agent chemo followed by excision of the persistent mass in the retroperitoneum.

Q 88. What are the alternative drugs for chemotherapy? (PG)

Ifosfamide/Doxorubicin.

Q 89. What is the prognosis of nonseminomatous germ cell tumor? (PG)

Stage II – 90% cure rate at 5 years
Stage III – 70% cure rate at 5 years
Choriocarcinoma – 35% at 5 years

Q 90. What is the management of the given case?

In this patient the tumor is arising from intra-abdominal testis. It should be removed transabdominally and the further management depends on the histopathology. Considering his age, the pathology is likely to be seminoma and therefore he requires radiotherapy.

Case

20 Portal Hypertension

Case Capsule

A **55-year-old male patient** presents with **melena of one week duration**. He is a **chronic alcoholic** and gives history of **three bouts of hematemesis** in the last 2 months. He complains of **distension of the abdomen, abdominal discomfort, and lethargy** for the last 6 months. He gives **history of jaundice in the childhood**. His sleep pattern is not altered. There is no history of treatment with NSAIDs, paracetamol and anti- tuberculous drugs. There is **no history of omphalitis** in the newborn period. There is no history of chronic pancreatitis or history of convulsions.

On general examination, the patient is **ill looking, poorly nourished and there is obvious muscle wasting**. He is **fully oriented**. There is no memory impairment. The speech is normal. There is **pallor and mild icterus**. Both **lower limbs show pitting type of edema. Clubbing of the fingers and toes** are seen. About **10 spider nevi spots** are present in the **front of the chest, face and arms** (1 mm size bright red spots with radiating small branches spreading to 2 mm diameter. They fade completely when compressed with finger and refill as soon as the pressure is released). Patient has got **bilateral gynecomastia**. There is **loss of pubic and axillary hair**. There is no evidence of palmar erythema. **Skin bruising** is noted in the right forearm of about 5 × 4 cm size. There is no flapping tremor and there is no fetor hepaticus.

On examination of the abdomen, there is **generalized distension of the abdomen** and the umbilicus is everted. There are no caput medusae. There is **shifting dullness and fluid thrill** demonstrated. Dipping palpation revealed **splenomegaly**. On auscultation a **venous hum** is heard **in the epigastrium** that is louder on inspiration. On examination of the genitalia, both testes are found to be small and soft suggestive of **testicular atrophy**. Central nervous system examination showed **no evidence of encephalopathy**. The cardiovascular system is normal and there are no features suggestive of constrictive pericarditis or tricuspid valve incompetence.

Read the checklist for abdominal examination.

Checklist for history

- History of alcoholism
- Previous jaundice
- Schistosomiasis
- Valvular heart disease, constrictive pericarditis
- Abdominal tumors—extrinsic compression
- Hematemesis and melena.

Checklist for examination

- Stigmata of liver disease (refer chapter on liver)
- Triad of portal hypertension namely esophageal varices, ascites and splenomegaly
- Look for jaundice
- Features of encephalopathy
- Look for anemia
- Look for pitting edema of lower limbs
- Look for ascites
- Look for hepatosplenomegaly
- Look for caput medusae
- Look for testicular atrophy
- Look for gynecomastia
- Look for Kenawy's sign—venous hum, heard louder on inspiration in the epigastrium in portal hypertension
- Look for Cruveilhier-Baumgarten syndrome—loud venous hum at umbilicus in case of portal hypertension.

Q 1. What is the probable diagnosis in this case?

Cirrhosis of liver with portal hypertension.

Q 2. What are the points in favor of portal hypertension?

1. History of alcoholism
2. History of upper GI bleed
3. Melena
4. Hepatosplenomegaly on examination
5. Mild icterus
6. Presence of ascites.

Q 3. What are the causes for ascites?

Causes for ascites are:

Hepatic causes
- Cirrhosis with portal hypertension
- Hypoalbuminemia of any cause

Malignant ascites
- Secondary to any primary or metastatic malignancy

Contd...

Infective
- Tuberculous peritonitis
- Bacterial peritonitis
- Primary peritonitis

Congestive
- Right sided heart failure
- Budd-Chiari syndrome
- Constrictive pericarditis

Miscellaneous causes
- Pancreatic ascites
- Chylous ascites
- Meig's syndrome
- Pseudomyxoma peritonei.

Q 4. What are the causes for general fullness of the abdomen?

It may be due to:

- Fat
- Fluid
- Flatus
- Feces
- Fetus.

Q 5. What is the minimum amount of fluid required to demonstrate free fluid in the abdominal cavity?

The minimum amount of fluid to demonstrate clinical ascites is 1500 mL.

Q 6. What is the minimum amount required radiologically to demonstrate fluid within the peritoneal cavity?

The minimum amount required radiologically to demonstrate ascites is 150 mL.

Q 7. What are the types of ascitic fluid?

May be transudate or exudates.

Q 8. What are the differences between transudate and exudates?

Differences between transudate and exudate

	Transudate	*Exudates*
Protein	Low—most of which is albumin < 1gm/dL	High—(2.5 – 3.5 gm/dL) High content of fibrinogen
Specific gravity	< 1.012	> 1.020
Glucose content	Same as plasma	Low < 60 mg/dL
pH	> 7.3	< 7.3
LDH	Low	High
Cellular debris	Few cells	More cells
Cause	Obstruction to the venous outflow from liver (ultrafiltrate of blood plasma and results from imbalance across the vascular endothelium) permeability of endothelium—normal	Inflammatory extravascular fluid formed by the escape of fluid, proteins and blood cells from the vascular system into the interstitial tissue or body cavities because of increased vascular permeability
SAAG (Serum ascites albumin gradient)	> 1.1 (Ascitic fluid has less albumin than serum)	< 1.1 (Ascitic fluid has more albumin than serum)

Q 9. What are the signs of ascites?

Signs of ascites

- Puddle sign—mild ascites
- Shifting dullness—moderate ascites
- Fluid thrill—severe ascites
- Tanyon sign—the umbilicus is pushed upwards in ovarian cyst and downwards in ascites

Q 10. What is puddle sign?

This is a clinical method to demonstrate minimum amount of fluid in the peritoneal cavity. The patient is positioned in the knee elbow position and the abdomen is percussed around the umbilicus that will reveal dullness.

Q 11. How will you demonstrate shifting dullness?

Ask the patient to turn on to his left side, wait for a minute so that the fluid gravitates. Start percussion from the right side to the left noting where the resonant area becomes dull and then mark the spot on the abdominal wall. Then the patient is asked to turn slightly on to his right side and after 1 minute if shifting dullness is present, the dull area will become resonant and vice versa.

Q 12. How will you demonstrate fluid thrill?

An assistant places the edge of his hand firmly on the center of the abdomen in order to damp down a fat thrill. The abdominal wall on one side is flicked and the hand on the other side of the abdomen feels the thrill.

Q 13. How will you differentiate ascites from ovarian cyst (Pelvic mass)?

Differences between ascites and ovarian cyst

	Ascites	*Ovarian cyst*
• *Dullness**	Is dull in the flanks and hypogastrium	Pelvic mass is dull in the hypogastrium only and flanks are resonant
• *Ruler test*—a flat ruler is placed on the abdomen just above the anterior superior iliac spine and pressed firmly backwards	Negative	In the case of ovarian cyst, the pulsations of the aorta are transmitted to the fingers through the ruler
• *Position of* umbilicus	The umbilicus is displaced downwards	The umbilicus is displaced upwards

Note: ***Mechanism of dullness**—The ovarian cyst displaces the loops of intestine to the flanks and occupies the middle of the abdomen. Hence, the dullness is felt over the mass in the hypogastrium while the flanks are resonant. Ascitis fluid displaces the loops of intestines to the middle of the abdomen. The flanks are occupied by the ascitic fluid that on percussion shows dullness while the floating loops of intestine are resonant over the middle of the abdomen (around the umbilicus).

Q 14. What is dipping palpation?

It is a special technique to palpate organs or tumors in cases of ascites. The pads of fingers are placed on the abdomen and then by a quick push, the abdominal wall is depressed. By this method an enlarged liver is felt easily so also a tumor mass.

Q 15. What is the definition of upper GI bleed?

Upper GI bleed is a bleeding located between the oropharynx and the ligament of Treitz (lower GI bleeding is a bleeding arising from distal to ligament of Treitz).

Q 16. What is hematemesis?

Vomiting of blood that is either fresh and unaltered or digested by gastric secretion.

Q 17. What is melanemesis?

Vomiting of altered blood is called melanemesis.

Q 18. What is the cause for coffee ground vomitus?

It is due to vomiting of blood that has been in the stomach long enough for gastric acid to convert hemoglobin to acid hematin.

Q 19. What is hematochezia?

Passage of bright red blood per rectum is called hematochezia. The bleeding source may be from colon, rectum or anus. If the intestinal transit is rapid during brisk bleeding in the upper intestine, bright red blood may be passed unchanged in the stool.

Q 20. What is melena?

It is defined as the passage of a black, tarry stool. Usually it is because of bleeding from the upper GI tract. But it can be produced by blood entering the bowel at any point from mouth to the cecum. The black color is because of the formation of hematin that is a product of oxidation of heme by intestinal and bacterial enzymes.

Q 21. What is the minimum amount of intestinal bleeding required to produce melena?

About 50 to 100 mL of blood in the stomach.

Q 22. How long it will take to clear a melena of a bleed of about 1000 mL of blood in the GI tract?

Three to five days.

Q 23. What is the minimum amount of blood required in the stool for a positive occult blood test?

More than 10 mL (normal subjects lose about 2.5 mL of blood per day in their stool from minor mechanical abrasion.

Q 24. What are the causes for upper GI bleeding?

Causes for upper GI bleeding

Common causes

1. Peptic ulceration—gastric ulcer, duodenal ulcer, stomal ulcer
2. Esophagogastric varices
3. Gastritis
4. Mallory-Weiss syndrome
5. Acute mucosal lesions—(erosions)—they do not extend through the muscularis mucosa and therefore called erosions, not ulcers
6. Stress ulceration (secondary to shock, sepsis following operation, trauma, etc.)—it is because of decreased splanchnic blood flow and not because of increased gastric secretion.

Uncommon causes

7. Reflux esophagitis
8. Gastric neoplasms
9. Curling's ulcer—erosion of stomach and duodenum in burns
10. Cushing ulcer—after head injury and cranial operations
11. Steroid induced—steroid ulcers
12. Hiatal hernia
13. Duodenal diverticulum
14. Miscellaneous
    - vascular lesions such as
    - Angioma
    - Rendu-Osler-Weber syndrome
    - Aortoenteric fistula
    - Hematobilia.

Q 25. What is the most important investigation for diagnosis in this case?

Esophagogastroduodenoscopy: It can be done in emergency situations when the patient's general condition is stabilized.

Q 26. What is the endoscopy finding for varices?

Varices appear as 3 or 4 large tortuous submucosal bulging vessels running longitudinally in the distal esophagus. The bleeding site may be identified. The lesion may be obscured by blood.

Q 27. What is the endoscopic grading of esophageal varices?

Grade 1—visible, nontortuous

Grade 2—tortuous, nonprotruding

Grade 3—protruding (normal mucosa in between the columns)

Grade 4—like grade 3, no normal mucosa.

Q 28. What is "varices upon varices"?

The small vessels seen on the surface of varices endoscopically are called varices upon varices.

Q 29. What are the endoscopic signs of prediction for bleeding?

Endoscopic signs of prediction for bleeding

- Varices upon varices
- Red wale marking
- Cherry red spot
- Hematocystic spot
- Blue varices
- Erosions on mucosa.

Q 30. Any role for upper GI barium series?

Barium studies are neither sensitive nor specific. A barium swallow outlines the varices in 90% of the cases. But they are difficult and dangerous in bleeding patients.

Q 31. Is it possible to have bleeding duodenal ulcer in patients with esophageal varices?

Yes. It is to be stressed that even in known patients of esophageal varices, it is important to repeat the upper GI endoscopy so as to exclude a bleeding peptic ulcer.

Q 32. What are the important investigations in upper GI bleeding?

Important investigations in upper GI bleeding

1. Endoscopy
2. LFT—bilirubin is usually elevated, serum albumin is often decreased
3. Hemoglobin—anemia may be as a result of bleeding, hypersplenism or nutritional deficiency
4. Coagulation profile—PT, APTT, INR, platelet count may be deranged in cirrhosis
5. Ultrasound abdomen—for identifying the size of portal vein, the status of liver (cirrhotic or not), for ascites, the amount of collaterals, etc.
6. Splenoportography—for identifying the site of obstruction
7. Ascitic fluid study
8. Liver biopsy—for confirming the cause of portal hypertension.

Q 33. What are the peculiarities of portal vein?

- It is unique in that it starts and ends in capillaries
- It has no valves.

Q 34. What is the normal portal pressure? What is the pressure in portal hypertension?

Normally it ranges from 7–10 cm of saline. In portal hypertension the portal pressure exceeds 10 cm of saline averaging around 20 cm of saline.

Q 35. How portal vein is formed?

It is formed in front of the inferior vena cava (IVC) and behind the neck of the pancreas by union of the superior mesenteric and splenic vein. This union occurs at the level of the second lumbar vertebrae. The vessel is 5–8 cm long and passes up and to the right in the gastrohepatic omentum (lesser) to enter the hilum of liver where it immediately divides into right and left branches. In the liver right branch is short and supplies the caudate lobe of the liver and then divides into anterior and posterior branch. The longer left branch of the portal vein runs to the left in the porta hepatis.

Q 36. What is the mechanism of development of collateral circulation in portal hypertension?

The obstruction to the flow of portal venous blood in the liver promotes expansion of collateral channels between the portal and systemic venous system. When the portal pressure reaches around 40 cm of water (30 mm of Hg) the hepatic resistance reaches a point of occlusion of the portal vein and diverts the flow through collaterals without significantly increasing in pressure.

Q 37. What are the sites of portosystemic anastomosis?

Sites of portosystemic anastomosis and the resulting manifestations are:

Sl. No	*Site*	*Portal*	*Systemic*	*Manifestation*
1.	Lower end of esophagus	Coronary vein from stomach	Esophageal vein draining to azygos and vena cava	Esophageal varices and hematemesis
2.	Around the umbilicus	Veins along the falciform ligament	Epigastric veins	Radiating veins from umbilicus—caput medusae

Contd...

Contd...

3.	At the lower end of rectum	Superior rectal vein	Middle and inferior rectal veins	Anorectal varices (they are submucosal veins extending upwards well above the level of hemorrhoids and are easily compressible)
4.	In front of the kidney at the back of the colon	Vessels of peritoneum and colon	Vessels of the kidney (Veins of Retzius)	
5.	Bare area of the liver	Liver veins	Diaphragmatic veins	–

(See Fig. 20.1)

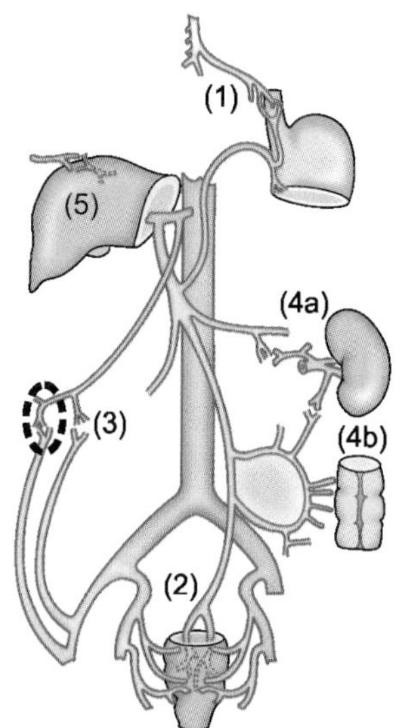

Fig. 20.1: Portosystemic anastomotic sites

Q 38. What are the sites of spontaneous bleeding in portal hypertension?

It is seen only from gastroesophageal junction. This place is rich in the submucosal veins that expands disproportionately in patients with portal hypertension.

Q 39. What is the pathogenesis of rupture of varices?

There are two theories.

1. Erosion from without (esophagitis)
2. Explosion from within (by increased pressure).

Q 40. Can you get isolated gastric varices without esophageal varices?

Yes. Isolated thrombosis of the splenic vein causes localized splenic venous hypertension. This will result in development of large collaterals from spleen to gastric fundus. From there the blood returns to the main portal system through the gastric coronary vein.

Q 41. How will you assess the functional status of the liver disease?

Many scoring systems are available. The Child - Pugh classification is one of the standard systems to assess the functional status in liver disease.

Child-Turcotte-Pugh classification of functional status in liver disease			
Parameter		*Numerical score*	
	1	*2*	*3*
	Class – A [Risk - Low]	*Class–B[Risk - Moderate]*	*Class – C [Risk- High]*
Ascites	Absent	Slight to Moderate	Tense
Encephal-opathy	None	Grade I - II	Grade III - IV
Serum albumin (g/dL)	> 3.5	2.8 – 3.5	< 2.8
Serum bilirubin mg/dL	< 2 - 0	2.0 – 3.0	> 3.0
Prothrombin time (seconds above control)	< 4.0	4.0 – 6.0	> 6.0

Total score	*Child - Turcotte-Pugh classification*	*Risk*
5 – 6	A	Low risk
7 – 9	B	Moderate risk
10 – 15	C	High risk

Q 42. What is Child's classification?

Child's classification of hepatocellular function in cirrhosis.

Q 43. What are the causes for portal hypertension?

A. May be because of increased resistance to flow:
- Prehepatic
- Hepatic
- Posthepatic.

B. Increased portal blood flow—(because of the tremendous reserve capacity of the liver to accommodate increased blood flow, this is uncommon).
- Banti's syndrome
- Tropical splenomegaly
- Myeloid metaplasia.

Prehepatic causes
- Thrombosis of portal vein
- Thrombosis of splenic vein
- Congenital stenosis or atresia
- Extrinsic compression by tumors.

Hepatic causes
- Cirrhosis—portal, postnecrotic, biliary, Wilson's disease, hemochromatosis
- Congenital hepatic fibrosis
- Idiopathic portal hypertension
- Schistosomiasis
- Chronic active hepatitis
- Acute alcoholic liver diseases.

Posthepatic causes
- Budd-Chiari syndrome (hepatic vein thrombosis)
- Veno-occlusive disease
- Cardiac diseases—constrictive pericarditis, valvular heart disease, right heart failure, etc.

Q 44. What are the important common causes for portal hypertension?

Common causes for portal hypertension

1. Cirrhosis
   a. Cirrhosis (alcoholic)—85%
   b. Postnecrotic cirrhosis
   c. Biliary cirrhosis
2. Extrahepatic portal venous thrombosis (children and younger patients)
3. Idiopathic portal hypertension (Southern Asia)
4. Schistosomiasis (Egypt).

Q 45. What is the cause of abnormal resistance in the portal system in cirrhosis?

The resistance is predominantly postsinusoidal thought to be because of:

- Distortion of the hepatic veins by degenerating nodules
- Fibrosis of perivascular tissue around the sinusoids and hepatic veins
- Centrilobular swelling and fibrosis produce portal hypertension in acute alcoholic hepatitis in the absence of cirrhosis.

Q 46. What is wedged hepatic vein pressure?

A catheter is wedged in a tributary of the hepatic veins that will permit estimation of the pressure in the afferent veins to sinusoids.

Q 47. What is the site of obstruction in schistosomiasis?

Schistosomiasis produces presinusoidal obstruction because of deposition of parasite ova in small portal venules. This produces inflammation followed by fibrosis.

Q 48. What is Budd-Chiari syndrome?

This is a condition affecting mainly young females. The obstruction is in the hepatic veins as a result of hepatic vein thrombosis or congenital webs (venous web). The liver becomes congested as a result of obstruction, resulting in impaired liver function and portal hypertension. The patient also develops ascites and esophageal varices. If chronic, the liver progresses to cirrhosis. It is important to rule out the cause for venous thrombosis such as:

- Procoagulant states such as protein C, protein S and antithrombin III, deficiencies
- Myeloproliferative disorders.

Q 49. What is the CT finding in Budd-Chiari syndrome? (PG)

- Ascites
- Large congested liver (early)
- Small cirrhotic liver (late) with gross enlargement of segment I (caudate lobe).

Q 50. What is the cause for enlargement of segment? (PG)

Segment I is having direct venous drainage to the IVC (inferior vena cava). When there is atrophy of the rest of the liver because of hepatic vein obstruction, there will be gross enlargement of this segment.

Q 51. How will you confirm the diagnosis of Budd-Chiari syndrome? (PG)

This is done by hepatic venography through a transjugular approach. This will reveal occlusion of the hepatic veins.

Q 52. What is the treatment of Budd-Chiari syndrome? (PG)

- If cirrhosis is not established—TIPSS or shunt surgery
- If cirrhosis is established—Liver transplantation
- Lifelong anticoagulation with warfarin may be required.

Q 53. What is TIPSS?

Transjugular intrahepatic portosystemic stent shunt (TIPSS) was introduced 1988 as an emergency treatment for variceal hemorrhage not responding to medical management and endoscopic sclerotherapy. The procedure is done under local anesthesia and sedation using fluoroscopic guidance and ultrasonography. A guide wire is inserted through the internal jugular vein and then via the superior vena cava, hepatic veins and hepatic parenchyma to a branch of the portal vein. The track in the parenchyma is then dilated with a balloon catheter and a metallic stent is inserted. This will produce satisfactory drop in portal venous pressure, by shunting blood from portal system to the inferior vena cava directly.

Q 54. What are the complications of TIPSS? (PG)

- Perforation of liver capsule and fatal intraperitoneal hemorrhage
- TIPSS occlusion—further variceal hemorrhage
- Post-shunt encephalopathy (40%)
- Stenosis of the shunt (50% at one year).

Q 55. What is the cause for post-shunt encephalopathy after TIPSS? What is the incidence? (PG)

The portal blood bypassing the detoxification effects of the liver will enter the systemic circulation resulting in a confusional state. It occurs in 40% of patients similar to the surgical shunts. The early manifestations are subtle and mental and personality changes may be overlooked in the postoperative period. Restlessness, irritability and insomnia are common. Neuromuscular signs of unsustained clonus, increased tendon reflexes and extensor plantar are seen. Blood ammonia determination is unreliable. Finally more obvious confusion, drowsiness, stupor and coma develop.

Q 56. What is Banti's syndrome? (PG)

It is defined as a liver disease secondary to primary splenic disease. It was erroneously considered as the cause of portal hypertension but now it is known that it is as a result of cirrhosis.

Q 57. What are the criteria by which you categorize a patient to low-risk category in upper GI bleed? (PG)

Low-risk—upper GI bleed

1. Age < 75 years
2. No unstable comorbid illness
3. No ascites evident on physical examination
4. Normal PT (prothrombin time)
5. Systolic BP above 100 within 1 hour after admission (with or without fluid resuscitation)
6. Nasogastric aspirate free of fresh blood.

Q 58. What is the management of variceal bleeding? (Flow chart 20.1)

Emergency admission and following management is carried out.

1. Monitor the patient for BP, pulse, CVP, hematocrit, hourly urine output
2. Peripheral and central venous access
3. Arrange adequate blood (initially 10 units)
4. Serial hematocrit determination—is best for monitoring continued blood loss and appropriate replacement of the lost blood
5. Nasogastric aspiration—look for the color of the aspirate (blood or altered blood is present or not)
6. Stabilize the patients
7. Endoscopy within 24 hours after admission (in 80% the bleeding source can be identified). Two lesions are identified in 15% of patients
8. Upper GI series if endoscopy is equivocal
9. Medical management—vasopressin, terlipressin, somatostatin analog (octreotide)
10. Mechanical—balloon tamponade
11. Interventional—endoscopic sclerotherapy/banding
12. Prevent encephalopathy
13. Injection vitamin K to correct emergent coagulopathy (fresh frozen plasma may be required to correct coagulopathy).
14. Maintain fluid and electrolyte balance
15. Surgical—emergency shunt
    - Esophageal transection and anastomosis
    - Devascularization procedures.

Q 59. What is the initial therapy of choice?

- Endoscopic sclerotherapy or banding
- Vasopressin or propranolol may or may not be included

Flow chart 20.1: The management of portal hypertension

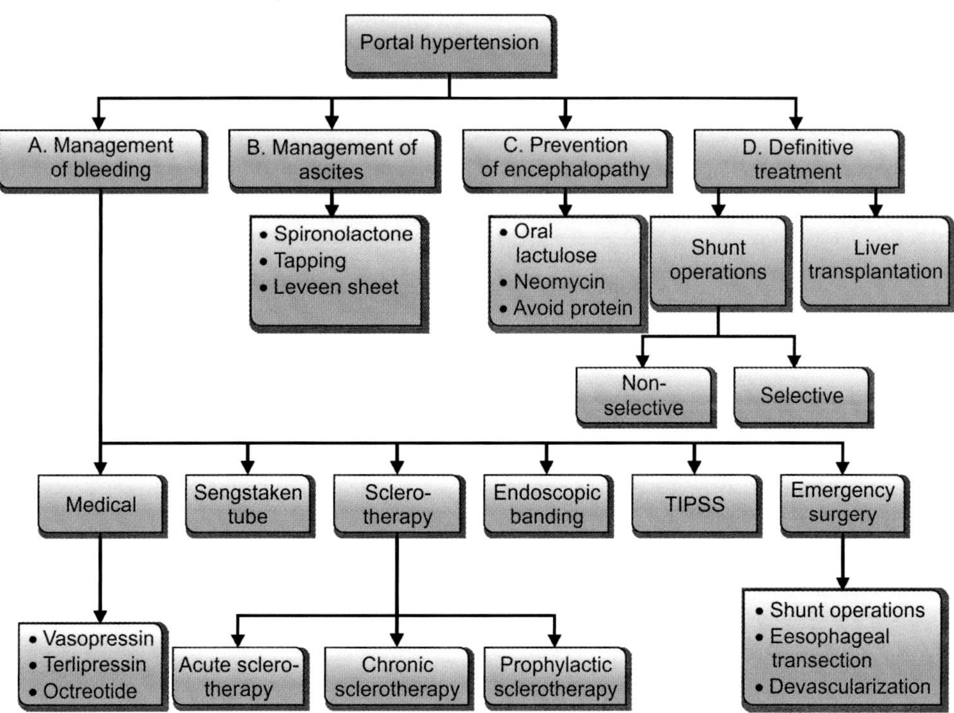

- Balloon tamponade (no longer used routinely)—reserved for special situations.

Q 60. What is sclerotherapy?

Through the fiberoptic endoscope 1–2 mL of the sclerosant solution is injected into the varix either intravariceally or paravariceally in a circumferential pattern at the gastroesophageal junction and subsequently also injected 3–4 cm proximal to the junction. Following the injection, the endoscope is advanced into the stomach and is kept there for 4–5 minutes in order to compress the varices. It may be done as emergency procedure or elective procedure.

Methods of sclerotherapy

a. Intravariceal—obliteration of varices
b. Paravariceal—perivascular cicatrization
c. Combined method of injection.

Q 61. What are the sclerosants used? (PG)

The commonly used sclerosants

- Fatty acid derivatives
  - Sodium morrhuate (5%)
  - Ethanolamine oleate (5%)
- Synthetic products
  - STD (Sodium Tetradecyl Sulphate)—1–3%
  - Polidocanol (Hydroxy Polyethoxy dodecan (HPD also called aethoxysklerol - 1%
- Other agents—Butyl cyanoacrylate
- Mixture of sclerosants.

Q 62. What is the mechanism of sclerotherapy? (PG)

It will cause:

- Intimal injury
- Thrombosis of submucosal vessels (in 24 hours)
- Superficial and deep ulceration (5–7 days)
- Submucosal fibrosis (1month).

Q 63. How often sclerotherapy is repeated? (PG)

During active bleeding:

- It is repeated on 3rd day and 7th day
- After resolving edema repeat the procedure 3–4 weeks after the last injection
- 5 to 6 procedures may be required for total obliteration
- Endoscopic evaluation is done 3 to 6 months after this.

Q 64. What is a successful sclerotherapy? (PG)

- If the aspirate is clear within 12 hours, it is considered successful
- If unsuccessful repeat sclerotherapy 3 times at an interval of 12 hours.

Q 65. What is the success rate of sclerotherapy? (PG)

Sclerotherapy controls bleeding in 80–95% of patients.

Q 66. What is prophylactic sclerotherapy? (PG)

- When sclerotherapy is given for a patient with esophageal varices without history of bleeding, it is called prophylactic sclerotherapy
- When sclerotherapy is given during bleed free intervals, it is called chronic sclerotherapy
- When it is given during hemorrhage, it is called acute sclerotherapy.

Q 67. What are the complications of sclerotherapy? (PG)

Complications may be classified as:

1. *Minor*
   - Substernal pain
   - Esophagitis (48 hours)
   - Fever—25%
2. *Major*

   Esophageal
   - Ulceration—(7 days)
   - Perforation (5 – 19 days)
   - Stricture (4 months)

   Pulmonary and mediastinal
   - Pleural effusion right side
   - Atelectasis
   - Chylothorax right side
   - ARDS
3. *Rare*—Superior mesenteric vein thrombosis.

Q 68. What is the treatment of gastric fundal varices? (PG)

- Injection sclerotherapy with butyl cyanoacrylate or
- Endoscopic banding.

Q 69. What is endoscopic banding?

The varix is lifted with suction tip and a small rubber band is slipped around the base. The varix necroses leaving behind a superficial ulcer. The rebleeding episodes are less in banding, so also the morbidity compared to sclerotherapy.

Q 70. What is the role of vasopressin?

The vasopressin will lower the portal blood flow and portal pressure by directly constricting splanchnic arterioles. This will reduce the portal flow. Vasopressin alone controls acute bleeding in 80% of patients and this is increased to 95% when used in combination with balloon tamponade.

Q 71. What are the complications of vasopressin?

Complications of vasopressin
1. Myocardial infarction
2. Cardiac arrhythmias
3. Intestinal gangrene
4. Reduction in cardiac output
5. Reduces hepatic blood flow
6. Reduces renal blood flow.

Q 72. How can one prevent the complications of vasopressin?

Simultaneous administration of nitroglycerin or isoproterenol along with vasopressin.

Q 73. What is the dose of vasopressin?

It is given as an IV infusion in the dose of 0.4 units/mt. The infusion is better than bolus injection. The nitroglycerine can be given IV or sublingually (20 units in 10 mL of 5% dextrose IV over 10 minutes initially).

Q 74. What is Terlipressin?

It is a synthetic vasopressin analog. It undergoes gradual conversion to vasopressin in the body. It causes fewer cardiac side effects than vasopressin.

Dose 2 mg bolus injection IV 6th hourly.

Q 75. What is the role of octreotide acetate?

It is a long-acting synthetic somatostatin analog. The action is similar to vasopressin but without significant side effects. This is the drug of choice for the pharmacological control of acute bleeding varices.

Dose: 100 µg initial bolus, followed by continuous infusion of 25 µg/h for 24 hours.

Q 76. What is the effectiveness of pharmacological control?

- Vasopressin alone is superior to placebo
- Vasopressin and nitroglycerine is superior to vasopressin alone.

Q 77. What is the role of Sengstaken-Blakemore tube?

It is used for temporary hemostasis initially (balloon tamponade). It has got 3 lumens with 2 balloons which can be inflated (esophageal balloon and gastric balloon). The balloons are inflated in the lumen of gut (gastric balloon is inflated with 250 ml of air, and esophageal balloon to a pressure of 40 mm of Hg). The third lumen is for aspiration of the gastric contents. The tube is introduced transorally. After inflating the two balloons, traction is applied to the tube so that gastric balloon compresses the collateral veins at the cardia of the stomach. The contribution of esophageal balloon compression is negligible. The balloon should be temporarily deflated after 12 hours to prevent pressure necrosis of the esophagus.

Q 78. What are the complications of this tube?

- Aspiration of pharyngeal secretions and pneumonia
- Esophageal rupture (this balloon is therefore infrequently used)
- Pressure necrosis of the esophagus.

Q 79. What is the success rate of balloon tamponade?

Above 75% of the actively bleeding patients can be controlled by balloon tamponade. When bleeding has stopped, it should be left in place for another 24 hours.

Q 80. What is Minnesota tube?

This tube has got a 4th lumen to aspirate the esophagus proximal to the balloon.

Q 81. What is the role of TIPSS in the management of portal hypertension (read the answer in the initial part of this chapter)? (PG)

- It is useful for the control of acute bleeding and to prevent rebleeding (the portal hypertension also is controlled)
- Patients with advanced liver disease are considered for TIPSS
- TIPSS is used as a bridge to transplantation
- It should not be regarded for definitive therapy (the shunt remains open for up to a year)
- Less severe cirrhosis patients—consider for shunt surgery/devascularization.

Q 82. What are the surgical options? (Flow Chart 20.1)

- Surgical procedures may be classified as:
  - Emergency procedures
  - Elective surgical procedures.

Q 83. What are the emergency surgical procedures? (PG)

- Surgical procedures are rarely considered for the acute management of variceal hemorrhage, since the morbidity and mortality are high
- The increasing availability of TIPSS and liver transplantation is another factor
- Initial bleeding is usually controlled with sclerotherapy/banding
- The main indication for surgery is a Child's grade—A cirrhotic patient in whom the bleeding has been controlled by sclerotherapy
  1. Emergency shunt operations
  2. Emergency esophageal transection (stapled transection)
  3. Emergency devascularization.

Note:All these procedures are usually done as elective procedures.

Q 84. What is the principle of shunt surgery and what are the types of shunt surgery?

They reduce the pressure in the portal circulation by diverting the blood into the low-pressure systemic circulation. The different types of shunts are:

Nonselective (portacaval)

1. Side-to-side—portacaval, mesocaval, reno-splenic, etc.
2. End-to-side—portacaval (total)
3. Mesocaval (H)

Selective

1. Distal splenorenal (lienorenal) (Warren shunt)—it is time consuming in emergency situations
2. Left gastric vena caval (Inokuchi).

Q 85. What are the advantages of selective shunt? (PG)

- They preserve blood flow to the liver while decompressing the left side of the portal circulation, that is responsible for esophageal and gastric varices.
- Selective shunts are associated with lower incidence of portosystemic encephalopathy (PSE).

Q 86. What is total shunt (Eck fistula)? (PG)

This is an end-to-side shunt that completely disconnects the liver from the portal system. The portal vein is transected near its bifurcation in the liver hilum and anastomosed to the side of the inferior vena cava. The hepatic stump of the vein is over sewn. This type of shunt gives immediate and permanent protection from variceal bleeding and somewhat easier to perform than side-to-side portacaval shunt. Encephalopathy is less compared to side-to-side shunt.

Q 87. What is mesocaval shunt?

A segment of prosthetic graft or internal jugular vein is anastomosed between the inferior vena cava and the superior mesenteric vein. It is useful in cases of portal vein thrombosis. The portal flow to the liver is lost in this procedure. The portal flow to the liver can be preserved by reducing the diameter of the graft to 8 mm (from 12–20 mm). This will decrease the incidence of encephalopathy, still preventing variceal hemorrhage.

Q 88. What is central splenorenal shunt? (PG)

Here splenectomy is performed and the splenic vein is anastomosed to the renal vein.

Q 89. What are the emergency shunt surgical procedures commonly performed? (PG)

1. End-to-side portacaval
2. H - mesocaval shunt.

Q 90. What is the contraindication for shunt procedure? (PG)

A good transplantation candidate should not be subjected to portosystemic shunt or other shunt. Generally, Child's class A, patients are candidates for portal decompression and class C patients are candidates for transplantation.

Q 91. How will you select a shunt procedure? (PG)

- For elective portal decompression—distal splenorenal shunt (Warren)
- If ascites is present—end-to-side portacaval shunt
- Severe ascites—side-to-side shunt
- Budd-Chiari syndrome
- Emergency decompression—end-to-side or H mesocaval.

Q 92. What are the results of portosystemic shunts? (PG)

- Incidence of recurrent variceal bleeding—10%
- 5-year-survival for alcoholic liver disease—45%
- Encephalopathy 15–25% (severe encephalopathy in 20% of alcoholic after total shunt)
- Patency of shunt—90%.

Q 93. What is esophageal transection (stapled transection)?

In many surgical units, it is the first choice when nonsurgical methods fail. It must be done as soon as a second attempt at sclerotherapy has failed. It must be viewed as an emergency procedure and not a definitive treatment.

Circular stapling device is used for resecting and reanastomosing a ring of the lower esophagus. This procedure is being replaced by TIPSS in centers where it is available.

Q 94. What are the devascularization procedures? (PG)

The devascularization procedures reduce proximal gastric blood flow.

These procedures are not done nowadays.

1. *Gastroesophageal decongestion and splenectomy of Hassab*—All the vessels except the left gastric vessels are ligated.
2. *Sugiura procedure*—it is done in two stages. The first stage is transthoracic and the dilated venous collaterals between esophagus and adjacent structures are divided. The esophagus is then transected and reanastomosed. The second stage is done by laparotomy after the first stage if the patient is bleeding (but deferred 4–6 weeks in the elective cases). The upper 2/3rds of the stomach is devascularized, selective vagotomy, pyloroplasty and splenectomy are performed.

Q 95. What is the definitive treatment for portal hypertension because of cirrhosis?

In cirrhosis the basic pathology is failing liver cells and none of these procedures will rectify the problem. Therefore, the definitive treatment is liver transplantation. Any young patient with cirrhosis who has survived an episode of variceal hemorrhage should be considered a candidate for liver transplantation. Any other form of treatment carries a much higher mortality rate within the subsequent 1–2 years.

Q 96. What are the contraindications for liver transplantation? (PG)

Contraindications for liver transplantation
1. Age > 65 years
2. Ischemic heart disease
3. Cardiac failure
4. Chronic respiratory disease
5. Continued alcohol use
6. Previous surgical shunt (relative).

Q 97. What is the procedure of choice during the preparation period for transplantation? (PG)

Transjugular intrahepatic protosystemic shunt (TIPSS).

Q 98. What is the treatment of nonbleeding varices (prophylactic therapy)?

There is a 30% chance for bleeding at some point for this group of patients. Of those who bleed 50% die. Patients who have bled once from varices have a 70% chance of bleeding again. The treatment of patients with varices that have never bled is referred to as prophylactic therapy. Thus, we have prophylactic sclerotherapy, prophylactic propranolol, etc. The therapy of patients who have bled before is referred to as therapeutic. The prophylactic therapy consists of the following:

a. Prophylactic sclerotherapy
b. Prophylactic propranolol.

Q 99. What is the action of propranolol?

This beta-adrenergic blocking agent decreases cardiac output and splanchnic blood flow and therefore reduces the portal blood pressure. Chronic propranolol therapy in a dose of 20–160 mg twice daily decreases the frequency of rebleeding by 40%. It also reduces the overall mortality.

Q 100. What is left sided portal hypertension?

It is caused by isolated splenic vein thrombosis.

Q 101. What are the causes of ascites in portal hypertension?

- Decreased colloid osmotic pressure (decreased proteins)
- Increased hydrostatic pressure
- Lymphatic blockage.

Q 102. What are the complications of ascites?

Complications of ascites
• Umbilical hernia
• Spontaneous bacterial peritonitis
• Respiratory embarrassment.

Q 103. What is the treatment of ascites in portal hypertension?

1. Medical
   - Spironolactone 25 mg bd orally
   - Limit sodium intake.
2. Ascitic tap—slow gradual tapping is done
3. Shunt operations
   - Leveen shunt (peritoneovenous shunt—peritoneal cavity to internal jugular vein)
   - Denver shunt—Peritoneal cavity to internal jugular vein with a subcutaneous chamber that can be milked when blocked.

Q 104. What is the management of encephalopathy?

1. Protein-free diet
2. Oral Lactulose—30 mL tid
3. Oral neomycin—1–2 g 6th hourly (not given in renal impairment)
4. Parenteral nutrition—(calories from carbohydrate sucrose is preferred over glucose)
5. Administration of 50% glucose in central vein.

Q 105. What is hepatorenal syndrome?

Acute renal failure without apparent cause may occur in patients with liver disease at any time during hospitalization. This is due to impaired renal perfusion. Other possible causes include infection, drug toxicity, etc. They usually succumb to hepatic failure.

Case

21 Mesenteric Cyst

Case Capsule

A **15-year-old girl** presents with **abdominal distension and recurrent colicky type of abdominal pain** of two months duration. There is no associated vomiting and no other complaints. There is no history of respiratory infection preceding the attack. There is no alteration in bowel habits.

On general examination, she is afebrile, not ill looking. There is no generalized lymphadenopathy and no icterus. There is **no circumoral pallor**. On examination of the abdomen, a **central abdominal fullness** is noticed on inspection. A **spherical swelling of 15 cm diameter** is situated **in the umbilical region**, all the borders of which are well-defined. The surface of the swelling is smooth. The **swelling moves freely at right angles to the line of attachment of the mesentery.** It is **dull to percussion**, however, the surrounding areas are resonant. On fixing the swelling with the help of the patient's hand, it appears to be **fluctuant**. The swelling cannot be pushed to the pelvis. There is neither **shifting dullness nor fluid thrill**. There is no organomegaly. The hernial orifices are normal. On digital rectal examination, it is not possible to feel the swelling from below. The supraclavicular nodes are not enlarged.

Read the checklist for abdominal examination.

Checklist for history
Checklist for examination

Look for

- Circumoral pallor—mesenteric adenitis
- Cervical lymph nodes—seen in mesenteric lymphadenitis
- Shifting tenderness, which is a sign of mesenteric adenitis
- Free movement in a plane at right angles to the attachment of mesentery (from left of the umbilicus to the right iliac fossa)
- A zone of resonance around the swelling.

Q 1. What is the probable diagnosis in this case?
Mesenteric cyst.

Q 2. What are the differential diagnoses?

Differential diagnoses of central abdominal cystic swelling

- Ovarian cyst
- Omental cyst
- Cyst of the mesocolon
- Tuberculous abscess in the mesentery
- Hydatid cyst of the mesentery

Contd...

Contd...

- Pancreatic pseudocyst
- Inflammatory cyst
- Serosanguinous cyst—may be traumatic in origin
- Retroperitoneal cyst.

Q 3. What are the characteristics of mesenteric cyst?

1. A cystic swelling in the center of the abdomen
2. It moves at right angles to the line of attachment of the root of the mesentery, but only slightly, parallel to the root of the mesentery
3. Fluid thrill will be present
4. It is dull to percussion
5. One can get below the swelling (unlike ovarian cyst)
6. There is a zone of resonance around the cyst.

Q 4. What is the line of attachment of mesentery?

It is attached to the posterior abdominal wall to the left of the 2nd lumbar vertebrae and passes obliquely to the right and inferiorly to the right sacroiliac joint and is 15 cm long.

Surface marking in the abdomen:

An oblique line starting 2.5 cm to the left of the midline and 2.5 cm below the transpyloric plane and extending downwards and to the right for about 15 cm.

Direction of movement of mesenteric cyst is showing in Figure 21.1.

Q 5. What is the "sign of mesenteric cyst"?

Tillaux Triad

1. Soft swelling at the level of umbilicus
2. Movement perpendicular to mesentery
3. Dull note over the swelling surrounded by resonance.

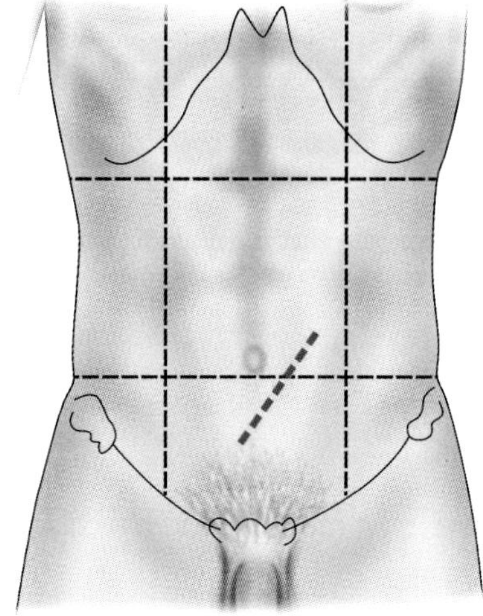

Fig. 21.1: Mesentery (small intestine) attachment direction of movement of mesenteric cyst

The lump moves in a plane from the right hypochondrium to the left iliac fossa, but not in the plane at right angles to this.

Q 6. What is mesenteric cyst and what is the classification?

- They are developmental lesions

Classification of mesenteric cyst

- Chylolymphatic (commonest variety)
- Enterogenous
- Urogenital remnant
- Dermoid (teratomatous cysts).

Q 7. What is the age group affected by mesenteric cyst?

- Most frequently in the second decade
- Less often 1 – 10 years
- Exceptionally in infants under 1year.

Q 8. What are the differences between chylolymphatic cyst and enterogenous cysts?

Differences between chylolymphatic cyst and enterogenous cysts	
Chylolymphatic cyst	*Enterogenous cysts*
• Arises from congenitally misplaced lymphatic tissue with no efferent communication with lymphatic system	• Arises from a diverticulum of the mesenteric border of the intestine which has become sequestrated from the intestinal canal or duplication of the intestine
• Wall is thin—connective tissue lined by endothelium	• Thicker wall—lined by mucous membrane (sometimes ciliated)
• Filled with clear lymph or chyle (milky)	• Content is mucinous (colorless or yellowish brown)
• Blood supply is independent of that of the adjacent intestines	• Common blood supply with intestine
• Usually enucleation is possible without resection of the gut	• Removal always entails resection of the related portion of intestine

Q 9. What is the cause for recurrent attacks of abdominal pain?

It may be due to—

1. Torsion of the mesentery
2. Temporary impaction of food bolus in the intestine narrowed by the cyst.

Q 10. What are the complications of the cyst?

Complication of mesenteric cyst
1. Torsion of the cyst
2. Rupture of the cyst
3. Hemorrhage into the cyst
4. Infection
5. Peptic ulceration (when it contains ectopic gastric mucosa)
6. Perforation

Q 11. How will you differentiate it from omental cyst?

A lateral radiograph or ultrasound or CT scan will show the cyst in front of the intestines, if it is an omental cyst.

Q 12. What are the investigations in a suspected case of mesenteric cyst?

1. Plain X-ray will show calcified lymph nodes in tuberculous mesenteric lymph nodes
2. Barium meal and follow through hollow viscera will be found to be displaced around the cyst or lumen of the intestine may be seen narrowed
3. Ultrasound abdomen will reveal the cystic nature and the origin of the cyst
4. IVU to rule out hydronephrosis if ultrasound is not done
5. CT scan
6. Needle aspiration and instillation of radio-paque water-soluble contrast media.

Q 13. What is the treatment of chylolymphatic cyst?

- Enucleation in toto
- After major portion of the cyst has been dissected free, a portion abutting on the intestine or a major blood vessel can be left attached after destroying its lining.

Q 14. What is the treatment of enterogenous cyst?

- Enucleation is contraindicated
- Resection of the cyst with adherent portion of the intestine followed by intestinal anastomosis

- If a very large segment of small intestine is implicated, an anastomosis should be made between the apex of the coil of small intestine and the cyst wall (the cyst wall will hold sutures well).

Q 15. What is the role of marsupialization?
This is an old form of treatment not recommended nowadays because of the fear of fistula and recurrence.

Q 16. What is the surgical treatment if it is an omental cyst?
Omentectomy.

Q 17. What are the neoplasms of the mesentery?
They are classified as benign and malignant.

Benign	*Malignant*
• Lipoma	• Lymphoma
• Fibroma	• Secondary carcinoma
• Fibromyxoma	

Q 18. What is the management of benign neoplasms?
Benign tumors are excised in the same way as mesenteric cyst, along with resection of the adjacent intestine.

Q 19. What is the management of malignant neoplasms?

- Biopsy confirmation
- Chemotherapy for lymphoma
- Chemotherapy for secondary carcinoma.

Q 20. How does tuberculous lymphadenitis occur?
The tubercle bacilli are usually ingested and they enter the mesenteric lymph node by way of Peyer's patches. The organism may be human or bovine. It can occur after ingestion of raw milk. It may affect a single lymph node or multiple lymph nodes presenting as massive abdominal swelling.

Q 21. What is pseudomesenteric cyst?
When tuberculous mesenteric lymph nodes break-down, the tuberculous pus may remain between the leaves of the mesentery and cystic swelling similar to mesenteric cyst is formed. When such a situation is found the pus is evacuated without soiling the peritoneal cavity and anti tuberculous treatment is instituted.

Q 22. What is the cause for yellow-colored lymph nodes in the ileocecal region?
Metastasis from carcinoid of the appendix will give rise to yellow color for the lymph nodes.

Q 23. What are the causes for calcified shadows in the plain radiograph of the abdomen?

Causes for radiopaque shadow in plain X-ray abdomen

1. Renal or ureteric stone (renal stones are uniform in density, take the shape of pelvicalyceal system and lies superimposed on the shadows of the vertebral column in the lateral view)
2. Gallstones are (less dense in the center and in front of the vertebral bodies on the lateral view)
3. Pancreatic calculi
4. Calcified tuberculous lymph node—usually in the ileocecal region and line of attachment of the mesentery—outline is irregular and the nodes are mottled like black berry
5. Phlebolith
6. Calcified costal cartilage
7. Fecolith
8. Stone in the appendix
9. Calcified renal artery
10. Calcified aneurysm of the abdominal aorta
11. Chip fracture of the transverse process of the vertebrae.

Q 24. How long it will take for calcification to occur in tuberculous lymph nodes?

Eighteen months.

Q 25. Will the nodes be noninfective in such a situation?

No. The node need not be defunct. So infection is still possible.

Q 26. What is the cause for acute non specific ileocecal mesenteric adenitis?

The etiology of this condition is unknown, it affects children and unusual after puberty. Some cases are associated with Yersinia infection of the ileum. In other situations unidentified virus is blamed. Respiratory infection precedes an attack of mesenteric adenitis. This is a self-limiting disease. It is called nonspecific in order to distinguish it from tuberculous mesenteric adenitis.

Q 27. What are the clinical manifestations of nonspecific mesenteric adenitis?

- Central abdominal pain lasting for 10–30 minutes
- Associated circumoral pallor
- Vomiting is common

Contd...

Contd...

- No alteration in bowel habits
- Intervals of complete freedom from pain
- The patient seldom looks ill
- Temperature may be elevated but never exceeds 38.5
- Tenderness along the line of mesentery
- Shifting tenderness (after the patient lies on the left side for a few minutes the tenderness shift to the left side)
- Pelvic peritoneum is tender to palpation.

Q 28. What will be the total leukocyte count like?

There is often leukocytosis in contrast to tuberculosis.

Q 29. What is the treatment of nonspecific mesenteric adenitis?

- Bed rest for a few days (if the diagnosis can be made with certainty).
- If appendicitis cannot be excluded do laparoscopy followed by appendectomy if required.

3

SECTION

Short Cases

Case 22 Non-thyroid Neck Swelling

Examination of non-thyroid neck swellings:

Diagnostic algorithm for a neck swelling

1. Identify the anatomical situation of the swelling (in relation to the triangle in the neck)

↓

2. Decide the **plane of the swelling**

↓

3. Recollect your anatomy (what are the normal anatomical structures situated in the region of the swelling in that plane)

↓

4. Check for **mobility/fixity** of the swelling

↓

5. Find out the **external** (size, shape, surface, edge, temperature, tenderness, etc.) and **internal features** of the lump (solid or cystic, compressible/ reducible, pulsation, transillumination) and **auscultation** of the swelling

↓

6. Find out its **effect on the surrounding tissue** (feel the superficial temporal artery, examine the relevant cranial nerves and look for Horner's syndrome)

↓

7. Look for regional nodes (if the swelling is a node look for another group and contralateral side of the neck)

↓

8. In the case of paired organs like salivary gland, look for contralateral pathology also

↓

9. Look for a primary lesion (scalp, oral cavity, pharynx, hidden areas, etc.)

↓

10. Come to an **anatomical diagnosis**

↓

11. Come to a **pathological diagnosis** (Decide whether it is **congenital /traumatic/inflammatory/neoplastic—primary or secondary)**

↓

12. If it is an organ concerned with function decide whether it is hyper functioning, normally functioning or hypo-functioning **(functional diagnosis). The final diagnosis = Anatomical + Pathological + Functional diagnosis.**

Q 1. What are the causes for non-thyroid neck masses?

All regions

- **Skin and subcutaneous tissue**
  1. Sebaceous cyst
  2. Lipoma
  3. Neurofibroma
- **Lymphadenopathy**
  1. Acute infection
  2. Chronic infection—tuberculosis
  3. Primary malignant—lymphoma
  4. Secondary malignant—metastasis

Midline

1. Sublingual dermoid
2. Thyroglossal cyst/fistula
3. Pharyngocele
4. Laryngocele.

Note: **3 and 4** do not lie in the midline but arise from the midline.

Lateral

1. Parotid swellings
2. Submandibular salivary gland
3. Branchial cyst
4. Carotid body tumor
5. Carotid aneurysm
6. Carotid tortuosity
7. Cystic hygroma
8. Subclavian aneurysm.

Triangles of the Neck

The neck is divided into **Anterior** and **Posterior** triangles (Fig. 22.1).

The boundaries of the anterior triangle are:

- Midline

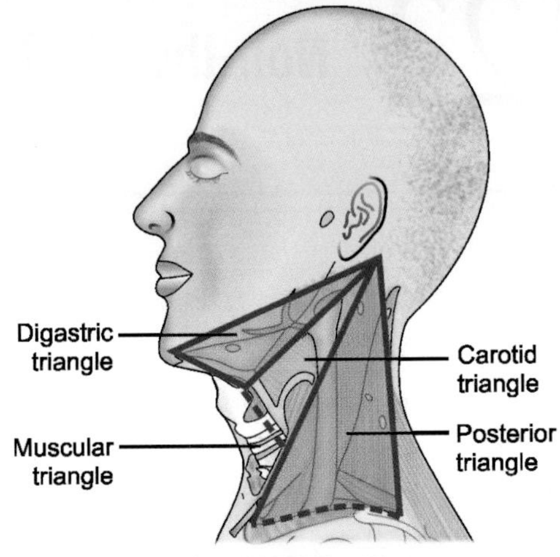

Fig. 22.1: Triangles of the neck

- Anterior border of the sternomastoid (oncologically the boundary is the posterior border of the sternomastoid)
- Inferior border of the ramus of the mandible.

The anterior triangle is further divided into:

- Digastric
- Carotid
- Muscular.

The boundaries of the posterior triangle are:

- Posterior border of the sternomastoid
- Anterior border of trapezius
- Upper border of the middle-third of the clavicle.

Table 22.1 showing the Triangles of the neck, its boundaries, contents and possible swellings in each area.

Table 22.1: Triangles of the neck

Triangle	*Boundaries*	*Contents*	*Possible swellings*
Digastric	• Inferior border of the ramus of the mandible • Anterior portion of the digastric muscle • Posterior portion of the digastric muscle • Midline	• Submandibular gland • Lymph node • Facial artery	• Submandibular swellings—sialadenitis, tumor • Lymph nodes swelling • Ranula (plunging) • Sublingual dermoid
Carotid	• Anterior belly of omohyoid • Anterior border of sternomastoid • Posterior belly of digastric	• Common carotid artery dividing to internal and external at the level of hyoid bone • Vagus nerve • Lymph nodes • Internal jugular vein	• Carotid body tumor • Branchial cyst • Carotid aneurysm • Pharyngocele
Muscular	• Anterior belly of digastric • Anterior belly of omohyoid • Midline	• Thyroid—may extend beyond this area including the posterior triangle • Laryngeal structures	• Thyroid swelling • Laryngocele • Innominate aneurysm
Posterior	• Posterior border of sternomastoid • Anterior border of trapezius • Upper border of middle third of clavicle	• Lymph nodes • Accessory nerve • Scalenus anterior muscle	• Thyroid swelling • Cystic hygroma • Lymph nodes • Subclavian aneurysm

**Note:* Skin and subcutaneous swellings like lipoma, sebaceous cyst and neurofibroma can occur in all the regions.

Remember the etiology of non-thyroid neck mass.

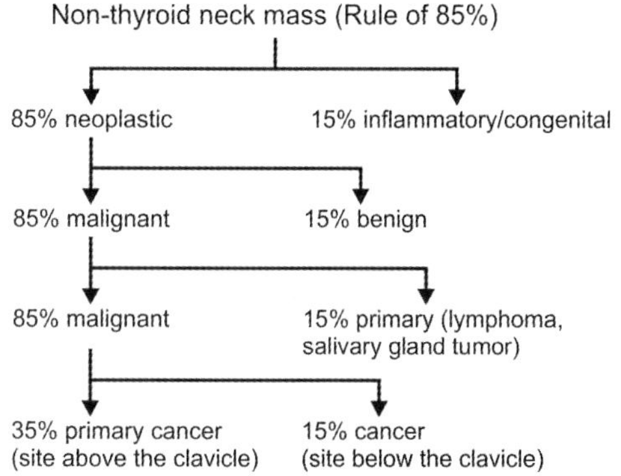

Non-thyroid neck mass (Rule of 85%)
- 85% neoplastic
  - 85% malignant
    - 85% malignant
      - 35% primary cancer (site above the clavicle)
      - 15% cancer (site below the clavicle)
    - 15% primary (lymphoma, salivary gland tumor)
  - 15% benign
- 15% inflammatory/congenital

Remember the midline swellings of the neck. They are from above downwards:

Midline swellings of the neck

1. Sublingual dermoid
2. Plunging ranula
3. Thyroglossal cyst
4. Pharyngocele
5. Laryngocele
6. Swellings from isthmus of thyroid
7. Prelaryngeal lymph node
8. Pretracheal lymph node
9. Lymph nodes in the space of burns.

Remember the hidden areas of primary for a metastasis in the neck.

Hidden areas for primary

- Pyriform sinus
- Vallecula
- Tonsillar fossa
- Base of tongue
- Fossa of Rosenmüller

Case

23 Tuberculous Cervical Lymph Node

Case Capsule

A **20-year-old male patient with** multiple swellings on the side of the neck **involving the** jugulodigastric **group of lymph nodes and** nodes on the anterior and posterior triangles **of neck. The nodes are of** varying consistency, **some are soft and some are firm. The jugulodigastric and upper deep cervical nodes are** matted together. **The patient complains of** evening rise of temperature.

Read the diagnostic algorithm for a neck swelling.

Read the checklist of case no. 15 of long cases

Checklist for history

- Family history of tuberculosis
- H/o exposure to tuberculosis
- H/o BCG vaccination
- H/o evening rise of temperature
- H/o loss of appetite and loss of weight

Checklist for lymph node examination:

1. Remember the pneumonic – **PALS (P** – Look for **P**rimary lesion in the drainage area, **A** – Look for **A**nother lymph node, **L** – Look for **L**iver, **S** – Look for **S**pleen) (Read case no.15 of long cases)

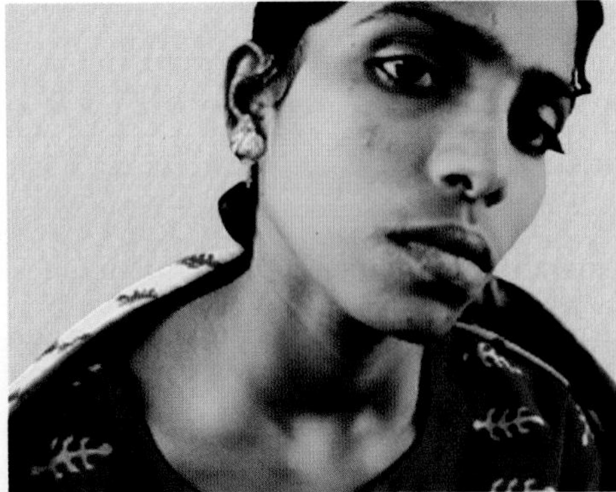

Tuberculous lymph node right supraclavicular

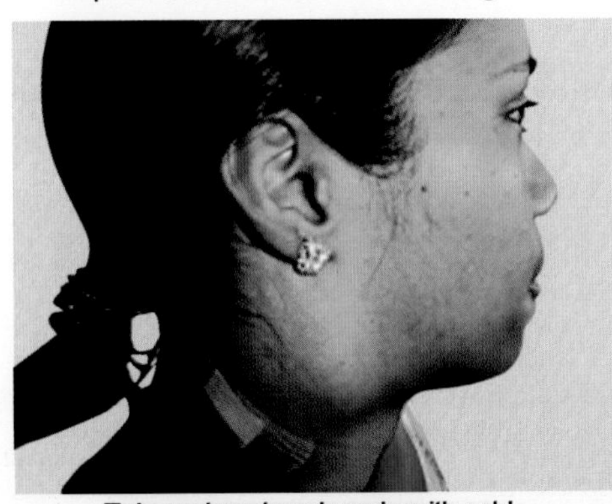

Tuberculous lymph node with cold abscess and biopsy incision

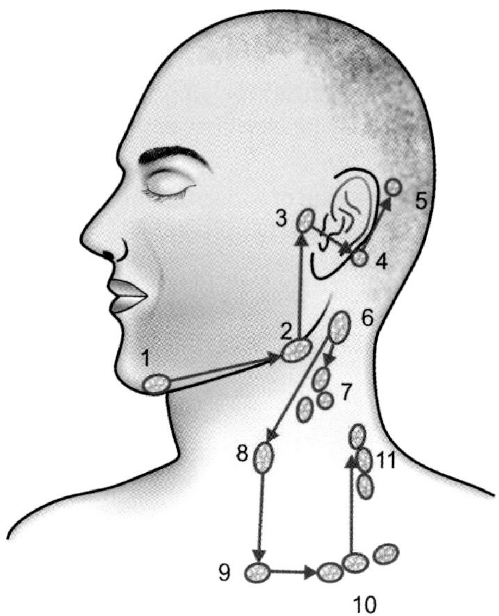

Fig. 23.1: Cervical lymph node examination

2. Remember the **3 lymphatic water sheds** in the body for the skin lymphatic drainage (**Read case no.15 of long cases**).
3. Remember the **order of palpation** of cervical lymph nodes (Fig. 23.1)
4. Remember the **causes for matting** of lymph nodes
5. Always **examine the oral cavity** including the tonsil
6. Examine the chest for evidence of **pulmonary tuberculosis**.

Q 1. What is the anatomical diagnosis in this case?
Lymph nodes.

Q 2. What are the diagnostic points in favor of lymph nodes?
1. Shape of the swelling
2. Plane of the swelling—deep to deep fascia.

Q 3. What is the plane of the cervical lymph nodes?
For all practical purposes majority of the **cervical lymph nodes are deep to deep fascia**.

Flow chart 23.1: Classification of cervical lymph nodes

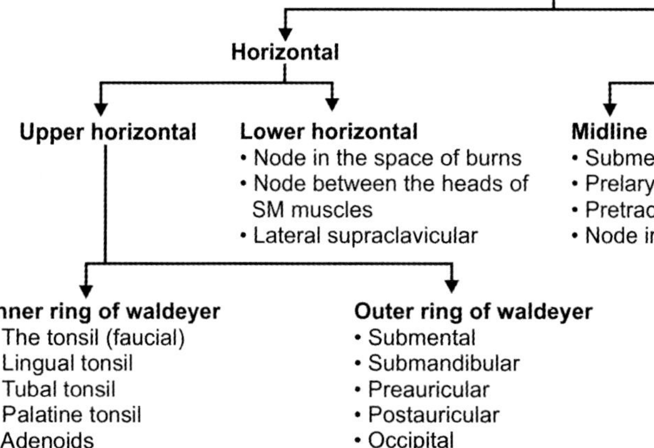

Q 4. What are the groups of lymph nodes which are superficial to the deep fascia in the neck?

1. The external jugular group of lymph nodes
2. The submental nodes
3. The occipital nodes
4. The facial nodes
5. Postauricular nodes.

Q 5. How many lymph nodes are there in the neck?

- Roughly **300** nodes (out of total **800** nodes in the human body)
- About 150 are in the mesentery.

Q 6. What are the functions of lymph nodes?

1. Filtration of **effete cells, bacteria and antigens**
2. Presentation of antigens to the lymphocytes
3. Regulation of protein content of efferent lymph.

Q 7. How will you classify cervical lymph nodes?

They may be classified as shown in Flow chart 23.1.

Note: SM muscle—sternomastoid muscle.

Q 8. What is the sequence of palpation of cervical lymph nodes?

The following sequence is recommended. Start palpitating **from above** from the submental node and **proceed backwards** (Fig. 23.1).

1. Submental
2. Submandibular
3. Preauricular
4. Postauricular
5. Occipital.

Then **proceed downwards** laterally from the jugulodigastric

6. Jugulodigastric
7. Deep cervical
8. Jugulo-omohyoid
9. Scalene
10. Supraclavicular.

Now **proceed upwards** to the external jugular nodes (superficial).

Q 9. What are the causes for lymphadenopathy?

The causes may be classified as shown in Flow chart 23.2.

Q 10. What is the plan of action for finding out the source of the enlarged lymph nodes?

Search for primary lesion in cervical lymphadenopathy.

Start from above and work downwards

1. Examine the skin of the scalp, face, ears and neck
2. Examine the nose
3. Transilluminate the air sinuses
4. Examine the oral cavity
5. Examine the nasopharynx and larynx (**ENT examination**)
6. Palpate the salivary glands (parotid and submandibular)
7. Examine the thyroid gland
8. Examine the breast
9. Examine the chest
10. Examine the abdomen and genitalia.

Q 11. What is the pathological diagnosis in this case?

Most probably this is a case of tuberculous cervical lymphadenitis.

Q12. What are the points in favor of tuberculosis of the lymph node?

1. Matting of lymph nodes
2. Varying consistency of the nodes
3. Jugulodigastric node is affected (which is the most common group affected in tuberculosis)
4. Evening rise of temperature.

Flow Chart 23.2: Classification of causes for lymphadenopathy

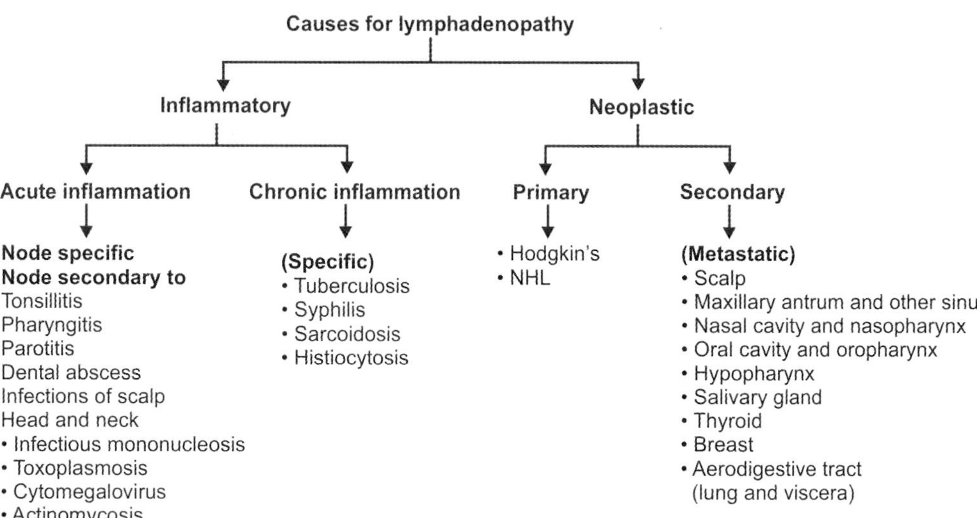

Q 13. What are the causes for matting?

Causes for matting of lymph nodes:

1. Tuberculous lymphadenitis
2. Acute lymphadenitis
3. Late stages of lymphoma
4. Late stages of metastasis neck.

Q 14. What is the cause for matting?

The organism will reach the lymph node from the primary focus via the **lymphatics**. The lymphatics are distributed along the periphery of the lymph nodes and from there it will reach the **subcapsular sinus**. The subcapsular sinuses of **adjacent lymph nodes** are involved subsequently and this will produce matting.

Q 15. Can you get tuberculosis of the nodes without matting?

Yes. In miliary tuberculosis there won't be any matting. The organisms coming via the blood vessels enter the medullary region directly and therefore there is no periadenitis and matting in miliary tuberculosis.

Q 16. What is the anatomy of the cut section of lymph node?

The lymph node is kidney-shaped and it has got a **hilum**. The **afferent and efferent vessels** enter and leave the hilum. It has got a **capsule** and beneath the capsule there is the **subcapsular space**. All around the lymph nodes you get the **lymphatics** reaching the capsule and sub-capsular space. Organisms coming to the lymph node thus reaches the subcapsular space initially. The lymph node has got a **cortex and a medulla**. The cortex has **lymph follicles** which is situated externally. Beneath the cortex you get the medulla where the **medullary cords** are seen. Organisms coming via the vessels reach directly the medulla in contrast to the lymphatics (Fig. 23.2).

Q 17. What is the primary focus for cervical lymph node tuberculosis?

The **tonsil** is usually the primary focus for the cervical node tuberculosis. This can lead to **jugulodigastric** node enlargement (the **tonsillar group of lymph nodes**) and from there it will reach other groups in the neck.

Q 18. If you get isolated posterior triangular group of nodes which are proved to be tuberculosis, what is the likely primary focus?

Adenoids.

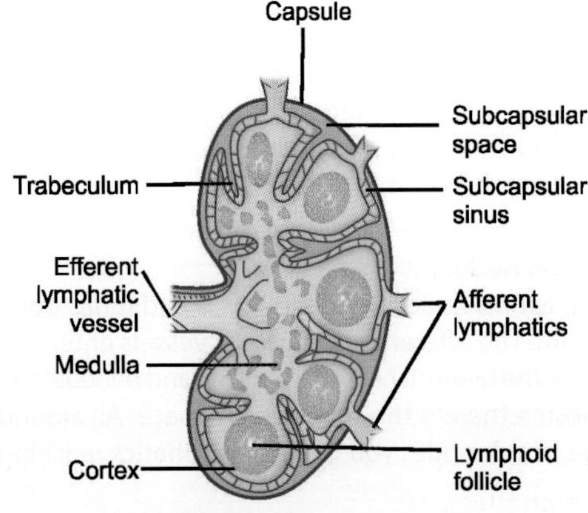

Fig. 23.2: Lymph node section

Q 19. What is the incidence of cervical node tuberculosis secondary to pulmonary tuberculosis?

- In 80% of cases the tuberculosis process is limited to the affected lymph nodes
- Primary focus in the lungs must always be suspected and investigated
- Atypical mycobacterial adenitis is seldom associated with pulmonary tuberculosis.

Q 20. What are the groups of lymph nodes affected by tuberculosis in the body?

1. Upper deep cervical
2. Supraclavicular
3. Mediastinal nodes
4. Axillary
5. Inguinal nodes.

Note:

a. Supraclavicular nodes represent the upward extension of hilar and mediastinal lymphadenopathy
b. Axillary and inguinal nodes are involved by hematogenous or retrograde lymphatic spread.

Q 21. What are the pathological stages of tuberculous lymph nodes?

There are five stages (Fig. 23.3):

Stage 1: The lymph nodes are **enlarged and solid**. There is no matting of lymph nodes (no periadenitis).

Stage 2: The lymph nodes are large, firm and matted together (fixed to each other) because of the **periadenitis**.

Stage 3: **Stage of caseation and cold abscess**—The lymph nodes breakdown, and liquefy. The pus will collect beneath the deep fascia. A fluctuant mass will be palpated **without any overlying skin inflammation** (cold abscess). In addition, nodes

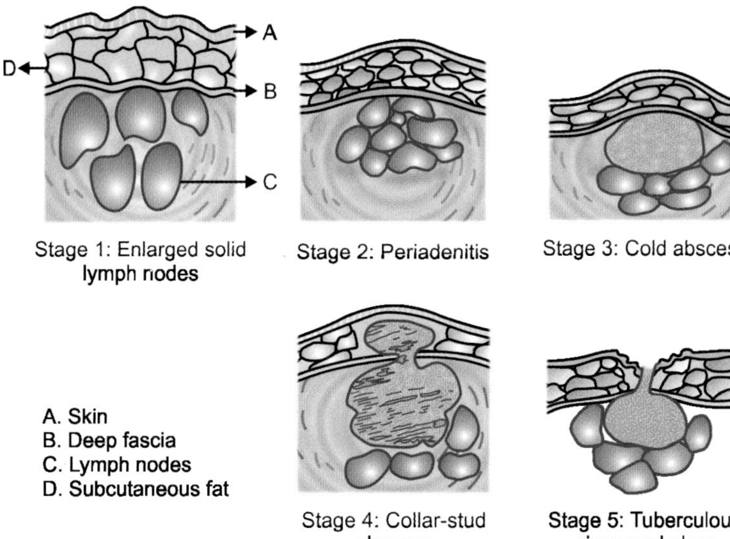

Fig. 23.3: Tuberculosis lymphadenitis stages in order

without softening will also be present which will give rise to **varying consistency**.

Stage 4: **Stage of collar-stud abscess**—The deep cervical fascia is eroded eventually resulting in the escape of pus beneath the superficial fascia which is a laborious space.

Stage 5: **Stage of sinuses and ulcers**—The pus will eventually burst through the skin resulting in a discharging sinus or ulcer.

Q 22. Will the cold abscess contain tubercle bacilli?

Yes. The abscess is lined by granulation tissue and caseous material.

Q 23. How a tuberculous ulcer is formed?

Once a sinus is formed the discharge will infect the surrounding skin and cause ulceration.

Q 24. What are the characteristics of tuberculous ulcer?

The tuberculous ulcer has got undermined edges, seropurulent discharge and pale granulation tissue.

Q 25. What is collar-stud abscess?

The pus is formed as a result of breakdown of a lymph node which will subsequently erode the deep fascia and come to the space beneath the superficial fascia. There is a superficial soft swelling, which is nothing but pus, and is communicating with the offending lymph node situated deep to the deep fascia. The **node, the connection and the superficial soft swelling** together will take the shape of a collar-stud.

Q 26. What are the clinical types of tuberculous lymphadenitis?

There are four types:

1. **Acute type**
   - Seen in infants and children below five years
   - Inflammatory signs may be there and may resemble acute lymphadenitis.
2. **Caseating type**—commonest type seen in young adults with typical matted nodes with caseation, cold abscess and sinuses.
3. **Hyperplastic type**—this is seen in patients with good resistance. The lymphoid hyperplasia is more predominant than caseation. The nodes are usually firm and discrete.
4. **Atrophic type**—seen in elderly where the lymph nodes undergo natural involution. The nodes are small and burst resulting in caseation.

Q 27. What is scrofuloderma?

The skin involvement as a result of tuberculosis is called scrofuloderma. The skin will be discolored bluish or hyperpigmented.

Q 28. How will you investigate and confirm your diagnosis?

1. ESR—will be raised
2. X-ray chest—evidence of pulmonary tuberculosis need not be there because majority of the cervical lymph node tuberculosis are primary (and not secondary to pulmonary tuberculosis)
3. Tuberculin test (Mantoux)—a positive test has no diagnostic value (because of BCG vaccination) a negative test is useful in excluding tuberculosis
4. FNAC of the lymph node
5. Biopsy of the lymph node **for pathology and microbiology**
6. Aspiration of the cold abscess for AFB staining.

Q 29. How Mantoux test is done?

One unit of PPD (**Purified Protein Derivative**) **is injected intradermally in the volar surface of the forearm.** After 48 hours, **look for area of induration surrounding the injection site. A positive test is one where the** induration exceeds12 mm. **A positive test is suggestive of prior or present infection with *M. tuberculosis*. Negative results do not always rule out tuberculosis** (immunosuppression, malnutrition and diseases like lymphomas suppress the test).

Q 30. Is FNAC of the node reliable?

For lymph node pathology biopsy of the intact lymph node is always superior because a pathologist can study the architecture of the lymph node (this is not possible with FNAC). If the needle is striking the granuloma in the lymph node, the pathologist will give a positive report. Therefore, **biopsy is always a superior investigation for lymph node**.

Q 31. What are the important points to be remembered while taking cervical lymph nodes for biopsy?

1. Always try to take an **intact node** for biopsy
2. If possible take **2 nodes** (1 node for the pathologist and 1 node for the microbiologist)
3. Send the lymph node for the pathologist in **formalin**
4. Send the lymph node for the microbiologist in **saline solution** (this is for AFB culture).

Q 32. What is the media used for culture and how long it will take to get a positive culture?

- Lowenstein—Jensen media
- Takes 6 weeks for positive culture
- Selinite medium—shortens the time of growth to 5 days.

Q 33. What are the new methods for the diagnosis of tuberculosis?

PCR – The result will be ready in one week.

BACTECT – (Using radioactive C14) Result will be ready in 4 days

Q 34. Suppose there is only one lymph node, would you attempt FNAC?

No. FNAC will induce changes in the lymph node, which are likely to alter the pathological picture if it is subsequently taken for biopsy study. This is called **WARF** (**W**orrisome **A**nomaly **R**elated to **F**NAC).

Q 35. What are the pathological changes in the lymph node?

Pathologically we get the **tubercle**, which consists of an **area of caseation surrounded by giant cells, epithelioid cells, lymphocytes and plasma cells.**

Q 36. What is the difference between caseous material and tuberculous pus?

Caseous material—dry, granular and cheese like material is called caseous material (granular structure less material).

Tuberculous pus—softening and liquefaction of the caseous material results in the formation of a **thick creamy fluid** called tuberculous pus. It is highly infective because liquefaction is associated with **multiplication of the organism.** In addition, it contains fatty debris in serous fluid with few necrotic cells.

Q 37. Can you start antituberculous treatment empirically without pathological or microbiological report?

No. Pathological or microbiological support is necessary for starting the antituberculous treatment.

Q 38. What are the organisms responsible for lymph node tuberculosis?

- Human tuberculosis
- Bovine tuberculosis.

Q 39. What are the organisms responsible for atypical *Mycobacterium tuberculosis*?

- *Mycobacterium avium intracellulare*
- *Mycobacterium scrofulaceum.*

Q 40. Is there any role for urine examination?

Yes. The renal and pulmonary tuberculosis occasionally coexist. Therefore, the urine should be carefully examined.

Q 41. Is it possible to get calcified cervical lymph node without prior symptoms of cervical lymph node tuberculosis?

Yes. In patients with natural resistance to the infection, the nodes may accidentally detected at a later date as calcified nodes.

Q 42. What is the treatment of choice in a proved case of cervical lymph node tuberculosis?

Antituberculous chemotherapy – **Triple Drug Therapy– Rifampicin, INH** and **Ethambutol**—(Read the chapter on *long cases*- right iliac fossa mass - abdominal tuberculosis).

Q 43. What are the indications for surgery in cervical lymph node tuberculosis?

Indications for surgery in tuberculous lymph-adenitis

1. Biopsy (the most important indications)
2. Excision of a group of nodes if it is **not responding** to antituberculous treatment
3. Excision of the offending lymph node in cases of **collar-stud** abscess
4. Excision of abscess if it is not responding to aspiration
5. Persistent sinus.

Q 44. What are the causes for persistent sinus?

Causes for persistent sinus:

1. Secondary infection
2. Considerable fibrosis
3. Necrotic and calcified material replacing the lymph node.

Q 45. If the cervical nodes are not responding to the antituberculous drugs what should be suspected?

Atypical mycobacterial adenitis.

Q 46. What is the treatment of cold abscess?

Aspiration. Incision and drainage is not recommended because it will result in sinus formation.

Q 47. How will you aspirate cold abscess?

Aspiration is done through the nondependent part.

Case

24 Cervical Metastatic Lymph Node and Neck Dissections

Case Capsule

A 65-year-old male patient **presents with** a hard lymph node **swelling of 3 cm size involving the** level III group **on right side. The swelling is mobile.** The superficial temporal artery is palpable. **The** cranial nerves are normal. **There are no abdominal, chest or ENT complaints. The patient is apparently healthy. Read the diagnostic algorithm for a neck swelling.**

Checklist for history

1. Alcohol and tobacco use in history
2. Pain around the eyes – referred from the nasopharynx
3. Otalgia—carcinoma base of tongue, tonsil, and hypopharynx can cause otalgia
4. Odynophagia—as a result of cancers of the base of the tongue, hypopharynx, cervical node metastasis, etc.
5. Bleeding from the nose (epistaxis)—cancers of the nasal cavity
6. Hemoptysis
7. Alteration of phonation
8. Difficulty in breathing
9. Difficulty in swallowing—late symptom of base of tongue, hypopharynx and cervical esophagus

Contd...

Contd...

10. Difficulty in hearing—from nasopharynx
11. Hoarseness of voice—carcinoma glottis and carcinoma thyroid
12. History of prior SCC.

Checklist for examination

1. Careful examination of oral cavity after removal of dentures
2. Bimanual palpation of the floor of the mouth
3. Check for nasal block
4. Check for sensory loss in the distribution of infraorbital nerves—maxillary sinus cancer
5. Examine the cranial nerves III–VII and IX–XII (involvement in nasopharyngeal cancer)
6. Look for Horner's syndrome—involvement of cervical sympathetic chain, extralaryngeal spread of laryngeal cancer and extracapsular invasion of cervical lymph node
7. Look for trismus
8. A thorough ENT examination
9. Examination of thyroid
10. Examination of salivary glands
11. Examination of breast
12. Examination of chest
13. Examination of abdomen.

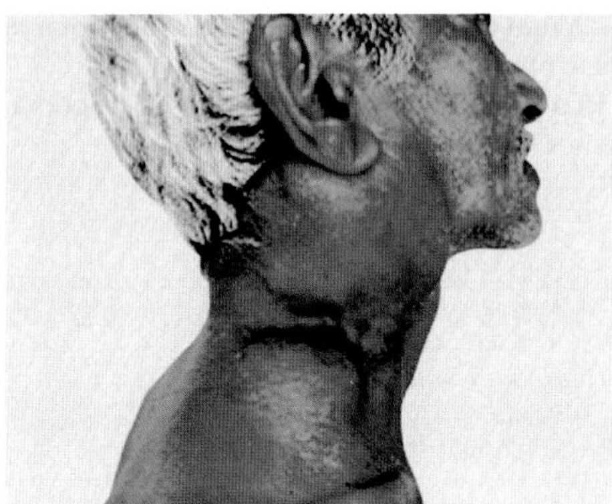
Metastatic cervical lymph node right side of neck

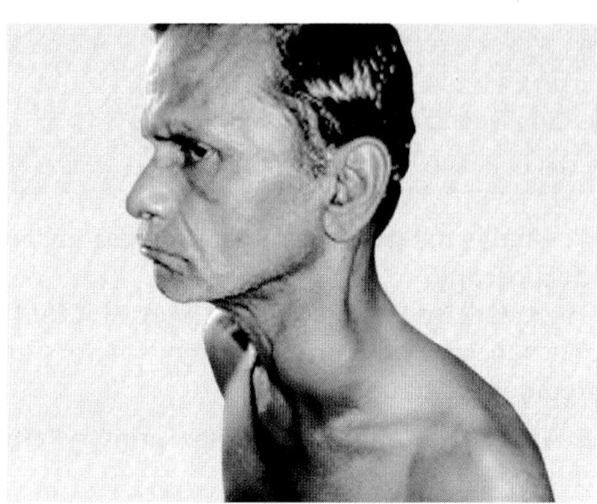
Metastatic lymph node in level IV

Q 1. What is the most probable diagnosis in this case?

Metastatic lymph node.

Q 2. Why metastatic lymph node?

- Since the lymph nodes are hard, one should suspect a malignant node
- It is a disease of old age (**mean age for male is 65 years and female 55 years**)
- Males are more affected than females (4:1)
- 85% of the malignant nodes are metastatic (only 15% are primary)
- 85% are likely to have a **primary in the supraclavicular region.**

Q 3. What is the most important clinical examination in such a patient?

A complete head and neck examination is required (since 85% are having a supraclavicular primary).

Q 4. What are the areas to be examined in the head and neck?

Checklist for evaluation of metastatic cervical lymph nodes
1. Clinical examination of ipsilateral and contralateral neck.
2. Palpation of thyroid gland and parotid gland
3. Examination of oral cavity
4. Examine the tonsillar region
5. Laryngoscopy (both direct and indirect)
6. Examination of nasopharynx
7. Examination of hypopharynx

Q 5. What are the other clinical examinations?

1. Examination of breast for a primary lesion
2. Examination of chest for a primary lesion
3. Examination of abdomen for visceral malignancy.

Q 6. If all these clinical examinations are negative what is the course of action?

An examination under anesthesia (**EUA**)—followed by **Panendoscopy.**

Panendoscopy

- Nasopharyngoscopy
- Esophagobronchoscopy
- Laryngoscopy (direct).

Q 7. What is the purpose of esophagoscopy and bronchoscopy?

In metastatic squamous cell carcinoma (**SCC**), **10-20%** chance for a **second primary** is there in the **aerodigestive tract**.

Q 8. What is the definition of a "new primary" after treatment of previous cancer?

One arising **more than 3 years** after previous cancer is considered a new primary.

Q 9. If nothing is found on panendoscopy, what next?

Surveillance biopsy: blind biopsies are taken from the following areas.

Areas for blind biopsy

- Tonsils
- Tonsillar beds
- Base of tongue (posterior 1/3rd)
- Pyriform sinus
- Subglottic region
- Fossa of Rosenmüller
- Adenoids
- Retromolar trigone.

Q 10. If surveillance biopsy is negative how to proceed?

Ipsilateral tonsillectomy.

Q 11. What is the purpose of surveillance biopsy?

In the absence of gross lesion, in **10–15%** of cases primary will be revealed by surveillance biopsy.

Q12. What is the order of frequency of primary in a case of metastasis?

- **Head and neck source of primary**: The primary sites in order of frequency are:

1. Nasopharynx
2. Tonsil
3. Base of tongue
4. Thyroid
5. Supraglottic larynx
6. Floor of mouth
7. Palate
8. Pyriform fossa

- **Nonhead and neck source of primary** (in order of frequency)

1. Bronchus
2. Esophageus
3. Breast
4. Stomach

Q 13. What is the contraindication for a preliminary lymph node biopsy in a metastatic lymph node? (PG)

- A biopsy will produce **scarring of subcutaneous tissue** and will **destroy the tissue planes**. This will affect the neck dissection if it becomes necessary because the scar tissue can not be distinguished from the tumor
- Biopsy will destroy **nodal or fascial barriers** holding the cancer in check and seedling of the soft tissues and lymphatics will occur
- Chances for **neck recurrence** will occur as a result of biopsy (recurrence is the major cause of death rather than metastasis in SCC)
- Chances for general spread is high.

Q 14. If nothing is found after pan endoscopy and blind biopsy, what next?

MRI of the neck is done.

Q 15. Why MRI is superior to CT for evaluation of a metastatic node of unknown primary?

- MRI can identify subtle changes in soft tissues
- Guided biopsy of the primary lesion is possible
- Extension of the primary to the surrounding soft tissues can be identified.

Q 16. If MRI is negative, what is the next step?
FNAC.

Q 17. If FNAC is negative, what is the next step?
An open biopsy is indicated now. If metastatic SCC is found on frozen section, it is immediately followed by a neck dissection if it is operable.

Q 18. Why not a delayed neck dissection?
The best chance for cure and time for dissection is when the normal tissue planes are intact. **Thus, the time to carry out a biopsy is when you are ready to carry out a dissection.**

Q 19. What are the possible FNAC or biopsy reports?
Histological types of metastasis (50% SCC, 25% poorly differentiated and 25% adenocarcinoma).

Histological type of metastasis

1. **Squamous cell carcinoma (SCC)**
2. **Nonsquamous cell carcinoma**
   - Adenocarcinoma
   - Poorly differentiated carcinoma
   - Poorly differentiated neoplasm.

Q 20. If the report is adenocarcinoma what are the possibilities?
Primary source for adenocarcinomatous deposits in the neck nodes:

- Salivary neoplasm
- Thyroid carcinoma
- Breast carcinoma
- Occult lung cancer
- Prostatic cancer
- Renal malignancy
- GI malignancy.

Q 21. What is the treatment of metastatic adenocarcinoma? (Flow chart 24.1)
There is no role for surgery because it is a disseminated malignancy. Patient will go in for chemotherapy (Paclitaxel and carboplatin).

Q 22. What is the management of poorly differentiated neoplasm? (Flow chart 24.1) (PG)
Repeat the FNAC. If this too turns out to be inconclusive, do a biopsy. If biopsy too proves to be inconclusive do **immunohistochemistry**.

Q 23. What is the purpose of immunohistochemistry?
Immunohistochemistry and electron microscopy is done to identify the **lymphomas** and other chemoresponsive neoplasms (about 60%).

Q 24. What is the management of poorly differentiated carcinoma? (Flow chart 24.1) (PG)
Again immunohistochemistry and electron microscopy are recommended in order to identify the chemoresponsive subgroups:

- Lymphoma
- Ewing's tumor
- Neuroendocrine tumors
- Primitive sarcomas.

Q 25. What is the commonest pathological type of neck node metastasis?
Squamous cell carcinoma—80%.

Flow chart 24.1: Management of occult primary

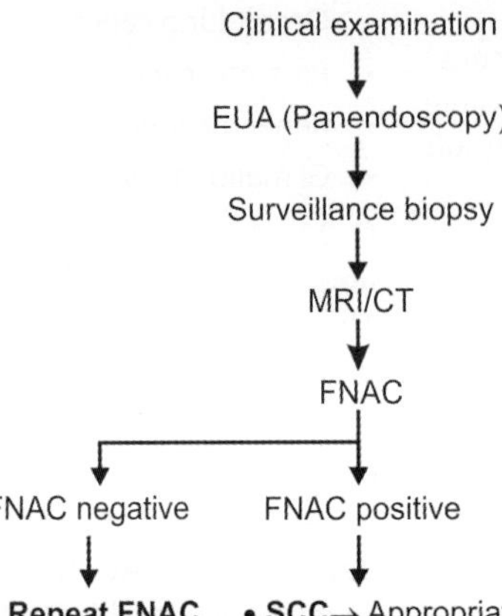

FNAC negative → **Repeat FNAC**

Open biopsy and frozen section (immunoperoxidase, electron microscopy, chromosome analysis) immediate neck dissection if **SCC**

FNAC positive →

- **SCC**→ Appropriate management
- **Non SCC**

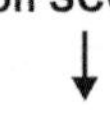

- Adenocarcinoma → empiric chemotherapy (neck dissection for salivary gland and thyroid)
- Poorly differentiated carcinoma (**immunoperoxidase staining electron microscopy**) → chemotherapy
- Poorly differentiated neoplasm (**immunoperoxidase staining electron microscopy, chromosome analysis**) → chemotherapy

Q 26. What are the squamous cell carcinomas which will metastasize bilaterally? (PG)

SCC with bilateral metastasis
1. Lower lip
2. Supraglottis
3. Soft palate.

Q 27. Which group of lymph node is involved in carcinoma nasopharynx? (PG)

Nodes involved in carcinoma nasopharynx
• Retropharyngeal nodes
• Parapharyngeal nodes
• Level II – V.

Q 28. What are the carcinomas which will metastasize to retropharyngeal lymph nodes? (PG)

Malignancies involving the retropharyngeal nodes
1. Nasopharynx
2. Soft palate
3. Posterior and lateral oropharynx
4. Hypopharynx.

Q 29. What are the primary sites below the clavicle?

Sites of the primary below the clavicle (15%)
• Lung (commonest)
• Pancreas

Contd...

Contd...

- Esophagus
- Stomach
- Breast
- Ovary
- Testis
- Prostate.

Q 30. Which group of lymph nodes are involved in infraclavicular primary?

The level **IV and V** (lower jugular chain and supraclavicular nodes).

Q 31. What are the other investigations recommended?

- X-ray chest
- Sputum cytology
- CT scan of the chest and abdomen
- Mammography
- PET scan (if required).

Q 32. What is the role of PET scan?

The 18-Fluorodeoxyglucose (18FDG) analog is preferentially absorbed by neoplastic cells and can be detected by positron emission tomography (PET) scanning. It is more sensitive than CT in identifying the primary lesion. But in the case of unknown primary the sensitivity is not more than 50%. This is because the unknown primary tumor may have spontaneously involuted.

Q 33. What is the definition of occult primary?

When the lymph node is found to contain metastatic carcinoma but the primary is unknown, even after all these investigations, then it is called occult primary.

Q 34. What are the levels of lymph nodes?

There are VII levels of lymph nodes

Level - I : Submental, submandibular

Level - II : Upper jugular

Level - III : Mid jugular

Level - IV : Lower jugular

Level - V : Posterior triangle (spinal accessory and transverse cervical) (upper, middle, and lower, corresponding to the levels that define upper, middle, and lower jugular nodes)

Level - VI : Prelaryngeal (**Delphian**), pre-tracheal, paratracheal

Level - VII : Upper mediastinal

Other groups: Suboccipital, retropharyngeal, parapharyngeal, buccinator (**facial**), preauricular, periparotid and intraparotid.

Q 35. What are the boundaries of each level?

The boundaries are as follows (Fig. 24.1):

Level - I : It is bounded by the anterior and posterior bellies of the digastric muscle

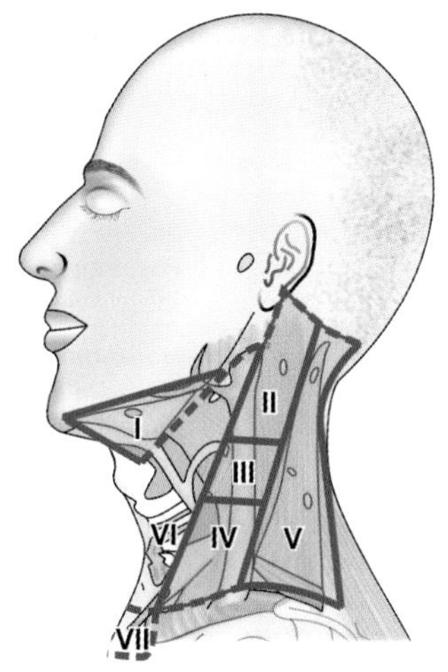

Fig. 24.1: Lymph node levels of neck

and the hyoid bone inferiorly and the body of the mandibles superiorly

Level - II : Contains the upper jugular lymph nodes and extends from the level of the **skull base** superiorly to **the hyoid bone** inferiorly (the nodes in relation to the upper third of the internal jugular vein – **upper jugular group**).

Level - III : Contains the middle jugular lymph nodes from the **hyoid bone** superiorly to the level of the lower border of the **cricoid** cartilage inferiorly (nodes in relation to the middle third of the internal jugular vein – **middle jugular group**)

Level - IV : Contain the lower jugular lymph nodes from the level of the **cricoid** cartilage superiorly to the **clavicle** inferiorly (nodes in relation to the lower third of the internal jugular vein – **lower jugular group**)

Level - V : Contains the lymph nodes in the posterior triangle bounded by the **anterior border of the trapezius** muscle posteriorly, the **posterior border of the sternocleidomastoid** muscle anteriorly, and the **clavicle inferiorly**. For descriptive purposes, Level V may be further subdivided into **upper, middle, and lower** levels corresponding to the superior and inferior planes that define Levels II, III, and IV.

Level - VI : Contains the lymph nodes of the anterior central compartment from the **hyoid bone** superiorly to the **suprasternal notch** inferiorly. On each side, the lateral boundary is formed by the medial border of the **carotid sheath**.

Level - VII: Contains the lymph nodes **inferior to the suprasternal** notch in the superior mediastinum.

Note: Further divisions as per AJCC 7th edition

Level	Superior	Inferior	Anterior (medial)	Posterior (lateral)
IA	Symphysis of mandible	Body of hyoid	Anterior belly of contra lateral digastric muscle	Anterior belly of ipsilateral digastric muscle
IB	Body of mandible	Posterior belly of digastric muscle	Anterior belly of digastric muscle	Stylohyoid muscle
IIA	Skull base	Horizontal plane defined by the inferior border of the hyoid bone	The stylohyoid muscle	Vertical plane defined by the spinal accessory nerve
IIB	Skull base	Horizontal plane defined by the inferior body of the hyoid bone	Vertical plane defined by the spinal accessory nerve	Lateral border of the sternocleidomastoid muscle

Contd...

Contd...

VA	Apex of the convergence of the sternocleidomastoid and trapezius muscles	Horizontal plane defined by the lower border of the cricoid cartilage	Posterior border of the sternocleidomastoid muscle or sensory branches of cervical plexus	Anterior border of the trapezius muscle
VB	Horizontal plane defined by the lower border of the cricoid cartilage	Clavicle	Posterior border of the sternocleidomastoid muscle	Anterior border of the trapezius muscle

Q 36. What are the probable primary sites for each level? (PG)

Primary sites for each level of cervical lymph nodes

Lymph node level	*Primary cancer sites*
Level I	Oral cavity, lip, salivary gland, skin
Level II	Oral cavity, nasopharynx, oropharynx, larynx, salivary gland
Level III	Oral cavity, oropharynx, hypopharynx, larynx, thyroid
Level IV	Oropharynx, hypopharynx, larynx, thyroid, cervical esophagus
Level V	Nasopharynx, scalp (Accessory nodes)
Level V	GI tract, breast, lung (supraclavicular)

Q 37. What is the area of drainage of suboccipital nodes?

Skin of the scalp.

Q 38. What is the drainage area of parotid nodes?

Parotid gland and skin.

Q 39. What is the N (regional lymph node) staging?

N staging as per AJCC 7th edition	
NX	Regional lymph nodes cannot be assessed
N0	No regional lymph node metastasis
*N1	Metastasis in a single ipsilateral lymph node, **3 cm or less** in greatest dimension
*N2	Metastasis in a single ipsilateral lymph node, **more than 3 cm but not more than 6 cm** in greatest dimension; **or** in multiple ipsilateral lymph nodes, none more than 6 cm in greatest dimension; **or** in bilateral **or** contralateral lymph nodes, none more than 6cm in greatest dimension.
*N2a	Metastasis in single ipsilateral lymph node **more than 3 cm** but not more than 6 cm in greatest dimension
*N2b	Metastasis in multiple ipsilateral lymph nodes, **none more than 6 cm** in greatest dimension.
*N2c	Metastasis in bilateral or contralateral lymph nodes, **none more than 6 cm** in greatest dimension
*N3	Metastasis in a lymph node **more than 6cm** in greatest dimension

* *Note:* **For Nasopharynx**

N1 is unilateral metastasis in cervical lymph node (s), 6 cm or less in greatest dimension, above the supraclavicular fossa, and or unilateral or bilateral retropharyngeal lymph nodes 6 cm or less in greatest dimension.

N2 – Bilateral metastasis in cervical lymph node (s), 6 cm or less in greatest dimension, above the supraclavicular fossa.

N3 – Metastasis in lymph node (s)* > 6 cm and/or to supraclavicular fossa*

Supraclavicular zone or fossa is relevant to the staging of nasopharyngeal carcinoma and is the triangular region which is defined by three points.

1. The superior margin of the sternal end of the clavicle
2. The superior margin of the lateral end of the clavicle
3. The point where the neck meets the shoulder.

Q 40. What is the importance of the "U" and "L"?

When the lower lymph nodes namely **level 4 and 5**, below the lower border of the cricoid cartilage are involved the prognosis is bad.

Q 41. What percentage of occult metastasis, the primary identification is possible?

Roughly in **1/3rd** cases primary can be identified.

Q 42. Why primary is nonidentifiable in some cases? (PG)

Possibly because of the **spontaneous involution** of the unknown primary.

Q 43. If primary is not identified in the given case would you recommend surgery if the report is coming as SCC?

- Yes. A neck dissection is recommended if the nodes are resectable
- A neck dissection removes additional ipsilateral cervical nodes.

Q 44. What are the conditions where neck dissections are valuable? (PG)

Conditions in which neck dissections are recommended

1. Squamous cell carcinoma
2. Salivary gland tumors
3. Thyroid carcinoma
4. Melanoma.

Q 45. What type of neck dissection is recommended?

Modified neck dissection may be appropriate.

Q 46. What are the indications for radiotherapy after a modified neck dissection?

Indications for radiotherapy after a modified neck dissection:

- If more than two lymph nodes contain metastasis
- Nodes at two or more levels contain metastasis
- Extracapsular spread of metastasis.

Q 47. What are the types of neck dissection?

The neck dissections may be classified as –

- Radical neck dissection (RND)—classical Crile procedure (level I–V nodes removed)
- Modified radical neck dissection (MRND) (described by **Bocca**) preserves one or more of the following structures—spinal accessory nerve, internal jugular vein and sternomastoid muscle—**type I, type II, type III**

  Type I—spinal accessory alone preserved

  Type II—spinal accessory and sternomastoid preserved

  Type III—spinal accessory, sternomastoid and internal jugular vein are preserved.
- **Functional neck dissection** (level II–V)—preserving sternomastoid, internal jugular vein and spinal accessory nerve
- Selective neck dissection—here one or more lymph node groups are preserved –
  1. Supraomohyoid neck dissection (removal of level I–III)
  2. Posterolateral neck dissection (removal of level II, III, IV, V)
  3. Lateral neck dissection (removal of level II, III, IV)
  4. Anterior compartment dissection (removal of level VI).

Q 48. What is the difference between modified radical neck dissection and functional neck dissection?

- Modified neck dissection always preserves spinal accessory nerve
- Functional neck dissection always preserves sternomastoid muscle, the internal jugular vein and spinal accessory nerve.

Q. 49 What are the structures removed in radical neck dissection?

En-bloc removal of fat, fascia, and lymph nodes from level I to level V.

They include the following:

- **Two muscles**—sternomastoid and omohyoid
- **Two veins**—internal jugular vein and external jugular vein
- **Two nerves**—spinal accessory nerve and cervical plexus
- Two glands—submandibular salivary glands and tail of parotid
- **Prevertebral fascia.**

Q 50. What is extended radical neck dissection? (PG)

This refers to the removal of one or more additional lymph node groups and/or nonlymphatic structures not encompassed by the radical neck dissection. This may include the parapharyngeal and superior mediastinal lymph nodes. The nonlymphatic structures may include the carotid artery, the hypoglossal nerve, the vagus nerve and the paraspinal muscles. This is not an operation for occult primary.

Q. 51. What is the prognosis if the primary tumor is never found? (PG)

This won't influence the prognosis. If the primary tumor is small or occult, it will be probably included in the field of the **postoperative irradiation** and cured by such treatment.

Prognosis is determined by whether or not the tumor recurs or whether it metastasizes (metastasis to lungs, bone or liver).

Q 52. How will you summarize the treatment for SCC occult metastasis? [*treatment of adenocarcinoma, poorly differentiated carcinoma and poorly differentiated neoplasms are already* given above]

Summary of treatment for squamous cell carcinoma metastasis from occult primary

It is treated according to the N stage:

N 1	–	MRND (surgery is the treatment of all N1 nodes) RT (radiotherapy) if positive margins, capsular invasion and multiple level nodes irradiate neck and all potential sites of primary
N 2a and N2b	–	Mobile → RND followed by RT, Fixed → RT followed by RND
N 2c	–	Bilateral RND followed by bilateral RT
N 3	–	**Resectable** → RND followed by RT + Chemo (controversy) **Unresectable** → RT followed by RND when it becomes resectable.

RND: Radical neck dissection
RT: Radiotherapy

Note: Regarding radiotherapy:

1. Radiotherapy is given for contralateral neck nodes if primary is nasopharyngeal carcinoma.
2. Level II lymph nodes alone—primary is likely to be nasopharynx and RT is preferred for such cases.

Q 53. What are the incisions used for neck dissection? (Fig. 24.2) (PG)

1. **Macfee incision**: It consists of 2 horizontal limbs. The first begins over the mastoid curving down to the hyoid bone, and up again to the chin, the second horizontal incision lies about

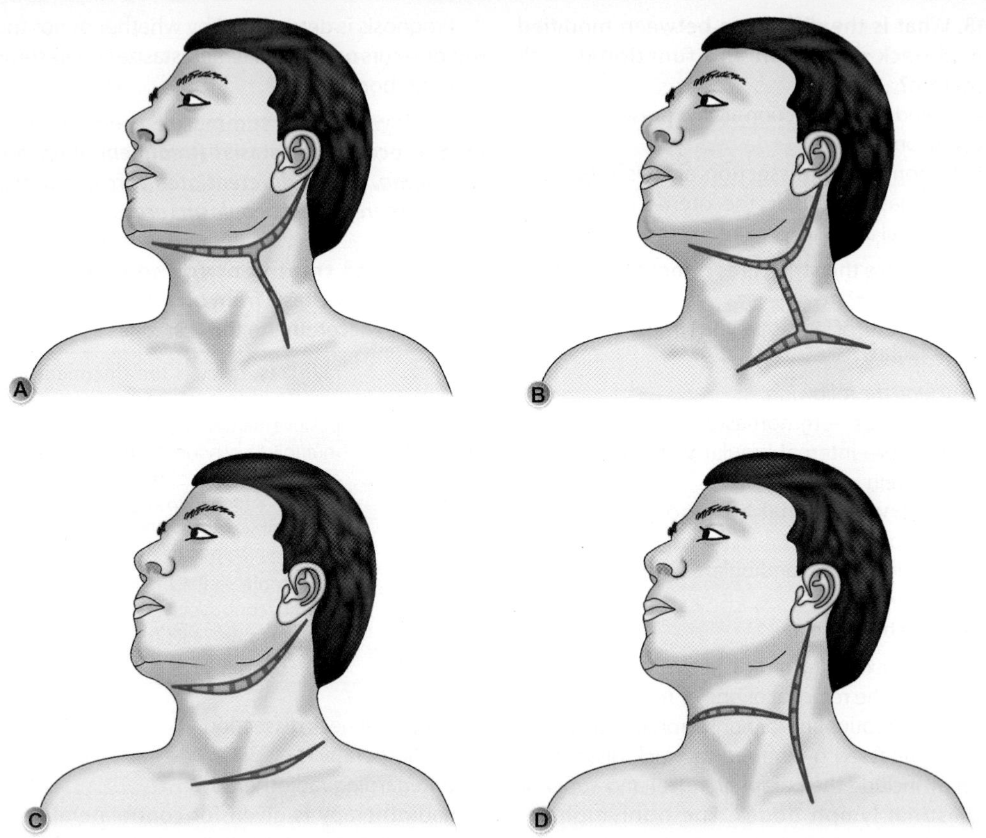

Fig. 24.2: Neck incision series (A) Modified Crile incision for neck dissection (B) Martin neck incision ('double Y') (C) MacFee neck incision (D) Schechter neck incision

2 cm above the clavicle from the anterior border of the trapezius to the midline.

2. **Schechter incision**: It has a vertical limb and horizontal limb. The vertical comes from the mastoid process to the point where trapezius meets the clavicle along the anterior border of the trapezius. The horizontal, starting from the middle of the vertical to the prominence of thyroid cartilage.
3. **The classical incision by Crile**: It is a Y-shaped incision with the upper limbs of the "Y" reaching posteriorly to the mastoid and anteriorly to the

chin. The stem of the "Y" reaches down to the middle of the posterior triangle.

4. **Martin incision:** "Double Y" incision.

Q 54. What is the most poorly vascularized area of skin in the neck and why? (PG)

- The middle of the neck laterally over the common carotid artery
- The blood supply to the skin **comes down** from the face, **up from the chest, around from trapezius** and from the external carotid on the other side
- Avoid a **vertical incision over this area** so that a carotid artery rupture can be avoided
- Avoid **three point junctions** in the center of the neck.

Q 55. What are the complications of neck dissection? (PG)

Complications of neck dissection
1. Bleeding
2. Pneumothorax
3. Raised intracranial pressure (avoid pressure dressings, use mannitol if required)
4. Wound breakdown
5. Infection
6. Necrosis of the skin flap
7. Seroma (use suction drain)
8. Rupture of the carotid artery
9. Chylous fistula (thoracic duct injury)
10. Frozen shoulder (due to accessory nerve damage) —difficulty to abduct the arm.

Q 56. What precautions are taken to prevent rupture of carotid artery? (PG)

- The carotid sheath should be protected either by a **muscle flap or a free dermal graft**
- The commonly used muscle flap is **levator scapulae**
- **Use horizontal incisions**
- **Avoid three point junctions in incisions.**

Q 57. What is the sequencing of bilateral neck dissection and its prognosis? (PG)

- The presence of bilateral neck nodes at presentation is a **bad prognostic** sign
- Five year survival rate falls to about 5%
- The usual practice of **staged neck dissection** is now changing to simultaneous bilateral neck dissection
- The most feared complication after bilateral neck dissection is **increased intracranial pressure**
- Tying one internal jugular vein produces three-fold increase in the intracranial pressure
- Tying the second side produces five-fold increase in intracranial pressure
- However, the pressure tends to fall over a period of 8 days (the pressure fall is rapid within the 1st 12 hours).

Q 58. How will you avoid this complication of increased intracranial tension? (PG)

1. Lumbar drain (removal of CSF)
2. Nursing the patient in the sitting position
3. Infusion of mannitol
4. Avoiding pressure dressings.

Case 25 Carcinoma Tongue with Submandibular Lymph Node

Case Capsule

A 65-year-old male patient who is addicted to **pan chewing and smoking** presents with nonhealing ulcer in the right lateral aspect of the tongue. He has **profuse salivation** and carries a handkerchief for wiping the saliva. There is a **pad of cotton wool** in the right ear, which he claims to take care of his earache. He has **difficulty in protruding the tongue** out. He has **slurring of speech**. There is **offensive smell** when he opens his mouth. The **submandibular lymph node** on right side is enlarged firm and mobile of about 2 × 1 cm size. The **jugulodigastric nodes** on both sides are enlarged, firm and mobile.

Checklist for history

1. History of chewing tobacco
2. History of smoking tobacco
3. History of alcoholism
4. History of tooth extraction followed by failure of the socket to heal
5. History of unexplained tooth mobility
6. History of difficulty in wearing dentures
7. History of difficulty in opening the mouth and protrusion of the tongue
8. History of difficulty in swallowing
9. History of excessive salivation
10. History of earache.

Checklist for clinical examination

1. Ask for ear pain or **otalgia** [Irritation of the lingual nerve is referred to the auriculotemporal nerve]—Cotton wool pad in the ear of the patient
2. **Slurring of speech**, when tongue is involved
3. Look for inability to protrude the tongue **[ankyloglossia]**
4. **Ulcer** *that bleeds* on touch
5. Look for **profuse salivation** which is due to the irritation of nerve fibers of taste and as a result of difficulty in swallowing
6. Look for **deviation of the tongue** indicating involvement of the nerve supply to half of the tongue [hypoglossal nerve]
7. Look for **induration** of the tongue when the tongue is inside the mouth
8. Palpate the back of the tongue while the patient sits on a stool
9. Tumors of **posterior 3rd of tongue will spread to tonsil and pillars** of the fauces
10. Examine the cheek, gums, floor of the mouth, trigone [retromolar] area and tonsils for a second primary
11. Infiltration of the mandible causes pain and **swelling of the jaw**

Contd...

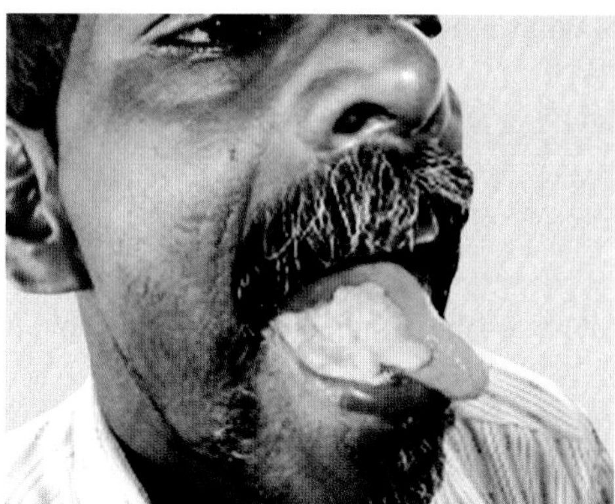

Carcinoma tongue lateral margin extending to the floor

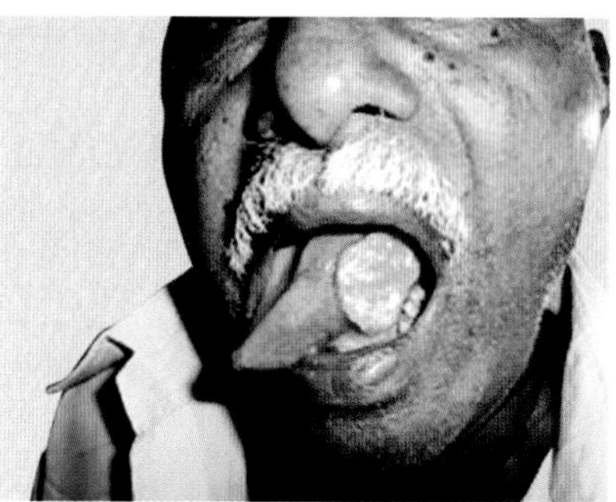

Carcinoma lateral margin left side of tongue

Contd...

12. **Look for lymph nodes** of the tongue namely, tip to the submental and jugulo-omohyoid, margin to the submandibular and upper deep cervical and from the back to the jugulodigastric and jugulo-omohyoid
13. Remember the decussation of lymphatics of the tongue and therefore the nodes of the other side of the neck may be involved
14. Carcinoma tongue is a systemic disease, and therefore look for metastasis especially pulmonary
15. Look for precancerous conditions and lesions.

Q 1. Why this is carcinoma tongue?

a. Elderly patient with an ulcer in the tongue having raised and everted margins
b. There is induration on palpation which is in favor of malignancy
c. Profuse salivation
d. Ankyloglossia
e. Offensive smell of malignant ulcer
f. Significant metastatic lymph node in the submandibular region.

Q 2. What are the differential diagnoses?

Differential diagnoses of carcinoma tongue
a. Dental ulcer [caused by irritation of tooth/denture]
b. Tuberculous ulcer—multiple small-grayish yellow ulcers with undermining edges
c. Aphthous ulcer—small painful ulcer seen on the under surface of the side of the tongue
d. Gumma—[very rare nowadays]
e. Chancre
f. Nonspecific glossitis.

Q 3. What is the most common malignancy of the tongue?

Squamous cell carcinoma.

Q 4. What are the other malignancies possible in the tongue other than squamous cell carcinoma?

a. Malignant melanoma
b. Adenocarcinoma.

Q 5. What are the investigations for the management?

Investigations for oral carcinoma

1. **Incisional biopsy** of the ulcer under local anesthesia for confirmation of the diagnosis—biopsy should include the **most suspicious area** along with normal adjacent mucosa. Areas of necrosis and gross infection should be avoided
2. **FNAC** of the lymph node
3. **Radiography**—Orthopantomogram (*OPG*)—provides information regarding the entire mandible, but limited in its ability to evaluate the symphysis and lingual cortex
4. OPG may be supplemented with **dental occlusal** and **intraoral X-rays**
5. **CT**
    - Indicated in patients with trismus
    - Lesions abutting the mandible
    - Where marginal mandibulectomy is planned
    - To evaluate the clinically negative neck
    - Patients with large nodes to look for carotid artery involvement
    - It is very useful for the assessment of pterygoid regions
6. **MRI** scan for assessing the soft tissue spread and perineural involvement. It is very **useful** *for tongue* for assessing the extent of cancer. It is also useful for other oral and **oropharyngeal** cancers. Its great advantage over CT is that the image is not degraded by the presence of metallic dental restoration
7. **Ultrasound of the neck and abdomen**—ultrasound guided aspiration of the neck is useful in surveillance of patients with clinically NO neck after treatment
8. **X-ray chest** for all patients
9. **Dental consultation if radiation is planned**
10. **Assessment of the performance status (See chart section)**
11. Hb, full blood count, nutritional status, LFT and RFT.

Q 6. What are the macroscopic types of oral cancers?

Macroscopic types of oral cancers

- Exophytic—less aggressive
- Ulcerative
- Combination.

Q 7. What are the pathological types of squamous cell carcinoma?

Types of squamous cell carcinoma

- Verrucous—No lymph nodes
- Basaloid SCC—Advanced disease (Metastasis may be there)
- Sarcomatoid—Lethal (Rapidly growing polypoidal cancers).

Q 8. What are the peculiarities of verrucous carcinoma?

- It is a controversial subject
- Presents as exophytic, whitish warty or cauliflower-like growth
- Radiotherapy in verrucous carcinoma results in a recurrence with anaplastic pattern than the original primary
- **Radiotherapy induces anaplastic transformation**
- It seems that verrucous carcinoma already contain foci of more malignant cells before radiotherapy
- There is minimal invasion and induration.
- The lesions is densely keratinized and presents as soft white velvety area
- **Lymph node metastasis is late**
- It is a **low grade squamous cell carcinoma**
- Most verrucous carcinomas are suitable for **excision** and that **is the treatment of choice.**

Q 9. What are the modes of spread of oral cancer?

1. Local spread to adjacent structures—soft tissues, muscles, bone and neurovascular structures
2. Lymphatic spread—the **first echelon lymph nodes** of primary SCC of the oral cavity are in the **supraomohyoid triangle** of the neck (Level **I, II, III**)
3. Distant metastasis—exceedingly rare (lungs and bones).

Note: Skip metastasis from primary carcinoma may occur in 15% of patients of carcinoma tongue without involvement of first echelon lymph nodes.

Q 10. Which oral cancer is having highest incidence of nodal metastasis?

Carcinoma of the tongue, followed in descending order by:

- Tumors of the floor of the mouth
- Lower alveolus
- Buccal mucosa
- Upper alveolus
- Hard palate.

Q 11. What is the mechanism of involvement of mandible?

- It is involved by infiltration through its dental sockets
- Through dental pores on the edentulous alveolar ridge.

Q 12. What are the etiological factors for oral cancer?

Etiological factors for oral cancer

A. Lifestyle habits
  a. Tobacco (smoked or smokeless)
(Synergistic effect of smoking and chewing of tobacco)
  b. Betel nut
  c. Alcohol

Contd...

Contd...

  d. Human papilloma virus (HPV)
    – Detected in 60–90% cases of oral cancer
    – Present in 40% of normal oral cavity (direct link between HPV and oral cancer remains to be established)
  e. Epstein-Barr virus

B. Dietary factors
  a. Vitamin A (protective role)
  b. Fresh fruits and vegetables
  c. Iron deficiency anemia (Plummer-Vinson syndrome) (SCC of hypopharynx and oral cavity)

C. Other risk factors
  a. Poor dental hygiene
  b. Ill-fitting dentures (chronic irritation).

The six **S—Spices, Sprit, Sepsis, Sharp tooth, Syphilis and Smoking**.

Q 13. What is the risk of tobacco chewing for oral cancer?

- Tobacco chewing, the risk is **8 times for buccal cancer**
- With **quid** it increases to **10 times**
- If the quid is kept **overnight**, the risk increases to **30 times**
- **Alcohol has synergetic** effect with tobacco.

Q 14. What are the ingredients of tobacco chewing?

It contains the following:

- Betel leaf
- Areca nut
- Smoked lime
- Catechu
- Condiments.

Note: It is commercially available as Pan masala.

Q 15. What is quid (Night quid)?

The above ingredients are kept in the gingivolabial sulcus during night gives kick throughout night. This is called a night quid.

Q 16. Which component of the chewing is responsible for the premalignant lesions?

The chewing habits vary from place-to-place. The usual ingredients are: betel leaf, lime, betel nut and tobacco. The **most important carcinogen** is **tobacco**. The betel nut has got two alkaloids namely, **arecoline** and **tannins**. The arecoline stimulate collagen synthesis and proliferation of fibroblasts. The tannins stabilizes collagen fibrils.

Q 17. What is the action of alcohol?

The following actions are there for the carcinogenesis:

- Promoter
- Irritant
- Solvent—increases the solubility of carcinogen
- Alcohol suppresses the efficiency of the DNA repair after exposure to nitrosamine compounds.

Q 18. What are the premalignant lesions of the oral cavity?

Lesions of the oral cavity associated with an increased risk of malignancy:

Precancerous lesions
- a. Leukoplakia
- b. Erythroplakia
- c. Chronic hyperplastic candidiasis

Precancerous conditions
- a. Oral submucous fibrosis
- b. Syphilitic glossitis
- c. Sideropenic dysphagia

Doubtful association
- a. Oral lichen planus
- b. Discoid lupus erythematosus
- c. Dyskeratosis congenita.

Note:

- **Precancerous lesions**—These are morphologically altered tissue in which cancer is more likely to occur than in its apparently normal counterpart.
- **Precancerous conditions**—These are generalized states associated with significantly increased risk of cancer.

Q 19. What is the WHO definition of leukoplakia?

Any white patch or plaque that cannot be characterized clinically or pathologically as any other disease.

Clinically present as white or gray/soft or crusty lesion.

Q 20. What is the natural course of leukoplakia?

It may:

- Persist
- Regress
- Progress
- Recur.

Q 21. Which type of leukoplakia is dangerous?

There are two types of leukoplakia:

- Nodular
- Homogenous.

Speckled or nodular leukoplakia, which are the most likely ones that will turn malignant.

Q 22. What are the pathological changes in leukoplakia?

Pathological changes in leukoplakia

- Hyperkeratosis
- Parakeratosis
- Acanthosis.

Q 23. What is the incidence of malignant change in leukoplakia?

Incidence of malignancy in leukoplakia		
• Overall 5% risk of malignant transformation		
• More than 10 years duration	–	2.4%
• More than 20 years duration	–	4%
• Less than 50 years of patient's age	–	1%
• Between 70 and 89 years	–	7.5%

Note: Leukoplakia of the **floor of the mouth and ventral surface of the tongue** has high incidence of malignant change due to the **pooling of carcinogens** in the floor of the mouth.

Q 24. What are the early clinical features of malignancy in leukoplakia?

Clinical features of malignancy in leukoplakia
• Nodularity and thickness
• Ulceration
• Rolled margins
• Growths
• Indurated areas.

Q 25. What is the management of leukoplakia?

- Most of cases of **leukoplakia will disappear** if alcohol and tobacco consumption ceases—ask the patient to **stop tobacco**
- 1 year after the patient stops smoking and drinking alcohol, leukoplakia will disappear in 60% of cases
- All lesions are biopsied (Biopsy from suspicious area—**ulceration, induration and hyperemia**)
- If required **surgical excision/CO_2 laser** may be used and the small defects are closed and the larger defects are left to epithelialize
- Regular **follow-up at 4 monthly intervals.**

Q 26. What is hairy leukoplakia?

White friable lesions of the tongue seen in *AIDS* are called hairy leukoplakia.

Q 27. What is the WHO definition of erythroplakia?

Any lesion of the oral mucosa that presents as bright red velvety plaques, which cannot be characterized clinically or pathologically as any other recognizable condition.

Q 28. What is the management of erythroplakia?

All lesions are excised because of the high incidence of malignancy.

Q 29. What is chronic hyperplastic candidiasis?

Dense **chalky plaques** of keratin which are more opaque than noncandidal leukoplakia. These lesions are seen commonly in **commissures.** Here, there is invasive candidal infection with an immunological defect, there is high incidence of malignant change.

Q 30. What is oral submucous fibrosis?

In this condition, **fibrous bands form beneath the oral mucosa** and these bands progressively contract ultimately resulting in restriction of opening of the mouth and tongue movements. This entity is **confined to Asians**. The etiology is obscure. **Hypersensitivity to chilli, betel nut, tobacco and vitamin deficiencies** are implicated. Slowly growing **squamous cell carcinoma** is seen in 1/3rd of patients.

Q 31. What are the features of oral submucous fibrosis (SMF)?

Features of oral submucous fibrosis
• SMF is a high-risk precancerous condition
• There is strong association between SMF and chewing areca nut
• It can affect any part of the oral mucosa

Contd...

Contd...

- Palpable fibrous bands over the buccal mucosa, retromolar area and rima oris
- Restriction of mouth opening—Trismus (in severe case impossible to open the mouth)
- It will not regress with cessation of areca nut chewing
- It may spread to involve wider areas.

Q 32. What is the histology of oral submucous fibrosis?

- Juxta epithelial fibrosis with atrophy or hyperplasia of the overlying epithelium (fibroelastic transformation initially)
- Areas of epithelial dysplasia are seen.

Q 33. What is the treatment of oral submucous fibrosis?

- Intralesional injection of steroids
- Surgical excision and grafting (*Note:* this will not prevent squamous cell carcinoma).

Q 34. What is syphilitic glossitis?

Syphilitic glossitis will produce the following changes:

Syphilitic glossitis
↓
Endarteritis
↓
Atrophy of overlying epithelium
↓
More vulnerable to irritants
↓
Squamous cell carcinoma (even in the absence of leukoplakia)

Note:

- These changes are irreversible
- There is no specific treatment for syphilitic glossitis
- The syphilis must be treated.

Q 35. What are the causes for glossitis?

Causes for glossitis

- Median rhomboid glossitis
- Geographic tongue
- Hairy tongue—It is only the appearance and not the presence of hair
- Pernicious anemia—Hunter's glossitis
- Agranulocytosis
- Pellagra (deficiency of B2).

Q 36. What are the causes for hairy tongue?

- Black hairy tongue occurs in response to some antibiotics and antiseptics
- There is overgrowth of filiform papillae which become stained black by bacteria, medication or tobacco.

Q 37. What is median rhomboid glossitis?

It is characterized by the appearance of a rhomboid or oval mass in the midline of the tongue, immediately in front of the foramen cecum. The mass is slightly raised, smooth and devoid of papillae. It is probably as a result of **candidal infection**.

Q 38. What is geographic tongue?

- It is a condition of unknown etiology
- Red patches with yellow borders form a pattern on the dorsum of the tongue
- The pattern will change from day-to-day
- The condition starts in childhood and continues throughout life
- Some cases remit spontaneously.

Q 39. What is sideropenic dysphagia (Plummer-Vinson syndrome/Paterson-Kelly syndrome)?

- Common in Swedish women
- Higher incidence of cancer of the upper alimentary tract in this group
- It is the cause for higher incidence of oral cancer in women in Sweden

- Of women with oral cancer 25% are sideropenic
- The pathogenesis may be similar to syphilitic glossitis (as a result of epithelial atrophy)
- The iron deficiency anemia seen will respond to treatment with iron supplements (the risk of subsequent malignant change may not be altered).

Q 40. In which type of oral lichen planus, there is more risk for malignant transformation?

Atrophic and erosive lichen planus.

Q 41. What is dyskeratosis congenita?

This syndrome is characterized by:

a. Reticular atrophy
b. Nail dystrophy
c. Oral leukoplakia.

Q 42. What is the most common site of squamous cell carcinoma in the tongue?

Middle third of the lateral margin of the tongue.

The incidences at various sites in the tongue are given below:

- 25%—Anterior 1/3rd (lateral margin) × 2 (on each side = 50%)
- 10%—Tip of the tongue
- 10%—Under surface of the tongue
- 5%—Dorsum of the tongue
- 25%—Posterior 3rd of the tongue (posterior 3rd is not oral tongue).

Q 43. What are the clinical features of carcinoma of the tongue?

Clinical features of carcinoma of the tongue
• Exophytic lesion with areas of ulceration
• Ulcer in the depth of fissure
• Superficial ulceration with infiltration
• Ankyloglossia (inability to protrude the tongue)
• Hypoglossal nerve palsy
• Regional node enlargement
• Earache
• Profuse salivation (inability to swallow and increased salivation because of irritation of the nerves of taste)
• Difficulty in speech
• Dysphagia
• Offensive smell (fetor).

Contd...

Contd...

Q 44. What is the lymphatic drainage of tongue?

Lymphatic drainage of the tongue
• Lymphatics from the tip of the tongue—to the submental nodes and jugulo-omohyoid
• Lymphatics from the margin—to the submandibular nodes and upper deep cervical
• From the back of the tongue—to the jugulo-digastric and jugulo-omohyoid
• There is decussation of lymphatic vessels.

Note: The lymph nodes of **both sides of the neck** must be examined, even if the lesion is unilateral since the lymphatic vessels are decussating.

Q 45. What is the AJCC staging of the oral cavity tumors?

AJCC staging	
Primary	
Tis	Carcinoma *in situ*
T1	Tumor< 2 cm
T2	Tumor> 2 cm to < 4 cm
T3	Tumor > 4 cm
T4a	*Moderately advanced local disease*. Tumor invades through cortical bone, inferior alveolar nerve, floor of mouth, skin of face, that is chin or nose. Tumor invades adjacent structures only.

Contd...

Contd...

	For example, Cortical bone (mandible or maxilla) into deep extrinsic muscle of tongue (genioglossus, hyoglossus, palatoglossus and styloglossus), maxillary sinus, skin of face
T4b	*Very advanced local disease* – Tumor invades masticator space, pterygoid plates or skull base and or encase internal carotid artery

Note: Superficial erosion alone of bone/tooth socket by gingival primary is not sufficient to classify as T4.

Neck

N0	No clinically palpable node
N1	Single ipsilateral node < 3 cm
N2a	Single ipsilateral node > 3 cm to 6 cm
N2b	Multiple ipsilateral nodes < 6 cm
N2c	Bilateral or contralateral nodes < 6 cm
N3	Nodes > 6 cm

Distant Metastasis

MX	Distant metastasis cannot be assessed
M0	No distant metastasis
M1	Distant metastasis

Stage Grouping

Stage 0	Tis	N0	M0
Stage I	T1	N0	M0
Stage II	T2	N0	M0
Stage III	T3	N0	M0
	T1	N1	M0
	T2	N1	M0
	T3	N1	M0
Stage IV A T4a	N0	M0	
(moderately T4a	N0	M0	
advanced T4a	N1	M0	
disease) T1	N2	M0	
T2	N2	M0	
T3	N2	M0	
T4a	N2	M0	
	Any T	N2	M0
Stage IVB	Any T	N3	M0
Very advanced T4b	Any N	M0	
Stage IVC *Metastatic* Disease	Any T	Any N	M1

Contd...

Q46. What is the surgical management of carcinoma of the tongue?

- It consists of treatment of the **primary lesion** and treatment of the **metastatic nodes**.
- **Three dimensional excision is the treatment of choice for the primary**

a. *Small lesions less than 2 cm size*:
   - Excise the lesion and the defect is left to granulate and epithelialize
   - Resection of **less than one third** of the tongue does not require reconstruction
   - It can also be treated by **Brachytherapy** by iridium wires (this will **preserve the tongue**)
   - CO_2 laser also can be used for partial glossectomy.

b. *Lesions of more than 2 cm size:*
   - **Hemiglossectomy** is the minimum treatment
   - **Preserve one hypoglossal nerve** (this will give reasonable speech and the patient will learn to swallow)
   - For T1 and T2 lesions after glossectomy, simple **quilted splint skin graft** is enough

c. *Extensive lesion involving the floor of the mouth and alveolus:*
   - Major 3 dimensional resection by **lip split** and **mandibulotomy** is required

- **Marginal mandibular resection** may be required
- **Dissection of the neck** on the same side is also carried out
- This is followed by reconstruction with a **Radial forearm flap** with microvascular anastomosis (**radial forearm flap is the work horse of oral reconstruction**). This flap is useful if the volume defect is less than 2/3rd of the original tongue
- A bulky flap may be required after total glossectomy for a very large defect

Q 47. What is marginal mandibular resection?

Marginal mandibulectomy involves an in-continuity excision of tumor with a margin of mandible and overlying gingiva. Mandibular continuity is maintained and a much better cosmetic and functional end result is achieved. **A segment of bone at least 1 cm thick must be left inferiorly.** Marginal mandibular resection is done if the tumor reaches but does not **invade the alveolus**.

This is because of the peculiarity of the mode of involvement of the mandible. It is involved by infiltration through its **dental sockets or dental pores** on the edentulous alveolar ridge. These cells proceed along the root of the tooth into the **cancellous part of the mandible** and then along the **mandibular canal**.

Q 48. What are the contraindications for marginal mandibulectomy?

- Radiological involvement of the bone
- Previous radiotherapy—cause osteoradionecrosis and fracture
- Retromolar primary lesion
- Deeply infiltrating gingivobuccal lesion with paramandibular infiltration.

Q 49. What is commando operation?

It is an old operation where **combined (composite) excision** of the **primary tumor**, block dissection of the cervical **lymph nodes** and removal of the intervening body of the **mandible** is done (it was presumed previously that the spread to the mandible is by lymphatics on its way to the regional nodes. But now we know the method of spread to the mandible and hence, the introduction of marginal mandibulectomy).

Q 50. What is the management of neck nodes?

(Read the block dissection part in *short case No:2)*

- A modified radical neck dissection (MRND) is recommended for N1 and N2 nodes.
- A supraomohyoid neck dissection (SOHND) (clearance of level I, II, III nodes with preservation of sternocleidomastoid, internal jugular vein and spinal accessory) and postoperative radiotherapy has been advocated by some authors for **N1, Level I disease**.

Q 51. Is there any role for elective lymph node dissection (ELND) in N0 neck (no neck nodes)?

Yes.

- Occult nodal metastatic disease is present in 5–40% of oral cancers depending on T status and grade of primary
- Clinical N0 neck should be treated by supraomohyoid neck dissection (SOHND), if the risk of occult nodal metastasis is greater than 15–20% in patients with T3/T4 primary
- Patient with T1/T2 tongue tumors and cancers of the floor of the mouth more than 2 mm thick.
- It is also indicated if it is necessary to enter the neck for resecting the primary
- In short neck individuals requiring bulky flap for oral reconstruction (to create space)

- If the patients are unreliable for follow-up.
- In patients undergoing elective SOHND 24 to 31% will have histological evidence of lymph node metastasis.

Q 52. If the neck nodes are pathologically positive after SOHND, what next?

- If detected positive on the operating table, then SOHND should be converted to RND/MRND
- If positive following surgery—subsequent RND or postoperative radiotherapy.

Q 53. How to tackle the skip metastasis to level IV which is seen in 15% patients with tongue cancer?

Extended SOHND is recommended by some group to tackle this problem where the level IV nodes are also removed.

Q 54. What is the management of bilateral nodal metastasis?

Bilateral neck dissection with preservation of internal jugular vein on one side.

Q 55. What are the indications for radiotherapy for primary?

Indications for radiotherapy

- For early lesions of the tongue
- Early lesions of the buccal mucosa
- Patient is medically unfit
- Patient is unwilling for surgery.

Q 56. How is radiotherapy given?

- External beam radiotherapy
- Interstitial radiotherapy
- Combination of both.

Q 57. What is the dose of radiotherapy?

The total dose is 65–75 Gy to the primary and neck.

Q 58. What are the complications of radiotherapy?

Complications of radiotherapy

- Xerostomia
- Tissue edema
- Erythema
- Skin sloughing
- Ulceration
- Dental caries
- Osteoradionecrosis.

Q 59. What are the causes of death in carcinoma tongue?

Causes of death in carcinoma tongue

- Inhalation and aspiration pneumonia
- Cachexia and starvation
- Hemorrhage from growth
- Hemorrhage from carotid artery when eroded by metastatic lymph nodes
- Asphyxia secondary to pressure from lymph nodes
- Edema glottis.

Case

26 Carcinoma of Gingivobuccal Complex (Indian Oral Cancer)

Case Capsule

A 60-year-old male patient addicted to chewing tobacco for the last 35 years and drinking alcohol presents with history of tooth extraction with subsequent **failure of the socket to heal** in the right **lower molar region** for the last 6 months. On examination there is an **indurated ulceroproliferative lesion** extending from the tooth extraction socket in the first molar region of the lower gingiva to the **gingivobuccal sulcus** of 5 × 3 cm size. This lesion involves the overlying **skin of the cheek resulting in 3 sinuses**. The patient has difficulty in opening the mouth (**trismus**). The anterior pillar of the fauces and retromolar trigone seems free. The **submandibular lymph node** is enlarged of about 2 × 1 cm size and hard in consistency. There are 3 leukoplakic patches seen on the buccal mucosa on left side.

Read the checklist for the history and examination of carcinoma tongue.

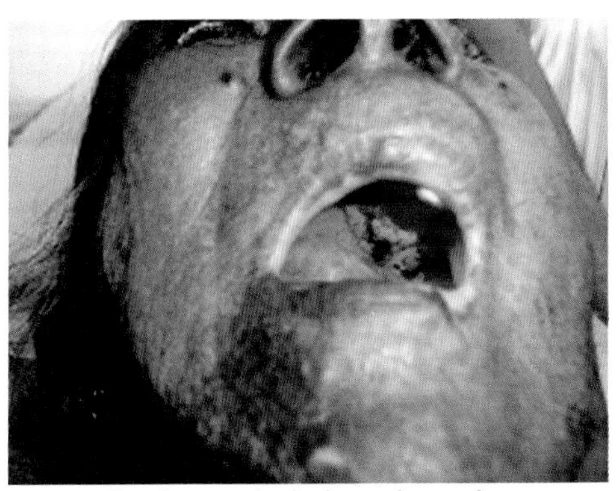

Carcinoma gingivobuccal complex

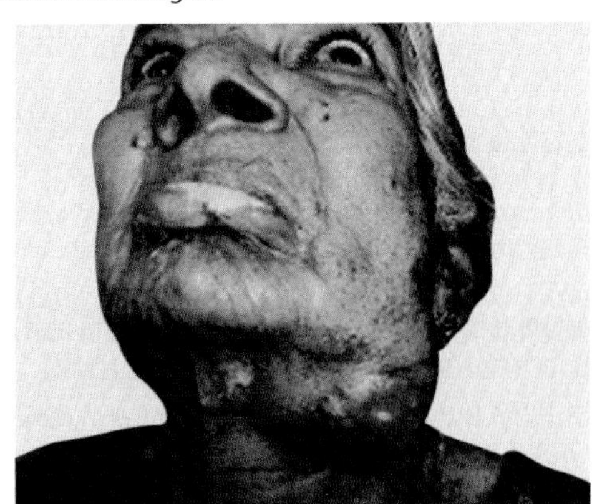

Carcinoma gingivobuccal complex with fungating left submandibular lymph nodes

Q 1. What is the most probable diagnosis in this case?

Carcinoma of the gingivobuccal complex.

Q 2. What are the clinical points in favor of carcinoma?

- History of tooth extraction followed by failure of the socket to heal
- The indurated ulceroproliferative lesion with everted margins
- Involvement of the overlying skin with sinuses
- Presence of hard submandibular lymph node
- Trismus
- Presence of leukoplakia
- History of pan chewing and smoking.

Q 3. What is the definition of oral cavity?

The term oral cavity refers to the following:

Oral cavity
• Lips • Buccal mucosa • Alveolar ridges (upper and lower gingiva) • Retromolar trigone • Hard palate • Floor of the mouth • Anterior two-thirds of the tongue (oral or mobile tongue).

Note: Cancer of the lip behaves clinically like skin cancer, and therefore not discussed with oral cavity lesion.

Q 4. What is the incidence of oral cancers in India?

About 16 to 28 per 100,000 population [ICMR].

Q 5. What is the commonest oral cancer in India?

In India, carcinoma of the **buccal mucosa** is the commonest oral cancer constituting about 50 to 83% of oral cancers. In the West, tongue and floor of the mouth are the commonest sites [30%].

Q 6. What are the areas involved by buccal cancers?

- The gingivobuccal sulcus
- Retromolartrigone
- Lower and upper alveolus
- Buccal mucosa.

Q 7. What is Indian oral cancer?

The buccal mucosa and gingiva are more often affected by cancer as a result of placement of the tobacco quid in the oral cavity. This cancer of the **gingivobuccal complex** is described as the **Indian oral cancer**.

Q 8. What is the commonest age group affected?

It is 5th to 7th decade.

Q 9. What is the extent of buccal mucosa?

The buccal mucosa extends from the **upper alveolar ridge** down to the **lower alveolar ridge, from the commissure** anteriorly to the **mandibular ramus and retromolar region posteriorly.**

Q 10. What is the cause for trismus in this case?

Infiltration of the muscles by carcinoma is responsible for trismus in this case. The following muscles may be involved in carcinoma of the buccal mucosa:

- Buccinator
- Pterygoid
- Masseter
- Temporalis.

Q 11. What are the causes for trismus?

Causes for trismus
• Submucous fibrosis • Invasion of muscles by carcinoma (mentioned earlier) • Tetanus—Risus sardonicus (painful smiling) • Parotitis • Dental abscess • Erupting wisdom tooth • Peritonsillar abscess.

Q 12. What is the grading of trismus? (PG)

Depending on the degree of mouth opening possible it is graded into 4 groups:

Grading of trismus		
• Grade I	–	more than 35 mm
• Grade II	–	26 to 35 mm
• Grade III	–	16 to 25 mm
• Grade IV	–	< 15 mm

Q 13. What is the cause for sinus in this case?

Orocutaneous fistula secondary to malignant infiltration.

Q 14. What is retromolar trigone?

- The retromolar trigone is defined as the anterior surface of the ascending ramus of the mandible
- It is triangular in shape
- The base is superior behind the 3rd upper molar tooth
- The apex is inferior behind the 3rd lower molar tooth.

Q 15. What are the special problems of carcinoma of the retromolar trigone? (PG)

- Tumors at this site may invade the ascending ramus of the mandible
- It may spread upwards to involve the pterygomandibular space
- A lip split and mandibulotomy are needed to gain access to this region
- Mandibulectomy is required for clearance of the pterygoid region
- The resultant defect is managed by masseter and or temporalis muscle flap.

Q 16. What is the staging in this case?

Read the staging of oral cancers given in Carcinoma Tongue Chapter.

It can summarized as:

In this case the staging is:

T4, N1, M0 $\rightarrow$ stage IV A.

Q 17. What are the investigations required?

Read the investigation chart for carcinoma tongue. **(Confirm the diagnosis by biopsy from the most suspicious area avoiding the areas of infection and necrosis).**

Q 18. What is the management of stage IV disease?

- Generally **stage I and II (Early)** diseases are managed by **Surgery/Radiotherapy** (Either surgery or radiotherapy)—*No radiotherapy* in gingivobuccal complex due to close proximity of the tumor to bone and **risk of radio necrosis.**
- Stage *III and IV* **(Advanced)** are managed by **Radical Surgery and Reconstruction and Radiotherapy** (Surgery and Radiotherapy are combined).
- Surgery is the treatment of choice for **all alveolar carcinomas** except for patients unfit for surgery.

Q 19. What is the surgical treatment if the carcinoma is confined to the buccal mucosa?

- It is excised widely including the underlying Buccinator muscle.
- This is followed by split—skin graft.

Q 20. What is the surgical management of more extensive lesion?

- Three dimensional excision and reconstruction.

Q 21. What are the flaps available for reconstruction after 3dimensional excision of oral cancer? (PG)

Flaps available for reconstruction
• Free radial forearm flap—is the work - horse of oral reconstruction
• Buccal fat pad—For small intraoral defects of upto 3 × 5 cm – Used for reconstruction of maxillary

Contd...

Contd...

defects, hard and soft palate defects, cheek and retromolar defects
- Temporalis muscle flap (for larger defects along with buccal fat pad)
- Forehead flap—now rarely used because of the poor cosmetic outcome.

Q 22. What is the management if the mandible is radiologically not involved?

Marginal mandibulectomy (Read carcinoma tongue).

Q 23. What are the contraindications for marginal mandibulectomy? (PG)

Contraindications for marginal mandibulectomy

- Gross clinical involvement of mandible
- Radiological involvement of the mandible
- Deeply infiltrating lesions of the gingivobuccal sulcus with paramandibular infiltration
- Previous radiotherapy (osteoradio necrosis)
- Retromolar lesions (clearance of the pterygoid region is not possible).

Q 24. In the present case there is gross clinical involvement of the mandible and paramandibular infiltration. What is the surgical management?

Hemimandibulectomy or **segmental mandibulectomy** is required, along with the *3 dimensional* **excision** and a modified radical neck dissection (*MRND*).

Q 25. What is the deformity produced by the resection of the anterior arch of mandible? (PG)

Andy Gump deformity.

Q 26. What are the bony substitutes available for reconstruction after mandibulectomy? (PG)

Reconstruction with **osteomyocutaneous flap or free microvascular bone graft immediately.**

- Radial forearm flap with a section of radius
- Compound groin flap based on the deep circumflex iliac vessels
- Free fibula flap
- Corticocancellous grafts harvested from iliac crest (packed into mesh trays—Titanium trays)
- Rib grafts.

Q 27. What is the soft tissue cover for the reconstructed bone? (PG)

- For the microvascular free flaps the associated skin is used (compound groin flap based on the deep circumflex iliac vessels)

Pectoralis major muscle flap (this is wrapped around the bone graft and sutured on the labial aspect).

Q 28. What are the indications for surgery in general for oral cancer?

Indications for surgery in oral carcinoma

1. Tumors on alveolar process
2. Very large mass when there is invasion of bone
3. Nodal involvement—primary and nodes are treated surgically
4. Multiple primary tumors—surgery is preferred
5. Verrucous carcinoma.

Q 29. Is there any role for radiotherapy as a primary modality in Early gingivobuccal complex?

No. (Because of the proximity to mandible)

Q 30. What is the role for preoperative radiotherapy in Advanced gingivobuccal complex?

Indications for preoperative radiotherapy in advanced gingivobuccal complex

- Inoperable diseases
- Patient is unfit for surgery
- Patient is unwilling for surgery
- Down staging is possible.

Q 31. What are the indications for postoperative radiation therapy to the primary?

Indications for postoperative radiation therapy to the primary
• T3/T4 primary • Residual microscopic tumor • Positive surgical margins • Gross residual tumor after resection.

Q 32. What are the indications for adjuvant radiation to the neck after radical neck dissection?

Indications for adjuvant radiation to the neck after radical neck dissection
• More than 2 positive nodes • 2 or more levels of nodes involved • Extracapsular spread.

Q 33. What are the indications for elective neck irradiation?

Elective neck irradiation is used for N0 or N1 neck if the treatment of primary with radiation therapy is effective.

Q 34. What is the survival for stage III and IV disease after treatment? (PG)

- With radiation or surgery alone the survival for stage III is 41% and Stage IV is 15%.
- *When* surgery is combined with postoperative radiation therapy these rates increase to 60% and 35%.

Q 35. What is the management of inoperable cases?

Inoperable cases are managed by radiation therapy with or without chemotherapy.

Q 36. What are the indications for chemotherapy? (PG)

Indications for chemotherapy
• Palliation for advanced oral cancer • Recurrent oral cancers • Verrucous carcinoma • Adjuvant • Neoadjuvant • Concurrently with radiation: chemoradiation.

Q 37. What is the advantage of chemoradiation?

- Improve the locoregional control
- Prevent metastasis.

Q 38. What is the disadvantage of chemoradiation?

- Significant treatment related morbidity.

Q 39. What is the contraindication for chemotherapy?

Poor performance status (Read the Chart and Table section).

Q 40. What are the chemotherapeutic agents used?

Cisplatin—based combination chemotherapy is more effective than single agent chemotherapy (Cisplatin and 5-FU).

The commonly used agents either alone or in combination are:

- Methotrexate
- 5-fluorouracil (5-FU)
- Cisplatin
- Bleomycin
- Ifosfamide.

Q 41. What are the poor prognostic factors?

Poor prognostic factors
• Stage at presentation (single most important) • Lymph node metastasis • Number of lymph nodes involved • Extracapsular spread in the node • Tongue cancer has poor prognosis compared to other subsites.

Q 42. What is the survival figure for early and advanced stages? (PG)

- Stage I and II (early)—5 year survival of 31–100%.
- Stage III and IV (advanced stages)—5 year survival of 7–41% depending on the site of the disease.

Case

27 Parotid Swelling

Case Capsule

A 45-year-old male patient presents with **painless enlargement of the right parotid gland**. On examination, there is a swelling of about **4 × 3 cm size** irregular in shape and occupying the hollow between the mandible and mastoid. It is firm in consistency, deep to the parotid fascia, and superficial to the masseter muscle. The swelling **raises the right ear lobule**. The **facial nerve is intact.** The superficial temporal artery is palpable above the swelling. There are no palpable ipsilateral nodes. The patient is apparently healthy.

Read the diagnostic algorithm for a neck swelling

Checklist for history

1. History of systemic diseases responsible for sialadenosis like—DM, drugs (antiasthmatic, Guanethidine) endocrine disorders, alcoholism, pregnancy, bulimia (eating disorders)
2. History of exposure to mumps
3. History of collagen diseases
4. History of salivary colic
5. History of increase in size during salivation

Contd...

Contd...

6. History of similar swelling on the contralateral side
7. History of recent illness and major surgery (acute parotitis)
8. History of exposure to HIV (HIV associated sialadenitis).

Checklist for examination

1. Look for obliteration of the hollow below the ear lobule
2. Look for fixity to masseter
3. Bimanual palpation of the deep lobe with one finger inside at the tonsillar region and other hand externally
4. Bidigital palpation of the Stensen's duct (thumb externally and index finger internally)
5. Look for lymph nodes—Preauricular, parotid and submandibular nodes
6. Look for movements of the jaw
7. Look for facial nerve palsy
8. Examine the oral cavity—Orifice of Stensen's duct, Tonsil (whether pushed medially or not)
9. Always examine other ipsilateral salivary glands and other contralateral salivary glands.

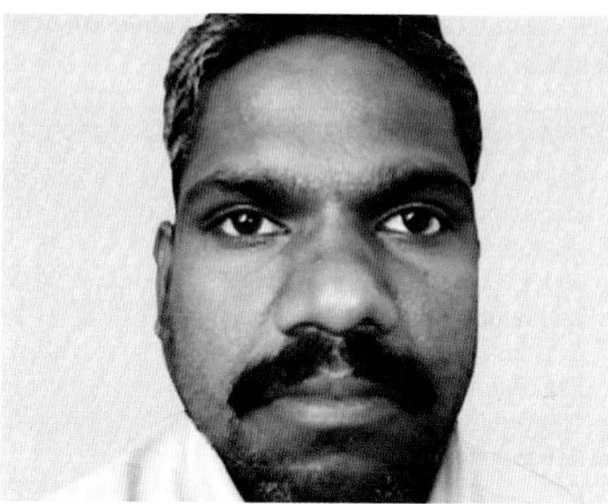
Bilateral parotid enlargement—Sjogren's syndrome

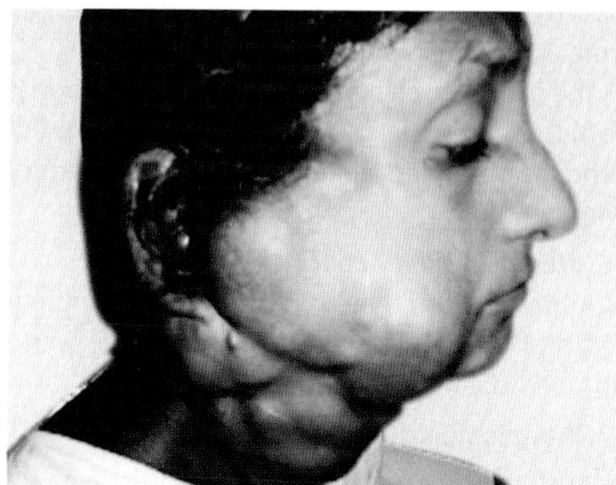
Malignant parotid with metastatic node

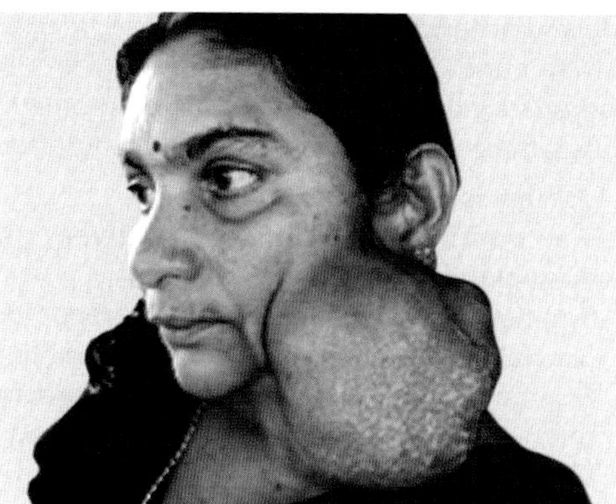
Pleomorphic adenoma turning malignant

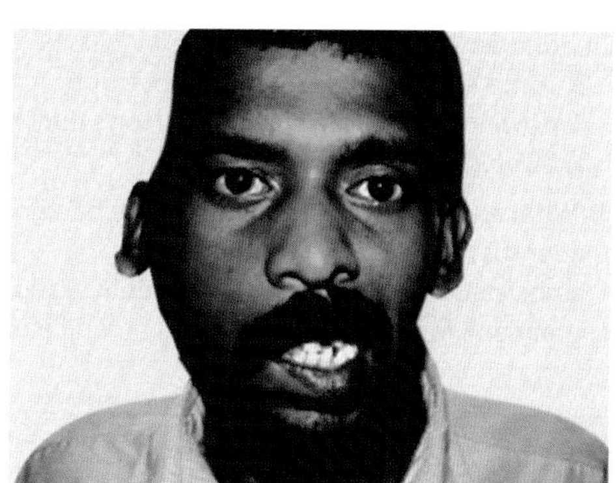
Malignant parotid with right facial palsy

Q 1. What is the most probable diagnosis?
Parotid swelling.

Q 2. What are the points in favors of parotid swelling?
The following points characterize the swelling:

1. Deep to the parotid fascia
2. It is superficial to masseter
3. It is raising the ear lobule
4. Occupying the normal anatomic area of the parotid.

Q 3. What is the classical site of parotid swelling?

- *Below, behind and slightly in front of the ear lobule*
- It obliterates the normal hollow below the lobule of the ear.

Q 4. What is the clinical test by which you say that the swelling is deep to parotid fascia?
The parotid fascia is stretched by asking the patient to open the mouth. If the swelling is deep to the parotid fascia, the swelling will become less prominent.

Q 5. Why do you say that the swelling is superficial to masseter muscle?

Ask the patient to clench the teeth. This will contract the masseter muscle. The parotid gland is superficial to the masseter and therefore it will become more prominent.

Q 6. What is salivary colic?

During salivation, there will be pain and increase in size of the swelling, which is typically seen in submandibular salivary duct stones.

Q 7. What is sialadenitis?

Inflammation of the salivary gland is called sialadenitis it may be classified as:

- Acute bacterial sialadenitis—Seen in elderly bedridden patients and neonates
- Chronic sialadenitis—Due to obstruction or narrowing of the Stensen's or Wharton's duct by a calculus or stricture.

Q 8. What are the manifestations of acute bacterial sialadenitis?

It is associated with poor oral hygiene, dehydration, general debilitation, etc. and clinically manifested as:

- Sudden painful (tender) swelling of the parotid gland
- Trismus
- Dysphagia
- Fever.

Q 9. What are the manifestations of chronic sialadenitis?

- Recurrent parotid swelling especially during eating
- Enlargement of the gland (rubbery hard)
- Stricture of the duct.

Q 10. What is the commonest cause of acute parotitis?

Mumps (caused by paramyxovirus) manifested by

- Bilateral or unilateral parotid swelling (double chin appearance due to the spreading down of the edema)
- Fever
- Arthralgia
- Orchitis (rarely)
- Pancreatitis
- Thyroiditis
- Sensory neural hearing loss.

Q 11. Why should you examine the contralateral side and other salivary glands?

Autoimmune diseases of the salivary gland like **Sjögren's syndrome and Mikulicz's syndrome** will cause symmetrical enlargement of the salivary glands.

Q 12. What is Mikulicz's syndrome?

It is a combination of bilateral salivary and lacrimal gland enlargement

- Symmetrical enlargement of salivary glands (one gland alone is involved initially for a quite long time)
- Enlargement of lacrimal glands (bulge below the outer end of the eyelids and narrowing of the palpebral fissure)
- Dry mouth.

Q 13. What are the causes for Mikulicz's syndrome?

- Sarcoidosis
- Leukemia
- Lymphoma
- Sjogren's syndrome.

Q 14. What is Sjögren's syndrome?

It is a rare autoimmune condition affecting the salivary glands and it can occur in combination with other autoimmune connective tissue disorders.

The manifestations and associated conditions seen in Sjögren's syndrome.

Manifestation	*Condition*
Deficient tear film	Keratoconjunctivitis sicca
Deficient salivation and gland enlargement	Xerostomia
Deficient tear and saliva	**Primary glandular sicca syndrome**
Deficient tear and saliva along with hyperglobulinemic **purpura, vasculitis, or Raynaud's** phenomenon or **B cell lymphoma**	Primary extra-glandular sicca syndrome
Any of the above occur-ring together with **rheumatoid arthritis, systemic lupus erythematosus** or other recognizable **connective tissue disorders**	Secondary Sjögren's syndrome

Q 15. What is the importance of oral cavity examination in parotid swelling?

- To look for the orifice of the Stensen's ducts which is situated opposite the crown of the **second upper molar tooth**—Look for **blood and pus**.
- To palpate the mouth of the duct for any **lumps and induration**.
- Gentle pressure on the gland externally may bring out purulent discharge.
- **The tonsil may be pushed medially** when the deep lobe of the parotid gland is enlarged.
- **Bimanual palpation of the parotid gland**—One finger externally behind the ramus of the mandible and one finger inside the mouth just in front of the tonsil and behind 3rd molar tooth internally.

Q 16. What is the anatomical position of the parotid duct?

It is deep to the anterior border of the gland and runs **superficial to the masseter muscle**. It then curves inwards by piercing the buccinator to open on the mucous membrane of the mouth opposite the crown of the upper second molar tooth.

Q 17. How would you palpate the Stensen's duct?

It is best done by a **bidigital palpation** by index finger inside the mouth and thumb over the cheek.

Q 18. What is the surface marking for Stensen's duct?

It lies about **one fingerbreadth below the inferior border of the zygomatic bone.**

Q 19. What is the most important differential diagnosis for a small parotid swelling?

Preauricular lymph nodes (enlargement secondary to infection or metastasis).

Q 20. What are the primary foci for enlarged preauricular lymph nodes?

Primary sites for preauricular node metastasis:

Drainage area for pre auricular node
• Forehead
• Scalp
• Eyelids
• Cheek
• External auditory meatus.

Q 21. What is the distinguishing clinical feature of the lymph node?

It is the mobility of the lymph node—The preauricular lymph node is outside the capsule of the gland and usually very mobile, unlike the tumor in the parotid which has got restricted mobility.

Q 22. What is parotid sandwich?

The facial nerve is passing through the substance of the parotid gland, dividing the gland into a **superficial lobe and deep lobe.** Therefore the gland is called **parotid sandwich.**

Q 23. What is faciovenous plane of Patey?

The facial nerve is seen, **superficial to the posterior facial vein** in the substance of the gland. This plane is called faciovenous plane of Patey.

Q 24. What is Pes anserinus?

Pes anserinus means **goose foot.**

In the parotid gland the facial nerve divides into—

1. The temporofacial (runs sharply upwards)—**two divisions** (temporal, zygomatic)
2. The cervicofacial—continues the course of the parent trunk downwards, forwards and outwards—**three divisions** (buccal, mandibular and cervical).

These divisions in turn divide to form the goose's foot (Pes anserinus).

Q 25. What is sociaparotidis?

It is nothing but **accessory lobe** of the parotid seen just above the Stensen's duct.

Q 26. Which type of facial palsy is seen in parotid tumors?

Lower motor neuron type of facial palsy is seen (involvement of both lower and upper half of the face).

Q 27. What are the tests for facial palsy?

The tests for facial palsy are:

Test	*Manifestations*
1. Ask the patient to show his teeth	Angle of the mouth drawn to the healthy side
2. Ask the patient to puff out the cheeks	The paralyzed side bellows out more than the normal side
3. Ask the patient to shut his eyes	Will not be able to close the eyes on the affected side and on attempting to do so to the eyeball will be seen to roll upwards
4. Ask the patient to move his eyebrows upwards	The paralyzed side remains immobile

Note: The nasolabial fold and furrows of the eyebrow are less marked on the affected side. The angle of the mouth is drawn to the sound side.

Q 28. Will all the malignant tumors produce facial palsy?

No.

Q 29. What are the clinical features of malignancy in the parotid?

Clinical features of malignancy

a. Pain
b. Rapid increase in size
c. Very hard consistency
d. Facial palsy
e. Enlarged metastatic regional node
f. Skin involvement (skin tethering)
g. Fixity
h. Trismus—involvement of pterygoid muscle by deep parotid lobe malignancy

Q 30. What is the commonest parotid swelling?

Pleomorphic adenoma (mixed parotid tumor).

Q 31. What percentage of tumors are benign in parotid?

Site	*% of benign*	*% of malignant*
Parotid	80%	20%
Submandibular	50%	50%
Minor salivary gland	10%	90%
Sublingual	5%	95%

Q 32. What are the other benign tumors of the parotid gland?

- **Warthin's tumors** (papillary cyst adenoma lymphomatosum)
- **Oxyphylic adenoma** (Oncocytoma).

Q 33. What are the features of Warthin's tumor?

Clinical features of Warthin's tumor

- 2nd most common benign tumor
- It is soft and sometimes fluctuant (cystic)
- Seen usually in males
- Seen after 40 years
- May be bilateral (10% bilateral)
- This tumor has no malignant potential.

Q 34. What is the origin of Warthin's tumor?

The tumor probably arises from **parotid tissue included in the lymph nodes** which are usually present within the parotid sheath. Microscopically it is lined by columnar epithelial cells supported by **lymphoid stroma**.

Q 35. Is there any method of confirming Warthin's other than FNAC? (PG)

Yes. Tc ^{99}m scintigraphy will reveal a **hot spot.** This is due to the high mitochondrial content within the cell.

Q 36. What is oncocytoma? (PG)

They arise from oncocytes which are derived from intralobular ducts or acini. They are usually seen in minor salivary glands, nasopharynx and larynx in the elderly males.

Q 37. What is the investigation of choice in parotid tumors?

Fine needle aspiration cytology (FNAC).

Q 38. Why biopsy is contraindicated in parotid tumors?

Biopsy is contraindicated because of the following reasons:

1. Seedling of the tumor will occur
2. Chance for parotid fistula is there
3. Chance for facial nerve injury.

Q 39 What are the other investigations?

1. **CT/MRI** is taken to rule out deep lobe involvement
2. **Chest X-ray to rule out metastasis.**

Indications for CT

1. If deep lobe tumor is suspected
2. If extension to deep lobe is suspected
3. Trismus.

Indication for MRI

When facial nerve is involved.

Q 40. What is the WHO classification of parotid neoplasms?

1. Adenomas – Pleomorphic
   Monomorphic – Warthin's tumor
2. Carcinoma:

   Low grade
   - Acinic cell carcinoma
   - Adenoid cystic carcinoma
   - Low grade mucoepidermoid carcinoma.

   High grade
   - Adenocarcinoma
   - Squamous cell carcinoma
   - High grade mucoepidermoid carcinoma.
3. Nonepithelial tumors:
   - Hemangioma
   - Lymphangioma
   - Neurofibroma.
4. Lymphomas:
   - Primary—NHL
   - Lymphoma in Sjögren's syndrome.
5. Secondary:
   - Local—tumors of head and neck
   - Distant—skin and bronchus.

6. Unclassified tumors
7. Tumor-like lesions:
   - Adenomatoid hyperplasia
   - Salivary gland cysts.

Q 41. Why pleomorphic adenoma is called mixed parotid tumor?

It is called mixed parotid tumor because it has got both epithelial and mesodermal elements.

Q 42. Can pleomorphic adenoma occur bilaterally?

Yes.

Q 43. What are the peculiarities of pleomorphic adenoma?

- It is considered a benign tumor with long quiescent periods and short periods of rapid growth
- Potential for recurrence
- Potential for malignant change.

Features of pleomorphic adenoma

1. The **capsule is incomplete** and the tumor will have extensions beyond the capsule
2. **Recurrence** can occur if tumor excision is not complete
3. 10% of the tumors are **highly cellular** and more liable to recur
4. Tumor contains both **epithelial and mesodermal elements** (myoepithelial cells surrounding the tubules)
5. After surgery for recurrence, **radiotherapy** is indicated even though it is benign
6. Benign pleomorphic adenomas **metastasize inexplicably**—metastatic pleomorphic adenoma—it is not malignant
7. It is a tumor readily implanted during removal in the residual parotid.

Q 44. What are the malignant parotid tumors in order of frequency?

- Mucoepidermoid carcinoma (most common)
- Malignant mixed tumor
- Acinic cell carcinoma
- Adenocarcinoma, polymorphous type of adenocarcinoma (Indian file appearance)
- Adenoid cystic carcinoma—10% (2/3rd in minor salivary gland)
- Epidermoid carcinoma (squamous cell carcinoma).

Q 45. Which is the carcinoma parotid with worst prognosis? (PG)

- Carcinoma arising in pleomorphic adenoma
- There is accelerated recurrence rate and high incidence of metastasis
- Five year survival is less than 40%.

Q 46. What is the type of malignancy in pleomorphic adenoma? (PG)

1. Carcinoma originating from pleomorphic adenoma **(carcinoma ex-pleomorphic adenoma) 15 years** after the original swelling–9.5% chance for carcinoma.

Q 47. What are the peculiarities of adenoid cystic carcinoma?

- Propensity for perineural invasion
- Regional lymph node involvement uncommon
- Distant metastasis occur within 5 years (however they remain asymptomatic for years)
- The malignancy will start as pain in the parotid region.

Q 48. What is the difference between low grade and high grade mucoepidermoid carcinoma?

High grade lesions have propensity for both regional and distant metastasis.

Q 49. What is the staging of parotid tumors? (PG)
TNM staging as per AJCC 7th edition is recommended.

TX	–	Primary tumor cannot be assessed
T0	–	No evidence of primary tumor
T1	–	Tumor 2 cm or less in greatest dimension without extraparenchymal extension
T2	–	Tumor more than 2 cm but not more than 4 cm in greatest dimension without extraparenchymal extension
T3	–	Tumor more than 4 cm and/or tumor having extraparenchymal extension
T4a	–	**Moderately advanced disease**—Tumor invades skin, mandible, ear canal, and/or facial nerve
T4b	–	**Very advanced disease**—Tumor invades skull base and/or pterygoid plates and/or encases carotid artery

Note: N stage is same for all head and neck malignancies.

Staging

Stage 1	–	T1	N0	M0
Stage 2	–	T2	N0	M0
Stage 3	–	T3	N0	M0
		T1	N1	M0
		T2	N1	M0
		T3	N1	M0
Stage 4A	–	T4a	N0	M0
		T4a	N1	M0
		T1	N2	M0
		T2	N2	M0
		T3	N2	M0
		T4a	N2	M0
Stage 4B	-	T4b	any N	M0
		Any T	N3	M0
Stage 4C	-	Any T	Any N	M1

Q 50. What is the difference between staging for major salivary gland tumors and minor salivary gland tumors? (PG)
The minor salivary gland tumors are located in the lining of upper aerodigestive tract and they are staged according to the anatomic site of origin (e.g. oral cavity, sinuses, etc.).

Q 51. What are the major salivary glands?
They include **parotid, submandibular and sublingual glands.**

Q 52. What is the regional node spread in parotid tumor?
Intraglandular node → Periparotid node → Submandibular node → Upper and mid-jugular nodes (occasionally to retropharyngeal nodes).

Q 53. What are the causes for bilateral parotid tumors?

1. Warthin's tumor
2. Acinic cell carcinoma—2% bilateral.

Q 54. What is the CT sign of inoperability in parotid carcinoma? (PG)
Involvement of the masseteric space (pre masticator space) is suggestive of inoperability. It is divided by zygoma into supratemporal (contains temporalis muscle) and infra temporal space (contains lateral and medial pterygoid muscles).

Q 55. What is the CT sign of skull base involvement in parotid tumor? (PG)
Widening of foramen ovale is suggestive of lower cranial nerve involvement. Involvement of the pterygoid plate is another sign.

Q 56. What is the test for temporomandibular joint involvement? (PG)

a. The little finger is introduced to the external auditory meatus with the pulp of finger forwards and simultaneously assess the difference in range of movement.

b. Inter incisor distance measurement.

Q 57. What is the treatment of pleomorphic adenoma?

- Superficial parotidectomy is the minimum surgical procedure
- There is no role for enucleation and excision (because of the reasons mentioned above)
- Facial nerve should be spared if a plane exists and when it is not involved
- Facial nerve is scarified only if it is involved or it is totally encased as in cases of carcinomas.

Q 58. If the facial nerve is involved what is the treatment option?

The nerve is excised and a nerve graft is done with **Great auricular nerve.**

Q 59. What is the management of facial nerve injury? (PG)

1. Nerve transection is managed by nerve suturing
2. Loss of a segment is managed by cable graft using great auricular or sural nerve
3. If the proximal end of the nerve is not available for suturing, hypoglossal nerve transposition or redirection is done.

Q 60. If facial palsy is identified postoperatively. What is the management?

1. Give steroids (prednisolone) and wait for improvement.
2. If there is no improvement re-exploration and repair is an option.
3. Masseter transfer can be done for the deviation of the angle of mouth.
4. Temporalis transfer can be done for the orbicularis oculi function.

Q 61. Is nerve grafting a contraindication for radiotherapy?

No.

Q 62. What is the timing of radiotherapy? (PG)

3–6 weeks after surgery.

Q 63. What are the indications for radiotherapy? (PG)

Indications for radiotherapy (50–70 Gy given in 1.8–2.0 Gy in 5–8 weeks time)
1. T3 and T4 tumors
2. High grade tumors
3. Deep lobe involvement
4. Perineural spread
5. Vascular invasion
6. Multiple lymph node involvement
7. Close margins

Q 64. Is there any indication for chemotherapy? (PG)

No.

Q 65. What is the surgical treatment of nodes?

Comprehensive neck dissection in the form of **Radical neck dissection** is done.

Q 66. What are the important anatomical points to be remembered in parotid surgery?

1. The gland is situated in the space behind the ramus of the mandible, below the base of the skull and in front of mastoid process.
2. Deeply it is applied to the styloid process and its muscles.
3. The upper pole lies just below the zygomatic arch and wedged between the meatus and mandibular joint.
4. *Upper pole*—The superficial temporal vessels, the temporal branches of the facial nerve and

the auriculotemporal nerve are found entering or leaving the gland near the upper pole.

5. *Lower pole*—The cervical branch of the facial nerve and the two divisions of the posterior facial vein emerge from its lower pole.
6. *Anterior border*—Overlies the masseter. The parotid ducts, the zygomatic, buccal and mandibular branches of facial nerve emerge from the anterior border.
7. **The external carotid artery,** the **facial nerve** and the **retromandibular vein pass through the substance of the gland** (the external carotid artery terminates behind the neck of the mandible by dividing into maxillary and superficial temporal arteries). **Intraparotid lymph nodes** are also seen in the substance of gland.
8. The facial nerve is seen in the **faciovenous plane of Patey** (the nerve is seen superficial to the posterior facial vein which is formed within the substance of gland by the continuation of the superficial temporal vein and emerges usually into two branches at the lower pole of the gland).
9. The nerve is dividing the gland into a **superficial lobe and deep lobe.** 80% of the gland lies superficial to the nerve and 20% deep to the nerve.
10. An **accessory lobe** is present in less than 50% of the population.

Q 67. What is the incision used for superficial parotidectomy?

A lazy '*S*' incision is used—**Preauricular—Mastoid - Cervical incision.**

Q 68. What are the essential steps of superficial parotidectomy?

1. Surgery is done under general anaesthesia with endotracheal intubation.
2. Lazy 's' incision is used as mentioned above.
3. Infiltration with local anesthetic and adrenalin for better delineation of the plane.
4. Reflect the skin flaps anteriorly just superficial to the parotid fascia upto the anterior border of the gland.
5. Back of the parotid gland is identified, and dissection is carried out to expose the facial nerve.
6. The sternomastoid is retracted and great auricular nerve divided in the avascular plane along the anterior border of the muscle.
7. Identify the posterior belly of digastric.
8. Identify the avascular plane along the anterior border of cartilaginous and bony external auditory meatus immediately anterior to the tragus.
9. *Landmarks for identification of facial nerve*—(always identify the trunk of the nerve first rather than tracing the branches from the periphery).
   a. *Conley's pointer*—The inferior portion of the cartilaginous canal. The facial nerve lies 1cm deep and inferior to its tip.
   b. The upper border of the **posterior belly of digastric muscle**—The facial nerve is usually located immediately superior to it.
   c. The **stylomastoid artery** lies immediately lateral to the nerve.
10. Identify the two main divisions.
11. Dissect the gland off branches of the facial nerve.
12. With the exception of buccal branch, all transected nerves are repaired with cable graft from **great auricular nerve.**
13. The desired amount of gland is removed.
14. A suction drain is applied and wound is closed.

Q 69. What is radical parotidectomy?

Radical parotidectomy involves removal of **all parotid gland** tissue and elective **sectioning of the facial nerve** usually through the main trunk. The surgery removes ipsilateral masseter muscle in addition. If there is clinical, radiological, and cytological evidence of lymph node metastasis a simultaneous radical neck dissection is carried out. It is done for:

- High grade malignant tumors
- Squamous cell carcinoma.

Q 70. What are the complications of parotid surgery?

Complications are
Complications of parotidectomy 1. Seroma 2. Wound infection 3. Permanent facial palsy (transection of the nerve) 4. Temporary facial nerve weakness 5. Facial numbness 6. Permanent numbness of the ear lobe (due to great auricular nerve transection) 7. Sialocele 8. Frey's syndrome (Gustatory sweating) 9. Parotid fistula.

Q 71. What is Frey's syndrome?

This is due to inappropriate regeneration of the damaged parasympathetic autonomic nerve fibers to the overlying skin. Salivation resulting from smell or taste of food, will stimulate the sweat glands of the over lying skin instead of the parotid. The clinical features are:

1. Sweating over the region of parotid gland
2. Erythema over the region of parotid gland.

Q 72. What is the clinical test to demonstrate Frey's syndrome? (PG)

Starch iodine test—Paint the affected area with iodine and allow it to dry. Apply dry starch over it. The starch turns blue on exposure to iodine in the presence of sweat. The sweating is stimulated after painting starch.

Q 73. What is the management of Frey's syndrome? (PG)

Prevention

It can be prevented by placing a barrier between the skin and parotid bed to prevent inappropriate regeneration of autonomic nerve fibers. The following methods are useful—

1. Temporalis fascial flap
2. Sternomastoid muscle flap
3. Artificial membrane between the skin and parotid bed.

Management of established syndrome:

1. Tympanic neurectomy
2. Injection of botulinum toxin into the affected skin. (simple and effective method)
3. Antiperspirants—Aluminium chloride.

Case 28 Submandibular Sialadenitis

Case Capsule

A 35-year-old female patient presents with **right submandibular swelling** of **4 × 2.5 cm size**, firm in consistency and has pain and **increase in size** of the swelling **during salivation** (eating) for 6 months. The swelling is **bidigitally palpable**.

Read the diagnostic algorithm for a swelling.

Checklist for history

1. History of systemic diseases responsible for sialadenosis like—DM, drugs (antiasthmatic, guanethidine), endocrine disorders, alcoholism, pregnancy, bulimia (eating disorders)
2. History of salivary colic
3. Increase in size during salivation
4. History of collagen diseases
5. History of similar swelling on the contralateral side.

Checklist for examination

1. Bidigital palpation with a gloved finger inside the oral cavity
2. Palpation of the Wharton's duct for stones in the floor of the mouth
3. Examine the opening of the duct (sublingual papillae on the side of the frenulum) for inflammation and for purulent discharge

Contd...

Contd...

4. Look for regional lymph nodes
5. Look for induration/ulceration of the overlying skin—suggestive of malignancy
6. Look for other salivary glands on both sides.

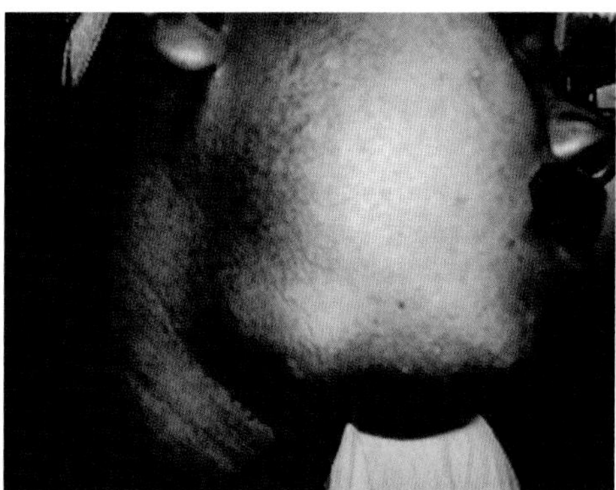

Submandibular sialadenitis

Q 1. What is your diagnosis? What is the differential diagnosis?

- Chronic submandibular sialadenitis (It is bi-digitally palpable)
- DD—Submandibular lymph nodes.

Q 2. How to differentiate them?
- If the swelling is bidigitally palpable, it is submandibular salivary gland
- Lymph nodes are not bidigitally palpable.

Q 3. Why salivary gland is palpable bidigitally?
The submandibular salivary gland has a portion above the myelohyoid muscle (deep lobe) in the floor of mouth. Therefore, the gland is bidigitally palpable.

Q 4. What are your points in favor of submandibular salivary gland?
1. Salivary colic—pain induced by salivation as a result of obstruction to the outflow from the gland (may be a stone in the duct).
2. Increase in size during salivation (above reason)
3. Decrease in size of the swelling or disappearance **1 to 2 hours after the meal** is completed
4. Positive bidigital palpation
5. Solid nature of the swelling.

Q 5. If the swelling is cystic, what are the possibilities?
If it is cystic, one has to rule out a **sublingual dermoid**.

Q 6. What is the importance of palpating the Wharton's duct and its opening (sublingual papillae)?
- Palpation in the **gingivolingual sulcus** will reveal stones in the Wharton's duct.
- Inspection of the **sublingual papillae** reveals inflammation and discharge (purulent).

Q 7. Why stones are more common in the submandibular salivary gland compared to the parotid?
- The gland and duct system has a shape similar to the **retort.**
- The duct is above and the gland is below. The gland has **antigravity drainage.**
- The secretion is thicker in the submandibular salivary gland.

Q 8. What are the types of inflammation in the submandibular gland?
The inflammation of the gland is called sialadenitis. The types of sialadenitis are:
- Acute
- Chronic
- Acute on chronic.

Q 9. What are the causes for acute sub- mandibular sialadenitis?
- Viral—mumps
- Bacterial—secondary to obstruction.

Q 10. What are the causes for chronic sialadenitis?
- Obstruction by stone formation, which may be within the gland **(sialolithiasis)**, within the duct system
- Trauma to the floor of mouth by denture—subsequent inflammation and stricture of the duct.

Q 11. How many percentage of the submandibular are radio opaque?
- 80% are radio opaque
- It can be identified in plain radiograph.

Q 12. Which is the commonest site of the submandibular stone—gland or duct?
About 80% of the stones are situated in the sub mandibular gland.

Q 13. Which type of sialadenitis is more common—bacterial or viral?
Bacterial.

Q 14. How will you manage this case?
- Investigations for diagnosis
- Investigations for surgery.

Investigations for diagnosis
1. *Plain X-ray:* Occlusive view using dental film. This will demonstrate radioopaque calculus in the duct and salivary gland.

2. *USG:* Ultrasound is a very useful tool for the demonstration of stones.
3. *FNAC:* To rule out a tumor of the salivary gland and to rule out lymph node.

Investigations for surgery

1. X-ray chest
2. ECG
3. Hemogram
4. Blood sugar
5. Renal status.

Q 15. If no stone is demonstrated and it is found to be sialadenitis, what is the management?

Bacterial sialadenitis has a poor capacity for recovery following infection and the gland becomes chronically inflamed. Therefore, the gland has to be removed—**Sialadenectomy**.

Q 16. If stone is demonstrated radiologically, what is it called?

Sialolithiasis.

Q 17. If the stone is clinically and radiologically demonstrated in the Wharton's duct, what is the management?

If the stone is lying **anterior** to a point at which the **duct crosses the lingual nerve** (second molar region), the stone can be removed by **incising longitudinally** over the duct. This is done under the **local anesthesia**.

Q 18. Will you close the duct after removal of the stone?

- No
- The duct should be left open for free drainage of saliva
- Suturing will lead to stricture formation and recurrence of obstructive symptoms.

Q19. When the stone is proximal to the crossing of lingual nerve, what is the management? (PG)

- Intraoral approach is avoided because it leads to injury to the lingual nerve
- **The gland is removed** by external approach—**Sialadenectomy** along with removal of the stone from the duct and ligation of the duct.

Q 20. What are the indications for excision of submandibular salivary gland? (PG)

1. Sialadenitis
2. Stones in the gland
3. Stones in the duct proximal to the lingual nerve
4. Salivary tumors.

Q 21. What is the difference between sialadenectomy for inflammatory condition and tumor of the submandibular salivary gland? (PG)

- **Intracapsular dissection** is done for inflammatory condition
- Extracapsular dissection with a cuff of normal tissue around is done for tumor. This may be combined with **suprahyoid neck dissection**.

Q 22. What is the incision for sialadenectomy and what precautions are taken?

It is important to avoid injury to the **marginal mandibular branch** of the facial nerve and therefore the incision is placed **3 to 4 cm below the lower border of the mandible.** A 6 cm long incision is cited within the skin crease.

Q 23. In which plane you get marginal mandibular branch of the facial nerve? (PG)

Subplatysmal plane. The skin flaps are raised at subplatysmal level.

Q 24. Is it necessary to close the platysma at this situation? (PG)

- Yes. It is sutured with continuous absorbable suture.

- Platysma muscle has direct contribution to the depressor activity of the corner of the mouth.

Q 25. What are the important anatomical relationships of the submandibular gland?

- **Three cranial nerves are at risk:**

1. Marginal mandibular branch of the facial nerve
2. The lingual nerve
3. The hypoglossal nerve.

- **Two vessels need ligation**
  1. Anterior facial vein running over the surface of the gland
  2. Facial artery.
- **Two Muscles are related to the gland**
  1. **Mylohyoid muscle**—around its posterior border **the large superficial lobe** becomes the small deeper lobe
  2. The deep part of the gland lies on the **hyoglossus muscle** closely related to the **lingual nerve and hypoglossal nerve.**

Q 26. What is the anesthesia of choice for sialadenectomy?

General anesthesia—with endotracheal intubation.

Q 27. What are the peculiarities of the facial artery in this situation? (PG)

- The course of the artery is variable here
- The artery lies in the groove on the deeper aspect of the gland
- Sometimes the artery will penetrate the substance of the gland
- Passes around the gland sometimes
- The artery has to be ligated doubly, superiorly and inferiorly.

Q 28. What is the landmark for identification of the deep lobe?

- Posterior border of the myelohyoid
- Once the muscle is retracted forwards the deep lobe can be identified.

Q 29. Is there any attachment of the gland to the lingual nerve? (PG)

The gland is attached to the lingual nerve **through parasympathetic secretomotor fibers.** These parasympathetic nerve fibers are divided, protecting the lingual nerve.

Q 30. How do you tackle the submandibular duct? (PG)

It is identified and ligated as anteriorly as possible.

Q 31. Is there a need for a wound drain after surgery?

It is better to put a continuous suction drain for 24 hours. There are numerous veins encountered on the deeper aspect of gland, which are coagulated or ligated.

Q 32. What are the complications of sialadenectomy?

Complications of submandibular sialadenectomy

1. Injury to the marginal mandibular nerve
2. Hematoma
3. Wound infection
4. Injury to the nerve to mylohyoid producing submental anesthesia
5. Lingual nerve injury
6. Hypoglossal nerve injury.

Q 33. What are the clinical features of malignancy in the gland?

Signs of malignancy in submandibular salivary gland

- Rapid increase in size
- Induration
- Ulceration of the overlying skin
- Cervical node enlargement.

Q 34. What is the incidence of malignancy in submandibular salivary gland?

About 50% are malignant in contrast to the parotid where only 20% are malignant. **The chances of malignancy increase from parotid to submandibular to sublingual and minor salivary glands.**

Q 35. What are the investigations for diagnosis in suspected tumors of the submandibular salivary gland?

- FNAC—It is the investigation of choice.
- CT/MRI—If required to know the nature of surrounding invasion.

Q 36. Is there any contraindication for open biopsy?

Open biopsy is **contraindicated** because of the tumor seedling.

Q 37. What is "Stafne Bone Cyst"? (PG)

It is an **ectopic lobe** of the submandibular salivary gland presenting as **asymptomatic radiolucency** of the angle of the mandible, below the inferior dental neurovascular bundle. **Edward C Stafne** a dental surgeon from Mayo clinic described this condition. No treatment is required for this condition.

Case 29 Ranula, Plunging Ranula, Sublingual Dermoid and Mucous Cyst

Case Capsule

A 20-year-old male patient presents with a **bluish tinged spherical cystic swelling** 5 × 3 cm size in the **floor of the mouth** on one side of frenulum lingulae (sublingually). It is **translucent**. Externally there is no visible swelling.

Read the diagnostic algorithm for a neck swelling.

Checklist for history

1. History of trauma
2. History of long duration.

Checklist for examination

1. Look for color—blue or opaque white
2. Decide whether it is solid or cystic
3. Decide whether the swelling is purely intraoral or it is extending down to the neck
4. Look for swelling beneath the chin
5. **Bimanual palpation,** if there is swelling beneath the chin decide whether the intraoral part is continuous with the swelling beneath the chin
6. Decide whether it is **midline or lateral**
7. Look for the **submandibular duct traversing** the dome of the cyst in the floor of the mouth
8. Look for **translucency.**

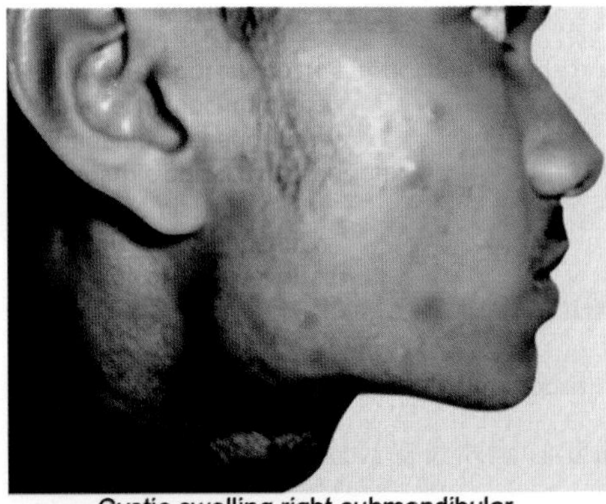

Cystic swelling right submandibular region- dermoid

Q 1. What is your diagnosis?

Ranula.

Q 2. What are the diagnostic points in favor of ranula?

1. Tense cystic swelling in the floor of the mouth
2. It is blue in color
3. It is translucent
4. It is situated to one side of frenumlingulae
5. The submandibular duct can be seen traversing the dome of the cyst.

Q 3. What is the most important differential diagnosis?

Sublingual dermoid cyst.

Q 4. What are the clinical points against sublingual dermoid in this case?

- Translucency is a point against sublingual dermoid
- Sublingual dermoid may be placed in the mid-line unlike ranula which is to one side of the frenum
- Sublingual dermoid is not blue in color. It is white and opaque.

Q 5. What is ranula?

It is a **mucous extravasation cyst** arising from the sublingual salivary gland.

Q 6. Why it is called ranula?

It is called ranula because of its resemblance to frog's belly.

Q 7. Who gave this name?

Hippocrates.

Q 8. What is plunging ranula?

Here the cyst penetrates the mylohyoid diaphragm to enter the neck. Therefore, there will be a swelling in the floor of the mouth along with a swelling in the neck, resembling a dumbbell. This **retention cyst** may be arising from **sublingual or submandibular salivary gland**. The neck swelling may be in the submental or submandibular region of the neck.

Q 9. What is the clinical test for plunging ranula?

Here one should elicit the **Bidigital palpation** – with index finger of one hand in the mouth and fingers of the other hand exerting upward pressure externally from the below the lower jaw over the neck swelling. In case of plunging ranula it will be positive.

Q 10. How to confirm the diagnosis of ranula?

1. Ultrasound examination
2. MRI (for plunging ranula)
3. Plain X-ray to rule out stones.

Q 11. What are the complications of ranula?

1. Infection
2. Mechanical interference with speech
3. Difficulty in eating.

Q 12. What is the surgical treatment of ranula?

Excision of the cyst and the affected sublingual gland.

Q 13. What is the approach for surgery?

Intraoral approach is preferred.

Q 14. Why not incision and drainage of the cyst?

It is not recommended, because it will result in recurrence of the cyst.

Q 15. What is the surgical approach for plunging ranula?

Excision is performed via cervical approach.

Q 16. What is the incision for cervical approach?

- The incision is similar to submandibular sialadenectomy
- The cyst together with submandibular and sublingual salivary glands are excised.

Q 17. What is mucous cyst?

It is an **extravasation/retention cyst** in relation to minor salivary gland.

Q 18. What is the commonest site for mucous cyst?

Lower lip.

Q 19. What is the cause for mucous cyst?

It is as a result of trauma to the overlying mucosa.

Q 20. What is the transillumination finding in mucous cyst?

It may or may not be translucent.

Q 21. What is the surgical treatment?

- Formal surgical excision is required along with the affected minor salivary gland under local anaesthesia.
- Some may resolve spontaneously.

Q 22. How many minor salivary glands are there in the oral cavity?

Around **450** (They contribute 10% of the salivary volume).

Q 23. What is the distribution of minor salivary gland?

Sites of minor salivary glands
• Cheek • Palate • Floor of the mouth • Lips • Retromolar area • Upper aerodigestive tract: – Oropharynx – Larynx – Trachea – Sinuses.

Q 24. Is it possible to get a tumor in the sublingual salivary gland?

Yes. They are extremely rare. They present as firm or hard painless swelling in the floor of mouth. **95% are malignant.**

Q 25. What is the surgical management of this malignancy?

Wide excision along with overlying mucosa combined with suprahyoid neck dissection.

Q 26. What are the types of sublingual dermoid?

There are two types:

1. Median—in the midline
2. Lateral:
   - It may be situated above the mylohyoid—**supramylohyoid variety** (floor of the mouth)
   - It may be below the mylohyoid—**infra-mylohyoid variety** (swelling beneath the chin)—double chin appearance.

Q 27. What are the diagnostic points in favor of sublingual dermoid?

Diagnostic points for sublingual dermoid

1. Color-opaque white cyst in contrast to ranula
2. Content—sebaceous material
3. May present as swelling in the floor of the mouth or swelling beneath the chin
4. No attachment to the covering mucosa or skin
5. Do not transilluminate.

Q 28. What are the two most important examinations in suspected sublingual dermoid cyst?

1. Examination of the neck to rule out an extension beneath the chin or laterally in the submandibular region in the case of the lateral variety
2. Bimanual palpation—positive bimanual palpation suggests extension beneath the mylohyoid.

Q 29. What are the other differential diagnoses of a swelling beneath the chin?

- Thyroglossal cyst
- Subhyoid bursa.

Q 30. What is the incision for excision of a median sublingual dermoid?

1. If there is extension beneath the chin, consider **external incision** in the submental region. **Division of mylohyoid** may be required. The cyst is then **enucleated**.
2. If there is no extension beneath the chin, **intraoral approach** will suffice for the enucleation.

Q 31. How a sublingual dermoid cyst is formed?

During the process of **fusion of the facial processes**, a piece of the **skin may get trapped** deep in the midline just behind the jaw and later form the dermoid cyst. The cyst may be **midline or lateral.**

Q 32. What is the age group affected?

It is 10–25 years (Both sexes equally affected).

Q 33. What are the complications of sublingual dermoid?

1. Infection (painful)
2. Interfere with eating (when it is big)
3. Interfere with speech.

Case 30 Thyroglossal Cyst, Lingual Thyroid, Ectopic Thyroid Subhyoid Bursa and Carcinoma Arising in Thyroglossal Cyst

Case Capsule

A **15-year-old girl** presenting with a **spherical cystic swelling** in front of the neck beneath the hyoid bone of **1.5 cm diameter**. There is **movement with protrusion of the tongue**. The swelling is moving up and down with deglutition.

Read the diagnostic algorithm for a swelling.

Checklist for history

- Family history of goiter
- History of radiation to the neck
- History of dysphagia
- History of dysphonia
- History of dyspnea
- History of pain over the swelling
- History of rapid increase in size of the swelling
- History of discharge from the swelling
- History of operations for the swelling.

Checklist for examination

1. Elicit **fluctuation by Paget's method** : it may appear as firm or tense cystic. Some cysts are too small to fluctuate
2. Look for **transillumination**
3. Look for **movement with protrusion of the tongue** and movement with deglutition

Contd...

Contd...

4. Always **examine the oral cavity** : Base of the tongue for ectopic thyroid/lingual thyroid
5. Always **palpate for the presence of normal thyroid** and cervical ectopic thyroid
6. Look for **regional lymph node** enlargement.

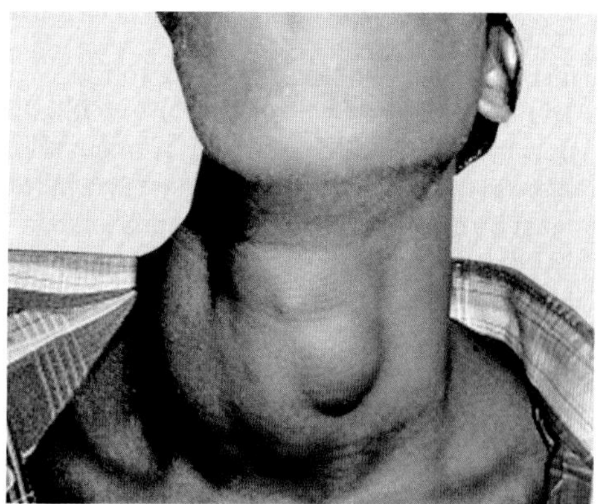

Thyroglossal cyst

Q 1. What is the most probable diagnosis in this case?

Thyroglossal cyst.

Q 2. What are the diagnostic points in favor of thyroglossal cyst?

1. The most important sign of thyroglossal cyst is the **upward movement of the swelling when the tongue is protruded**. This is because of its connection via the thyroglossal duct with the base of the tongue. It will also move up and down with deglutition. In addition, there will be **horizontal movement** but no vertical movement.
2. The presence of a small cystic swelling in the midline of the neck (seldom large enough to exhibit fluctuation).
3. May or may not be translucent (when the content is thick as a result of past infection, the cysts do not transilluminate).

Q 3. How will you demonstrate the upward movement during protrusion of the tongue?

a. Request the patient to open the mouth
b. Grasp the swelling between the finger and thumb
c. Instruct the patient to put out the tongue
d. The positive test will give an **unmistakable upward tug** (certain amount of movement will be there in this region for all swellings). **The mouth must be open** when the tug is appreciated.
e. The patient may be instructed to put the tongue in and out again if required.

Q 4. What are the differential diagnoses?

Differential diagnoses of thyroglossal cyst
1. Median sublingual dermoid
2. Enlarged submental lymph node
3. Subhyoid bursa
4. Enlarged Delphian node
5. Solitary thyroid nodule
6. Thyroid cyst
7. Dermoid cyst
8. Collar—stud abscess in connection with a **lymph** node
9. Ectopic thyroid
10. Sebaceous cyst
11. Lipoma

Q 5. What are the other midline swellings in front of the neck?

Midline swellings in front of the neck (in addition to the differential diagnoses given above).

- **Ludwig's angina** in the upper part
- **Retrosternal and plunging goitre** in the lower part
- Swellings from the **Space of Burns** in the lower part **(lymph node and lipoma)**
- Dermoid cyst in the lower part
- **Thymic swellings**
- **Aneurysm** of innominate artery.

Q 6. What are the causes for enlarged submental lymph node?

1. **Inflammatory**—**Specific** like tuberculosis
   —Nonspecific
2. **Neoplastic**—**Primary**—Hodgkin's and NHL
   —**Secondary** from carcinoma of **lower lip, tip of tongue, floor of mouth**.

Q 7. What is sublingual dermoid?

It is a sequestration dermoid cyst secondary to sequestration of surface ectoderm at the **site of fusion of mandibular arches**. The swelling is situated in the midline in the floor of the mouth. The lateral variety of sublingual dermoid arises from second branchial cleft. It is soft, cystic and lined by **squamous epithelium**. It contains **sebaceous material** and therefore **not translucent**.

Q 8. How will you differentiate solitary thyroid nodule from thyroglossal cyst?

The sign of upward tug during protrusion of the tongue is absent in the case of the thyroid nodule.

Q 9. What are the positions of the thyroglossal cyst?

1. **Suprahyoid:** Here the swelling is situated immediately above the hyoid bone and the differential diagnosis is median sublingual dermoid.
2. **Subhyoid:** It is the **commonest** site of thyroglossal cyst.
3. **At the level of the thyroid cartilage** (second commonest position): At this level the cyst is usually to one side of the midline (left side) because the thyroid cartilage is shaped like the prow of a ship and may be because of the levator glandulae thyroide muscle
4. **At the level of the cricoid cartilage:** The thyroglossal cyst at this level is less common and the differential diagnosis of thyroid nodule comes here.
5. **Beneath the foramen cecum**
6. **In the floor of the mouth.**

Q 10. What are the complications of thyroglossal cyst?

1. *Infection:* The overlying skin will be hot and red.
2. *Thyroglossal fistula* (**Result from bursting or incision for infection**): **The thyroglossal fistula is always acquired in contra-distinction to the Branchial fistula which is always congenital.**
3. *Rarely carcinoma:* Malignant potential of dysgenetic thyroid tissue causes papillary thyroid cancer in 1% of cases (Papillary carcinoma develops more frequently in ectopics than normal thyroid).

Q 11. Why there is more chance of infection in thyroglossal cyst?

The wall of the **cyst contains lymphatic tissue** and with attacks of respiratory infection, the cyst will get infected.

Q 12. Once an abscess is formed, what is the treatment?

Incision and drainage is the treatment. Formal excision of the tract is done (Sistrunk's operation) **after 6 weeks.**

Q 13. What is the classification of cyst in general?

Cysts are classified into congenital cyst and acquired cyst.

Congenital cysts—examples	Acquired cysts—examples
• Thyroglossal cyst	• Sebaceous cyst
• Branchial cyst	• Mucous cyst of mouth (retention)
• Urachal cyst	• Cystadenoma (neoplastic)
• Hydatid of Morgagni	• Teratoma (neoplastic)
• Dermoid cyst	• Hydatid (parasitic)
• Enterogenous cyst	• Implantation dermoid
• Cystic hygroma	• Traumatic cyst (Hematoma)
• Lymphatic cyst of greater omentum	

Q 14. What are the complications of cysts in general?

Complications of cysts anywhere

1. Hemorrhage—breathing difficulties in **thyroglossal cyst**
2. Infection—pain
3. Torsion—present as acute abdomen in **ovarian cyst**
4. Pressure effects on adjacent structures—abdominal fullness in abdomen
5. Obstruction to pelvic veins—manifest as varicose veins in the case of large **ovarian cyst**
6. Calcification.

Q 15. What is the typical appearance of a thyroglossal fistula?
The skin surrounding the opening has a peculiar **crescentic appearance** due to the uneven rate of growth of the thyroglossal tract (**semilunar sign**).

Q 16. What is the lining of thyroglossal fistula?
It is lined by columnar epithelium.

Q 17. What is the nature of discharge of thyroglossal fistula?
Mucus (because of the lining)—**in tuberculous sinus, the discharge will be purulent**.

Q 18. What is the differential diagnosis of thyroglossal fistula?
Tuberculous sinus—especially when the fistula is situated low in the neck (**the discharge will be purulent**).

Q 19. What is the commonest site for thyroglossal fistula?

1. Just below the hyoid bone
2. Thyroglossal fistulas originating in the infancy tend to be situated lower in the neck.

Q 20. What is the development of thyroid?
The thyroid gland is **endodermal** in origin and develops from the **median bud of the pharynx between 1st and 2nd pharyngeal pouch** and descends along the midline of the neck to lie anterior to the second, third and fourth tracheal rings. Each thyroid lobe amalgamates with the **ultimobranchial body (neuroectodermalin origin)** arising as a diverticulum of the fourth pharyngeal pouch on each side. The parafollicular cells (C cells) from the neural crest reach the thyroid via the ultimobranchial body. The line of descent of thyroid is called the thyroglossal tract. The thyroglossal tract extends from the **foramen cecum** (**vestigial remnant of the duct**) of the tongue to the isthmus of the thyroid gland. Usually the tract will completely atrophy by **5th week. If any portion of this tract remains patent**, it can form a cyst. Theoretically, thyroglossal cyst can occur anywhere between the bases of the tongue and the isthmus of the thyroid gland (**between the chin and second tracheal ring**). The tract descends through the 2nd branchial arch anlage, i.e. **hyoid bone** prior to fusion in the midline.

Q 21. What is the treatment for thyroglossal cyst?
Sistrunk's operation.

Q 22. What is Sistrunk's operation?
It consists of removal of the **thyroglossal cyst** along with the **entire thyroglossal tract up to the foramen cecum**. The central part of the body of the hyoid bone (**1cm**) is excised during the process of excision of the tract (In majority of the cases the tract will be going behind the body of the hyoid bone). It is important to **core out the entire tract** in the floor of the mouth up to the foramen cecum.

Q 23. If the thyroglossal cyst is low down, can you core out the entire tract through a single incision?
No. Initially a **skin line horizontal incision** is put over the cyst and the tract is dissected up to the hyoid bone. At this level, **another skin line incision** may be put so that the entire tract can be cored out up to the base of the tongue. The same technique is used for the surgical treatment of **thyroglossal fistula**.

Q 24. What are the clinical features of carcinoma arising in the thyroglossal cyst? (PG)

Features of malignancy in thyroglossal cyst

- Recent rapid increase in size of the cyst
- Hard consistency
- Fixity
- Irregularity
- Presence of enlarged lymph node.

Q 25. What is the treatment of carcinoma arising in the thyroglossal cyst? (PG)

- The usual surgery performed is **Sistrunk's operation** if the thyroid is found to be normal (**Routine thyroidectomy is not recommended** in all patients with carcinoma in thyroglossal cyst). **The indications for thyroidectomy** are:
  1. Nodular thyroid with cold nodule
  2. Presence of enlarged neck nodes
  3. History of irradiation to the neck.

  Following thyroidectomy radioiodine ablation is recommended:
- **Thyroid suppression is recommended for all patients with papillary carcinoma of the thyroglossal duct cyst regardless of the status of thyroid**
- Long-term follow-up is mandatory.

Q 26. What is ectopic thyroid?

Presence of residual thyroid tissue along the course of the thyroglossal tract is called ectopic thyroid. The ectopic thyroid may be:

1. Lingual
2. Cervical
3. The whole gland may be ectopic.

Q 27. What is the manifestation of lingual thyroid?

- It will present as a swelling at the back of the tongue in the region of foramen cecum.
- **Always palpate the neck and make sure that the normal thyroid is present** (If bare tracheal rings are palpated in the midline, one should suspect absence of thyroid in the normal position. It may also be due to absence of the isthmus of the thyroid).

The symptoms of lingual thyroid

- Dysphagia
- Dysphonia

Contd...

Contd...

- Dyspnea
- Hemorrhage
- Pain
- Carcinoma (develops more frequently in ectopic thyroid tissue than in normal thyroid gland).

Q 28. What are the differential diagnoses of lingual thyroid? (PG)

Differential diagnoses of lingual thyroid

1. Hypertrophied lingual tonsil
2. Carcinoma of the tongue
3. Fibroma
4. Angioma
5. Sarcoma
6. Ranula.

Q 29. What is athyreosis?

Athyreosis

- Absence of palpable lateral lobes
- Absence of isthmus
- Hypothyroidism.

Q 30. What is the investigation of the choice in lingual thyroid?

1. FNAC
2. Radioiodine scintiscan—to find out whether it is the only functioning thyroid and to find out the presence of normal thyroid.

Q 31. What is the treatment of choice in lingual thyroid?

The treatment options are:

1. **Thyroid suppression** with thyroid hormone—it should get smaller.

OR

2. Ablation with radioiodine.

OR

3. **Excision** if it is causing symptoms and replacement therapy with thyroid hormone (if it is the only functioning thyroid).

Q 32. What is median ectopic thyroid?

It forms a swelling in the upper part of the mid- line of the neck and it is one of the differential diagnoses of thyroglossal cyst. It may be the only functioning thyroid and therefore rule out presence of normal thyroid before excision.

Q 33. What is lateral aberrant thyroid?

This is a misnomer. Any normal tissue found laterally separate from the thyroid gland must be considered as lymph node metastasis from occult papillary thyroid cancer and treated as such.

Q 34. What is struma ovarii?

This is nothing but ovarian teratoma with thyroid tissue. Rarely, it can produce hyperthyroidism or neoplastic change.

Q 35. Can agenesis of thyroid occur?

Yes. Usually agenesis is seen on left side.

Q 36. How to make a diagnosis of subhyoid bursa?

1. Clinically
   - The swelling is located below the hyoid bone
   - In front of the thyrohyoid membrane
   - Transversely oval swelling
   - Moves up with deglutition
   - Soft and cystic
   - Not translucent (turbid fluid).
2. FNAC.

Q 37. What is the treatment of subhyoid bursa?

Excision.

Case 31 Branchial Cyst, Branchial Fistula, Cystic Hygroma

Case Capsule

A **25-year-old male** presenting with a **cystic swelling of about 5 × 3 cm size** at the **anterior border of the sternomastoid muscle** at the **junction of upper and middle third** on the right side of the neck. It is **cystic and fluctuant**. There is no transillumination.

Read the diagnostic algorithm for a swelling.

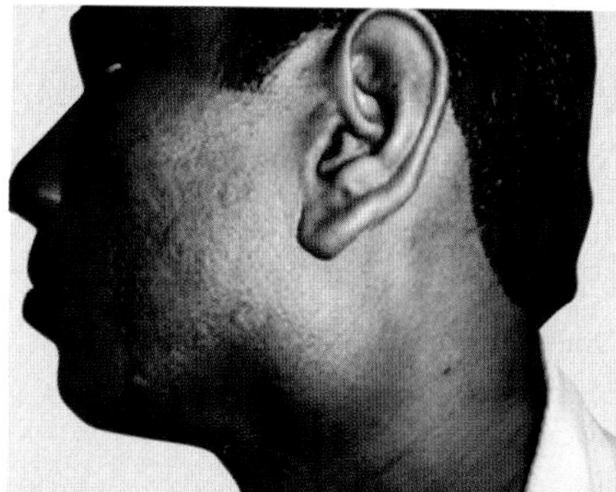

Branchial cyst on left side

Checklist for history

- Present from birth or not
- History of intermittent swelling
- History of attacks of inflammation
- The nature of discharge
- History of previous surgery.

Checklist for examination

1. Assess the plane of the swelling
2. Look for fixity to surrounding structures
3. Look for **fluctuation**
4. Look for **translucency**
5. Look for **compressibility**
6. Examine the **contralateral side** for similar swellings
7. Look for other arch problems like **accessory tragi and periauricular sinuses and cysts**
8. Look for lymph nodes
9. Look for the **nature of discharge from fistula**
10. Rule out **pharyngeal communication.**

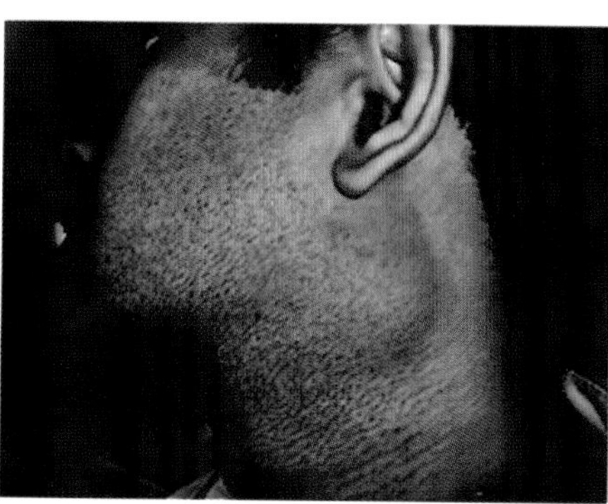

Left branchial cyst

Q 1. What is the probable diagnosis in this case?
Branchial cyst.

Q 2. What are the characteristic features of branchial cyst?

Clinical features of branchial cyst
1. It is situated at the junction of upper and middle third of the anterior border of the sternomastoid
2. 2/3rd of the swelling is anterior to the sternomastoid and 1/3rd deep to the sternomastoid
3. The cyst is a **loose cyst (It is not a tense cyst)**—the consistency is compared to that of a **half filled hot water bag**
4. May or may not be translucent.

Q 3. What are the theories of origin of branchial cyst?
There are two theories:
1. Arising from the cervical sinus of His (**Developmental origin**)
2. **Epithelial inclusion** within a lymph node.

Q 4. What is cervical sinus of His?
In the 3rd week of embryonic life, a series of **mesodermal condensations** known as branchial arches appear in the walls of the primitive pharynx. The second arch over grows and joins with the 5th arch producing the buried space lined by squamous epithelium. This space is called **cervical sinus of His**. Normally, it disappears entirely. **Should a part of the space persist**, it will form a **branchial cyst** (Fig. 31.1).

Q 5. How many branchial arches are there?
Six branchial arches with five pharyngeal pouches internally and five branchial clefts externally. The branchial pouches are lined by endoderm and the clefts are lined by ectoderm.

Q 6. What is the supporting evidence for the epithelial inclusion in the lymph node?
Most branchial cysts have **lymphoid tissue** in their walls.

Q 7. What is the most common age group affected?
Even though it is a congenital abnormality the most common age group is **3rd decade** (suggesting a different pathogenesis).

Q 8. How to explain the late appearance of the cyst if it is congenital?
Initially the cyst is an empty sac of embryological tissue. The **epithelial debris accumulates for**

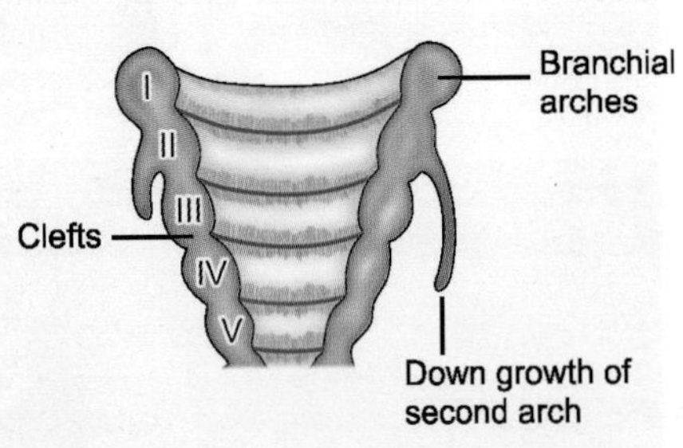

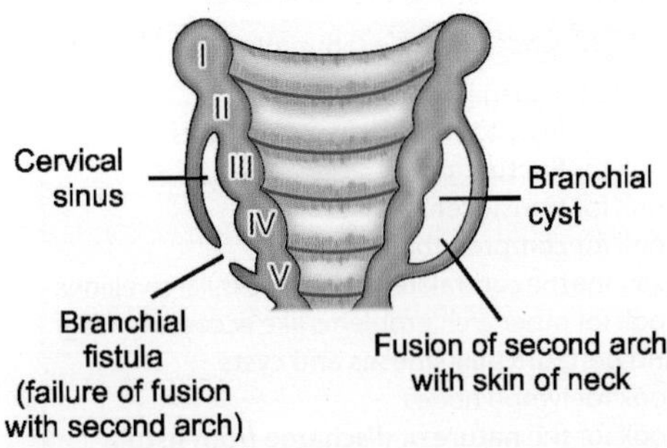

Fig. 31.1: Branchial arch pathology

number of years with super added infection making the appearance of the cyst.

Q 9. Why branchial cysts do not transilluminate?
The cyst contains yellow fluid with cholesterol crystals and epithelial debris, therefore, it will not transilluminate.

Q 10. How a branchial fistula is formed?
Should the **second arch fail to fuse with the 5th arch**, an opening will be found on the neck at birth along the anterior border of the sternomastoid muscle at the junction of the middle and lower third.

Q 11. Is there any communication of the fistula to the pharynx?
Usually, they are separated from the pharynx by a septum, which represents the remains of the cleft membrane (**ending blindly on the lateral pharyngeal wall like a sinus**). If the fistulous tract is complete, it will open **just behind the tonsil** on the affected side (On the anterior aspect of the posterior faucial pillar). There may be small amount of mucus or mucopurulent discharge coming out through the fistulous opening. If the tract is communicating into the oral cavity the liquids taken during meals will come out through the fistulous opening.

Q 12. What is the lining of the branchial cyst?

1. Branchial cyst—stratified squamous epithelium
2. Branchial fistula—stratified squamous or pseudosquamous epithelium externally and non-ciliated columnar epithelium inside
3. Thyroglossal cyst—pseudostratified ciliated columnar epithelium
4. Thyroglossal fistula—columnar epithelium.

Q 13. What is the lining of branchial fistula?
The fistula is lined with **squamous epithelium** up to the partition (cleft membrane). Internal to the partition it is lined with **ciliated columnar epithelium**.

Q 14. What is the course of the branchial fistula?
It is below the 2nd arch structures and above the 3rd arch structures.

Q 15. What is the nerve and artery of 2nd and 3rd arches?

- The nerve of 2nd arch is facial nerve
- The artery of the 2nd arch is external carotid artery
- The nerve of 3rd arch is 9th
- The artery of 3rd arch is internal carotid.

Q 16. What is the time of clinical presentation of branchial fistula?
The opening is present at birth (It is always congenital).

Q 17. What is the clinical feature other than the opening?
Mucoid discharge is noticed in children after a hot bath.

Q 18. What is the exact course of the branchial fistula?
The external opening is usually seen in relation to the lower 3rd of the anterior border of sternomastoid muscle. From its opening on the skin it passes **subcutaneously** to the level of the **upper border of the thyroid cartilage** where it **pierces the deep fascia.** The fistula then passes **beneath the posterior belly of the digastric** muscle and the stylohyoid muscle, **crosses the hypoglossal nerve** and **internal jugular vein**, to traverse the **fork of the carotid bifurcation.** Here the external carotid artery is superficial and the internal carotid deep to the tract. It then **crosses the glossopharyngeal nerve and the stylopharyngeus muscle to pierce the superior constrictor** and to open on the **posterior pillar of the fauces** behind the tonsil.

Q 19. Can the fistula be bilateral?

Yes. In 30% of cases.

Q 20. Can the branchial cyst be bilateral?

Yes. In 2% of cases it is bilateral.

Q 21. On which side the branchial cyst is more commonly seen?

It is seen 60% on left side.

Q 22. Which sex is more affected?

Males are more affected – 60%.

Q 23. Can the cyst be intermittent?

Yes. In 20% of the patients, the cyst will be intermittent.

Q 24. If the cyst is disappearing at the time of surgery? What is the course of action?

There is no place for exploration in this situation. The cyst may not be found at exploration. Partial excision will lead on to sinus formation.

Q 25. What are the other associated congenital anomalies?

Associated anomalies in branchial cyst

- Preauricular sinuses
- Periauricular cysts
- Accessory tragi
- Subcutaneous cartilaginous nodules.

Q 26. The branchial fistula is congenital or acquired?

- The branchial fistula is always congenital (the position of the cyst is in the upper part and the fistula is in the lower part due to the developmental reasons already mentioned)
- The thyroglossal fistula is always acquired.

Q 27. Can similar swellings occur in relation to other cleft apparatus?

Yes. It can occur in relation to first branchial cleft.

Q 28. What is bronchogenic carcinoma?

It is controversial whether this entity is a malignancy in branchial cyst or it is a cystic degeneration in a lymph node containing deposit from squamous cell carcinoma. The latter is more possible. The primary growth may not be apparent and it may be situated in the nasopharynx, tonsil, base of tongue, pyriform fossa or supraglottic larynx. Therefore, it is important to rule out an occult primary in such conditions.

Q 29. What are the other cysts having cholesterol crystals?

- Hydrocele
- Dental cyst
- Dentigerous cyst.

Q 30. What are the most important differential diagnoses for a branchial cyst?

Other cystic swellings on the lateral side of the neck like.

Cystic swellings on the side of the neck

- Branchial cyst
- Cystic hygroma (Lymphangioma)
- Hemangioma
- Cold abscess
- Dermoid cyst
- Laryngocele
- Pharyngocele
- Sebaceous cyst.

In addition, the following solid swellings form differential diagnoses for branchial cyst.

Solid swellings on the side of the neck

1. Reactive lymphadenitis
2. Lipoma
3. Neurofibroma
4. Chemodectoma (potato tumor)
5. Paraganglioma
6. Lymphoma
7. Metastatic carcinoma in node from thyroid
8. Tuberculous lymph node.

Q 31. How to differentiate clinically cystic hygroma from branchial cyst?

- Cystic hygroma is **brilliantly translucent**
- Cystic hygroma is **partially compressible**
- Usually seen in the **neonate and early infancy**
- Increase in size when the child cries or coughs.

Q 32. Why cystic hygroma is brilliantly translucent?

- The cysts are filled with clear fluid
- Lined by single layer of epithelium (with a mosaic appearance).

Q 33. How a cystic hygroma is formed?

Cystic hygroma develops from the primitive lymph sac called **jugular lymph sac** (they are situated in the neck between the jugular and subclavian veins). Sequestration of a portion of jugular lymph sac will result in the formation of cystic hygroma.

Q 34. What are the other situations where you get cystic hygroma?

Sites for cystic hygroma

- Axilla
- Groin
- Mediastinum
- Cheek
- May involve salivary glands
- Tongue
- Floor of the mouth.

Q 35. What are the complications of cystic hygroma?

- Infection
- Increase in size and respiratory embarrassment
- Obstructed labor during delivery.

Q 36. What are the treatment options for cystic hygroma?

1. Meticulous conservative neck dissection with excision of all lymphatic tissue
2. Injection of sclerosing agents (Picibanil or OK432 is a recent sclerosant).

Q 37. What are the problems of sclerotherapy for cystic hygroma?

- Extracystic injection can produce inflammation of adjacent tissue
- Usually they are multicystic and extensive and therefore difficult to eradicate
- Recurrence is common after sclerotherapy.

Q 38. What are the investigations in branchial cyst?

- Ultrasound
- FNAC
- Aspiration and examination under microscope for cholesterol crystals
- CT/MRI if paraganglioma is suspected.

Q 39. What are the complications?

- Infection
- Abscess formation.

Q 40. What will happen if formal excision is carried out during the stage of inflammation?

- It will result in fistula formation
- Do the surgery only when the lesion is quiescent **(2 to 3 months later)**.

Q 41. What is the treatment of branchial cyst?

Excision of the cyst under general anesthesia is the treatment. If the cyst is large and tense, it may be decompressed with a large bore needle to facilitate the dissection.

Q 42. What are the structures to be taken care of during surgery?

- The cyst may be passing backwards and upwards through the carotid fork and reach as far as the pharyngeal constrictors.
- It passes superficial to the hypoglossal and glossopharyngeal nerves and deep to the posterior belly of the digastric.
- The spinal accessory nerve must be identified and protected.

Q 43. What is the most important investigation for branchial fistula?

Fistulogram (this will provide information regarding the nature, whether it is sinus or fistula). The entire tract must be removed to prevent recurrence.

Q 44. What is the covering of the fistula external to the epithelial lining?

Muscle fibers and lymphoid tissue.

Q 45. What is the surgical treatment for branchial fistula?

Complete excision of the tract.

Q 46. What is the incision used for excision of the tract?

Elliptical and Step ladder

1. Initially an **elliptical** incision around the opening and the tract is dissected through the deep cervical fascia.
2. **Step ladder** incisions later on and tract is followed towards the pharyngeal wall (any mucosal breach of the pharynx is repaired).

Q 47. If the fistula is asymptomatic, is there any need for surgical treatment?

- There is no need to treat asymptomatic fistula other than cosmetic reasons
- Once there is discharge, it should be excised because patient is likely to get repeated infections.

Case 32 Soft Tissue Sarcoma

Case Capsule

A **50-year-old male** patient presents with swelling in **front and lateral part of right thigh** of about **15 × 10 cm size, hard in consistency, deep to deep fascia** with **restricted mobility**. The regional nodes are not palpable. There is **no distal neurovascular deficit**. The movements of right knee joint are normal. The flexion of right hip joint is restricted due to the size of the swelling. Abdominal and chest examination are normal.

Read the diagnostic algorithm for a swelling.

Checklist for history

- History of radiation
- History of chemical exposure—Arsenic, vinyl chloride
- History of lymphedema
- History of familial lymphedema
- History of neurofibromatosis
- History of retinoblastoma
- History of familial polyposis coli.

Checklist for examination

1. Look for other swellings
2. Look for **pigmented lesions** in the body
3. Local rise of temperature and tenderness
4. Look for **dilated veins** over the swelling

Contd...

Contd...

5. Assessment of the **plane of the swelling**
6. Involvement of muscle groups
7. **Involvement of neurovascular bundle** with distal neurovascular deficit—check for distal pulsations and sensations
8. Look for **movement of the swellings** (whether it is fixed to the bone or not)
9. Check for movement of the joints both proximal and distal
10. Look for **wasting of muscles**
11. Look for **regional nodes**
12. Examine the **chest for metastasis.**

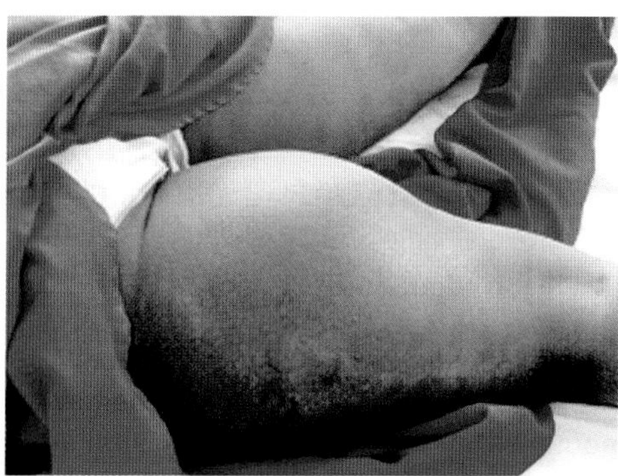

Soft tissue sarcoma back of right thigh

Soft tissue sarcoma medial part of left thigh

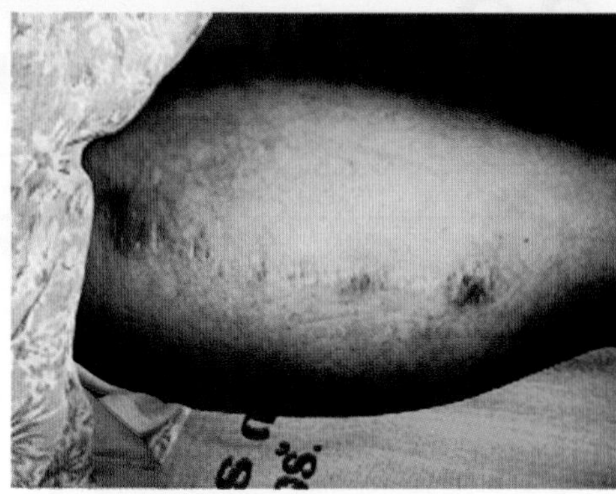

Recurrent soft tissue sarcoma of back of thigh

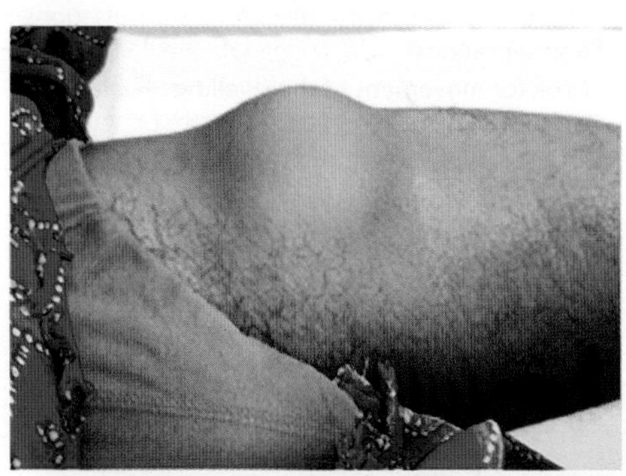

Soft tissue sarcoma of left thigh

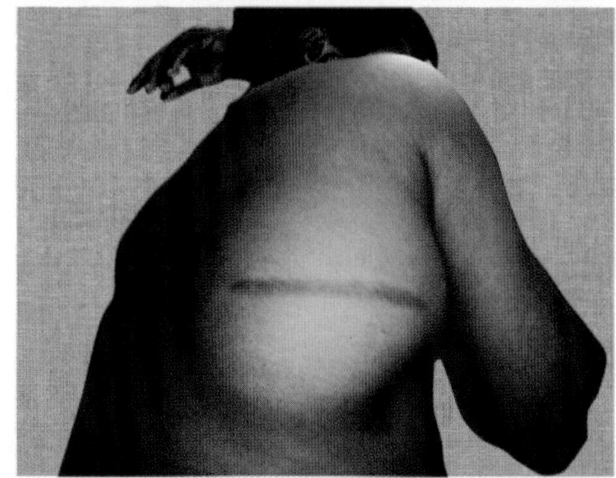

Soft tissue sarcoma of right infrascapular region

Q 1. What is the most probable diagnosis in this case?

Soft tissue sarcoma (*STS*).

Q 2. What is soft tissue sarcoma?

They are malignant tumors that arise from skeletal and extraskeletal connective tissue, mesenchymal cells including adipose tissue, bone, cartilage, smooth muscle and skeletal muscle. As per the new definition they are thought to arise from **undifferentiated mesenchymal stem cells** that may be found virtually anywhere. This will explain the origin of a sarcoma from smooth muscle where anatomically smooth muscle is not present.

Q 3 .What are the differential diagnoses?

Benign soft tissue swelling such as:

- Lipoma
- Myositis ossificans

- Angiomyolipoma
- Hematoma
- Angiomyxoma.

Q 4. What are the etiological factors for soft tissue sarcoma?

1. *Genetic predisposition*
   - Neurofibromatosis – Von Recklinghausen's disease
   - Li-Fraumeni syndrome
   - Retinoblastoma
   - Gardner's syndrome (familial adenomatous polyposis)
2. *Radiation exposure*
3. *Lymphedema*
   - Postsurgical
   - Postirradiation
   - Parasitic infection (filariasis)
4. *Trauma*
5. *Oncogene activation*
   - MDM2, C-erB$_2$, C-KIT
6. *Chemical*
   - 2, 3, 7, 8 – Tetrachlorodibenzodioxin
   - Polyvinyl chloride
   - Chlorophenols
   - Phenoxy acetic acid.

Q 5. What is the pathogenesis of soft tissue sarcoma (STS)?

- Specific genetic alterations—fusion genes due to reciprocal translocations and specific point mutations
- Nonspecific genetic alterations—genetic losses and gains
- The tumor suppressor genes—p53 and RB1.

Q 6. What is the order of investigation in this case?

Imaging is the first investigation of choice which may be either **CT or MRI for extremity and CT for retroperitoneum**. This is followed by carefully planned biopsy—**Core biopsy or incisional biopsy**. The entry point of the core needle biopsy must be carefully placed such that it does not compromise subsequent radical excision. The incision is placed along the future resection axis, i.e. longitudinal for extremity soft tissue sarcoma.

Q 7. Why not FNAC?

There is **no role for FNAC** in a suspected case of soft tissue sarcoma. By FNAC you get a report of spindle cell neoplasm which is not going to guide the further management. The core biopsy will give the following:

1. Histopathological confirmation
2. Evaluate the grade
3. Identify the prognostic factors.

The only role of FNAC is for the confirmation of recurrence rather than the primary diagnosis.

Q 8. If the core biopsy is negative, is there any role for biopsy and what are the precautions to be taken?

Yes. A carefully planned incision biopsy is done with following precautions:

Precautions for biopsy

1. The incision must always be vertical and not horizontal centerd over the mass in its most superficial location (An elliptical incision to include the scar of the biopsy is used for formal wide excision later on). No tissue flaps are raised
2. Hemostasis is very important at the time of biopsy (hematoma can distort anatomy)
3. Use drains only if it is absolutely necessary. (Should not be used lateral to the vertical incision). The drain site should be as close to the incision as possible
4. If the swelling is less than 3 cm size, **excisional biopsy** is recommended.

The biopsy should establish the grade and the histologic subtype.

Q 9. What are the soft tissue sarcomas where lymph node metastases are seen? (PG)

Soft tissue sarcomas with nodal metastasis (< 3% of adult STS)
1. Synovial sarcoma
2. Ewing's sarcoma
3. Embryonal rhabdomyosarcoma
4. Epithelioid sarcoma
5. Lymphangiosarcoma
6. Angiosarcoma
7. Kaposi sarcoma
8. Malignant fibrous histiocytoma (MFH).

Nodes are markers of systemic disease and need radical node dissection.

Q 10. What are the common sites of soft tissue sarcoma and what is the incidence?

It forms 1% of adult human malignancy and 15% of pediatric malignancy.

Extremities – 50% (35% in lower limb and 15% in upper limb)
Trunk – 31%
Head and Neck – 9%
Others –

Q 11. What are the most common histopathological subtypes?

1. MFH (the new terminology as per WHO is **High grade undifferentiated pleomorphic sarcoma** – 24%
2. Liposarcoma – 19%
3. Leiomyosarcoma – 21%
4. Synovial sarcoma – 12%
5. Nerve sheath tumors – 6%
6. Fibrosarcoma – 11%
7. Other types – 7%

Cell of origin	*Sarcoma type*
Adipocyte	Liposarcoma
Fibrohistiocyte	Malignant fibrous histiocytoma (High grade undifferentiated pleomorphic sarcoma)
Fibroblast	Fibrosarcoma
Smooth muscle	Leiomyosarcoma
Skeletal muscle	Rhabdomyosarcoma
Vascular	Angiosarcoma, Kaposi's
Synovial	Synovial sarcoma
Unknown	Ewing's sarcoma, Epithelioid sarcoma

Q 12. What is the age group affected?

- Childhood – Embryonal rhabdomyosarcoma
- Less than 35 years – Synovial sarcoma
- Older patients – MFH and liposarcoma

Q 13. Why the grade is important in STS?

Grade of the tumor is included in stage grouping.

Q14. What are the factors considered for grade?

They include:

- Cellularity
- Differentiation
- Pleomorphism
- Necrosis
- Number of mitosis.

Q 15. Based on mitotic activity how is grading done?

- Mitotic activity 0–9 / high power field
- 10 – 19
- 20 or more.

Q 16. What are the imaging studies of choice?

- **Plain radiograph**—underlying skeletal deformities, callus and bony exostosis can be identified
- **CT** is preferred for intra-abdominal lesion because one can identify both primary and potential metastasis

- **MRI**—Best suited for accurate anatomical localization
  - Whether lesion is intra or extra compartmental
  - Can diagnose lipoma and hemangioma with reasonable accuracy
  - Identify the relationship of the sarcoma to neurovascular structures.
- **MR angiography** (The role of arteriography has decreased markedly after MR angiography)
- **Ultrasound**—can guide biopsy.

Useful under certain circumstances

1. **PET CT scan** may be useful for targeting biopsy, in prognostication, grading and determining response to preoperative chemotherapy. **MR spectroscopy is coming up in a big way for grading of the tumor.**
2. Consider **abdominal/pelvic CT** for the following types of extremity soft tissue sarcoma:
   - Myxoid liposarcoma
   - Epithelioid sarcoma
   - Angiosarcoma
   - Leiomyosarcoma
3. **MRI** of spine for myxoid round cell liposarcoma
4. **CNS imaging for alveolar** sarcoma and angiosarcoma.

Q 17. What is the timing of imaging?

Imaging is done prior to core biopsy and incision biopsy. The core biopsy will produce architectural alterations in the lesion.

Q 18. What is the metastatic work up?

- **X-ray chest** – 70% of the extremity sarcomas metastasize to the lungs
  - Retroperitoneal or visceral lesions metastasize to the liver parenchyma
- **CT scan of the chest** is recommended for high grade tumors and for all tumors > 5 cm size. Metastases are seen in the periphery of the lung. It is superior to chest X-ray for identifying metastasis for low grade tumors.

Q 19. What is the staging of soft tissue sarcoma? (PG)

TNM Staging: AJCC 7th Edition.

- **Grading has been reformatted from a four grade to a 3 grade system as per the criteria recommended by the College of American Pathologists**
- **N1 disease has been reclassified as stage III rather than stage IV.**

Primary Tumor (T)

TX – Primary tumor cannot be assessed
T0 – No evidence of primary tumor
T1 – Tumor *5 cm or less* in greatest dimension
T1a – *Superficial tumor*
T1b – *Deep tumor*
T2 – Tumor *more than 5 cm* in greatest dimension
T2a – *Superficial tumor*
T2b – *Deep tumor*

Regional Lymph Nodes (N)

NX – Regional lymph nodes cannot be assessed
N0 – No regional lymph node metastasis
N1* – Regional lymph node metastasis

Note:* **Presence of positive nodes (N_1) is considered Stage IV (the outcome of patients with N1 disease is similar to those with M1 disease).

Distant Metastasis (M)

MX – Distant metastasis cannot be assessed
M0 – No distant metastasis
M1 – Distant metastasis

Histologic Grade

GX – Grade cannot be assessed
G1 – Grade 1
G2 – Grade 2
G3 – Grade 3

Stage Grouping				
Stage	T size	N size	M	Grade
IA	T1a T1b	N0 N0	M0 M0	G1, Gx G1,Gx
IB	T2a T2b	N0 N0	M0 M0	G1, Gx G1,Gx
IIA	T1a T1b	N0 N0	M0 M0	G2, G3 G2,G3
IIB	T2a T2b	N0 N0	M0 M0	G2 G2
III	T2a, T2b Any T	N0 N1	M0 M0	G3 Any G
IV	Any T	Any N	M1	Any G

Q 20. What are the immunohistochemical markers for soft tissue sarcoma? (PG)

IHC marker	*Type of sarcoma*
Desmin	Sarcoma from smooth, skeletal muscle
CD 31, CD 34	Vascular sarcomas
S 100	Sarcoma with neural, lipomatous, chondroid differentiation
Vimentin	Many sarcomas—non specific
CD 117	Gastrointestinal stromial tumor
CD 57, Vimentin	Chondrosarcoma
CD 99, S 100, NET. Vimentin	PNET/Ewing's sarcoma
Cytokeratin, CD 99, NET Desmin	Desmoplastic round cell tumors
CD 57, EMA, Vimentin	Osteosarcoma

Q 21. What is the staging proposed by Memorial Sloan Kettering Cancer Centre (MSKCC)? (PG)

This is a simple staging system based on the three important prognostic factors namely:

1. High grade – 1 point
2. Tumor size > 5 cm – 1 point
3. Deep tumor – 1 point
4.

Good prognostic factor	*Poor prognostic factor*	*Staging*
Low grade	High grade	Stage 0 - no poor prognostic feature
Tumor size < 5cm	Tumor size > 5cm	Stage 1 – 1 poor prognostic feature
Superficial tumor	Deep tumor	Stage 2 – 2 poor prognostic feature Stage 3– 3 poor prognostic feature Stage 4 – metastatic sarcoma

Q 22. What you mean by superficial and deep in staging? (PG)

Superficial lesions—lesions not involving the **superficial fascia**.

Deep:

a. Lesions deep to, or involves the superficial fascia
b. All intraperitoneal visceral lesions
c. Retroperitoneal lesions
d. Mediastinal (Intrathoracic lesions)
e. Pelvic sarcomas
f. Head and neck tumors.

Q 23. What is the metastatic potential of low grade and high grade STS? (PG)

- Less than 15% risk of metastasis for low grade tumors
- More than 50% risk for high grade tumors

Note: For retroperitoneal sarcoma liver is the principal site of metastasis. For extremity sarcoma, lung is the principal site of metastasis.

Q 24. What are the sarcomas excluded from this staging system? (PG)

- Kaposi's sarcoma
- Dermatofibrosarcoma protuberans
- Infantile fibrosarcoma
- Angiosarcoma
- Sarcomas arising from the dura mater including brain
- Sarcoma arising in the parenchymatous organs
- Hollow viscera
- Inflammatory myofibroblastic tumor
- Fibromatosis (Desmoid tumor)
- Mesothelioma.

Q 25. What is fibromatosis?

Original fibrosarcoma grade I is now mentioned as fibromatosis (Desmoid) and they are not in soft tissue sarcomas.

Q 26. What is the staging in this case?

T2b, N0, M0 (*Stage 3*).

Q 27. What is the management of soft tissue sarcoma?

Multidisciplinary approach is recommended comprising expertise in the following specialties:

- Radiology
- Clinical oncology
- Surgical oncology.

Note: Limb sparing surgery is preferred. Amputation is performed in < 5–10% of cases.

Q 28. What is the surgical management of this tumor?

Limb sparing, function preserving, margin free (microscopically negative) **wide excision** is the treatment of choice.

Q 29. What is wide excision?

It is a wide en-bloc resection to obtain **1 cm uninvolved** tissue in all directions for low grade tumors and **2 cm** in all directions for high grade tumors (**3-dimensional**). A 3-dimensional clearance without seeing the tumor is achieved.

Note: All earlier scars, fine needle aspiration tracts and biopsy areas with hematoma should be excised en-bloc with the underlying tumor.

Q 30. What is "Pseudocapsule" in soft tissue sarcoma? (PG)

The sarcomas grow in an expansive fashion, flattening the normal soft tissue structures around them in a concentric manner and creating a **compression zone** of condensed and atrophic tissue. Outside this zone lies edematous neovascularized tissue called **reactive zone.** Together the compression and reactive zones comprise the **pseudocapsule**.

Small tentacles (small finger-like extensions) **extend for variable distance from the parent lesion** perforating the pseudocapsule to form clinically occult deposits beyond the pseudocapsule. **Therefore, tumor masses will be seen outside the pseudocapsule.**

Q 31. What are the barriers for the infiltrative growth of the sarcomas? (PG)

The expansive growth stops at the following boundaries:

1. Fascial boundaries
2. Periosteal structures
3. Adventitia of the vessels
4. Nerve sheaths.

Note: Gross involvement of these structures is seen early (may become infiltrated).

Q 32. What is intralesional excision? (PG)

When you leave behind the pseudocapsule and remove the lesion, it is called intralesional excision. **It is not recommended.**

Q 33. What is marginal excision? (PG)

Removal of tumor along with its pseudocapsule is called marginal excision (Not recommended).

Q 34. What is compartment excision? (PG)

Compartment excisions are done for soft tissue sarcomas of the extremities. Removal of muscle bundles from origin to insertion and all other structures in the compartment is called compartment excision. This is also given up in favor of wide excision.

Q 35. What is the role of amputation in soft tissue sarcoma?

There is a paradigm shift from radical amputation to limb salvage procedure in the treatment of soft tissue sarcoma.

- Amputation as an initial treatment did not decrease the probability of regional metastasis and did not improve the disease specific survival and therefore, a limb sparing attitude is taken
- Patient preference when gross total resection of the tumor is expected to render the limb non-functional
- Sarcomas involving bone or joint.

Note: Amputation should be performed one joint above the tumor.

Q 36. When complete encirclement of major neurovascular bundle occurs what should be the surgical approach? (PG)

1. **Nerve resection**: It may be necessary to sacrifice these structures and give **braces for footdrop** after **sciatic nerve resection, knee brace for joint stability** after loss of quadriceps function secondary to **femoral nerve resection.**
2. Resection **of a major artery** followed by saphenous vein graft or prosthetic graft for restoration of arterial flow.
3. If 1 and 2 are not feasible do **amputations.**

Q 37. In the given patient what will be the treatment option?

In the given case the wide excision will involve removal of part of the quadriceps muscle, resection of femoral nerve followed by knee brace for stability of the knee. The femoral vessels are unlikely to be encircled by the tumor.

Q 38. What is the role of adjuvant radiation therapy?

Radiotherapy is not a substitute for suboptimal surgery. There are three types of radiotherapy:

- Brachytherapy
- IORT
- XRT

The indications for radiotherapy are:

- High grade lesions
- Low grade lesions > 5 cm
- Margin positive
- Close soft tissue margin < 1 cm
- Recurrent sarcomas.

Q 39. What are the advantages and disadvantages of preoperative radiotherapy and the indications? (PG)

Preoperative radiotherapy is indicated for stage II and III disease. **The advantages are:**

- Reduces seeding in surgical manipulation
- Pseudocapsule may thicken and become acellular, easing resection
- To tackle occult micrometastasis
- To do less radical surgery later on
- In patients with unresectable tumors for limb sparing surgery later on

The disadvantages are:

- Wound healing problems—may need the help of plastic surgeon
- Resection is possible only after 3–6 weeks

The dose of radiotherapy is 50 Gy.

Q 40. What is the role of brachytherapy? (PG)

Adjuvant brachytherapy is being used increasingly nowadays. Brachytherapy will treat the **tumor bed**, within 2 cm of the margin. **Radioactive wires** are placed into the operative bed to improve local control. It will not treat large margins, overlying skin, and scar or drain site. It has got a short duration of treatment (*4–6 days*) compared to the external beam therapy consisting of **6–8 weeks duration**.

Q 41. What are the indications for chemotherapy? (PG)

- High grade liposarcoma
- High grade synovial sarcoma
- Ewing's sarcoma
- Rhabdomyosarcoma.

Q 42. What is rationale for preoperative chemotherapy? (PG)

- Preoperative chemotherapy is indicated for stage II and III
- To limit the spread of tumor at the time of surgery.

Q 43. What are the chemotherapeutic regimens?

- The single agents used are:
  - Doxorubicin, Ifosfamide and Dacarbazine
- Combination
  - Gemcitabine and Docetaxel combination
  - MAID: **M**esna, **A**driamycin, **I**fosfamide, **D**acarbazine

Q 44. What is the treatment protocol for the various stages?

It is managed by multidisciplinary team—Surgeon, Radiation Oncologist and Medical Oncologist. The diagnosis is established by a carefully planned biopsy which is done after imaging. Establish the grade of the tumor and histological type before treatment. Limb sparing, function preserving, margin free wide excision is the surgical procedure of choice.

Treatment protocol based on the staging:

Stage 1A (T1a - 1b N0, M0) /Stage IB:

- Wide excision—final margin > 1cm or intact fascial plane—follow-up.
- Final margin < 1cm or without intact fascial plane—consider radiotherapy
- Follow-up evaluation for rehabilitation, chest imaging every 6–12 months
- Stage II and III Resectable/potentially resectable disease
- Surgery/preoperative radiotherapy/preoperative chemotherapy, preoperative chemoradiation followed by surgery
- RT/ consider RT boost/ consider adjuvant chemotherapy
- Follow-up.

Unresectable primary disease:

- RT/Chemotherapy/Chemoradiation/**isolated regional limb therapy**
- Changes to resectable—surgery
- Unresectable—definitive RT/Chemotherapy/ Palliative surgery
- Follow-up.

Stage IV–Metastasis:

- Single organ/limited tumor bulk – primary tumor management and **metastatectomy** and RT/ chemotherapy and follow-up
- Disseminated metastasis—palliative chemo/ palliative surgery/palliative RT.

Case 33 Neurofibroma, von Recklinghausen's Disease

Case Capsule

A 14-year-old mentally retarded boy presents with **2 subcutaneous swellings of anterior chest wall, multiple café-au-lait macules** (CALMs) and thoracic **scoliosis**. There is a soft subcutaneous nontender **hanging swelling in the left mammary region** of 20 × 15 cm size, freely mobile over the pectoralis major muscle. The second swelling is of the size of **3 × 4 cm in the region of the right 5th rib in the anterior axillary line**. The plane of this swelling is also subcutaneous. There is no axillary, cervical or inguinal lymph adenopathy. There is a bony deformity involving the 3rd**, 4th and 5th ribs on right side**. Ophthalmologic examination showed **Lisch nodules**. Radiology revealed **hypoplastic sphenoid wings**, posterior scalloping of vertebral bodies, **twisted ribbon-like ribs** and mediastinal swelling.

Read the diagnostic algorithm for a swelling.

Checklist for history

- Family history of similar swelling, involvement of 1st degree relative with NF1
- History of rapid increase in size suggestive of malignancy
- History of headache

Contd...

Contd...

- History of seizures
- History of learning disabilities
- History of precocious puberty
- History of pain radiating down the swelling (tingling and numbness).

Checklist for examination

Read checklist for examination of the swelling.

1. Look for **café-au-lait macules** (CALMs)—6 or more in number each having > 1.5 cm size during post pubertal period
2. Look for **freckling of axilla and groin**
3. Look for more swellings
4. Rule out **short stature**
5. **Examination of the spine** for scoliosis and other vertebral anomalies
6. Examination of the long bones for bony abnormalities-**pseudoarthrosis,** etc.
7. Examination of the abdomen for **pheochromocytoma**
8. Record the **blood pressure** to rule out pheo
9. Complete neurological examination—both central nervous system and peripheral nervous system (including cognitive impairment, headache, etc.)
10. **Ophthalmological examination** to rule out Lisch nodules in Iris—2 or more Lisch nodules
11. Rule out hydrocephalus.

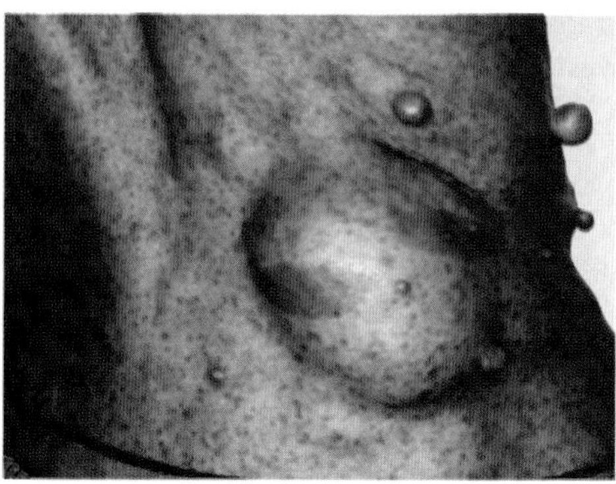
von Recklinghausen disease—
sarcomatous change

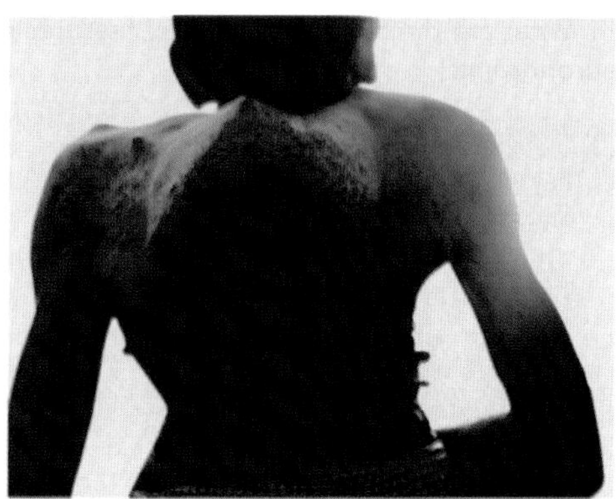
von Recklinghausen disease—
spinal deformity

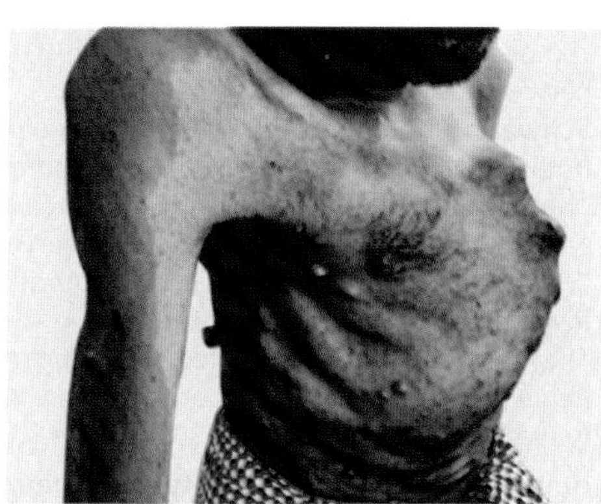
von Recklinghausen disease with
anterior chest wall deformity

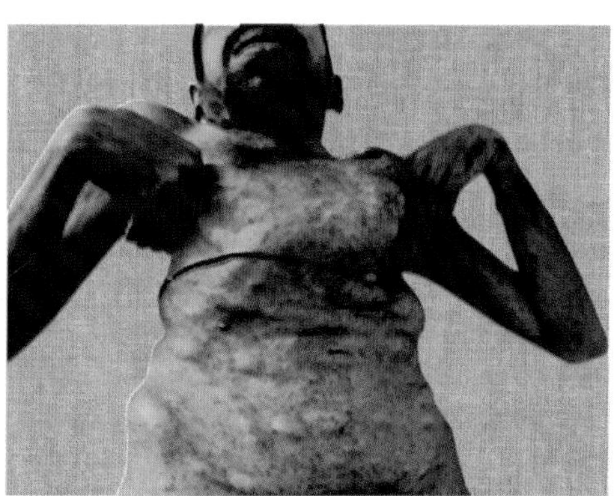
von Recklinghausen disease
with multiple swellings

Q 1. What is the most-probable diagnosis in this case?

von Recklinghausen's disease (neurofibromatosis)

Q 2. What is neurofibroma?

Neurofibromas are benign tumors which contain a mixture of neural (ectodermal) and fibrous (mesodermal) elements.

Q 3. What is the histology of neurofibroma?

There is a **generalized neoplastic activity** within the nerve sheath. Histologically **connective tissue** and **endoneural cells** intermixed with **axons** are seen.

Q 4. What are the diagnostic clinical features of neurofibroma?

Diagnostic features of neurofibroma

- They are seen in relation to a nerve (Need not be in relation to named nerve)
- Patients may get tingling sensation in the distribution of the nerve
- They are usually seen in the subcutaneous tissue and skin (Deep swelling can occur)
- Usually fusiform in shape
- Long axis of the swelling is along the length of the limb
- Firm or rubbery in consistency
- Mobile side-to-side (not longitudinally)
- Moves at right angles to the course of the nerve
- No nodal involvement
- Skin is not involved
- Nerve compression symptoms may be there.

Note: Deep neurofibromas in the extremities and intra-abdominal neurofibromas may not be showing the classical features.

Q 5. When neurofibromas are multiple what is it called?

- Neurofibromatosis
- When they are multiple and congenital and familial and transmitted by autosomal dominant gene, it is called von Recklinghausen's disease.

Q 6. What are the manifestations of neurofibroma?

It can be classified as:

- Irritative—pain distributed along the course of the nerve
- Paralytic
- Sensory dysfunction
- Motor dysfunction—weakness and muscle atrophy.

Q 7. What are the investigations for neurofibroma?

Investigations for neurofibroma

1. MRI—showing **Gadolinium enhancing mass** within a peripheral nerve
2. Nerve conduction studies
3. Electromyography.

Q 8. What is the treatment of neurofibroma?

- Neurofibromas **cannot be excised without resecting a segment** of the involved nerve.
- True neurofibromas should only be **biopsied** to ensure that they are not malignant and should be left in place unless the parent nerve can be sacrificed without producing significant neurological deficits.

Q 9. What is neurilemmoma? What is schwannoma?

- Tumors which are derived from the sheath of the nerve are called neurilemmoma.
- **Schwannoma**—When the tumor is arising from the Schwan cells it is called **schwannoma**. They are benign, painless firm nodules of 1–2 cm size seen along the peripheral nerves. They are usually asymptomatic with **no nodal involvement or malignant potential**.
- They can be carefully enucleated by incising the nerve sheath vertically without sacrificing the nerve.

Q 10. What are the clinical features of neurilemmoma and schwannoma?

They are having the same clinical features as neurofibroma.

Q 11. What is the treatment of schwannoma?

- Generally they are small and benign and they can be enucleated by incising the nerve sheath.
- Amputation may be required for malignant schwannoma.

Q 12. What are the types of neurofibromas?

Three types of neurofibromas are there:

1. Peripheral neurofibromas
2. Diffuse or plexiform neurofibromas – 5% undergo malignant transformation resulting in MPNST.
3. Malignant peripheral nerve sheath tumors (**MPNSTs**).

Q 13. What are the types of plexiform neurofibromas?

There are 3 types of neurofibromatosis:

1. *Plexiform neurofibromatosis*—It is an excessive over growth of neural tissue in the subcutaneous fat and makes the tissue look edematous. They are usually seen in connection with the branches of **5th cranial nerve.** This will present as mass of soft tissue hanging down in folds.
2. *Elephantiasis neuromatosis*—It is a variant of the above condition affecting the lower limb where the subcutaneous fat is replaced by fibrous tissue. It is often mistakenly diagnosed as lymphedema, but the lymphatics are normal.
3. *Pachydermatocele*—It is a type of neurofibromatosis in which coils of soft tissue hang around the root of the neck.

Q 14. What is amputation neuroma?

A tumor similar to neurofibroma occurring at the end of the divided nerve in amputation is called amputation neuroma. Such neuromas may also be seen where a divided nerve has failed to unite.

Q 15. What are the types of neurofibromatosis?

They are classified as:

A. *Isolated neurofibromas*

B. *Multiple neurofibromas (Neurofibromatosis)*—further classified as—
   1. *Neurofibromatosis*—Type I (NF - I) (von Recklinghausen's disease),
   2. *Central neurofibromatosis*—NF Type II.

Q 16. What is central neurofibromatosis (type II)?

- It is characterized by bilateral acoustic neuromas and spinal neuromas
- Always check the hearing
- Always check nerve root compression when you suspect spinal neuromas
- This condition also shows autosomal dominant inheritance.

Q 17. What is dumbbell tumor?

Spinal tumors may be dumbbell shaped and part of it may be inside and part of it outside the vertebral canal. It may cause nerve root compression.

Q 18. What is café-au-lait spot?

They are patches of pale brown pigmentation. The diagnostic criterion for café-au-lait spot is that they should be **greater than 6 in number and more than 1.5 cm size** across. **They are characteristic and diagnostic of von Recklinghausen's disease.**

Q 19. What are the diagnostic criteria for von Recklinghausen's disease (NF-1)?

The **NIH consensus criteria** are used. The diagnosis of NF-1 is rendered when **2 or more** of the following are present.

Diagnostic criteria for von Recklinghausen's disease (2 or more must be there)

1. **Six or more** café-au-lait spots. Each **1.5 cm or larger** in postpubertal individuals, **0.5 cm or larger** in prepubertal individuals
2. Two or more neurofibromas of any type OR one or more plexiform neurofibromas
3. Freckling of armpits or groin
4. Optic glioma (tumor of the optic pathway)
5. Two or more Lisch nodules (benign iris hamartomas)
6. A distinctive bony lesion—Dysplasia of the sphenoid bone/dysplasia or thinning of long bone cortex
7. First degree relative with NF-1.

Q 20. What are the pigmentary abnormalities in NF-1?

a. Café-au-lait macules (CALMs)
b. Skin fold freckling
   - < 5 mm in size, not apparent at birth
   - appears later in childhood.
c. Lisch nodules—(pathognomonic).

Q 21. What is skin fold freckling?

The second most common pigmentary abnormality NF-1 is skin fold freckling seen in the **axilla, groin** and **intertriginous non sun exposed areas**. It is also seen **under the chin and inframammary regions** in adults. Unlike café-au-lait spot these are < 5 mm in size and not apparent at birth.

Q 22. What is Lisch nodule?

It is pathognomonic for NF-1. Lisch nodules are raised, pigmented hamartomas of the iris. They do not interfere with vision and are not associated with any clinical symptoms.

Q 23. What are the malignancies associated with NF-1?

1. Optic gliomas (the most commonly recognized tumor)
2. Astrocytomas
3. Pheochromocytoma—**Check BP, do ultrasound abdomen and urinary VMA** for excluding pheo in all cases of NF1.
4. Non CNS malignancies—Leukemias (juvenile chronic myeloid leukemia, and myelodysplastic syndromes)

Among individuals with NF-1 pheo is rare, however in patients with pheo the incidence of NF-1 is estimated to be between 4–23%.

Q 24. What are the other neurological complications? (PG)

Other neurological complications of von Recklinghausen's disease

- Macrocephaly
- Hydrocephalus—Aqueductal stenosis
- Cognitive impairment
- Headaches
- Seizures (5–7%)
- Cerebral ischemia
- Learning disabilities
- Mental retardation (IQ < 70)
- Diffuse cerebral dysgenesis—10%
- Cerebrovascular abnormalities producing strokes.

Q 25. What are the bony abnormalities? (PG)

Bony abnormalities in von Recklinghausen's disease

- Dysplasia of sphenoid
- Scoliosis—10% of the affected individuals
- Short stature
- Vertebral defects—hemivertebrae
- Long bone deformities **Tibial dysplasia** (anterolateral bowing)—**thinning of the cortex** leading to **pathological fracture and** non union—**pseudoarthrosis**
- Twisted ribbon-like ribs.

Q 26. What is the genetics of von Recklinghausen's disease? (PG)

- It is a disease having autosomal dominant inheritance pattern.
- 30–50% do not have an affected parent (spontaneous mutation)
- The penetrance of NF1 is essentially 100% in individuals who have reached adulthood.
- The protein product of the NF1 gene is called **Neurofibromin**
- The gene is located in chromosome 17q 11.2. **(The NF2 gene is called Merlin)**.

Q 27. What is the management of von Recklinghausen's disease? (PG)

The NF1 management is teamwork of physicians, ophthalmologists, neurologists, orthopedic surgeons, dermatologists, oncologists, otolaryngologists, plastic surgeons, neurosurgeons, psychiatrists, social workers and child psychologists. This is better accomplished by *NF clinic.*

Optic pathway gliomas

- Serial neurologic and ophthalmologic examination
- MRI scan once tumor is identified (**ophthalmic examination should be performed on all children starting at 1 year and continuing annually for at least the first decade**).

Plexiform neurofibromas

- Needs regular follow-up because of the malignant transformation.

Scoliosis

- Requires orthopedic evaluation/bracing/surgery

Tibial dysplasia

- Orthopedic management

Learning disabilities

- Early intervention

Precocious puberty

- Requires management by endocrinologists.

Q 28. What is the role of genetic counseling? (PG)

Issues about genetic transmission, emotional aspect and what can be expected to come in future are discussed with the family.

Q 29. What is likely to be the future management? (PG)

Development of **targeted treatment** is likely to be the future treatment. The application of drugs that interfere with RAS proto-oncogene activity would be predicted to have beneficial effects.

Q 30. What surgical treatment you offer for the given patient?

The two chest wall swellings (Plexiform neurofibromas) will be excised under general anesthesia and the patient will be kept for regular follow-up.

Diagnostic algorithm for a swelling anywhere

1. Identify the anatomical situation of the swelling (In relation to the triangle in the neck)

↓

2. Decide the **plane of the swelling**

↓

3. Recollect your anatomy (What are the normal anatomical structures situated in the region of the swelling in that plane?)

↓

4. Check for **mobility/fixity** of the swelling

↓

5. Find out the **external** (size, shape, surface, edge, temperature, tenderness, etc.) and **internal features** of the lump (solid or cystic, compressible/ reducible, pulsation, transillumination) and **auscultation** of the swelling.

↓

6. Find out its **effect on the surrounding tissue**

↓

7. Come to an **anatomical diagnosis**

↓

8. Come to a **pathological diagnosis** (Decide whether it is **congenital/traumatic/ inflammatory / neoplastic**)

↓

9. **If it is an organ concerned with function decide whether it is hyperfunctioning, normally functioning or hypofunctioning** (functional diagnosis). The final diagnosis = Anatomical + Pathological + Functional diagnosis.

Case

34 Lipoma (Universal Tumor)

Case Capsule

A 40-year-old female patient presents with a swelling of the size of **5 × 4 cm** on the right side of the back of 3 years duration. On examination, the swelling is **soft and lobulated** with a **slipping edge** situated in the **infrascapular region**. The swelling is mobile. There are no signs of inflammation or malignancy. No axillary node involvement is noted. No other swellings detected clinically.

Read the diagnostic algorithm for a swelling.

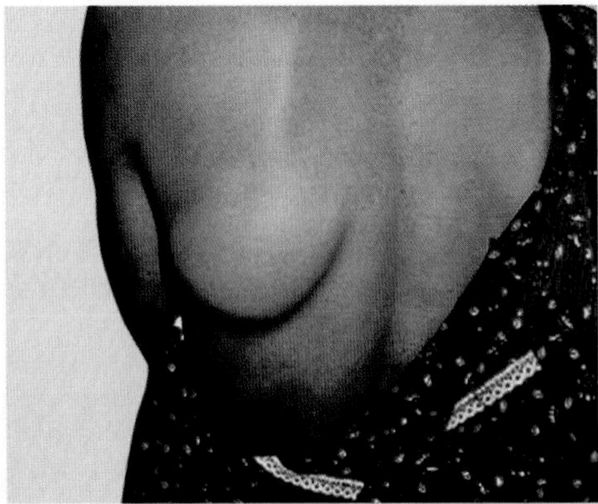

Lipoma back

Q 1. What is your clinical diagnosis in this case?

Lipoma.

Q 2. What is lipoma?

It is a benign tumor arising from **adult fat cells.**

Lipoma back

Q 3. What are the diagnostic points for lipoma?

1. Lobulation
2. Slip sign
3. Soft swelling with pseudofluctuation
4. Transillumination positive if it is subcutaneous
5. The overlying skin may show prominent veins when the lesions are large.

Q 4. What is the cause for pseudofluctuation?

Intracellular **fat is fluid at body temperature**. Therefore, the swelling will be soft and fluctuation will be elicited in one plane. For a true cyst one should elicit fluctuation in two planes at right angles to each other that is not possible in the case of lipoma and therefore, it is called pseudofluctuation.

Q 5. What is slip sign?

If the edge of the lump is pressed, the swelling slips from beneath the finger. This can be easily demonstrated in the case of a subcutaneous lipoma and it is said to be pathognomonic.

Q 6. How will you demonstrate lobulation?

The swelling is compressed between the finger and thumb of one hand, while its surface that is now made more prominent, is stroked firmly by the fingers of the other hand.

Q 7. What is the cause for lobulation?

The lobulation is because of the intervening **fine strands of fibrous septa** seen between the **fat lobules** (collection of overgrown fat cells). The lobules bulge out between the fibrous strands when pressure is applied.

Q 8. Why it is called universal tumor or ubiquitous tumor?

Lipomas can occur anywhere in the body where fat is present and therefore, it is called universal tumor. The aphorism "**When in doubt hedge on fat**" is still true. Whenever you do not have a diagnosis for a given swelling, lipoma is one of the differential diagnoses.

Q 9. Depending on the plane, how will you classify lipomas?

Lipomas can be classified as:

- Subcutaneous
- Subfascial
- Intermuscular
- Intramuscular
- Paraosteal
- Subperiosteal
- Subsynovial
- Intra-articular
- Subserous
- Subperitoneal
- Subpleural
- Subpericardial
- Extradural (type of spinal tumor)
- Submucous
- Intraglandular—seen in breast, pancreas, under renal capsule, etc.

Q 10. What is the commonest plane of lipoma?

Subcutaneous (between the deep fascia and skin).

Q 11. Is it possible to demonstrate all the classical signs of lipoma when the swelling is deep?

No. The classical signs of lipoma such as slip sign, lobulation and pseudofluctuation, etc. are demonstrated in subcutaneous lipoma. It is not possible to demonstrate, slip sign and lobulation in deep lipomas.

Q 12. What will be the finding in transillumination test?

In subcutaneous lipomas transillumination may be positive. Big lipomas and deep lipomas are not transilluminant.

Q 13. What are the diagnostic points for intermuscular lipoma?

On contraction of the concerned muscle the lipoma becomes more prominent, if it is intermuscular. If it is deep to the muscle, the lipoma will become less prominent.

Q 14. What is Nevolipoma?

When a lipoma contains dilated capillaries, it is called Nevolipoma. These swellings will be partially compressible.

Q 15. What is Dercum's disease (Adiposis dolorosa)?

It is a condition where multiple painful or tender subcutaneous lipomas are seen. It is called **adiposis dolorosa**. It is also called **neurolipomatosis**.

Q 16. What is fibrolipoma?

When lipoma contains much fibrous tissue it is called fibrolipoma.

Q 17. What are the symptoms of lipoma?

1. Swelling (lump)
2. Cosmetic (unsightly swelling)
3. Interfere with movement
4. Pain (due to trauma and fat necrosis).

Q18. What are the complications of lipoma?

1. Myxomatous degeneration
2. Calcification
3. Pressure effects

4. Fat necrosis (if they are situated over prominent areas and subjected to trauma)
5. Ulceration (repetitive friction cause ulceration)
6. Intussusception in submucous lipoma.

Note: Lipomas never turn malignant. Liposarcomas arise de novo and not in a benign lesion.

Q 19. Which are the areas where liposarcomas are commonly seen?

1. Proximal thigh
2. Retroperitoneum
3. Mediastinum.

Q 20. What are the investigations required?

1. FNAC from the swelling
2. Radiology of the part
3. If the swelling is big and sarcoma is suspected, **core biopsy and MRI** are done.

Q 21. What is the surgical treatment recommended in the given case?

Excision of the swelling under general anesthesia (if the swelling is small excision is done under local anesthesia using 1% lignocaine with or without adrenaline).

Case

35 Sebaceous Cyst/Epidermoid Cyst/ Wen/Dermoid Cyst

Case Capsule

A 45-year-old male patient presents with a swelling of size of **3 × 2 cm** on the **occipital region** of the scalp of 4 years duration. On examination, the swelling is **soft and cystic**. The **sign of indentation** is present. A **punctum** is visible at the summit of the swelling. The swelling is mobile. The skin can be pinched all over the swelling except at the punctum. There are no signs of inflammation or malignancy. No lymph node involvement. No other swellings detected clinically.

Read the diagnostic algorithm for a swelling.

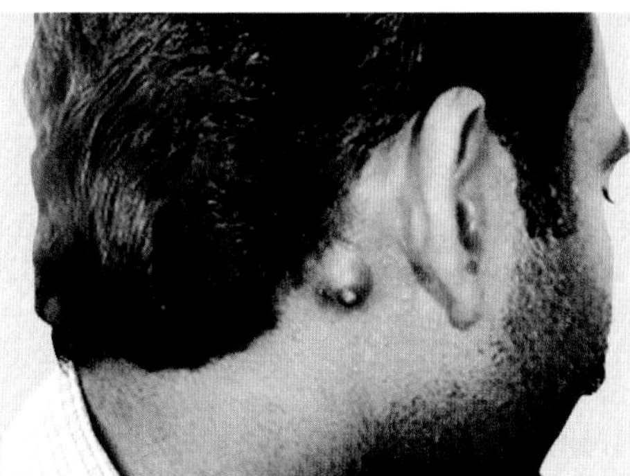

Sebaceous cyst with ulceration

Checklist for examination

- Look for **punctum**
- Pinch the skin and decide whether the skin is free or not (decide the plane)
- Look for **fluctuation**
- Try transillumination
- Look for the **sign of indentation**
- Decide whether it is **cystic or solid**
- Decide whether the swelling is **pulsatile or not**
- Look for a **depression in the bone** or defect in the bone
- Look for **cough impulse** (to rule out intracranial communication)
- Check the mobility (if it is bony it will not be mobile)
- Look for regional nodes.

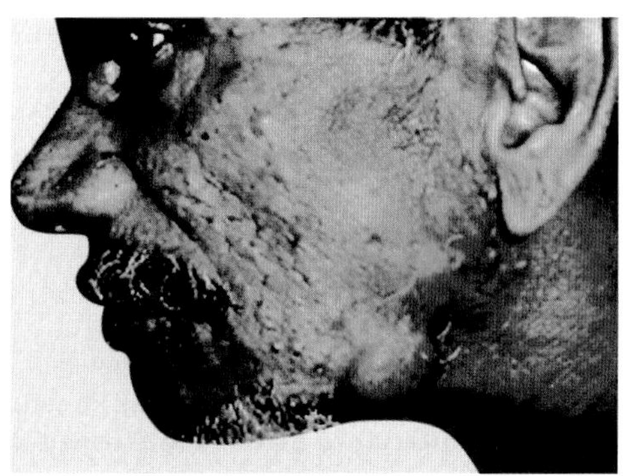

Sebaceous cyst on left side of cheek

Q 1. What is your clinical diagnosis in this case?
Sebaceous cyst.

Q 2. If the punctum is not there, what are the differential diagnoses?
1. Dermoid cysts.
2. Pulsatile bony swelling—primary/secondary.

Q 3. What are the primary pulsatile bony swellings?
1. Solitary plasmacytoma
2. Telangiectatic variety of osteogenic sarcoma.

Q 4. What are the causes for pulsatile bony metastasis in this region?
1. Metastasis from follicular thyroid cancer
2. Renal cell carcinoma metastasis.

Q 5. What is sebaceous cyst?
The skin is normally kept soft and oily by the **sebum** secreted by the sebaceous glands, **mouth of which open into the hair follicles.** If the mouth of a sebaceous gland is **blocked**, the gland will get distended by its own secretions producing sebaceous cyst.

Q 6. What is the plane of sebaceous cyst?
- All sebaceous cysts are attached to the skin
- The area of attachment may be small
- There is no independent movement of the cyst of the skin
- Part of the cyst will lie in the subcutaneous tissue.

Q 7. What is wen? Is there any other synonym for wen?
- It is a synonym for the sebaceous cyst of the scalp
- The other synonym is epidermoid cyst.

Q 8. Do the punctum exist in all cases?
Only 50% will have visible punctum. However all sebaceous cysts are attached to the skin. Punctum is some time **difficult to demonstrate especially in the scalp.**

Q 9. What is the "sign of indentation"?
Cysts containing pultaceous material can be moulded. When the swelling is indented with a finger, it stays indented in contradistinction to the sign of emptying.

Note: Pultaceous (Latin) = porridge.

Q 10. What are the conditions producing sign of indentation?

Conditions producing sign of indentation
- Lax sebaceous cyst
- Large dermoid
- Solid feces in sigmoid in the left iliac fossa.

Q 11. What is punctum?
The cyst is arising basically from a skin structure (sebaceous gland). The mouth of the sebaceous gland will open into the hair follicle or through a fine duct directly into the skin surface. **This point of fixation** is pulled inwards as the cyst grows to form the punctum. Gentle squeezing of the skin over the cyst will demonstrate the punctum.

Q 12. What are the classical sites for sebaceous cyst?
- It can occur wherever there are sebaceous glands
- They are found in the hairy parts of the body.

The sites are:

Classical sites for sebaceous cyst
- Scalp
- Scrotum
- Back
- Shoulders
- Neck
- Face.

Q 13. What is the age group affected?

- Rare before adolescence
- May appear suddenly during adolescence
- Most of them are seen in early adulthood and middle age.

Q 14. Mention two sites where sebaceous cyst will not occur?

- Palms
- Soles.

Note: There are no sebaceous glands in these regions.

Q 15. What is the syndrome associated with sebaceous cyst?

Gardner's syndrome

- Osteomas
- Intestinal polyposis
- Sebaceous cyst.

Q 16. What is the content of the cyst?

Toothpaste like, whitish, granular material with unpleasant smell (pultaceous).

Q 17. What are the complications of sebaceous cyst?

Complications of sebaceous cysts

- Infection
- Sebaceous horn
- Cock's peculiar tumor.

Q 18. What is sebaceous horn?

The slow discharge of sebum from a **wide punctum** hardens to form the horn. This will take the shape of a **conical spike**. Normally horn is not formed because soap and water and friction from cloths will remove the secretion of the gland. **Failure to wash the skin** over the cyst will result in horn. Wide punctum (opening) is seen after an infected cyst has ruptured. The horn can be broken off.

Q 19. What is Cock's peculiar tumor?

Suppurating and ulcerating sebaceous cyst is called Cock's peculiar tumor. It looks like a squamous cell carcinoma (SCC). This eponym is still used by surgeons for sentimental reasons.

It is an open, granulating and edematous sebaceous cyst. The granulation tissue arises from the lining of the cyst giving the lesion an everted edge. Because of the infection, the whole area is edematous, red and tender. The regional nodes may be enlarged unlike sebaceous cyst.

Q 20. What will be the history in such a case?

The usual history will be a long duration of swelling, followed by pain and discharge of pus from the swelling or history of inadequate incision of the swelling.

Q 21. How will you manage a sebaceous cyst?

1. FNAC
2. X-ray especially, if it is situated in the scalp (to rule out bony defect that will be seen in dermoid cyst or to rule out bone destruction seen in metastasis)
3. Rule out diabetes mellitus by doing blood sugar estimation.

Q 22. What is the surgical treatment of sebaceous cyst?

Excision under local anesthesia, using 1% or 2% lignocaine.

Q 23. What is the incision recommended?

An elliptical incision. The ellipse will encircle the punctum, so that the area of skin bearing the punctum is removed, along with the cyst. Try to remove the cyst intact along with the entire cyst wall.

Q 24. What is the treatment of infected sebaceous cyst?

- If frank pus is formed, incision and drainage is recommended, like any other abscess

- If it is inflammation alone, give a course of antibiotics and do elective excision.

Q 25. What will happen to the cyst after incision and drainage?

It will recur and need formal excision later on.

Q 26. What will be the histopathological feature of sebaceous cyst?

The content will be toothpaste like and fowl smelling and it will be lined by squamous epithelium.

Q 27. What are the differences between sebaceous cyst and dermoid cyst?

Sl. No.	*Features*	*Sebaceous cyst/Epidermoid cyst/Wen*	*Dermoid cyst*
1.	Cause	Due to blockage of duct of sebaceous gland	Congenital—sequestration of epithelial elements deep to the skin surface
2.	Site	Hair bearing site on the body—back, face, neck, scalp, scrotum	Along the lines of embryological skin fusion. External and internal angular dermoids, sublingual (superficial/deep), postauricular, pre and postsacral
3.	Skin-involvement	Present (tethering)	Not involved
4.	Punctum	Present	Absent
5.	Lining	Sebaceous cells/squamous epithelium	Skin with appendage, i.e. sebaceous glands, hair follicles and hair-(keratinized, stratified squamous epithelium)
6.	Content	Toothpaste like, whitish, fowl smelling material	Hair and sebaceous material
7.	Intracranial communication	No communication	Communication may be present
8.	Bony defect	No bony defect	Bony defect may be seen
9.	Palms and soles	No hair follicles and do not occur	Occur, e.g. implantation dermoid

Q 28. What are the classical sites of dermoid cysts?

- Dermoid cysts may be **congenital or acquired**.
- The example of **acquired dermoid** cyst is **implantation dermoid**, seen in the **hands and feet** as a result of trauma
- Congenital dermoid cysts are seen along the lines of embryological fusion:

Sites where congenital dermoid cysts are seen

- Midline of the body
- Sites where two embryonic processes meet:
  a. Outer angle of the orbit (frontonasal process and maxillary process fuse in this region)—**External angular dermoid**
  b. Behind pinna (**Postauricular**)
  c. Below the tongue (**sublingual dermoid**)
  d. **Pre and postsacral dermoid.**

Q 29. Why is the dermoid cyst at the outer angle of the orbit called external angular dermoid?

That is because it lies behind the outer end of the eyebrow, over the **external angular protuberance** of the skull. This is a congenital dermoid cyst.

Q 30. Can dermoid cyst occur at the inner end of the eyebrow (medial end of the eyebrow)?

Yes. It is called **internal angular dermoid.**

Q 31. What are the complications of external angular dermoid?

1. Bony depression—by pressure
2. Dumbbell extension into the orbit
3. Erosion of the orbital plate of frontal bone and getting attached to the dura.

Q 32. What is the peculiarity of postsacral dermoid?

It may expand within the spinal canal causing compression of the **cauda eqina.** The lesion may be present at birth but usually noted in the first two years and occasionally may be seen in adulthood.

Q 33. What is the cause for implantation dermoid?

They are usually traumatic. The surface ectoderm is being driven inside as a result of trauma (small cut or stab injury) and this will result in implantation dermoid. They are usually seen in fingers and toes. They may be sometimes **tense and hard.** History of **old injury or presence of a scar** will give the clue.

Q 34. What are the classical features of dermoid cyst?

Diagnostic features of dermoid cyst

1. Cystic swelling
2. Not transilluminant
3. The skin can be pinched (no punctum and therefore no tethering)—They are seen deep to the skin in the subcutaneous tissue
4. A bony depression or defect may be felt
5. Intracranial communication may be there.

Case

36 Ulcer

Case Capsule

A 20-year-old **male athlete** presents with an **ulcer** of size of **6 × 3 cm** over the shin of the leg of 6 months duration. He gives **history of trauma** to the shin region while playing followed by the development of ulcer. On examination, the floor of the ulcer is covered with red granulation tissue **surrounded by a blue line outer to the granulation** and white line further outside. There is minimal **serous discharge**. The ulcer is mobile and there is **no fixity** to the deeper structures. The vertical group of inguinal **nodes are enlarged and tender**. On examination, there is no evidence of varicose veins. The peripheral pulsations are normal. There are no sensory deficits and no other neurological problems. Systemic examination is normal.

Checklist for examination of ulcer

1. Examine the **site, edge floor, base and surrounding tissue (SEFBS)**
2. Look for **fixity** to underlying structures (check the movements of the ulcer)
3. Look for **peripheral pulsations** (arterial ulcer)

Contd...

Contd...

4. Look for **varicose veins** (venous ulcer)
5. Check for **sensations** (neuropathic ulcers)
6. Look for **nerve thickening**, hypopigmented patches and other stigmata of Hansen's disease (to rule out **Hansen's disease**)
7. Look for **movements of the joints** and **deformities** (deformity of the foot in DM equinus deformity in venous ulcer and deformity of Paget's disease of the bone)
8. Examine the **regional nodes** (vertical group of inguinal nodes are involved in lower limb ulcers)
9. Look for **stigmata of syphilis**
10. Examine for lymph nodes of neck, axilla, and inguinal region
11. Examination of the chest, to **rule out tuberculosis**
12. Rule out **diabetes mellitus**
13. Exclude anemia (including **sickle cell anemia**) and leukemia
14. Look for features of **rheumatoid arthritis**
15. Exclude **Paget's disease of the bone**
16. General neurological examination to **rule out nervous diseases**, spinal injuries, sciatic nerve injuries, etc.

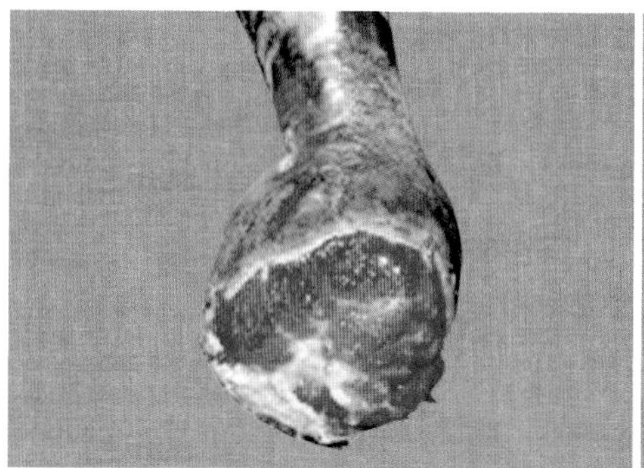
Diabetic foot after midtarsal amputation

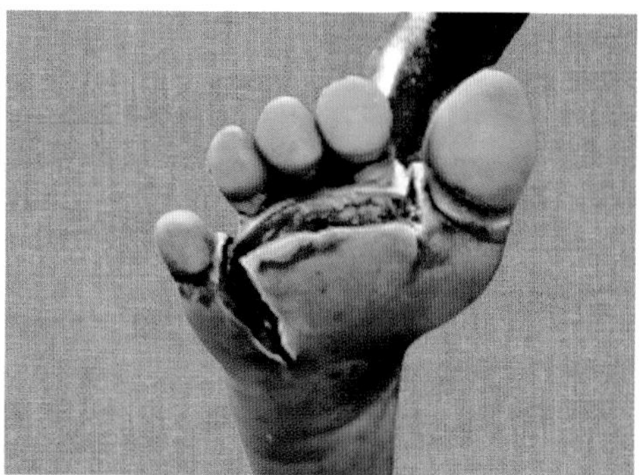
Diabetic foot after slough cutting

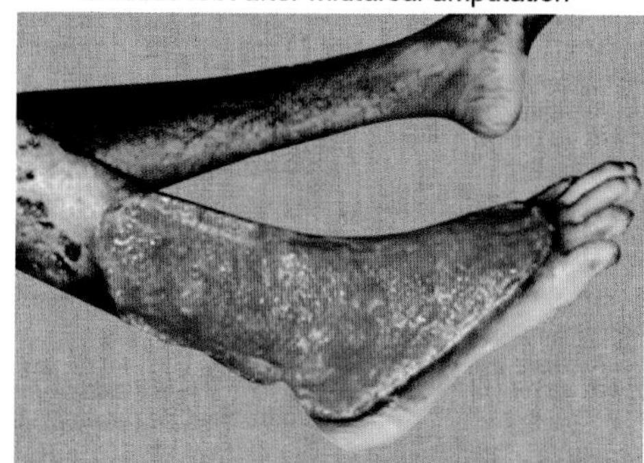
Healing ulcer on right dorsum of foot and leg with red granulation tissue

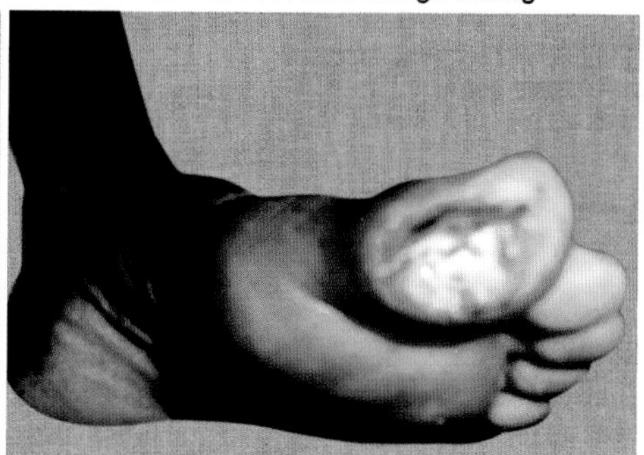
Ulcer of big toe

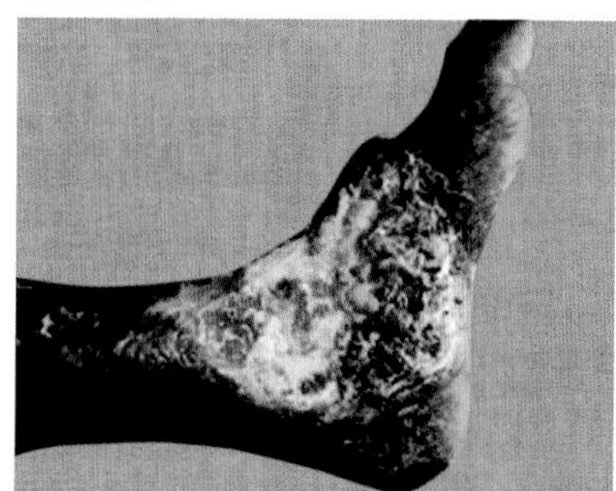
Venous ulcer with Marjolin's (malignant change)

Q 1. What is your diagnosis?

A healing traumatic ulcer.

Q 2. Why healing ulcer? Why traumatic?

Healing ulcer because:

- The floor is covered with red granulation
- The blue line outside the granulation is suggestive of growing epithelium
- The white line is suggestive of fibrous tissue
- There is no evidence of infection.

Traumatic because:

- No evidence of arterial, venous, neurological and other systemic problems
- Young athlete
- History of trauma is present.

Q 3. What is ulcer?

The ulcer is a break in the continuity of an epithelial surface that can occur in the skin or mucosa of the alimentary or respiratory passages.

Q 4. What is slough?

Slough is a piece of dead tissue.

Q 5. What is the classification of ulcer?

Ulcer may be classified as:

1. **Acute** or **chronic**
2. **Painful** or **painless** (malignant ulcers are painless in the early stages)
3. **Spreading ulcer** or **healing ulcer** or **callous ulcer**
4. **Nonspecific ulcer** or **specific ulcer** or **malignant ulcer**.

Q 6. What are the characteristics of healing ulcer?

Characteristics of healing ulcer

- The surrounding skin is not inflamed
- The edge shows **blue zone** (bluish outline of growing epithelium) and a **white zone** (fibrosis of the scar)
- Floor will have reddish granulation tissue
- Minimal serous discharge may be there.

Q 7. What are the characteristics of spreading ulcer?

Characteristics of spreading ulcer

- The surrounding skin of the ulcer is inflamed and edematous
- The floor is covered with slough
- No evidence of granulation tissue
- Discharge of pus will be there.

Q 8. What are the characteristics of callous ulcer?

Characteristics of callous ulcer

- Induration of the edge and surrounding tissue
- The floor will have pale granulation tissue
- No tendency towards healing
- Copious serous discharge.

Q 9. What are the causes for nonspecific ulcers?

The causes for nonspecific ulcers are:

1. **Traumatic**—(Footballers ulcer)
   - Physical—Electrical
   - Chemical—Caustics
   - Mechanical—Dental ulcer, pressure from splint, etc.
2. **Arterial**—Atherosclerosis, TAO, Raynaud's disease
3. **Venous**—Venous ulcer, postthrombotic ulcer, gravitational ulcer
4. **Neuropathic—(Neurotrophic** *or* **Perforating)** Diabetes, leprosy, tabes dorsalis, spina bifida, paraplegia, syringomyelia
5. **Tropical ulcers**—Tropical countries
6. **Metabolic**—Diabetes gout
7. **Secondary to diseases like:**
   - Rheumatoid arthritis
   - Erythrocyanosis frigida
   - Osteitis deformans (Paget's disease of the bone)
   - Avitaminosis

8. **Ulcers complicating blood diseases:**
   - Sickle cell anemia
   - Mediterranean anemia
   - Felty's syndrome (**look for spleen**)
9. **Ulcer occurring on paralyzed leg**—usually seen in anterior poliomyelitis
10. **Factitious ulcer** (artefact ulcer)
11. Diphtheritic desert sore
12. Yaws
13. Decubitus ulcer
14. Iatrogenic ulcer—extravasation of IV fluid
15. Ulcers in congenital **arteriovenous fistula**
16. Miscellaneous—**Martorell's ulcer.**

Q 10. What are the specific types of ulcers?

Examples of specific ulcers

- Tuberculosis
- Syphilitic
- Actinomycosis (bacterial)
- Soft sore
- Herpes simplex
- Fungal.

Q 11. What are the types of ulcers seen in syphilis?

- **Hunterian chancre (hard chancre)—Seen in primary syphilis**
  - About **3–4** weeks after exposure in the external genitalia
  - Ulcer is painless
  - **Lymph nodes are enlarged**
- **Gumma (lymph nodes are not involved)—Seen in tertiary syphilis**
  - Seen in subcutaneous bones like tibia, sternum, skull, and ulna
  - In relation to the testis
  - In the leg.

Q 12. What are the lesions in the secondary syphilis?

- Mucous patches—Sodden thickened epithelium
- Condylomas—Raised flat, white hypertrophied epithelium at the mucocutaneous junction (angles of mouth, anus, and vulva)
- Enlarged lymph nodes—**Epitrochlear**, and **sub-occipital nodes.**

Q 13. What is soft sore or soft chancre?

It is also called **Ducrey's ulcer**. They are multiple acute ulcers with yellowish slough seen in the external genitalia appearing 3 days after infection. They have copious purulent discharge. The regional lymph nodes are enlarged.

Q 14. What are the types of edges for the ulcer?

Edges may be:

Various types of edges of ulcer with examples

Sl no	*Type of edge*	*Examples*
1.	Sloping edge	Healing ulcers, venous ulcers
2.	Punched out edge	Syphilitic, trophic, ischemic and leprosy
3.	Undermined edge	Tuberculosis, bedsore, carbuncle
4.	Raised edge	Rodent ulcer (basal cell carcinoma)
5.	Everted edge	Squamous cell carcinoma (old name–epithelioma)

Q15. What is the cause for undermined edge in tuberculosis?

The tuberculosis destroys the subcutaneous tissue faster than it destroys the skin. The overhanging skin in this case is blue and unhealthy.

Q 16. What are the differences between floor and base?

- The **floor** is what you see and the **base** is what you feel
- The floor is the exposed surface of the ulcer.
- The base is on which the ulcer rests
- Pick up the ulcer between the thumb and index finger for feeling the base
- Slight induration is seen normally for any ulcer
- Marked induration is a feature of squamous cell carcinoma.

Q 17. What are the classical sites for the commonly seen ulcers?

Classical sites for commonly seen ulcers

Type of ulcer	*Site*
Venous ulcer	Just above the medial malleolus (**Gaiter area**)
Arterial ulcer	**Tips of toes and between the toes** (where the pressure is lowest), over the malleoli and heel (pressure areas)
Neuropathic ulcer	Over the **heads of the first and second metatarsal.**
Traumatic ulcer (footballer's ulcer)	**Shin** (the tibia is subcutaneous and there is lack of underlying muscle with resultant reduced blood supply)
Rodent ulcer (BCC)	**Above a line joining the angle of the mouth to the lobule of the ear**
Tuberculous ulcer	Seen in **neck, axilla and groin** (where tuberculous lymph nodes are seen)
Gummatous ulcer	Over the **subcutaneous bones** such as sternum, skull, tibia, etc.
Trophic ulcers	On the heel and ball of the foot.

Q18. What are the stigmata of Hansen's disease?

Stigmata of Hansen's disease

There are **three types of leprosy**—the lepromatous, tuberculoid and mixed

Lepromatous leprosy

- Leonine facies (subcutaneous tissue becomes infiltrated with granulomatous masses)
- Loss of outer half of the eyebrow hair
- Destruction of nasal cartilages—saddle nose deformity
- Testicular atrophy
- Gynecomastia

Tuberculoid

- Nerve paralysis
- Look for tender thickening of the following nerves
  - Ulnar nerve at the elbow
  - Great auricular nerve in the posterior triangle below the ear
  - Lateral popliteal nerve around the neck of fibula
- Ulnar claw hand
- Claw foot
- Trophic ulcers.

Q 19. What are the stigmata of syphilis?

Syphilitic stigmata

- Alopecia (loss of hair)
- Bossing of the skull
- Depression of the bridge of the nose
- Interstitial keratitis
- Otitis interna
- Perforation of the nasal septum
- Perforation of the hard palate
- Chronic superficial glossitis
- Hutchinson's teeth
- Mucous patches
- Condylomas
- Enlarged occipital lymph nodes
- Enlarged epitrochlear lymph nodes
- Gummatous orchitis
- Clutton's joints
- Sabre tibia.

Q 20. What is the peculiarity of venous ulcer in relation to the depth of penetration?

The venous ulcers usually do **not extend beyond the deep fascia**, unlike ischemic ulcers, which destroys the deep fascia and exposes the tendons, bones and joints.

Q 21. What are the types of discharges from the ulcer?

Types of discharges and the probable causes

Discharge	*Cause*
• Serous discharge	In healing ulcer
• Serosanguinous discharge	Tuberculous ulcer
• Greenish/bluish pseudomonas	Ulcer infected with
• Yellow discharge and creamy pus	Staphylococci
• Watery and opalescent	*Streptococcus*
• Yellow granules	Actinomycosis

Q 22. What is the significance of granulation tissue?

Granulation tissue signifies healing. It is usually pink with red dots. The red dots are seen at the sites of capillary loops.

Q 23. What is the significance of bluish granulation tissue in the floor?

It is suggestive of tuberculosis (*Apple-jelly granulation*).

Q 24. What is Wash-leather appearance (wet chamois leather)?

It is suggestive of syphilitic ulcer—gummatous ulcer.

Q 25. If the floor is covered with black mass what is the inference?

It is suggestive of malignant melanoma.

Q26. What is neurotrophic ulcer (perforating)?

Neurotrophic ulcers are seen in the following conditions:

Causes for neurotrophic ulcer

1. Diabetic neuropathy (peripheral neuritis)
2. Transverse myelitis
3. Syringomyelia
4. Tabes dorsalis
5. Spina bifida
6. Injury to spinal cord
7. Sciatic nerve injury
8. Hansen's disease (Leprosy).

Q 27. What are the characteristic features of tuberculous ulcer?

The tuberculous ulcer results as a result of bursting of caseous lymph node. It is seen in places where tuberculous lymph nodes are seen-neck, axilla and groin.

The characteristic features are as follows:

Features of tuberculous ulcer

1. Undermined edge
2. Sites—axilla, neck and groin (where tuberculous nodes are seen)
3. Floor is covered with blue granulation tissue (**Apple - jelly** *granulation)*
4. Serosanguinous discharge from the ulcer.

Q 28. What is lupus vulgaris?

It is nothing but cutaneous tuberculosis seen in the face and hand. The ulcer heels at the center and spreads at the periphery (**like a wolf**) and hence the name **lupus means wolf**.

Q 29. What are the characteristic features of venous ulcer (Named by John Gay in 1867)?

- They are seen in the **Gaiter area** of the leg (between the two malleoli and the tibial tuberosity)—usually above and behind the medial malleolus
- The ulcer is painless
- Ulcer never penetrates the deep fascia
- Surrounding skin will be pigmented and thickened (**lipodermatosclerosis**)
- One or more large feeding veins can be seen proceeding towards the edge of the ulcer
- Varicose veins affecting the long saphenous, short saphenous and perforating veins will be visible.

Q 30. What are the precursors of venous ulcer?

- Dermatitis (eczema)
- Pigmentation (sign of venous stasis)
- Splay of venules from the medial malleolus (**flare sign**).

Q 31. What is post-thrombotic ulcer?

Venous ulcer may be secondary to **deep vein thrombosis** and subsequent valvular incompetence resulting in chronic venous hypertension **or** it may be secondary to the **superficial system incompetence**. When it is secondary to deep vein thrombosis, it is called post-thrombotic ulcer. The peculiarity of this ulcer is it will be **painful**. In such cases, **varicose veins are lacking** in spite of careful search. Extensive **induration** is a remarkable feature in this case. The skin appears to be tethered to the underlined structures, which may extend half way up of the calf.

Q 32. What is gravitational ulcer?

It is another name for venous ulcer.

Q 33. What are the characteristic features of arterial ulcer?

- They are usually seen at the tips of toes and between the toes (heel and malleoli).
- Seen in usually older age group
- Destroys the deep fascia and expose the tendons
- Ulcers are punched out
- Peripheral pulsations will be absent.

Q 34. What is Meleney's ulcer?

It is also called **synergistic ulcer (symbiotic)**. It is due to symbiotic action of **microaerophilic nonhemolytic streptococci** and **hemolytic** *Staphylococcus aureus.* This was originally described in relation to the infected **abdominal and thoracic operation wounds**. However, it can occur in the leg and hands, arising either *de novo* are as a complication of preexisting ulcers. The characteristic feature of the ulcer is burrowing with a resultant **undermined edge**, which may extend for 2 cm. The ulcer is **painful and tender** and shows a tendency to spread. There will be a **central purplish zone surrounded by red inflammation** initially. This purplish zone becomes gangrenous producing an ulcer.

Q 35. What is factitious ulcer (Artefact ulcer)?

It is also called **automutilation ulcer**. This is a **self-induced** ulcer of the leg seen in highly neurotic individuals or in a litigant desirous of obtaining compensation. The mode of producing the ulcer varies. The ulcer is situated always in **accessible places** like anterior and lateral surface of the leg. Usually the ulcer will have clean pink healthy look with unusual shapes. If the ulcer is covered with, plaster cast so that the wound cannot be tampered the wound will heal.

Q 36. What is the feature of ulcer associated with Erythrocyanosis frigida (Bazin's Disease)?

This is usually seen in **young women** with plump legs and thick ankles living in cold climates. The patients are troubled by **chilblains**. Small superficial painful nodules will be felt in the legs, which are areas of fat necrosis, which will breakdown to form the ulcers. In addition, the blood supply to the lower third of the leg will be diminished producing ischemia of the leg. The skin is abnormally sensitive to temperature changes.

Q 37. What is the cause for ulcer in rheumatoid arthritis?

This is seen in 20% of the patients. It is due to **breakdown of a nodule**. The ulcers may be more than one having punched out edge seen in the **lateral surface of the lower third of the leg**.

Q 38. What is the situation of the ulcer secondary to osteitis deformans (Paget's disease)?

These small deep ulcers are situated right over the convexity of the anteriorly bowed tibia. The base of the ulcer is bone and the edges are densely adherent to the bone.

Q 39. What is tropical ulcer?

This ulcer is due to infection by **Vincent's organism** (**Bacteroides fusiformis**) together with many pyogenic bacteria, secondary to trauma or insect bite. It commences as a papulo pustule which in a matter of hours becomes surrounded by a zone of inflammation and induration. This is accompanied by tender lymphadenitis. In two or three days the pustule bursts and ulcer forms. The edges are undermined. There is copious serosanguinous discharge. The ulcer will remain indolent for a long time. Pain is a constant feature.

The classical features are:

- Profuse serosanguinous discharge
- Over powering vile odor
- Unremitting pain
- Minimal constitutional symptoms
- Extreme tenacity of the slough.

On healing it leaves a permanent scar which is circular, parchment like and faintly pigmented.

Q 40. What is the feature of ulcer due to Yaws?

The causative organism is *Treponema pertenue*. The primary sore may be found on the **legs or foot or buttocks** (of children before they walk). They are painless and in the course of healing form **tissue paper like scars**. In the tertiary stage multiple deep ulcers are seen.

Q 41. What is diphtheritic desert sore?

As the name implies it is seen in the desert. The organism responsible is *Corynebacterium diphtheriae*. It begins as a **papulo-pustule**. Within a few days it will form an ulcer reaching the size of 1–2 cm. The floor will be covered by **diphtheritic membrane**, which will be difficult to remove. Rarely the patient shows **signs of peripheral neuritis** due to toxins produce by diphtheria.

Q 42. What is Martorell's ulcer (hypertensive ulcer)?

This is seen in **old age group with atherosclerosis**. A patch of skin on the outer side of the calf suddenly becomes gangrenous and sloughs away producing a punched out ulcer. Even though it is an ischemic ulcer **all the peripheral pulses will be normal**.

Q 43. What is decubitus ulcer?

It is a synonym for **bedsore**. It is a type of direct traumatic gangrene. The bedsores are predisposed by factors like:

- Pressure
- Injury
- Moisture
- Anemia
- Malnutrition.

They typically appear over areas subjected to pressure like sacrum, gluteal region and heel in bedridden patients.

Q 44. What is the warning signal for bedsore?

The bedsore is to be expected over an erythema, which does not change color on pressure.

Q 45. How will you prevent bed sore?

Prevention of bedsore

- Skilled nursing
- Frequent change of position (2 hourly change of posture)
- Use of adhesive films such as Opsite
- Water bed—ripple bed
- Keep the area dry.

Q 46. Is there an entity called diabetic ulcer?

No diabetic ulcers are of multiple etiologies and therefore it is important to identify the cause of the ulcer in diabetes. The various causes for ulcer formation in diabetes mellitus are:

1. *Arterial*
   - Atherosclerosis (10 years earlier than the normal population)
   - Microvascular.
2. *Neuropathy*
   - Sensory—glove and stocking type of peripheral neuropathy
   - Motor (Intrinsic muscle paralysis with resultant unopposed action of long flexor tendons → shortening of the longitudinal arches → heads of metatarsals are subjected to additional load during walking).
   - Autonomic—Dry skin due to the absence of sweating
3. *Deformity* in diabetic foot.

Therefore in a given case the ulcer may be purely neuropathic or arterial or it may be a combination of factors, which the student has to identify.

Q 47. What is the commonest site for neuropathic ulcer in diabetes?

Over the heads of the first and second metatarsals.

Q 48. What is Marjolin's ulcer?

It's a **malignant ulcer** developing in **burns scar or venous ulcer** or edge of any **chronic ulcer** or **chronic discharging sinuses** such as osteomyelitis is called **Marjolin's ulcer**. Malignant change can occur in the tuberculous skin scarring of lupus vulgaris. It is nothing but a **squamous cell carcinoma** of skin with everted edges or **rolled out edges.** These changes can be easily missed and the **clinician must always be on the look out for any changes in the edge**. The peculiarity of this malignancy is the absence of involvement of regional lymph nodes. The scarring process in this condition destroys the lymphatics in the ulcer area.

Q 49. What is the management of the ulcer?

The principles of management of the ulcer are as follows:

1. Identify and correct the **comorbid factors** like **DM, anemia, leukemia, etc.** by doing:
   - FBS—If diabetic, control the diabetes
   - PPBS
   - Peripheral smear
   - Hemoglobin
   - Total leukocyte count
   - X-ray chest—to rule out tuberculosis.
2. **Determine the etiology of the ulcer:**
   - Biopsy from the edge of ulcer
   - If pus is present, send for culture and sensitivity and give appropriate antibiotic
   - X-ray of the part to rule out osteomyelitis.
3. **Adequate drainage and de sloughing**

4. **Care of the ulcer:**
    - Daily dressing
    - **Avoid antiseptic solutions**—impair capillary circulation
    - Use normal saline for cleaning
    - Use nonadherent and nonallergic dressing
    - Use microporous polyurethane film which are permeable to gases and water and impermeable to microorganisms.
5. **Treat the underlying cause:**
    - For example, Antituberculous drugs in the case of tuberculous ulcer
    - Treat the varicose veins in the case of venous ulcer
    - Revascularization in the case of arterial ulcers.
6. **Excision of the ulcer and skin grafting:** If the ulcer is not healing.

Case

37 Malignant Melanoma

Case Capsule

A 65-year-old male patient presenting with an **ulcer over the right heel** of size **5 cm** diameter of 8 months duration. On examination, the floor of the ulcer is covered with **black-colored granulation tissue**. The ulcer is not mobile and there is fixity to the deeper structures. The vertical group of **inguinal nodes are enlarged**, firm in consistency, discrete and mobile. Two horizontal group (medial) of nodes are also enlarged, which are firm discrete and mobile. Systemic examination is normal.

'Beware of the patient with a glass eye, and missing toe'

Read the checklist for examination of the ulcer.

Checklist for history

1. Family history of malignant melanoma
2. History of risk factors—**Sun exposure**
3. History of nonmelanoma skin cancer
4. History of **change in size, shape, color, inflammation, crusting, bleeding,** etc. of the mole
5. History of **increase in size**
6. History of **enucleation of the eye** and operations on the skin.

Checklist for examination

1. Look for the **ABCDE** of melanoma that is mentioned below
2. Look for **satellite nodules** and intransit metastasis
3. Look for **regional lymph nodes**
4. Look for **missing toes and glass eyes**
5. Intense search is made for the primary when the patient is presenting with metastatic nodes
6. Examine the abdomen to rule out **hepatomegaly**
7. Examine the chest for evidence of metastasis.

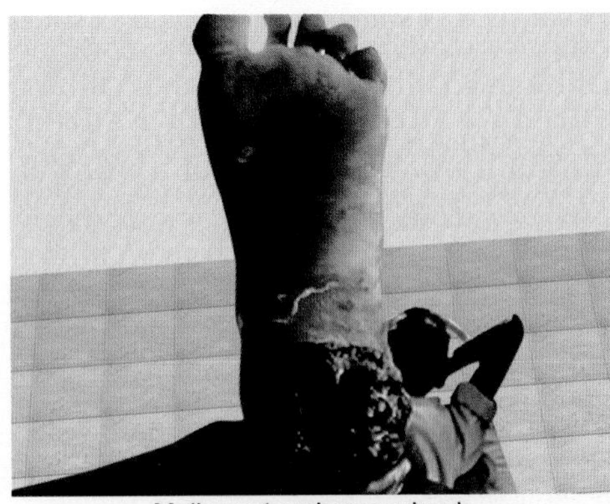

Malignant melanoma heel

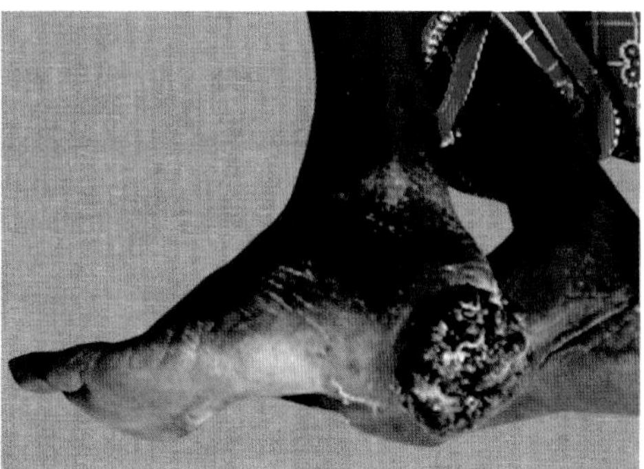

Malignant melanoma of left heel

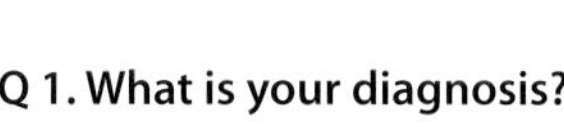

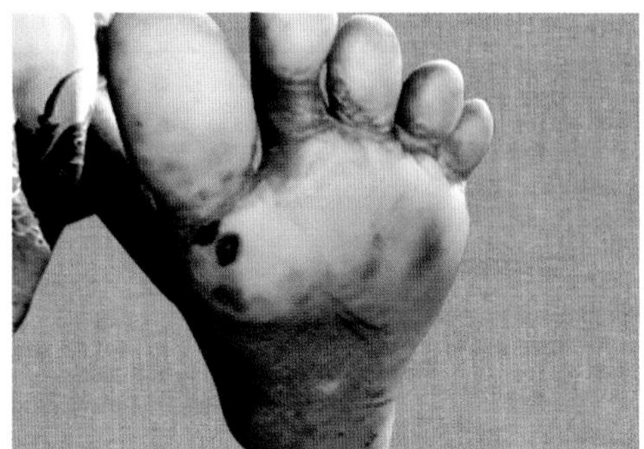

Two pigmented lesions in the forefoot — malignant melanoma

Q 1. What is your diagnosis?

Malignant melanoma.

Q 2. Why malignant melanoma?

An ulcer with black pigmented floor and enlarged inguinal nodes is in favor of diagnosis of malignant melanoma.

Q 3. What is malignant melanoma?

It is a skin neoplasm arising from **melanocytes**, a cell of **neural origin**.

Q 4. What are the differential diagnoses?

Differential diagnoses for malignant melanoma

1. Pigmented basal cell carcinoma
2. Junctional nevus
3. Seborrheic warts
4. Thrombosedangioma
5. Hemangioma
6. Telangiectasis
7. Granuloma.

Q 5. What are the organs where melanoma can occur?

Organs involved in malignant melanoma

- Skin
- Eye:
  a. Uveal tract – Iris
     – Ciliary body
     – Choroids
  b. Retina
- Meninges
- Mucocutaneous junction
- Conjunctiva.

Q 6. What are the modes of spread of malignant melanoma?

Modes of spread of malignant melanoma

1. Direct extension
2. Lymphatic—embolism and permeation
3. Hematogenous
   – Lungs
   – Liver

Contd...

Contd...

- Brain
- Bones
- Intestines
- Breast.

Q 7. What is the spread of malignant melanoma of the uveal tract?

There are no lymphatics in the uveal tract. They rarely metastasize to lymph nodes.

Q 8. What is a nevus?

The word nevus means a lesion that is present since birth.

Q 9. What is a mole?

Benign melanin producing lesions are called moles.

Q 10. What is the average number of moles a person will have?

About 80–100 moles in most Caucasians.

Q 11. In which area of the body moles are commonly seen?

They are most common in **limbs, face and mucocutaneous junctions** (the mouth and anus).

Q 12. What are the layers of the skin?

The skin has got **epidermis** and **dermis**.

The epidermis has got five layers.

The five layers of the epidermis are:

- Stratum corneum
- Stratum lucidum
- Stratum granulosum
- Stratum spinosum (prickle cell layer)
- Stratum basale (Basal layer).

Q 13. In which layer of the skin the melanocytes are seen?

They are normally found in small numbers among the cells of the **basal layer of epidermis**.

Q 14. What is melanoblast? (PG)

They are believed to originate in the neural crest. They have the power of forming the pigment and they are seen in the basal layer of epidermis. The cells are **Dopa positive and Fontana positive.**

Q 15. What are melanophores? (PG)

They are dermal macrophages carrying the pigment. They are Dopa negative and Fontana positive.

Q 16. What is the pathology of a mature adult mole? (Intradermal mole)

They consist of clusters of melanocytes in the dermis and therefore, they are called **intradermal mole**. Macroscopically the mole can be **flat or raised, smooth or warty, hairy or nonhairy**. They hardly ever turn malignant.

Q 17. What is a junctional mole?

If the movement of the melanocytes stop before they have all migrated into the dermis, there will be clusters of cells at various stages of maturity **in the epidermis and dermis**. This lesion is called junctional mole. **Junctional moles are immature and unstable and can turn malignant.** The majority of the malignant melanomas begin in junctional moles.

Q 18. In which part of the skin you get junctional moles?

- Palms of the hands
- Soles of the feet
- External genitalia.

Note: Higher incidence of malignant melanoma is seen in these sites.

Q 19. What is a compound mole?

When **intradermal and junctional features** are both present in one mole, it is called compound mole.

Q 20. What is juvenile mole (spitz nevus)?

A mole showing junctional activity before puberty is

called juvenile mole (**pigmented spitz nevus**). They finally become mature intradermal moles.

Q 21. What is a blue nevus?

When the melanocytes migrate to the bottom of the dermis and into the subcutaneous tissue, the lesion will get a blue appearance and it is called a blue nevus.

Q 22. In which ethnic group malignant melanoma is more common?

It is more common in Caucasians living in hot countries such as Australia (because of the greater quantity of UV light exposure). It is less common in Negroes.

Q 23. What is the incidence of malignant melanoma?

- The incidence of malignant melanoma is rising
- It forms 3% of all malignancies
- It forms 5% of the cutaneous malignancy
- 7% present as occult metastasis
- 10 – 20% occur in pre-existing nevi
- Seen 20 times more in whites
- Lowest incidence in Asia
- The incidence has doubled in Britain, Norway, Canada and America
- The incidence has quadrupled in Australia.

Q 24. What are the types of malignant melanoma?

Types of malignant melanoma
• Superficial spreading
• Nodular
• Lentigo malignant
• Acrolentigenous
• Amelanotic.

Q 25. What are the growth phases of malignant melanomatous lesions?

It has two types of growth:

1. *Radial growth phase*, e.g. the superficial spreading type (all melanomas show radial growth phase **except nodular melanoma**. Radial growth is an **intraepidermal growth**).
2. *Vertical growth phase*, e.g. the nodular melanoma (The vertical growth is the **tumor growth in dermis** leading to nodule formation).

Q 26. What are the features of superficial spreading type of malignant melanoma?

- It forms 70% of the lesions
- Peak incidence in the 5th decade
- Common in legs and back
- Long radial growth phase
- May arise in pre-existing nevus
- Wood's lamp can identify radial growth phase
- Dark brown, blue, black, pink or gray, white in color.

Q 27. What are the features of nodular melanoma?

- It is the most malignant type of melanoma
- Forms 15% of the lesions, twice common in men
- Predominant growth phase is vertical
- Common in trunk, head and neck
- Twice common in men
- Ulceration of the lesion is seen
- Crust formation also seen.

Q 28. What are the features of lentigo malignant melanoma?

- It forms 5–10% of the lesions
- It is an in situ variant with less metastatic potential
- It arises in Hutchinson's melanotic freckle
- Seen in old age (women more)
- Seen in sun exposed skin (prolonged and intense exposure)
- Lesions are mainly seen in head and neck
- 5 mm margin is enough for excision.

Q 29. What is Hutchinson's lentigo?

1. This is a term used to describe a large area of dark pigmentation, seen commonly on the face and neck in late adult life. It has got two special features:

2. Late development
3. High incidence of malignant change.

Some pathologists consider this as **pre-cancerous**. The surface is smooth with some raised areas suggesting the sites of junctional activity.

Q 30. What is Hutchinson's halo?

- This is a halo of brown pigment in the skin around the melanoma and satellite nodules. The halo is suggestive of malignant change in a pre-existing mole.

Q 31. What are the features of acral lentiginous?

- It affects the palms, soles, and beneath the nails (subungual)
- More seen in dark skinned group—70% of melanomas in black, 46% in Asians (It will affect any ethnic group)
- No history of sun exposure
- It forms 2–8% of the melanomas in white
- 46% of melanomas in Asians
- Usually > 3 cm in size
- Late presentation is a common feature
- The melanoma is more aggressive.

Q 32. Why the amelanotic melanoma is called so?

About 25% are amelanotic.

Here the malignant melanomatous lesion is not black and they appear as white. Therefore, it is called amelanotic melanoma.

Q 33. What are the features of amelanotic melanoma?

- The prognosis of this type is worse than nodular melanoma
- The lesions appear pink
- There will be delay in the diagnosis
- In GI tract it will produce obstruction.

Q 34. What is the ABCDE system for evaluation of pigmented skin lesion?

Look for the following things in a pre-existing pigmented lesion. If they are present it is suggestive of malignancy.

ABCDE system for evaluation of malignant change in a pigmented lesion
A – Asymmetry
B – Border irregularity
C – Color – variegation
D – Diameter > 6 mm
E – Elevation

Q 35. What is the Glasgow seven point checklist?

Glasgow seven point checklist
1. Change in size
2. Change in shape
3. Change in color
4. Inflammation
5. Crusting and bleeding
6. Sensory change
7. Diameter > 6 mm.

Q 36. What is satellite lesion?

Intralymphatic metastatic lesion within 2 cm of the primary tumor is called satellite lesion. This is considered as an extension of the primary and is categorized as N_2C (stage III C) in the new AJCC 7th edition.

Q 37. What is intransit metastasis?

Intralymphatic metastasis more than 2 cm from the primary lesion but not beyond regional lymph node basin is called intransit metastasis (N_2C).

Q 38. What are the risk factors incriminated in malignant melanoma?

The various risk factors are:

1. Sun exposure—most common (50%)—sun exposure before the age of 10 years and significant adult exposure
2. Multiple atypical nevi
3. Multiple benign nevi > 100
4. GCPN—Giant congenital pigmented nevus – 3–5% life time risk for malignant melanoma
5. Dysplastic nevus syndrome
6. Xeroderma pigmentosum
7. Nonmelanoma skin cancer (NMSC)
8. Previous malignant melanoma skin cancer
9. Immunosuppression (HIV, Hodgkin's)
10. Use of tanning lamps/photochemotherapy
11. Family history of malignant melanoma (8–12%)
12. Red hair
13. Tendency to freckle.

Q 39. What is the role of heredity in malignant melanoma?

- Familial malignant melanoma
- When three first degree relatives are affected it should be suspected
- There will be mutation in CDKN2A gene
- Genetic predisposition
- 8 – 12% of all melanomas are hereditary
- Second primary will be seen in 3–5% of cases.

Q 40. What is Breslow's thickness?

The thickness of the melanomatous lesion is measured from the top of the granular cell layer, to the base of the tumor with the help of **ocular micrometer**. This is called Breslow's thickness, that is the **most important prognostic factor** for malignant melanoma. **The original dimensions described by Breslow are not considered now for classification.**

Q 41. What is a thin melanoma?

A melanoma that is **less than 1 mm** is called thin melanoma. The survival of patients with this lesion is 95%.

Q 42. What is intermediate thickness lesion?

Lesions of thickness between **1 – 4 mm** are called intermediate thick lesions.

Q 43. What is thick melanoma?

Lesion with thickness more than 4 mm is called thick melanoma.

Q 44. What are the bad prognostic factors for melanoma? (PG)

The bad prognostic factors are:

Bad prognostic factors
1. Tumor thickness in mm is the most important prognostic indicator
2. LDH
3. Mitotic rate
4. Tumor infiltrating lymphocytes (TIL)
5. Ulceration—more than 3 mm ulcer
6. Vertical growth phase
7. Regression.

Q 45. What is the new AJCC staging system for malignant melanoma (7th edition)? (PG)

The summary of changes in 7th edition are:

- Mitotic rate is an important primary tumor prognostic factor and replaces level of invasion
- Nodal micrometastasis can be defined by H & E or immunohistochemical staging
- Metastatic melanoma in LN, skin, and s/c tissue from an unknown primary site is categorized as stage III rather than stage IV
- Sentinal LN biopsy is recommended for indentifying occult stage III disease in patients with clinical stage IB or II melanomas
- Thickness and ulceration in contrast to level of invasion used in T-category are still used
- Satellite mets and intransit metastasis grouped into stage IIIc disease.

T–classification

TX: Primary tumor cannot be assessed (e.g. curettaged or severely regressed melanoma)
T0: No evidence of primary tumor
Tis: Melanoma in situ.

T Classification	Thickness (mm)	Ulceration status/mitoses
T1	Tumor < 1 mm	a = without ulceration and mitosis < 1/mm^2 b = with ulceration or mitosis ≥ 1/mm^2
T2	Tumor 1 – 2 mm	a = without ulceration b = with ulceration
T3	Tumor 2 – 4 mm	a = without ulceration b = with ulceration
T4	Tumor > 4 mm	a = without ulceration b = with ulceration

Note:
- Ulceration is defined pathologically as full thickness epidermal defect including absence of stratum corneum and basement membrane
- 1 mm^2 is approximately 4 high power fields at 400 X in most microscopes.

Regional lymph nodes

NX	Regional lymph nodes cannot be assessed
N0	No regional lymph node metastasis
N1	Metastasis in **one lymph node** (**a**) micrometastasis, (**b**) macrometastasis
N2	Metastasis in **two to three regional nodes or intralymphatic** regional metastasis without nodal metastases **(a)** micrometastasis, **(b)** macrometastasis, **(c)** in transit mets/sat mets without metastatic LN
N3	Metastasis in **four or more** regional nodes, or matted metastatic nodes, **or intransit metastasis or satellite (s) with metastasis in regional node**

Distal metastasis (M)

M0	No distant metastasis
M1	Distant metastasis
M1a	Metastasis to distant skin, subcutaneous tissues or distant lymph node metastasis with **normal LDH**
M1b	Metastasis to lung with **normal LDH**
M1c	Metastasis to all other visceral sites or distant metastasis to any site combined with an **elevated serum lactic dehydrogenase (LDH).**

Clinical stage grouping (used after complete excision of the primary melanoma with clinical assessment for regional and distant metastasis).

Stage	*Tumor size*	*N*	*M*
0	Tis	N0	M0
IA	T1a	N0	M0
IB	T1b	N0	M0
	T2a	N0	M0
IIA	T2b	N0	M0
	T3a	N0	M0
IIB	T3b	N0	M0
	T4a	N0	M0
IIC	T4b	N0	M0
IIIA	Any T	1 – 3 lymph nodes with microscopic metastasis Primary melanoma not ulcerated	
IIIB	Any T	1 – 3 lymph nodes with macroscopic mets and non-ulcerated primary or 1 – 3 microscopic lymph nodes with ulceration or intralymphatic regional mets without nodal mets	

Contd...

Contd...

IIIC	Any T	1 – 3 macroscopic lymph nodes + ulcerated primary melanoma or Patients with satellite/intransit of ulcerated melanoma or Any patient with N3 regardless of T status	
IV	Any T	Any N	M1

Q 46. What is Clark's level?

This is used for the pathological assessment of the **depth of invasion** of the malignant melanoma. Because of the discrepancy in assessment of the pathological depth among pathologists Clark's level is used only for **T1 lesions.**

Clark's levels for depth of invasion	
Level I	Lesion confined to the epidermis
Level II	Lesion extending to the papillary dermis
Level III	Lesion filling the papillary dermis
Level IV	Lesion involving the reticular dermis
Level V	Lesion extending to the subcutaneous tissue

Q 47. What is the confirmatory investigation for the diagnosis of this lesion?

Biopsy.

Q 48. What type of biopsy is recommended and what are the precautions taken?

- **Excision biopsy is the procedure of choice,** elliptical incision is preferred.
- Consider definitive therapy before choosing technique
- 1 to 3 mm margin preferred
- Avoid wider margin to permit accurate subsequent lymphatic mapping
- Orientation of incision and specimen are important
- Biopsy up to the subcutaneous tissue
- There is no role for shave biopsies
- Incision biopsy is done only for large lesions—The incision biopsy may be taken from the thickest part as the last resort. It will interfere with the accurate Breslow's thickness determination that decides the ultimate excision margin (some areas may be thicker than others and therefore, full histological examination is not possible). It is also done for lesions of the face and ear
- Thickness of the lesion should be reported
- The deep fascia is not excised, unless involved
- In other places it is better to consider a split skin graft or fasciocutaneous flap.

Note: Original excision margin recommended by Handley in 1907 was 5 cm, that is having no clinical evidence support.

Q 49. What are the current guideline for the margin of excision?

- In situ – 0.5 cm
- Less than 1 mm thickness lesion – 1 cm margin and primary closure
- 1 – 2 mm thickness lesion – 2 cm margin is recommended
- More than 2 mm thickness lesion – 2 cm margin

Q 50. What is the margin of excision recommended for subungual melanoma?

1 cm margin is not possible in this situation without excision of the terminal phalanx. In general amputation of the digit is recommended.

Q 51. What are the diagnostic immunohistochemical markers for malignant melanoma? (PG)

Immunohistochemistry must include at least one melanoma specific marker. They are:

- HMB—45 (Premelanosomal protein)
- Melan—A
- Mart 1

Q 52. What is the management of lymph node?

- If clinically enlarged FNAC is preferable to excision biopsy for confirmation
- Open biopsy may increase the risk of tumor spillage
- If open biopsy is required the incision should be placed in such a way that it can be excised in continuity with lymph node field.

Q 53. What is the management of positive node?

- Therapeutic radical lymph node dissection is recommended
- For the lower limb it is radical ilioinguinal block dissection
- Limited dissections such as superficial femoral dissection and node picking are not recommended.

Q 54. What is the role of elective lymph node dissection—ELND (means managing the nodes, which are not involved)? (PG)

- Only 25% of the patients will show histological occult metastasis in such dissection
- It is unnecessary, therefore, in 75% of patients
- There is no survival advantage for ELND
- Thus, it is not recommended routinely.

The arguments in favor of ELND are:

- Incidence of positive nodes is 25–65%
- Survival rate are lower in patients who develop nodes
- The recurrence rate is higher when there is extracapsular spread or multiple nodes
- Patient may fail to attend regular follow-up
- The node dissection carries negligible morbidity.

Q 55. What is sentinel lymph node biopsy? (PG)

Indications are T_1b, T_2, T_3 and T_4 melanoma with clinically or radiologically uninvolved lymph nodes. It is done **prior to wide excision.** The anatomical concept is that lymphatics from defined regions of skin drain specifically to an initial node or nodes (sentinel nodes) prior to disseminating to other nodes in the same or nearby basins.

Sentinel lymph node biopsy is a technique initially described by **Cabanas** in **1974** for penile carcinoma. This was popularized by **Morton** in **1994** for melanoma. The aim of this technique is to identify those patients in whom it may be appropriate to carry out elective lymph node dissection by identifying the micrometastasis in the sentinel node.

Preoperative method—lymphoscintigraphy

The technique is to identify the first **echelon lymph node** (sentinel node) by **lymphoscintigraphy** following intradermal injection of **radioactive technetium^{99} sulfur colloid** around the primary site. A **hand held gamma probe** helps to locate the node. The position of this node is marked on the skin surface.

Perioperative method

The lymph node is identified intra-operatively by injecting **patent blue dye** around the site of the primary lesion. The node is removed and subjected for frozen section examination. If the node is found to be, pathologically positive radical lymph node dissection is carried out.

Q 56. What are the advantages of sentinel lymph node biopsy? (PG)

The node is send for frozen section, routine H and E staining and immunohistochemical staining.

- The pathologist can study 1 to 2 nodes fully rather than 10 to 30 nodes.
- Routine H and E staining can identify 1 tumor cell/10,000 normal size.
- **Reverse transcriptase PCR** will identify tumor protein production and one tumor cell per 1 million is identifiable.
- Histology negative but PCR positive tumors are having worse prognosis than histology negative.
- PCR status of the lymph node is the **most significant predictor of survival** even over tumor thickness.

Q 57. What are the investigations for melanoma?

1. Since wide excision is not possible in this case because of the fixity, take **incision biopsy** from the thickest part of the lesion (**excision biopsy is the investigation of choice normally**).
2. USG examination of the regional lymph nodes
3. FNAC of lymph node
4. LDH
5. Sentinel lymph node biopsy for stage Ia and II
6. CT/PET/MRI—abdomen/chest/pelvis (stage II to IIc) if clinically indicated.
7. Sentinel node positive and clinically stage III disease—CT/PET/MRI.

Q 58. What is the staging in the given case?

Since there is inguinal lymph node enlargement it is **Stage III.**

Q 59. What is the recommended surgical treatment in the given case?

Since, it is a big ulcer with fixity to the calcaneum he needs a below knee amputation for the primary along with ilioinguinal block dissection for the nodes.

Q 60. What is desmoplastic melanoma? (PG)

In desmoplastic melanoma the following features are seen:

- Histologically spindle cells are seen in fibrotic stroma with lymphocytic infiltration
- There is high rate of recurrence
- Wider margins are desirable
- Minimum of additional 1 cm margin is recommended
- They are rare and can arise de novo.

Q 61. What is neurotropic melanoma? (PG)

Neurotropic melanoma is characterized by:

- Peri/Intraneural infiltration
- It forms > 30% of desmoplastic melanoma
- High rate of recurrence
- Additional 1 cm margin is recommended.

Q 62. Any special form of treatment recommended for childhood melanoma? (PG)

- Melanoma in childhood is rare
- The differential diagnosis is pigmented spitz nevus (juvenile melanoma) that is a compound naevus in childhood
- Same treatment is recommended as in adults.

Q 63. What is the management of melanoma in pregnancy? (PG)

- Same treatment as in nonpregnant patient
- Early termination of pregnancy when the diagnosis is made
- Delay pregnancy for 2 years after treatment for melanoma
- Placental and fetal metastasis can occur in advanced melanoma.

Q 64. What is the incidence of mucosal melanomas? (PG)

- It forms < 1% of all melanomas
- Commonest site is oral cavity.

Q 65. What are the locations where you get mucosal melanomas?

Mucosal melanomas are seen in the following situations:

Sites of mucosal melanoma

- Oral cavity
- Rectum
- Anal canal
- Female genital tract
- Larynx
- Oropharynx
- Hypopharynx
- Nasopharynx
- Paranasal sinuses
- Esophagus (less common).

Q 66. What are the features of oral melanomas? (PG)

The characteristic features of oral melanoma

- Age incidence is between 40 and 60 years
- 50% are on hard palate
- 25% are on the upper gingiva
- 30% are preceded by an area of hyperpigmentation
- Pigmentation varies black to brown
- Red color indicates nonpigmented melanoma
- It may be flat or raised or nodular, later become ulcerated and may bleed
- It is notorious for rapid growth and poor prognosis
- Destruction of the underlying bone is a feature
- 50% will have metastasis at the time of presentation.

Q 67. What is the prognosis of mucosal melanomas? (PG)

They are having poor prognosis. The five-year survival rate appears to be about **5%.**

Q 68. What is the treatment of mucosal melanomas? (PG)

- **Wide excision** and reconstruction followed by **radical dissection of the nodes and radical radiotherapy**
- In the case of anal canal an abdominoperineal resection is recommended.

Q 69. What is the origin of melanoma in the eye?

It originates from the pigment cells of the choroid, ciliary body or iris.

Q 70. What are the clinical presentations of melanoma of eye?

It can present as:

- Reduction in vision
- Vitreous hemorrhage
- Elevated pigmented lesion in the eye.

Note: The more posterior the lesion in the eye the more malignant it is likely to be.

Q 71. What is the spread of melanoma of the eye?

The spread is often **delayed for many years** and often goes to the **liver**. Therefore, the aphorism:

'Beware of the patient with a glass eye, and an enlarged liver'—There will be history of enucleation of the eyeball years back for melanomatous lesion followed by use of glass eyes. The enlarged liver may be due to metastasis.

Q 72. What is the treatment of melanoma of the eye?

The following options are available:

Treatment options in melanoma of the eye

- Laser coagulation
- Radioactive plaques
- Radiotherapy
- Local excision using hypotensive anesthesia
- Enucleation.

Q 74. What is the investigations of choice for the diagnosis of melanoma of choroid? (PG)

Ultrasound examination that will show a solid tumor.

Q 73. What is the role of adjuvant chemotherapy after surgery in melanoma of the skin? (PG)

- It is the standard of care in the US
- In UK and rest of the World close follow-up followed by clinical trial in selected cases

- At present chemotherapy as an adjuvant modality is being given for high-risk patients with no evidence of systemic metastasis on clinical trial basis.
- The only approved agent for therapy is **interferon alpha – 2b (considerable toxicity is there).**

Q 74. What you mean by high-risk group?

High-risk group consists of **stages IIb, IIc and III. (node positive and thick node negative).**

Q 75. What are the other chemotherapeutic agents used in melanoma?

- Tumor response is < 20%
- Dacarbazine (DTIC) is the single most important drug with a response rate of 15–30%
- Temozolamide—oral analog—crosses blood brain barrier and it is used for cerebral metastasis.
- Combination chemotherapy—CVD regimen is used usually—cisplatin, vinblastine and dacarbazine.
- Tamoxifen – Given along with combination chemotherapy

Q 76. What is the treatment of local recurrence? (PG)

Wide excision with 2 cm margin is recommended.

Q 77. What is the treatment of intransit metastasis? (PG)

a. If they are few in number surgical excision with a margin of surrounding normal cutaneous and subcutaneous tissues (**excised en bloc with primary if possible and closure of the defect with flap or graft**).
b. Intralesional therapy with **granulocyte macrophage colony stimulating factor** (GM-CSF)
c. Laser therapy
d. Radiotherapy
e. Hyperthermic isolated limb perfusion.

Q 78. What is hyperthermic isolated limb perfusion? (PG)

It is introduced by Sydney Melanoma Unit in 1993.

Isolating blood circuit to the extremity and administering chemotherapeutic agent regionally at a concentration of 15–25 times higher without side effects is called **hyperthermic** isolated limb perfusion. A small bore vascular catheter is introduced into the femoral vessel from contralateral limb. A pneumatic tourniquet above the limb is applied and a small bore vascular catheter is used for introducing the agent.

- Melphalan and Actinomycin D in 400 mL of saline
- Gives significant palliation of locoregional symptoms
- No improval in survival is noted.

Q 79. What are the monoclonal antibodies available for treatment?

- Trametinib
- Dabrafenib.

Q 80. How do you stage metastatic melanoma of unknown primary?

- It is considered as stage III rather than stage IV
- Visceral metastasis is stage IV

  It may be as a result of:

  1. Previously biopsied and regressed
  2. From ocular primary
  3. From mucosal melanoma
- Look for primary
- Do surgery for the metastatic lymph node.

Q 81. Is there any role for radiotherapy in malignant melanoma?

Even though melanoma was considered to be resistant to radiotherapy, it is indicated in certain special situations with the dose mentioned below.

- More than 4 Gy dose-high response rate

- Large facial lentigo malignant melanoma
- Medically inoperable, those refusing surgery, thick melanoma, desmoplastic melanoma
- Incomplete excision of regional nodes especially head and neck
- For metastasis in lung, bone, brain, LN and subcutaneous nodule
- Lower recurrence rate following adjuvant XRT (10–25%)
- 50% Response rate for skin lesions and 30% for brain.

Q 82. What are the sites of metastasis?

- Can metastasize to any organ or site
- Skin, soft tissues
- Lung
- Liver
- Brain
- Bone
- GI tract.

Q 83. What is the management of metastatic disease?

- Interferon alpha and interleukin 2 are used
- < 5% of patients with metastasis survive 5 years (6–10 months)
- Resection of solitary mets can increase 5 years survival to 30%
- Lung → lobectomy
- Liver → lobar resection

Q 84. What is melanuria? (PG)

- Presence of melanin in urine is called melanuria
- It is seen in cases of extensive visceral involvement
- It is a terminal feature of malignant melanoma.

Q 85. What is targeted therapy for malignant melanoma? (PG)

Two-third of melanomas show activating mutation in BRAF. There is elevated Raf kinase activity. Blocking the Raf pathway using BAY 43 – 9006 is being tried as targeted therapy.

Q 86. What is spontaneous regression?

Spontaneous regression is an immunological phenomenon. Melanoma is considered an immunogenic human solid tumor. There will be no physical evidence of primary in **3 to 15% of patients** and the patients may present with lymph node metastasis. In such cases, **intense search should be made for the primary.** If primary is not found, treat the metastasis. The regression may be:

- **Partial/complete regression**
- Presenting as variation in color and irregular borders
- It is a host antitumor phenomenon
- Antimelanoma antibodies are found in blood
- Regression is associated with risk of metastasis.

Q 87. What are the pathological types of regression? (PG)

Pathologically the regression may be early, intermediate or late:

- *Early* – Lymphocytes are seen disrupting nests of melanoma cells
- *Intermediate* – There is loss of continuity of the lesion with mild fibrosis
- *Late* – There is extensive horizontal fibrosis.

Q 88. Why there is increased chance for metastasis in cases of spontaneous regression? (PG)

A subpopulation of melanoma cells **escaping immune recognition** is responsible for metastasis.

- Look for primary and excise
- Surgery for the metastatic lymph node.

Q 89. What is melanoma vaccine? (PG)

Unlike other vaccines the melanoma vaccine is used for treatment and not for prevention.

- Irradiated, allogenic cultured melanoma cells with or without BCG is used for treatment (polyvalent melanoma vaccine—3 melanoma cell line—cancerVax)
- The vaccine is prepared from the melanoma cells of the patients (autologous tumor vaccine) large amount of tumor is necessary for the production of vaccine.
- Vaccines prepared from viruses are also used - Vaccinia melanoma oncolysates—melacin
- GM2 ganglioside-based vaccine
- DNA immunization.

Q 90. What is the recommended follow-up for malignant melanoma? (PG)

- Every 3 months for 3 years
- Every 6 months for 2 more years
- Then yearly
- CXR annually.

Q 91. What are the preventive measures for melanoma?

- Genetic—autosomal dominant mode of transmission
- Sun exposure—intermittent intense exposure to UV is responsible for melanoma
- Monthly skin self-examination is recommended
- Clinical skin examination once or twice a year in high-risk areas
- Low threshold for simple excision of pigmented lesions
- Use of sunscreen.

Case

38 Basal Cell Carcinoma/Rodent Ulcer

Case Capsule

A 60-year-old male patient presenting with **pigmented ulcerated lesion** of 2 years duration at the region of **nasolabial fold** of the face on the right side of 1.5 cm size. The ulcer is having **raised and rolled edge** which is pigmented. The center of the ulcer is covered with a scab. The lesion is arising from the skin and it is mobile. There is no fixity to the deeper structures. There is **no regional lymph node enlargement**. Systemic examination is normal.

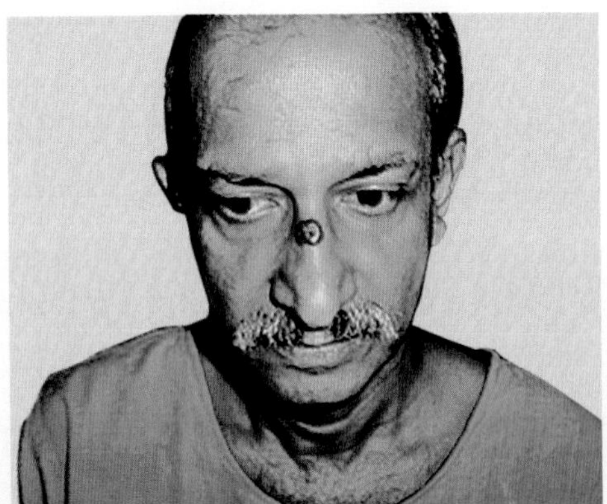

Basal cell carcinoma of nose

Read the checklist for examination of the ulcer.

Read the checklist for examination of melanoma.

Q 1. What is your diagnosis?

Basal cell carcinoma (Rodent ulcer).

Q 2. What is the commonest type of skin malignancy?

Basal cell carcinoma (BCC).

Q 3. Mention one hereditary syndrome associated with basal cell carcinoma?

Hereditary **Gorlin's syndrome**. This syndrome presents with **numerous BCC tumors**.

Q 4. What is the origin of basal cell carcinoma?

It is a malignant tumor of **pluripotential epithelial cell** arising from **basal epidermis** and hair follicle—affecting the **pilosebaceous skin**.

Q 5. What are the predisposing factors for basal cell carcinoma?

- UV light (most important)
- Arsenical compounds
- Coal tar
- Aromatic hydrocarbons
- Infrared rays
- Genetic skin cancer syndromes.

Q 6. What is the commonest age group affected?

It is 40–80 years (95% are seen in this age group).

Q 7. What are the diagnostic points for basal cell carcinoma?

1. Ulcerated lesion in the right side of the face with raised and rolled edge
2. Central part of the ulcer is covered with a scab
3. No regional lymph node enlargement.

Q 8. What are the characteristics of BCC?

Characteristics of BCC
1. It grows very slowly (over the course of many years)
2. No lymph node involvement
3. Local destruction by infiltration is the hallmark
4. The edge will be raised and rolled
5. The lesion may be pigmented or nonpigmented
6. It is seen in the classical area above a line joining the angle of the mouth to the ear lobule.

Q 9. What is the relationship of the BCC to arsenic?

Multiple basal cell carcinomas are seen in persons who have **arsenical dermatitis** following the administration of arsenic.

Q 10. Which sex is affected more by BCC?

- Men more than women
- Fair skinned more than dark skinned.

Q 11. What are the differential diagnoses in this situation?

1. Malignant melanoma (regional lymph node will be enlarged)
2. Keratoacanthoma just beginning to slough
3. Squamous cell carcinoma
4. Seborrheic keratosis.

Q 12. What is seborrheic keratosis?

This also called **senile wart, senile keratosis**, or **basal cell papilloma** or **verruca senilis** or **seborrheic wart.**

It is a **benign** over growth of epidermis containing swollen abnormal epithelial cells which raise it above the level of the normal epidermis giving a semitransparent oily appearance. It is seen on any part of the skin except those areas subjected to regular abrasions such as palms and sole. The majority are found on the back of the trunk. They have a rough and papilliferous surface.

Q 13. What is keratoacanthoma?

- This is a cup-shaped growth
- The central crater is filled with a plug of keratin
- Seen in the face of 50–70-year-old group (more common in men)
- Papilloma virus infection, smoking and chemical carcinogen exposure are etiological factors
- Lesions can grow upto 1 to 3 cm over 6 months and then, they spontaneously resolve
- Excision is recommended
- It is also called adenoma sebaceum or molluscum pseudo carcinomatosum.

Q 14. What are the types of basal cell carcinoma?

There are about 26 varieties of basal cell carcinoma. The important types are:

Important types of basal cell carcinoma
1. Nodular
2. Nodulocystic
3. Ulcerative
4. **Morpheic** (Sclerosing)
5. Pigmented
6. Superficial
7. Field - fire
8. Cystic
9. **Nevoid**
10. **Infiltrative.**

Note: Nodular and nodulocystic variants account for 90% of BCC.

Q 15. What are the sites for basal cell carcinoma?

They are usually seen on the face above a line drawn from the angle of the mouth to the ear lobule.

- Medial canthus of the eye
- Lateral canthus of the eye
- Nasolabial fold
- Nose
- Eyelid
- Cheek
- Ear.

It can also occur in other sites like scalp, neck, arms and hands.

Q16. Can you get multiple basal cell carcinomas?
Yes.

Q 17. What is the usual evolution of a basal cell carcinoma (BCC)?

- Usually it will start as a **small nodule.**
- The center of the nodule will die resulting in **ulcer formation with rolled edge.**
- If the center does not necrose and ulcerate the nodule will **look cystic** (but actually it will be solid).

Q 18. Why it is called rodent ulcer?
The main mode of spread is **local infiltration.** The longstanding ulcers **erode deep into the face destroying the bone** and exposing the nasal cavity, nasal sinuses, the eye and even the brain. Because the ulcer is eroding into deeper structures like a rodent, it is called a rodent ulcer. The BCC will kill the patient by local infiltration.

Q 19. What is geographical type of BCC?
The central area of the lesion is healing and the peripheral area is spreading and advancing. This is called the geographical type of BCC or a **Forest Fire type.** The edge will be irregular and rolled out with a white scar in the center.

Q 20. What is pearly edge?
When the nodule is getting ulcerated, the edge will appear as pearly white nodules just below the epidermis and therefore it is called pearly edge.

Q 21. What are the bad prognostic types? (PG)

- Infiltrative
- Morpheic.

Q 22. Why morphoeic type spread rapidly?
They synthesis type IV collagenase.

Q 23. What is high risk BCC?

- Lesions larger than 2cm situated near the eye, nose and ear
- Recurrent tumors
- Presence of immunosuppression.

Q 24. What is the macroscopic classification?
It is divided into:

- Localized (Nodular, nodulocystic, cystic, pigmented and nevoid)
- Generalized: **Superficial** (multifocal or superficial spreading).

Infiltrative (morpheic, ice pick and cicatrizing).

Q 25. What is the microscopic pathology of basal cell carcinoma? (PG)

- The characteristic finding is **ovoid cells in nests** with an outer **palisading** layer perpendicular to the surrounding connective tissue. Only the **outer layer of cells will actively divide.** This is the reason for the **slower growth rate.**
- Mitotic figures are absent.

Q 26. What are the modes of spread of BCC?

- Local infiltration—It is the predominant mode of spread.
- Perineural invasion is seen in morphea form of BCC—It is associated with high rate of recurrence and incomplete excision.

Q 27. What are the options for treatment?
The treatment options are:

1. *Surgical excision*
2. *Destructive Treatments*—
   a. Electrodesiccation and curettage (EDC)

b. Cryosurgery
c. Carbon dioxide laser
d. Radiotherapy.

Q 28. What is the margin of excision recommended?

Most authors currently recommend a margin of **2– 15 mm** depending on macroscopic variant.

Q 29. What is Mohs micrographic surgery? (PG)

This involves:

- Excision of all visible tumors in horizontal slices while mapping the exact size and shape of the lesion
- Horizontal frozen sections are taken from the under surface of the excised lesion
- They are examined microscopically
- Incompletely excised areas of tumor are mapped and marked for further excision
- This process is repeated until the entire tumor is removed.

Q 30. What are the advantages of this technique? (PG)

- High cure rate
- Decreased morbidity
- Tissue conservation.

Q 31. What are the disadvantages of this technique? (PG)

The only disadvantages is the need for two separate procedures when reconstruction is required.

Q 32. What is electrodesiccation and curettage? (PG)

- **This form of treatment is effective only for very small and superficial tumors**
- Lesions less than 2 mm are completely removed in 100%
- Lesions 2–5 mm are removed in 85% of cases
- Tumors more than 3 cm recur in 50% of cases.

Q 33. What is the role of cryosurgery?

This is also a form of treatment for small tumors.

Q 34. What are the complications of cryosurgery? (PG)

- Marked edema
- Permanent hypopigmentation
- Increased morbidity.

Q 35. What is the role of carbon dioxide laser?

- Useful for treatment of multiple tumors
- Useful in patients with hereditary Gorlin's syndrome
- Useful only for superficial BCCs confined to the epidermis and papillary dermis
- Treatment of deeper lesions will produce scarring
- Laser produces superficial vaporization of tissue
- Usually requires 3 passes on clinically visible tumor.

Q 36. What is the role of radiotherapy?

The BCC is radiosensitive with overall cure rate of 92%. *The advantages of radiotherapy are*:

- Can be used in areas which are difficult to reconstruct, e.g. eyelids, tear ducts, nasal tip, etc.
- Less traumatic than surgical excision
- No need for hospitalization
- Wide margin of tissue can be treated.

Q 37. What are the disadvantages of radiotherapy? (PG)

- Expensive facilities are necessary
- Radiation dermatitis
- Osteitis and chondritis
- Scarring
- Ulceration
- Ectropion

- Epilation
- Repeated is treatments are required over a period of 4–6 weeks
- Usually not used in age group less than 40
- Cannot be used if not responding to radiotherapy.

Radiation is therefore used only for elderly patients who are not suitable candidates for surgery.

Q 38. What is the role of topical agents?

5FU and imiquimod are used as topical agents in elderly who are reluctant to undergo surgery.

Q 39. What is the cause of death in BCC?

- Direct intracranial extension by infiltration
- Erosion of major blood vessels.

Q 40. What is the treatment of recurrence?

Immediate re-excision of all lesions.

Case 39 Squamous Cell Carcinoma—SCC (Epithelioma)

Case Capsule

A 65-year-old male patient presents with **ulcero-proliferative lesion** of **4 cm** size on the **dorsum of the left foot** of 8 months duration. He is a **farmer** by profession. The lateral half of the lesion is ulcerated having **everted edge**. The medial half of the lesion is showing **cauliflower-like proliferation**. There is copious, purulent and bloody **foul smelling discharge** from the ulcerated region. The floor of the ulcer is showing unhealthy granulation tissue. The base is indurated; however, the ulcer is mobile with no fixity to the underlying structures. The ulcer **bleeds to touch**. There are three discrete, mobile and **firm lymph nodes** in the vertical group of inguinal lymph nodes. The examination of the abdomen and chest are normal.

Read the checklist for examination of the ulcer.

Read the checklist for examination of melanoma.

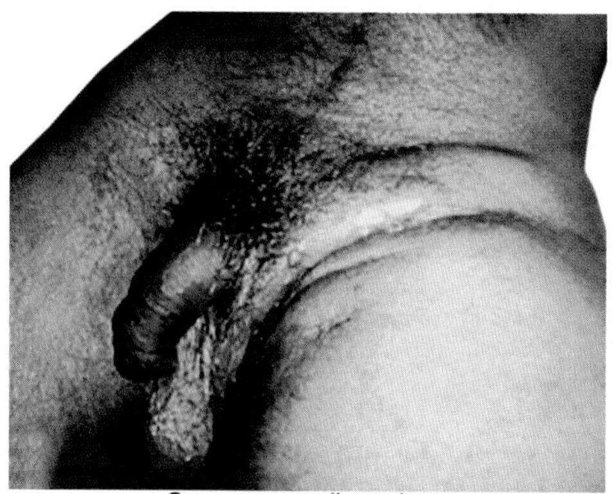

Squamous cell carcinoma with inguinal node metastasis

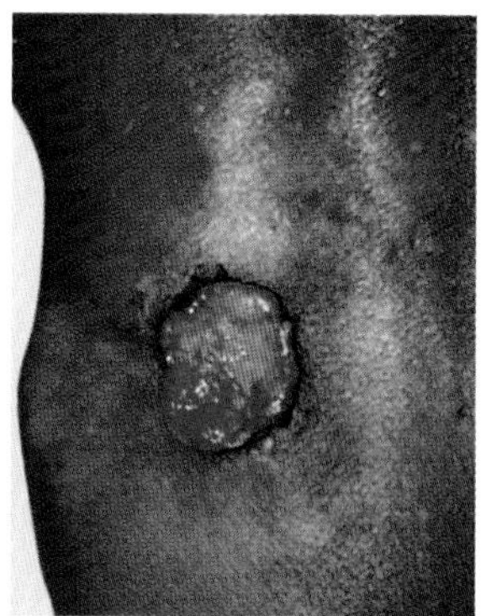

Squamous cell carcinoma on the back

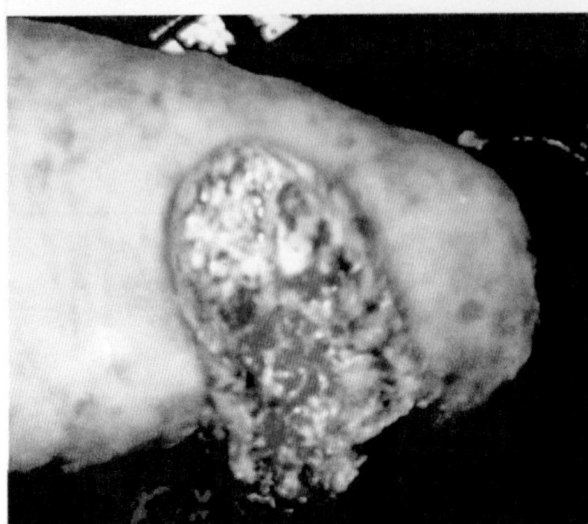

Squamous cell carcinoma—
right heel

Q 1. What is the probable diagnosis in this case?

Squamous cell carcinoma (SCC) of the dorsum of the foot.

Q 2. What are the diagnostic points in favor of SCC?

- Ulceroproliferative lesion
- The ulcer is having everted edges of SCC
- The proliferative area has cauliflower-like appearance
- The copious bloody foul smelling discharge
- Induration of the base
- Enlarged regional lymph nodes.

Q 3. What is the origin of SCC?

- It is a **malignant tumor of the keratinizing cells** of the epidermis or its appendages
- It can also arise from the stratum basale of the epidermis
- It expresses **cytokeratin 1 and 10.**

Q 4. Are these nodes really metastatic?

The lymph nodes are not very hard in this case. When the lymph nodes are palpable, in about **1/3rd of the patients the adenopathy may be secondary to infection, that** will subside after treatment of the primary lesion. Until proved otherwise, it should be assumed that they are metastatic.

Q 5. What are the differential diagnoses of a small lesion?

- Solar keratosis (Actinic keratosis)
- Basal cell carcinoma
- Keratoacanthoma
- Pyogenic granuloma
- Seborrheic warts.

Q 6. What are the premalignant (precancerous) conditions of the skin?

Precancerous lesions of the skin

- Senile keratosis
- Arsenic dermatitis
- Leukoplakia
- Solar keratosis (Actinic keratosis)
- Radiation dermatitis
- Kraurosis vulvae
- Xeroderma pigmentosum
- Junctional nevus
- Albinism
- Cutaneous horn
- Keratoacanthoma—Papilloma virus infection, smoking are associated—seen in old age
- Bowens disease—this is SCC in situ (HPV 16 is implicated)
- Extramammary Paget's disease—intraepidermal adenocarcinoma
- GCPN (Giant Congenital Pigmented Nevus)—for malignant melanoma.

Q 7. How about Paget's disease, Bowen's disease and Erythroplasia of Queyrat?

Paget's disease, Bowen's disease and Erythroplasia of Queyrat are **carcinoma** in situ (**Paget's disease is seen in nipple, erythroplasia of Queyrat is seen in penis**).

Q 8. What is the difference between precancerous lesion and carcinoma in situ?

The precancerous lesions will lead on to *in situ* cancer and finally cancer.

Precancerous lesion
↓
In situ carcinoma (preinvasive)
↓
Carcinoma

Q 9. What are the features of solar keratosis (Actinic keratosis)? (PG)

They are **discrete, scaly, irregular patches**, which may project occasionally.

Q 10. What is the treatment of actinic keratoses? (PG)

They are treated with:

- Cryotherapy
- Topical 5 Fu—(5 fluorouracil)
- Electrodesiccation and curettage
- CO_2 Laser
- Dermabrasion.

Q 11. What are the features of Bowen's disease? (PG)

They are irregularly shaped, well-defined **plaques** resembling a patch of eczema having **beefy red, erythematous** raised scaly crust on the surface.

Q 12. What are the features of erythroplasia? (PG)

They are having the same features as Bowen's disease, except for the fact that they are situated on the penis.

Q 13. Which part of the ultraviolet ray is responsible for skin damage?

Ultraviolet B is thought to be the form of radiation responsible for the damage by sunlight.

Q 14. What are the mechanisms by which the UV radiation affects the skin? (PG)

It affects the skin in two ways:

1. Direct carcinogenic effect on dividing keratinocytes in the basal layer of the epidermis.
2. Depression of the cutaneous immune surveillance response.

Q 15. What are the sites of SCC other than skin?

The SCC is seen in the following sites other than skin.

- Lips
- Mouth
- Pharynx
- Esophagus
- Anal canal
- Glans penis
- Uterine cervix
- Metaplastic areas of respiratory epithelium.

Q 16. What are the other predisposing factors?

Predisposing factors for SCC

1. Sunlight
2. Susceptible phenotype
3. Compromised immunity—(after 10 years of immunosuppression, 10% will develop malignancies—may be secondary to HPV virus)
4. **Chemicals**—For example, Hydrocarbons (soot), arsenical, tar, etc.
5. Infection—**HPV 5 and HPV 16**
6. Mineral oils
7. Arsenic
8. Chrome compounds
9. **Chronic inflammation**—Chronic sinus tract, pre-existing scars (Marjolin's ulcer), osteomyelitis, burns and vaccination points
10. Immunosuppression (organ transplant recipients)
11. Smoking—current and previous tobacco use.

Q 17. What is "Chimney sweeps" cancer?

The soot is one of the most important hydrocarbons responsible for **squamous cell carcinoma of the scrotum** in chimney sweeps. It is also seen in people who work in tar.

Q 18. What is "Khangri" cancer?

Khangri is an earthenware, filled with burning charcoal. The Kashmiris keep the Khangri on their abdomen to keep themselves warm. The patient will develop squamous cell carcinoma of the abdominal wall.

Q 19. What is Kang cancer?

This is a squamous cell carcinoma developing in the buttocks, back, heels and elbows. This is seen in Tibetans who sleep on the oven bed.

Q 20. What is countryman's lip?

This is nothing but SCC of the lower lip seen in farmers as a result of sun exposure.

Q 21. What are the macroscopic types of SCC?

Three types are seen:

1. Ulcerative
2. Proliferative (Cauliflower-like)
3. Ulceroproliferative.

Q 22. What is the microscopic pathology of SCC?

- Epithelial pearls (Cell nests)—Squamous cells arranged in concentric manner such as onion skin
- Plasma cell infiltration
- Positive for cytokeratins 1 and 10.

Q 23. What is the spread of SCC?

- Local spread—to the subcutaneous tissue, tendons, muscles, bone and vasculature (Involvement of the **local blood vessel** can cause thrombosis and ischemia. The subcutaneous spread may involve the nearby nerves causing **neuritis—perineural involvement)**
- The main spread is lymphatic reaching the lymph node
- Bloodstream spread occurs very rarely—(to the lungs).

Q 24. Can you get SCC without lymph node metastasis?

Yes. **Lymph node spread is absent** in the following situations.

- When the lesion is developing in scar and chronic ulcer (Marjolin's ulcer)
- SCC in old age.

Q 25. What are the characteristics of Marjolin's ulcer?

Characteristics of Marjolin's ulcer
• It arises from ulcer or scar
• The edge is not always raised and everted
• It is not very invasive
• The growth is very slow
• More aggressive than spontaneous SCC.

Q 26. What are the aggressive types of squamous cell carcinoma? (PG)

1. Squamous cell carcinomas seen in transplant patients
2. Squamous cell carcinomas developing in scars and ulcers
3. Anaplastic squamous cell carcinoma.

Note: Metastasis is more likely to arise from SCC in scars and ulcers even though the lymph nodes are not involved.

Q 27. What are the types of lesions prone for malignant change resulting in Marjolin's ulcer?

Lesions prone for Marjolin's
1. Venous ulcers
2. Chronic ulcers
3. Scar tissues—Postburn scarring
4. Scarring secondary to lupus vulgaris (tuberculosis)
5. Chronic discharging sinuses, e.g. osteomyelitis.

Q 28. How aggressive is SCC?

The SCC is **more aggressive than BCC** and therefore **wider excision margins** are required for local control.

Q 29. What is the type of biopsy recommended for SCC?

- Incision biopsy from the edge of the ulcer if the lesion is large (wedge biopsy from the edge)
- If the lesion is small excision is recommended.

Q 30. Why the edge of the ulcer is preferred for incision biopsy?

The edge of ulcer is the **growing part** which will show the malignant cells.

Q 31. What are the other investigations required?

- X-ray of the affected part to rule out bone involvement
- X-ray of the chest to rule out metastasis (very rare event)
- Other investigations required for anesthesia clearance.

Q 32. What is the staging of SCC? (PG)

The **TNM staging** is used (this is different from the TNM of the melanoma).

Primary tumor (T)

TX Primary tumor cannot be assessed
T0 No evidence of primary tumor
Tis Carcinoma in situ
T1 Tumor *2 cm or less* in greatest dimension with less than 2, high-risk factors
T2 Tumor greater than 2 cm, or tumor of any size with 2 or more high risk features
T3 Tumor with invasion of maxilla, mandible, orbit or temporal bone
T4 Tumor invasion of skeleton (axial or appendicular) or perineural invasion of skull base

Note: In case of multiple simultaneous tumors, the tumor with highest T category will be classified.

Regional lymph node (N)

NX Regional lymph nodes cannot be assessed
N0 No regional lymph node metastasis
N1, N2a, N2b, N2c & N3 as in head and neck malignancy **(Read case no: 24)**

Distant metastasis (M)

MX Distant metastasis cannot be assessed
M0 No distant metastasis
M1 Distant metastasis

Stage grouping			
Stage 0	Tis	N0	M0
Stage 1	T1	N0	M0
Stage II	T2	N0	M0
Stage III	T3	N0	M0
	T1	N1	M0
	T2	N1	M0
	T3	N1	M0
Stage IV	T1	N2	M0
	T2	N2	M0
	T3	N2	M0
	Any T	N3	M0
	T4	Any N	M0
	Any T	Any N	M1

Q 33. What is the importance of grade in SCC?

Grade has been included as one of the high-risk features within the T category and now contributes towards the final stage grouping. The grades are:

Gx – Grade cannot be assessed
G1 – Well differentiated
G2 – Moderately differentiated
G3 – Poorly differentiated
G4 – Undifferentiated

Q 34. What are the high risk features of SCC?

1. Histologic grade
2. Primary anatomic site—ear or hair bearing lip
3. More than 2 mm depth
4. Clark level more than IV
5. Perineural invasion.

Q 35. What are the bad prognostic factors for SCC? (PG)

Tumors of the following regions are having bad prognosis:

1. *Site of the tumor:* Ears and lips are having bad prognosis. Tumors of the **extremities fare worse than the trunk.**

2a. *Depth of invasion:* **Less than 2 mm** metastasis unlikely
More than 6 mm—15% will have metastasis

2b. *Surface size:* **Lesion more than 2 cm** have worse prognosis than smaller ones

3. *Histological grade:* Higher the Broder's grade the worse the prognosis
4. *Etiology:* SCC from burn scars, osteomyelitis, sinuses, chronic ulcers and areas that have been irradiated have a higher metastatic potential
5. *Immunosuppression:* Bad prognosis
6. *Perineural involvement:* Worse prognosis and require wider excision.

Q 36. What is the histological grading of SCC? (PG)

GX – Grade cannot be assessed
G1 – Well-differentiated
G2 – Moderately differentiated
G3 – Poorly differentiated
G4 – Undifferentiated

Q 37. What is the staging in this case? (PG)

It is stage II or III. (If the lymph node is positive).

Q 38. What are the options for treatment?

The treatment options are:

1. Surgical excision
2. Destructive therapy
3. Radiotherapy.

Q 39. What is the recommended excision margin for SCC?

- For lesions less than 2 cm diameter—4 mm margin is adequate
- For more than 2 cm lesions—1 cm margin is recommended.

Q 40. What would be the treatment of choice in this case?

- Wide excision with 1 cm clearance
- Split skin grafting of the raw area.

Q 41. What are the areas where a skin graft will not take? (PG)

The skin graft will not take in the following situations:

- Exposed cortical bone without periostium
- Cartilage without perichondrium
- Tendon without paratenon
- Irradiated tissue.

Q 42. What sort of cover is recommended in such situations?

A flap is recommended.

Q 43. What are the indications of the flap? (PG)

Flaps are indicated in the following situations:

1. Areas where graft will not take
2. Where there is risk of scar contracture especially across a joint
3. Where esthetic result is important
4. Where bulk or structural support is needed.

Q 44. What are the types of flaps? (PG)

It may be **Local flap**
Island flap
Free flap

Q 45. How do you manage the enlarged inguinal nodes?

- Give a course of antibiotics and see whether the nodes are subsiding or not
- If the nodes are remaining the same after 3 weeks, FNAC of the node is done
- If the FNAC of the node is positive for metastasis, an inguinal block dissection is carried out.

Q 46. If the lesion is involving the bone, what would be the treatment option? (In given case)

The primary needs **below knee amputation** and the inguinal nodes are managed as mentioned above.

Q 47. What are the indications for radiotherapy?

Radiotherapy has been shown to cure 90% cases of SCC:

It is recommended for the following situations:

- Debilitated patients
- Poor surgical risk candidates
- Those who refuse surgery.

Q 48. What are the problems of radiotherapy? (PG)

- Unpleasant side effects
- Protracted treatment.

Q 49. Is there any role for radiotherapy as an adjuvant treatment? (PG)

Yes. The indications are:

- High stage large tumors
- Recurrent tumors.

Q 50. Is there any role for topical 5-fluorouracil (5-FU)? (PG)

No, **it is not recommended for the primary treatment of SCC.**5-FU is an excellent method of treating, premalignant lesions associated with SCC such as actinic keratoses.

Q 51. What is the role of Mohs micrographic technique in SCC? (PG)

This technique is also used for the treatment of SCC. The advantages are:

- Tissue preservation
- Lower recurrence rate.

The disadvantages are:

- Patient inconvenience
- Expensive.

Q 52. What is the role of destructive techniques in the treatments of SCC (Cryosurgery and electro-desiccation and curettage)? (PG)

- They are best reserved for very small superficial lesions in noncritical areas
- The local failure rate is high
- They do not produce surgical specimen for histological examination and margin analysis
- The healing is by secondary intention
- It results in poor scars.

Q 53. Is there any role for prophylactic lymph node dissection? (PG)

No.

Case

40 Carcinoma Penis

Case Capsule

A 50-year-old **Hindu male** patient presents with **acquired phimosis of recent onset** with **seropurulent discharge** from beneath the prepuce. On examination, the penis is swollen at its tip. There is a **hard mass felt beneath the prepuce** on palpation. On forceful retraction, a part of the **ulceroproliferative lesion** is seen protruding from the glans. Palpation of the **corpora cavernosa** appear **normal**. There is no induration. On examination of the inguinal nodes, **two horizontal group of inguinal nodes** which are firm in consistency and mobile are felt on either side. There are no enlarged iliac nodes. The rest of the external genitalia and abdomen are normal.

Read the checklist for examination of the ulcer.

Checklist for examination

- Assess the location of the lesion
- Assess the size
- Decide whether it is mobile or fixed
- Palpate the penis for **involvement of the corpora** (induration)
- Check for **involvement of surrounding structures** like scrotum and perineum

Contd...

Contd...

- **Rectal examination** for involvement of perineal body and pelvic lymph nodes
- Examination of inguinal area for inguinal nodes and iliac nodes
- **Remember the three most important examinations in the male genitalia**
- Always retract the prepuce and see for any lesion
- Always examine the under surface of the penis for openings (hypospadias)
- Always examine the ventral surface of the scrotum for openings (hypospadias).

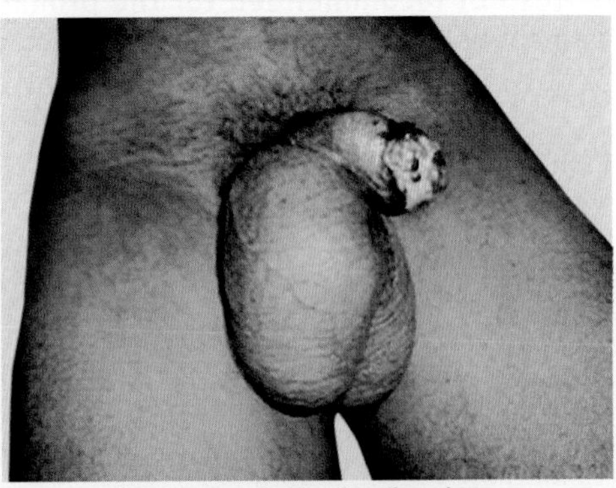

Carcinoma destroying the glans with right hydrocele

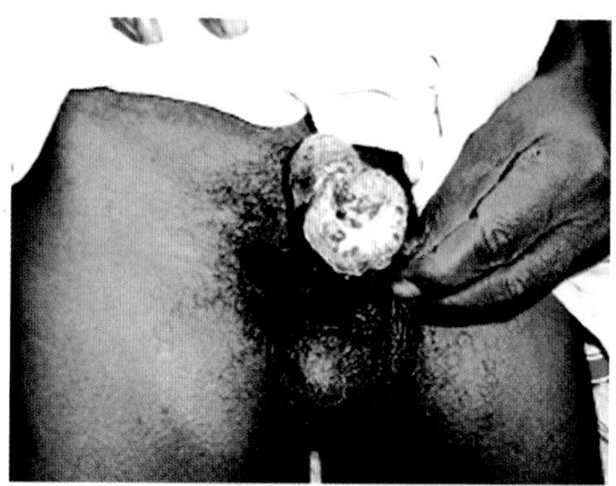

Carcinoma penis with involvement of body of penis

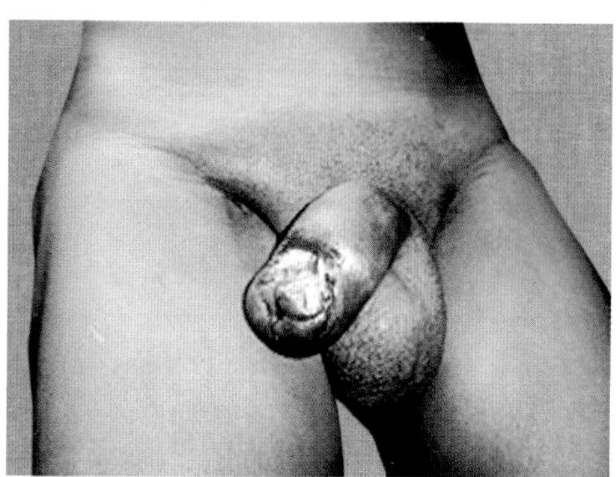

Dorsal slit showing carcinoma penis with edema of penis

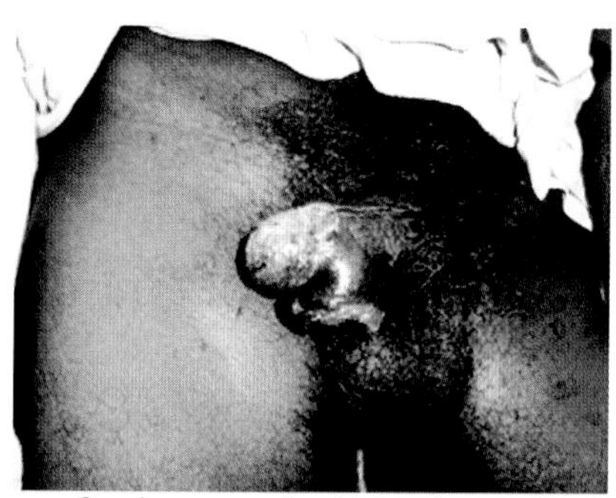

Carcinoma penis with involvement of body of penis

Q 1. What is the most probable diagnosis in this case?

Carcinoma penis with **acquired phimosis** and? Inguinal node metastasis.

Q 2. What are the differential diagnoses?

- Syphilitic chancre
- Soft chancre due to *Haemophilus ducreyi*
- Giant condyloma.

Q 3. What is phimosis?

Inability to retract the foreskin to expose the glans.

Q 4. What is paraphimosis?

Inability to reduce a previously retracted foreskin.

Q 5. What is the importance of religion in this case?

Hindus are usually not circumcised and therefore more prone for carcinoma of the penis.

Q 6. What is the commonest age group affected?

- 40% of the patients are under the age of 40 years.
- It is commonly seen in middle and old age.

Q 7. What is balanitis?

Balanitis is an infection of the glans penis.

Q 8. What is balanoposthitis?

It is commonly used to describe an infection within the preputial sac which, affects both the surfaces of the glans penis and the inner aspect of the prepuce.

Q 9. What are the causes for balanoposthitis?

Causes for Balanoposthitis
1. Carcinoma of penis
2. Nonspecific infection secondary to poor hygiene
3. Phimosis in diabetic patients
4. Primary chancre.

Q 10. What is the most important causative factor for carcinoma penis?

Human papilloma virus **16 (HPV 16)**.

Q 11. What are the other predisposing factors?

- Smoking
- Smegma
- Poor hygiene
- Chronic balanoposthitis.

Q 12. Will circumcision confer immunity against carcinoma penis?

- Circumcision soon after birth confers complete immunity against carcinoma
- Later circumcision does not have the same effect.

Q 13. What are the premalignant conditions?

- Leukoplakia of the glans (similar to the lesion seen in the tongue)
- Longstanding genital warts (chronic papilloma)
- Chronic balanitis.

Q 14. What is erythroplasia of Queyrat and Paget's disease?

They are nothing but in situ carcinoma presenting as persistent rawness of the glans.

Q 15. What is the appearance of leukoplakia?

It is identical to the appearance of leukoplakia of the tongue presenting as **patches of grayish white paint.**

Q 16. What are the sites where you can get leukoplakia?

- Oral cavity
- Tongue
- Vulva
- Vagina
- Penis.

Q 17. What is the appearance of erythroplasia of Queyrat?

It presents as a flat dark red slightly indurated patch.

Q 18. What is Balanitis xerotica obliterance (lichen sclerosus atrophicus)?

It is a condition with unknown etiology. The lesion appears as white plaques on the surface of glans and prepuce. The foreskin is thickened, fibrous and difficult to retract. It is seen in men aged **20-40 years** and they have higher incidence of associated **autoimmune disorders. Circumcision** is indicated in this condition. It may also cause meatal stenosis. This is **not a premalignant lesion**.

Q 19. What are the causes for acquired phimosis?

- Cancer
- Chancre
- Balanoposthitis.

Q 20. What is the management of acquired phimosis?

If retraction of the prepuce is not possible arrange for a **dorsal slit** of the prepuce and examine the inside or arrange for a **circumcision.**

Q 21. What are the macroscopic types of carcinoma penis?

- Flat type (infiltrative type)
- Papillary type with wide sessile pedicle
- Ulcerative type.

Q 22. What are the modes of spread of carcinoma penis?

1. Local spread
2. Lymphatic spread
3. Bloodstream spread (distant metastasis).

Q 23. What is the barrier for the local spread?

The fascial sheath of the corpora cavernosa.

Q 24. What is lymphatic drainage of penis?

- The superficial lymphatics drain to the inguinal nodes
- The deep lymphatics drain to the iliac nodes.

Q 25. What is the mode of transmission of HPV virus?

The HPV infection directly correlates with the number of life term partners (however carcinoma penis cannot be labelled as a sexually transmitted disease.

Q 26 . What are the locations for SCC of the penis?

- Glans (50%)
- Prepuce
- Coronal sulcus.

Q 27. What is Buschke-Loewenstein tumor?

Buschke-Loewenstein tumor has the following characteristics:

- It has got histological pattern of **verrucous carcinoma**
- It is locally destructive and invasive
- **No nodal metastasis** is seen
- **No distant metastasis**
- Treatment is surgical excision.

Q 28. How do you confirm the diagnosis?

- Incision biopsy from the lesion (if it is ulcerative take the biopsy from the edge)
- If acquired phimosis is there—do a dorsal slit of the prepuce and do incision biopsy from the lesion
- **Excision biopsy** for very small superficial lesions of the glans
- **Circumcision and biopsy** if the lesion is confined to the prepuce.

Q 29. What is the commonest pathological type?

Squamous cell carcinoma.

Q 30. Can you get metastasis in penis?

Yes. The usual sites for primary are **urinary bladder, prostate and rectum.**

Q 31. What are the other investigations required?

1. **Ultrasound of the penis**
   - To evaluate the depth of invasion
   - Detecting involvement of the corpus cavernosum.
2. **Contrast enhanced MRI**—for lesions suspected to invade corpora
3. **CT**—for evaluation of the inguinal and pelvic nodes (physical examination is enough in the ordinary circumstances)
4. **X-ray chest**.

Q 32. What is the staging of carcinoma penis? (PG)

The AJCC 7th edition TNM classification is used.

Summary of changes

1. T1 has been subdivided into T1a and T1b based on the **presence or absence of lymph vascular invasion** (LVI) or **poorly differentiated cancer.**
2. T3 is limited to urethral invasion.
3. Prostatic invasion is now considered T4.
4. Nodal staging is divided into both clinical and pathologic categories.
5. The distinction between superficial and deep inguinal nodes has been eliminated.
6. Stage II grouping includes T1b N0 M0 as well as T2–3 N0 M0
   - TX – Primary Tumor cannot be assessed
   - T0 – No evidence of primary tumors

- Tis – Carcinoma in situ
- Ta – Noninvasive verrucous carcinoma
- T1a – Tumor invades subepithelial connective tissue without lymph vascular invasion and is not poorly differentiated
- T1b – Tumor invades subepithelial connective tissue with lymph vascular invasion or is poorly differentiated
- T2 – Tumor invades corpus spongiosum or cavernosum
- T3 – Tumor invades urethra
- T4 – Tumor invades other adjacent structures

Regional Lymph Nodes (N)

- cNX – Regional lymph nodes cannot be assessed
- cN0 – No palpable or visibly enlarged inguinal lymph nodes
- cN1 – Palpable mobile unilateral inguinal lymph node
- cN2 – Palpable mobile multiple or bilateral inguinal lymph nodes
- cN3 – Palpable fixed inguinal nodal mass or pelvic lymphadenopathy unilateral or bilateral.

Note: Clinical stage definition based on palpation, imaging

Pathologic stage definition (based on biopsy or surgical excision)

pNX – Regional lymph nodes cannot be assessed.

pN0 – No regional lymph node metastasis.

pN1 – Metastasis in a single inguinal lymph node

pN2 – Metastasis in multiple or bilateral inguinal lymph nodes

pN3 – Extra-nodal extension of lymph node metastasis or pelvic lymph nodes(s) unilateral or bilateral.

Distant Metastasis (M)—lymph node metastasis outside the true pelvis in addition to visceral or bone sites

- MX – Distant metastasis cannot be assessed
- M0 – No distant metastasis
- M1 – Distant metastasis

Stage Grouping			
Stage 0	Tis	N0	M0
	Ta	N0	M0
Stage I	T1a	N0	M0
Stage II	T1b	N0	M0
	T2	N0	M0
	T3	N0	M0
Stage IIIa	T1-3	N1	M0
Stage IIIb	T1-3	N2	M0
Stage IV	T4	Any N	M0
	Any T	N3	M0
	Any T	Any N	M1

Q 33. What is the most important prognostic factor for survival in carcinoma penis?

Presence of metastasis to the inguinal nodes.

Q 34. What are the predictors for nodal involvement? (PG)

Predictors for nodal involvement

- Grade of the tumor (higher the grade more chance for involvement of nodes)
- Corporal involvement
- Vascular involvement
- Lymphatic embolization.

Q 35. What are the treatment options?

Treatment options for carcinoma penis
• Surgery (amputation of penis—partial or total) • Primary radiation therapy for the primary • Laser therapy—CO_2 laser/Nd: YAG laser (for very small non infiltrating lesions) • 5-FU cream (for early lesions) • Treatment of inguinal nodes—unilateral or bilateral lymph node dissection (inguinal) or bilateral inguinal irradiation • Adjuvant chemotherapy • Reconstruction of the penis if suitable.

Note: Stage 1 and 2 lesions can be treated with radiotherapy with a good cosmetic and functional result.

Q 36. What are the indications for radiation therapy for the primary?

Indications for radiotherapy
• Young patients with small lesions (2–4 cm) • Superficial lesions • Exophytic lesions • Noninvasive lesions on glans or coronal sulcus • Patients refusing surgery • Patients with inoperable tumors.

Q 37. What are the types of radiotherapy?

- External beam radiation
- Interstitial brachytherapy—Iridium 192 or Tantalum wire or Cesium 137
- Radioactive mould application (applied externally to the penis).

Q 38. What are the indications for organ preservation?

- Tis, Ta and T1 Infiltration of the shaft of the penis
- Large anaplastic growth
- Failure of radiotherapy.

Q 39. What are the indications for partial amputation of penis?

- T2 to T4-tumors
- If preservation of **2 cm penile stump** is possible after 2 cm clearance from the gross tumor.

Q 40. What are the advantages of partial amputation of penis?

- Less psychological trauma
- Ability to pass urine in standing position
- Preservation of sexual function.

Q 41. What is the minimum clearance required in carcinoma penis?

Well and moderately differentiated tumors need only 1cm margin.

Q 42. What is glansectomy? (PG)

- This is reserved for **verrucous carcinoma and minimally invading** T1 lesion
- It preserves more erectile tissue.

Q 43. What are the features of verrucous carcinoma and basaloid carcinoma?

Verrucous carcinoma	*Basaloid carcinoma*
They are well differentiated	Poorly differentiated
Presence of expansile border	Infiltrative
Non-metastatic	Frequently metastatic

Q 44. What is total amputation of penis?

- This is done for advanced lesions, and anaplastic lesions
- Perineal urethrostomy is done after total amputation.

Q 45. Is there any need for bilateral orchidectomy along with total amputation of the penis?

- The traditional arguments in favor of bilateral orchidectomy will not hold today (soiling of

scrotum during urination and edema scrotum after inguinal block dissection)
- The patient will loose his hormone (testosterone) and masculine features by doing orchidectomy
- Therefore, orchidectomy is not recommended.

Q 46. What are the indications for inguinal lymphadenectomy (inguinal block dissection)?

There are five groups of inguinal lymph nodes: Central, Superolateral, Inferolateral, Superomedial and Inferomedial. The superomedial is called Cabana's node. The indications for inguinal lymphadenectomy are:

- The nodes are usually managed after controlling the primary tumor and a course of antibiotics
- In palpable adenopathy, there is a higher likelihood of finding metastasis and a lower survival and therefore lymphadenectomy is justified
- T2 to T3 tumors without palpable inguinal adenopathy
- Tumors exhibiting lympho vascular invasion
- Poorly differentiated tumors even without invasion of corpora cavernosum or spongiosum.

Q 47. What are the situations where lymph-adenectomy is not required? (PG)

- Patients with Tis, Ta and T1 tumors without lympho vascular invasion and without poor differentiation and absence of palpable adenopathy.

Q 48. What is Cabana's node? (PG)

- Cabana described a procedure of **sentinel lymph node biopsy** for metastasis from carcinoma penis
- These nodes are situated superomedial to the junction of the long saphenous vein with femoral vein in the **area of superficial epigastric vein**
- If the sentinel nodes are negative for malignancy, then there is no need for inguinal block dissection
- The technique involves peri-tumoral injection of **Technetium ^{99}m and blue dye**
- It is not being used widely

Q 49. What is the lymphatic drainage of the corpora? (PG)

The corpora will drain directly to the **deep inguinal nodes (Rosenmüller's or Cloquet's node)**.

Q 50. What is the reason for recommending bilateral lymph node dissection when the nodes are positive? (PG)

It is because of the **anatomic cross over** the penile lymphatic.

Q 51. What type of inguinal dissection is recommended? (PG)

Initially a **superficial inguinal dissection** is recommended, which involves removal of the **nodes superficial to fascia lata**. These nodes are subjected for frozen section and if found to be positive the patient is subjected for **complete ilioinguinal and pelvic lymph node dissection.**

Q 52. What are the complications of inguinal block dissection?

Complications of inguinal block dissection
• Wound infection • Flap necrosis • Lymph edema of the lower limb • Lymph edema of the scrotum.

Q 53. What is the indication for bilateral inguinal irradiation? (PG)

- This is usually done for N0 nodes
- Not recommended for high-risk patients
- May be helpful in **fixed ulcerated inguinal nodes** as palliative procedure
- Preoperative radiation for down staging inguinal nodes.

Q 54. Is there any role for adjuvant chemotherapy? (PG)

Yes

- If more than two histological positive nodes
- If extra-nodal extension of cancer is present.

Q 55. What are the chemotherapeutic agents used? (PG)

- Cisplatinum based regimens are used (5-FU, bleomycin and methotrexate)
- Ifosfamide (new drug).

Q 56. Is there any role for penile reconstruction? (PG)

Reconstructions are being tried after total amputation of penis with various flaps. Restoration of phallus with tactile and erogenous sensation, creation of urethra and enough bulk are important for a successful reconstruction.

Q 57. What is the management of distant metastasis? (PG)

Chemotherapy with cisplatin and methotrexate.

Q 58. What is the cause of death in carcinoma penis?

It is usually by the metastatic nodes **eroding into the femoral or external iliac artery** with torrential hemorrhage

Q 59. What is the prognosis of carcinoma penis?

- The five year survival for lesions localized to the penis is 80%
- With nodal metastasis the five year survival is 50%
- With distant metastasis the five year survival is nil.

Case 41 Congenital Arteriovenous Fistula/ Hemangioma/Compressible Swelling

Case Capsule

A 25-year-old male presents with **dilated tortuous pulsatile vessels** on the **entire left lower limb** with **increased length and girth of the limb** suggestive of **local gigantism**. There is scoliosis of the spine. On examination there is **port wine discoloration** of the lateral part of the left thigh. Palpation revealed pulsations of the tortuous vessel and these vessels were **compressible** and clinically appearing to be veins. Palpation revealed **continuous thrill** over the vessels. The extremity is appreciably **warmer** and **moist** than the unaffected side. Auscultation revealed a **continuous machinery murmur** with systolic accentuation. Examination of the radial pulse revealed **collapsing radial pulse**. After occlusion of femoral artery, the **bradycardiac sign** was positive. There was no evidence of cardiac failure.

Read the checklist for examination of the swelling.

Checklist for history

- Find out whether the lesion is **present from birth or not**
- Find out whether there is rapid postnatal growth and slow involution (hemangioma)
- Find out whether the lesion is having **commensurate growth** as the age advances

Contd...

Contd...

- History of **hemorrhage (GI bleed)** and local bleeding
- History of ulceration of the limb or lesion
- History of stridor (subglottic hemangioma)
- History of sudden **increase in size** (bacterial infection, or secondary to hormonal changes).

Checklist for examination

- Examine the radial pulse and decide whether it is a **collapsing pulse** or not
- Look for skin discoloration
- Look for **compressibility** and decide whether it is partially compressible or completely compressible
- Check whether the swelling enlarges with dependency and **disappears with elevation** of the involved limb
- Palpate for increased **local warmth**
- Rule out increased moisture compared to the normal limb
- Check whether the overlying skin is normal or not (dystrophic changes in the skin)
- Look for **discrepancy in the limb length** and if it is there apparently, always take measurements
- Look for **increase in girth** by taking measurements in all segments of limb
- Look for atrophy of the affected area (**bone atrophy** as a result of reduction in distal circulation and hypoxia)

Contd...

Contd...

- Look for features of **platelet trapping**
- Look for **translucency**
- Look for **palpable thrill**
- Look for **continuous bruit**
- Look for **bradycardiac sign** after occluding the main feeding artery
- Always **examine the heart** especially for evidence of cardiac failure
- Look for hepatomegaly.

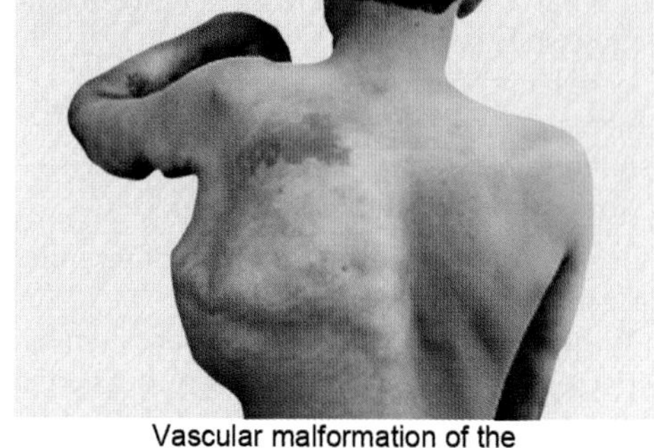

Vascular malformation of the upper back showing pink discoloration

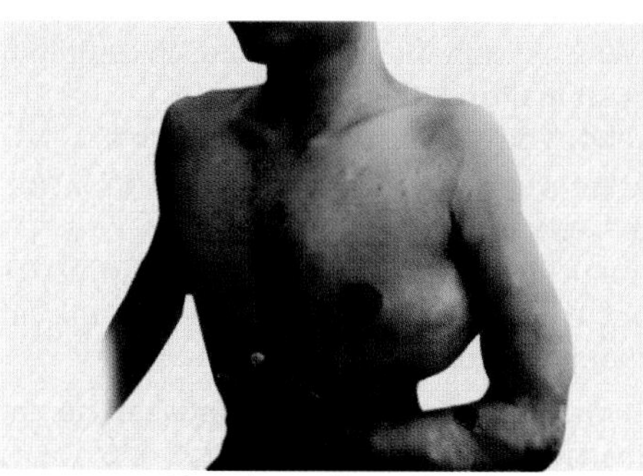

Vascular malformation of left side of chestwall and left upper limb

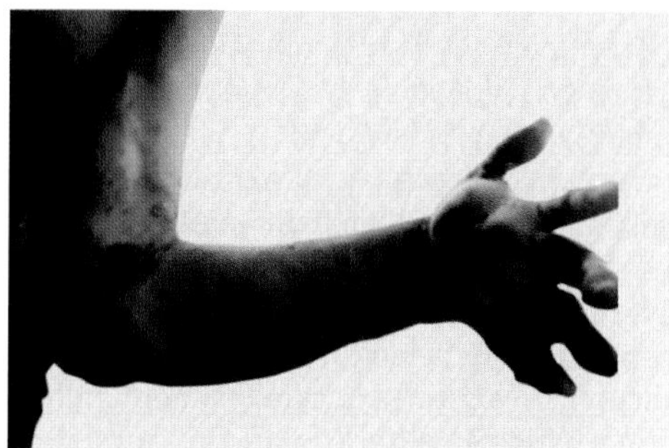

Vascular malformation involvement of the left upper limb

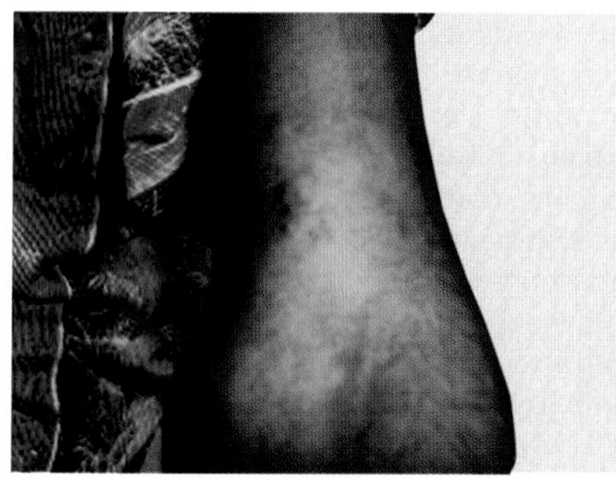

Vascular malformation in the left arm

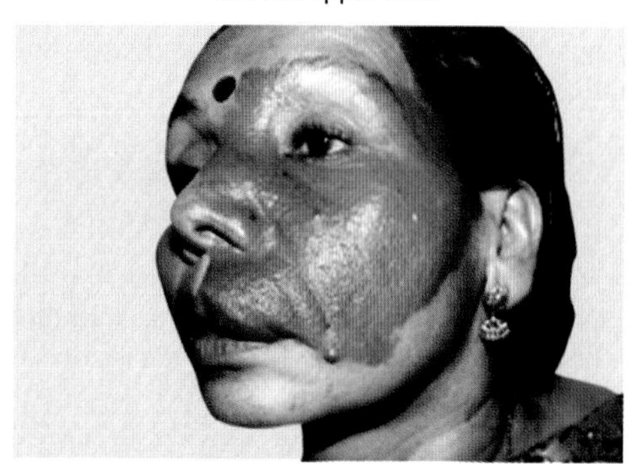

Port wine stain of left side of face

Q 1. What are the differential diagnoses for a compressible swelling?

1. Lymphatic cyst/lymphangioma
2. Hemangioma
3. Aneurysm
4. Arteriovenous fistula.

Q 2. What are the clinical points to differentiate these four conditions?

- The lymph cyst will be brilliantly transilluminant
- Hemangioma is not transilluminant, but partially compressible
- Aneurysm will show expansile pulsations and systolic bruit
- Arteriovenous fistula will show continuous thrill on palpation and continuous machinery murmur on auscultation.

Q 3. What is the difference between cavernous hemangioma and capillary hemangioma?

These are old terms and they are best avoided. **Cavernous hemangioma** is used to describe a **deep lesion** involving the deeper dermis or the subcutaneous tissue and **capillary hemangioma** is one which proliferates in the **superficial dermis**.

Q 4. What is the old classification of hemangioma?

They are classified into capillary and cavernous (not used now).

- Capillary hemangioma
  - Strawberry
  - Port wine stain
  - Spider nevi
- Cavernous hemangioma

Note: The term cavernous hemangioma is not there in the current terminology. Most of the lesions are actually venous malformations.

Q 5. What is the new classification?

The new classification distinguishes lesions as follows:

- Lesions that regress spontaneously— Hemangiomas
- Those that do not regress spontaneously—Congenital vascular malformations (Hamburg classification—Predominantly arterial, venous, lymphatic, arteriovenous shunting and mixed).

Another classification is

- Slow flow lesions
- Fast flow lesions—Arteriovenous fistula.

Q 6. Which channel is more affected in congenital vascular malformations?

- Venous defects are the most common
- Arteriovenous malformations makeup 1/3rd of the lesions
- About 90% of the arteriovenous malformations occur in the extremities, pelvis, trunk and shoulder girdle.

Q 7. What are the differences between hemangioma and vascular malformation?

- Hemangiomas result from cellular proliferation (It is a fibrofatty structure and the contained blood cannot be evacuated completely). The hemangiomas grow over the first six to eight months of life. After 1 year signs of involution appear until about 5–10 years old.
- Vascular malformations are embryonic and developmental abnormalities (error in vascular morphogenesis). These lesions grow parallel with the age, they may expand suddenly at times with associated infections. There is no involution. Limb hypertrophy or atrophy may occur.

Differences between hemangioma and vascular malformations

Hemangioma	*Vascular malformation*
• Usually present at birth	• Present at birth, may not be apparent
• Result from **cellular proliferation (Benign tumor)**	• **Embryonic and developmental** abnormalities
• Fibrofatty structure and contained blood **cannot be evacuated completely by compression**	• Easily evacuated by compression
• No enlargement with dependency and disappearance with elevation of the limb	• **Enlarges with dependency** and **disappears with elevation** of the limb
• Endothelial hyperplasia	• Flat endothelium
• **Female to male ratio 5:1**	• **Female to male ratio 1:1**
• Mast cells are increased	• Normal mast cells
• Multilaminated basement membrane	• Unilaminated basement membrane
• Platelet trapping present (Kasabach Merritt's syndrome)	• No platelet trapping
• Rapid postnatal growth with **slow involution**	• Commensurate growth **No spontaneous involution**
• No limb hypertrophy/ atrophy	• Limb hypertrophy or atrophy may occur
• **No treatment required** in majority	• Treatment may be required

Q 8. What are the examples of vascular malformations?

- Port wine stain (capillary malformation)
- Nevi
- Venous malformations
- Lymphatic malformation
- Arteriovenous fistula.

Q 9. What is the classical appearance of a strawberry hemangioma?

It looks like a raised, bright red patch with a textured surface like a strawberry. Veins radiating from the tumor may be seen beneath the skin. During proliferative phase the tumor enlarges and becomes brighter in color. Involution is heralded by softening and fading of color.

Q 10. What are the classical sites of hemangioma?

Sites of hemangioma

- Head and neck (60%)
  - Facial hemangioma
  - Eyelid hemangioma can cause astigmatism and amblyopia
  - Subglottic hemangioma causing biphasic stridor
- Trunk (25%)
- Limbs (15%)
- Liver
  - Multiple intrahepatic hemangiomas
  - Hepatomegaly
  - Heart failure
  - Anemia
- Intestines
- Lungs
- Brain.

Note: 80% are single tumors and 20% are multiple tumors.

Q 11. What are the complications of hemangiomas?

Complications of hemangiomas
• Platelet trapping – Kasabach—Merritt syndrome • Thrombocytopenia and hemorrhage – Gastrointestinal – Pleural – Intracranial – Intraperitoneal • Ulceration (5%) • Local bleeding • Infection • Visual problems by obstructing the vision • Stridor.

Q 12. What is the Kasabach-Merritt syndrome?
This was described by Kasabach and Merritt in 1940. It is characterized by:

Kasabach-Merritt Syndrome
• Hemangioma > 5 cm • Thrombocytopenia • Bleeding diathesis.

The thrombocytopenia is by platelet trapping. There is 37% mortality for this condition which is largely due to bleeding. The treatment is difficult and interferon, steroids and irradiation have all been tried with variable results.

Q 13. What is Hamburg classification?
Humburg classification is for vascular malformation based on the predominant nature of the malformation. They are classified into five types—predominantly arterial defects, predominantly venous defects, predominantly lymphatic defects, predominantly AV shunting defects and combined or mixed vascular defects.

Hamburg classification of congenital vascular defects

Type	*Forms*	
	Truncular	*Extra truncular*
Predominantly arterial defects	Aplasia or Obstructive dilation	Infiltrating or limited
Predominantly venous defects	Aplasia or Obstructive dilation	Infiltrating or limited
Predominantly lymphatic defects	Aplasia or Obstructive	Infiltrating or limited
Predominantly AV shunting defects	Deep or superficial	Infiltrating or limited
Combined/mixed vascular defects	Arterial and venous, no AV shunt Hemolymphatic, with or without AV shunt	Infiltrating hemolymphatic or limited hemolymphatic

Other classifications are:

A. **Schobinger classification:** Quiescent,
Expanding
Destruction
Decompensation

B. **International society on studies of vascular anomalies (ISSVA)**

Slow flow, Fast flow & Complex

Class I – Vascular tumors
- Infantile hemangioma
- Congenital hemangioma Rapidly Involuting Congenital Hemangioma **(RICH)** and Noninvoluting congenital hemangioma **(NICH)**
- Kaposiform hemangioendothelioma
- Dermatologically acquired vascular tumor like pyogenic granuloma

Class II – Vascular malformation
a. Slow flow—Capillary hemangioma and port wine stain
b. Fast flow—Arterial fistula, AV malformation and AV fistula
c. Complex

C. **Mulligan classification**
– Truncal, diffuse and localized

Q 14. What are the associations of congenital vascular malformations?

- Nevi
- Port wine stain
- Varicosities
- Arteriovenous fistula
- Hypertrophy and atrophy of the extremities
- Edema of the limbs.

Q 15. What is port wine stain (in old classification it was included with hemangioma)?

This is an extensive intradermal capillary malformations giving a deep purple color to the overlying skin. They are present at birth, commonly seen on the face, at the junction between limbs and trunk (shoulders, neck and buttocks). Sometimes they are seen distributed along sensory branches of the fifth cranial nerve. Microscopically they are formed by thin-walled capillaries in the dermis. They are non-involuting lesions like any other arteriovenous malformation (unlike hemangiomas).

Q 16. What are the treatment options of port wine stain?

- Camouflaging and Tattooing are the options for the management
- Flash lamp pulsed—dye laser (multiple sessions are necessary)
- Selective photo thermolysis
- If laser is unsuccessful, surgical excision and skin grafting.

Q 17. What is the age group for lymphatic malformations and what is the presentation?

They are seen in the first year of life and childhood. They present as lymphatic vesicles.

Q 18. What is lymphangioma/cystic hygroma?

It is a localized cluster of dilated lymph sac in the skin and subcutaneous tissues which do not connect into the normal lymph system (they are clusters of lymph sacs that fail to join into the lymphatic system during development). When they are large, cystic and translucent and confined to the subcutaneous tissue, they are called cystic hygroma.

Q 19. What are the manifestations of lymphangioma?

- Skin vesicles noticed by parent (may be clear or brown or black) as a result of the contained clotted blood—0.5 to 3 to 4 mm in diameter
- Some times the vesicles leak clear fluid
- May present with infected vesicles and pain
- The number and extent of the vesicles increases with age
- Multiple small lesions may not fluctuate and feel soft and spongy (one or two large cysts show fluctuation, fluid thrill and translucency)
- It may or may not be compressible
- When there is infection the regional nodes may be enlarged.

Q 20. What are the classical sites of lymphangioma?

Classical sites of lymphangioma
• Junction of the limb and neck • Junction of the limb and trunk • Around the shoulder • Axilla • Buttock • Groin.

Q 21. What is lymphangioma circumscriptum?

When the lesion is localized to a region like buttocks or side of the thigh it is called lymphangioma circumscriptum.

Q 22. What is Vin rose patch?

It is a congenital intradermal vascular abnormality in which mild dilatation of the vessels in the subpapillary dermal plexus gives the skin a pale pink color. It is associated with other vascular abnormalities like extensive hemangioma, arteriovenous fistulae and lymphedema. It can occur anywhere and causes no symptoms.

Q 23. What is Campbell de Morgan spot?

It is a bright red well-defined spot caused by the collection of dilated capillaries fed by a single or cluster of arterioles. They are usually seen in older age group above 45. One or more spots and some times a cluster may be seen. The usual site is upper half of the trunk and rarely in the limbs and face. They look like drops of dark red paint.

Q 24. What is spider nevus?

It is a solitary dilated skin arteriole, with visible radiating branches. They are usually associated with chronic liver disease and tumors producing estrogens. They appear on the upper half of the trunk, the face and the arms. They fade completely when compressed and refill as soon as the pressure is released.

Q 25. What is the age group for venous malformation?

The venous malformation may present at birth, childhood or adolescence.

Q 26. What is the clinical presentation of arteriovenous fistula?

- In early stages a pink stain and increased local temperature of the surrounding skin are the only signs
- Gradually distended veins occur and a thrill can be felt (followed by audible bruit). When varicose vein and skin discoloration over the lateral aspect of the thigh are present suspect congenital AV fistula
- Extensive dilated tortuous veins which are pulsatile (arterialized veins) are seen
- Limb hypertrophy and local gigantism will occur
- Blood is diverted from the arterial side to the venous side resulting in distal hypoxia.

Q 27. What is the commonest site for congenital AV fistula?

- The lower extremity is the most common site
- Upper extremity
- Congenital AV fistula in relation to the superficial temporal artery
- Congenital AV fistula in relation to the occipital artery.

Q 28. What are the signs of congenital AV fistula?

The following are the signs of congenital AV fistula

- Port wine discoloration and varicose veins—Suspect AV fistula.
- Local gigantism—Congenital arteriovenous fistula in the young patient will produce increase length and girth of the limb (the local gigantism may be associated with scoliosis).
- The lower limb is apparently warmer and moist than the unaffected side (in the case of head and neck the affected side will be warmer).
- Palpable continuous thrill in the dilated vessels.
- Continuous machinery murmur with systolic accentuation is obtained when the stethoscope is applied to the arterialized veins.
- Collapsing arterial pulse.
- Bradycardiac sign of Branham and Nicolodona—Digital occlusion of the main artery to the limb is followed by bradycardia indicating that considerable volume of blood is being short circuited.
- Leg ulceration due to hypoxia—These ulcers are known as **hot ulcers** (because the surrounding skin feels warmer than normal). These ulcers are very painful.

Q 29. What are the causes for acquired AV fistula?

- Trauma to the vessels
- Iatrogenic AV fistula (for dialysis).

Q 30. What are the differences between congenital and acquired AV fistula?

- The arteriovenous communications are innumerable in congenital
- The communications are one or two in acquired
- Congenital is difficult to treat
- Acquired is easily treated.

Q 31. What is Cirsoid aneurysm?

They are nothing but congenital arteriovenous malformations in relation to the superficial temporal artery or occipital artery. They may have intracranial extensions. It is very difficult to treat such lesions.

Q 32. What are the investigations in a case of vascular malformation?

Color Doppler and MR angiography are the two most useful investigations in the case of arterio-venous fistula.

- *Laboratory investigations*—No laboratory investigation can differentiate hemangioma from vascular malformation. However, estimation of fibroblastic growth factor secreted in the urine of patients with hemangioma may be useful.
- *Duplex scanning*—It is a useful noninvasive investigation.
- Tc-99 labeled human albumin is injected intra-arterially proximal to the AV fistula and measuring the radioactivity in the lungs with a gamma camera is a useful investigation for arteriovenous fistula (< 3% pass to the lungs normally).
- CT scanning with contrast enhancement
- *MRI*—Superior to CT (high and low flow lesions can be identified).
- *Magnetic resonance angiogram*—This will accurately distinguish hemangioma from vascular malformations. This is the most useful imaging study of choice.

- *Angiography*—It is not routinely done unless embolization is required prior to surgery.

Q 33. What is the treatment of hemangioma?

Treatment of hemangioma
• Most hemangiomas do not require any treatment because they resolve spontaneously • Avoid local trauma • Parents are direct to give local pressure in the event of bleeding • Corticosteroids (both systemic and **intralesional**) • Interferon a2a - used for life-threatening complications (interferon is an inhibitor of angiogenesis) • Lasers—Used to treat residual telangiectatic spots in after involution • Surgical excision—It is indicated when complications occur and also in the case of eyelids.

Q 34. What are the indications for corticosteroids?

- Life-threatening complications—Airway obstruction, bleeding
- Large facial hemangiomas
- Platelet trapping syndrome.

Q 35. What is the dose and duration of therapy?

Prednisolone 2 mg/kg/day are used orally. The treatment is continued for several months until the tumor is in its involuting phase.

Q 36. What is intralesional steroid therapy?

- This is used for localized facial hemangiomas
- Triamcinolone—3 to 5 mg/kg/procedure is injected directly into the lesion with a 26 gauge needle. The volume should not exceed 1 mL per injection.

Q 37. What are the management options in venous malformation?

Management options in venous malformation
• Elastic support • Low dose aspirin for preventing episodic thrombosis • Sclerotherapy—sodium tetradecyl sulphate injection locally followed by pressure • Laser therapy • Surgical treatment.

Q 38. What are the management options for arteriovenous fistula?

Management options for arteriovenous fistula
Emergency management of bleeding • Emergency ligation of feeding vessel or surgical packing—this will give temporary control (always recurrence should be anticipated and the recurrence is too difficult to treat owing to the recruitment of multiple new channels) • Transcatheter embolisation • Management of cardiac failure **Elective treatment** • Preoperative embolization followed by surgical excision (The resectability rate is < 20%) • The embolization should be done as near to the time of surgery as is feasible.

Q 39. What are the materials used for embolization?

Materials used for embolization
• Plastic particles • Foam pledgets • Stainless steel coils • Polymerizing adhesives.

Contd...

Contd...

- Ethanol - polyvinyl alcohol foam particles are available in graded sizes from 50–1000 micrometers diameter
- Sclerosing agents
- Acrylic adhesives.

Q 40. What is Klippel-Trenaunay syndrome?

They are combined vascular malformations (combined in the sense that they involve more than one type of channel). In this case, it is a combined capillary lymphovenous malformation. It is a slow flow lesion characterized by the following lesions:

Klippel-Trenaunay syndrome

- Geographic capillary stain
- Venous anomaly of the superficial and deep system
- Lymphatic abnormality
- Over growth of soft tissues and bones.

Q 41. What is Parkes-Weber syndrome?

This is a combined capillary and arteriovenous malformation. It is a flat blue lesion characterized by:

- Flat pink, (warm) stain
- Underlying multiple AV connections
- Venous malformation
- Tissue overgrowth.

Q 42. What is Maffucci syndrome?

The association of following constitutes Maffucci syndrome:

Maffucci syndrome

- Multiple enchondromas
- Venous malformations
- Bony deformities.

Case 42 Unilateral Lower Limb Edema

Case Capsule

A 45-year-old male patient presents with **swelling of the left lower limb** of 3 years duration. The **inguinal lymph nodes are enlarged**, firm, discrete and mobile. There is history of **recurrent attacks of fever, chills and pain** in the affected limb. The first episode of such attack started in early adult life. In the initial stages the swelling used to disappear in between the attacks of fever and chills. The frequency of such attack is increasing and the **edema is persistent nowadays**. The swelling does not reverse on elevation of the limb. The skin is **thickened and some warty nodules** are seen in the lower part of the leg anteriorly. The limb has attained enormous size in the last few months and it is now interfering with mobility of the limb and routine activities of the patient. The **edema is seen involving the dorsum of foot and toes.** On interrogation, it was found that he is coming from a **filarial belt.** There is no history of surgery and irradiation. Examination of the genitalia revealed **hydrocele of the TV sac** on left side. Abdominal examination is normal so also the digital rectal examination. There is no evidence of edema of the contralateral lower limb and upper limbs.

Checklist for history

- History of **geographical location** from where the patient is coming (endemic place for filariasis)
- Onset and duration of edema (congenital, adolescence, or adulthood)
- **History of injuries, wounds, abrasions, fissuring of the skin**, eczema and paronychia
- History of recurrent attacks of **fever, chills** and painful swellings
- Whether the swelling is initially **reversible or not**
- History of **tumors of the pelvic floor, prostate** cancer, etc.
- History of **surgical dissection** of lymph nodes
- History of **radiation therapy** for malignant tumors
- History of **podoconiosis** (cutaneous absorption of mineral particles)
- History of **venous diseases, venous surgery and venous thrombosis**
- History of **Hansen's disease**
- History of **Leishmaniasis**
- History of cardiac diseases
- History of hepatic and nutritional disorders
- History of amyloidosis.

Checklist for examination

- Decide whether the edema is unilateral or bilateral
- Look carefully for **thin red and tender streaks** on the skin suggestive of lymphangitis

Contd...

Contd...

- Check whether the edema is **pitting or non-pitting**
- Decide whether it is affecting the **entire limb or localized** to the ankle region or affecting the toes—ankle region is affected in DVT, entire limb is affected in iliac vein occlusion
- Decide whether the **skin is normal or hyperkeratotic** with nodules (hyperkeratotic skin is seen in **lymphedema**)
- Examine for **draining lymph nodes** (lymph nodes are enlarged in secondary lymph edema, but not in DVT)
- Examine the **genitalia to rule out hydrocele** and edema affecting the genitalia (both are seen in lymphatic filariasis)
- Examine the **breasts in females** to rule out edema of the breast (seen in filariasis)

Contd...

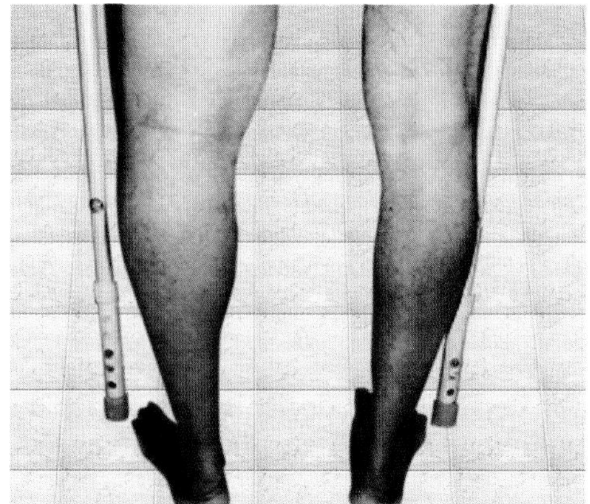

Left deep vein thrombosis affecting the leg segment

Contd...

- When there is evidence of **superficial thrombophlebitis**—If the episodes are transient, migrate and affect the arms in age group above 45 years suspect occult visceral carcinoma and examine the abdomen to rule out Ca
- **Examine the venous system** to rule out chronic venous insufficiency
- Examine the whole patient to **rule out cardiac causes** and **renal causes** for edema.

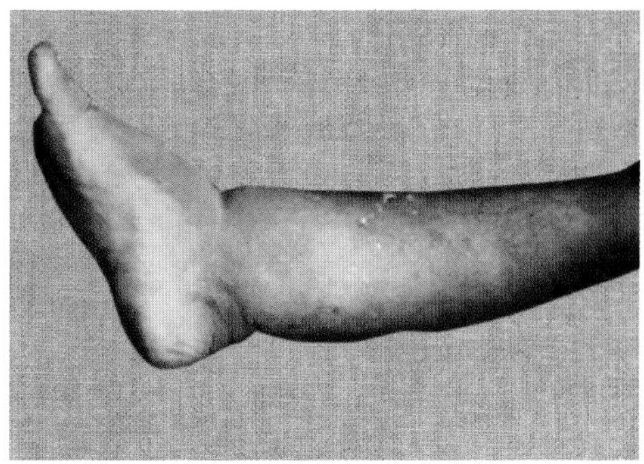

Lymphedema showing buffalo hump of the dorsum of foot

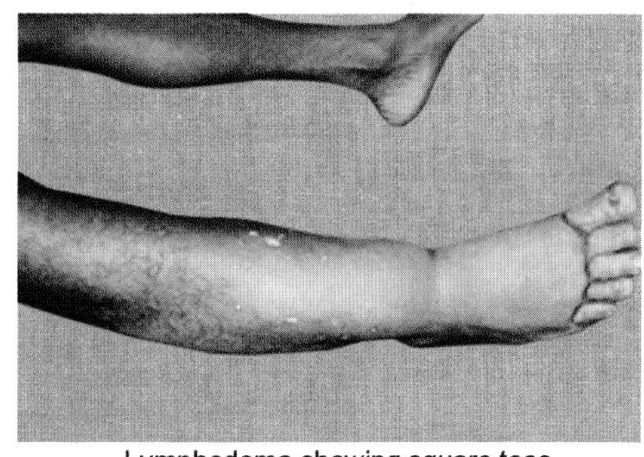

Lymphedema showing square toes

Q 1. What is your diagnosis?

Lymphatic filariasis with lymphedema.

Q 2. What are your points in favor of your diagnosis?

- Patient gives history of recurrent fever, chills and pain in the affected limb
- The edema is affecting the toes (a point in favor of lymphedema)
- The edema is nonpitting
- The swelling does not reverse on elevation of the limb
- The skin is thickened and warty nodules are seen
- The regional nodes are enlarged
- Patient is coming from an endemic area for filariasis.

Q 3. What are the differential diagnoses?

1. **Lower limb edema from lymphatic causes:**
   - Primary lymphedema
     - lymphedema congenita
     - lymphedema praecox: **2 to 35** years (sporadic or familial). The familial is called **Meige's** disease.
     - lymphedema tarda: **After 35** years (associated with obesity—the nodes replaced with fibrofatty tissue).
   - Familial lymphedema (**Milroy's disease**) — **familial form of congenital lymphedema**

     Two main types of familial (hereditary) lymphedema are recognized—**Nonne-milroy (type I) and Letessier-meige (type II)**. The incidence is 1 in 6000 live births and probably inherited as autosomal dominant with incomplete penetrance seen in chromosome IV. In Meige's disease lymphedema develops between puberty and middle age.
   - Secondary lymphedema—**Lymphatic filariasis**
     - Other infections: Tuberculosis, lymphogranuloma inguinale
     - Tumors of the pelvic floor (prostate cancer)
     - Surgical dissection of lymph nodes (block dissection)
     - Radiation therapy for malignant tumors
     - Podoconiosis (cutaneous absorption of mineral particles).
   - Lymphedema secondary to congenital vascular anomalies
     - Lymphatic angiodysplasia syndrome
     - Klippel-Trenaunay syndrome
     - Hyperstomy syndrome.
2. **Lower limb edema due to venous causes**:
   - Chronic venous insufficiency
   - Deep vein thrombosis
   - Post-thrombotic syndrome
   - Intravenous drug use
   - Phlegmasia alba dolens (**white leg or milk leg**)
   - Phlegmasia cerulea dolens.
3. **Cellulitis**
4. Endocrine disease—pretibial myxoedema
5. Immobility and dependency—Dependency edema (seen in cases of paralysis)
6. Hansen's disease
7. Dermal leishmaniasis
8. Mycetoma
9. Systemic causes
10. Factitious—Self harm.

Q 4. What is edema?

Edema represents an **imbalance between capillary filtration and lymphatic drainage** (the role of lymphatics in the development of edema is substantial. This does not mean that all edemas are lymphedemas).

Q 5. How the lymphatic system is formed and what is the function of lymphatic system?

It forms part of the microcirculation that helps to return **macromolecules like proteins**, cell debris and other particulate matter and **excess fluid** from the interstitial spaces to the venous system via large lymph vessels. The initial lymphatic capillaries in the skin **originate as blind ended tubes** formed by a single layer of endothelial cells with spaces in between for the entry of fluid and large molecules. They join to form larger vessel which **have smooth muscles in their walls**. The flow of lymph is unidirectional because of **the presence of valves** situated every 2 to 12 mm distance. The larger vessels are having smooth muscle in their walls. Gentle massage of the skin stimulates contractions. **Lymphatics are responsible for resorption of 10 to 20% of the tissue fluid. Two to four liters of lymph** with 70 to 200 gm of protein pass daily into the systemic circulation.

Q 6. What are the factors responsible for lymph flow?

- Contraction of muscles
- Pressure exerted by arterial pulsations
- Increase in fluid volume
- Elevation of the limb.

Q 7. What are the possible mechanisms for lymphedema?

1. When there is increased load of interstitial fluid—**high output failure**.
2. When the lymph vessels are absent, or abnormal or damaged due to acquired causes—**low output failure**.

Q 8. In which plane you get the lymphatics?

In the limbs they form:

- Superficial and deep **plexus in the dermis**—they drain to the subcutaneous lymph vessels following the course of superficial veins
- Subfascial plexus in the muscular compartments
- The lymphatics finally drain to the lymph nodes.

Q 9. What is the WHO grading of lymphedema?

WHO grading of lymphedema of the limbs (1992)	
Grade I –	Pitting edema **reversible on elevation** of the affected limb
Grade II –	Pitting or nonpitting edema which **does not reverse on** elevation of the affected limb, and there are no skin changes
Grade III –	Nonpitting edema that is not reversible, with thickening of skin
Grade IV –	Nonpitting edema that is not reversible, with thickening of skin **along with nodular or warty excrescences—the stage of elephantiasis.**

Q 10. What are the disadvantages of this grading?

- It does not differentiate the severity of skin changes
- Does not denote the magnitude of disability.

Q 11. What is the recent modification by the WHO?

Recent modification of WHO staging of lymphedema	
Stage 1 –	Same features as in grade I above
Stage 2 –	Same features as in grade II above
Stage 3 –	Presence of shallow skin folds
Stage 4 –	Presence of knobs or nodules
Stage 5 –	Presence of deep skin folds
Stage 6 –	Warty changes in the skin
Stage 7 –	Patient unable to move around due to enormous size of the swelling.

Q 12. What is Brunner's grading?

Grade (Brunner)	*Clinical features*
Subclinical (latent)	There is excess interstitial fluid and histological abnormalities in lymphatics and lymph nodes, but no clinically apparent lymphedema

Contd...

Contd...

I	Edema pits on pressure and swelling largely or completely disappears on elevation and bed rest
II	Edema does not pit and does not significantly reduce upon elevation
III	Edema is associated with irreversible skin changes, i.e. fibrosis, papillae

Q 13. What is the cause for primary lymphedema?

It is a **congenital pathology** affecting the lymphatic channels in the form of:

- Agenesis of lymphatics (Aplasia) – **lymphedema congenita**
- Hypoplasia—the commonest variety—**lymphedema praecox** and **tarda**
- Hyperplasia—lymphatics are enlarged, increased in number and tortuous
- Lymphangiectasia.

Q 14. What are the clinical subtypes of primary lymphedema?

The clinical subtypes are:

1. Congenital lymphedema
   - which appears shortly after birth
2. Lymphedema praecox
   - which starts during puberty
3. Lymphedema tarda
   - which usually starts in the 3rd decade.

Q 15. What are the clinical syndromes associated with primary lymphedema? (PG)

Syndromes associated with primary lymphedema

- Turner syndrome – XO karyotype
- Klinefelter syndrome – XXY
- Down's – Trisomy 21
- Noonan syndrome
- Yellow nail syndrome
- Intestinal lymphangiectasia.

Q 16. What is the commonest cause for lymphedema?

The commonest cause is **always secondary**. The commonest cause for secondary **lymphedema worldwide is lymphatic filariasis.** For the other causes for secondary lymphedema see answer of Q 3.

Q 17. What are the other cause for secondary lymphedema?

1. Malignant diseases
   - Lymph node metastasis
   - Lymphoma
   - Pressure from big tumors
   - Infiltrating tumors
2. Traumatic damage
   - Secondary to lymphadenectomy (block dissection)
   - Radiation to the lymph node area
   - Burns
   - Large circumferential wounds
   - Scarring
   - Varicose vein surgery: Vein harvesting
3. Infections
   - Lymphadenitis
   - Tuberculosis
   - Cellulitis
   - Other inflammatory conditions like rheumatoid arthritis and sarcoidosis.

Q 18. What is acute dermatolymphangioadenitis (ADLA)? (PG)

All cases of lymphedema whether primary or secondary are prone for acute dermato-lymphangioadenitis and **the manifestations are:**

- The draining lymph nodes are enlarged
- Fever and chills
- Painful swelling of the affected limb (initial stages the swelling of the limb will subside after an ADLA episode).

Q 19. What is the pathogenesis of filarial lymphedema?

- The adult parasites living in the lymph vessels initiate the damage
- Earliest pathology is the dilatation of the lymph vessel (**Lymphangiectasia**)
- This lymphangiectasia **is irreversible** even after treatment
- This will result in **stagnation of the lymph** and incompetence of the unidirectional valves
- Lymph stasis encourages the **growth of invading bacteria** as a result of trivial trauma
- The entry of organisms are through the so-called **entry lesions** namely:
  - Fissuring of skin
  - Paronychia
  - Eczema
- Secondary infection by microorganisms especially **streptococci** resulting in ADLA
- Each attack worsens the lymphedema as a result of **obstructive changes in the lymphatics**
- Finally **dermatosclerosis** with nodular and warty excrescences develops.

Q 20. What are the clinical features of filarial lymphedema?

- In the early stages the swelling is **reversible** on elevation of the limb and **will pit on pressure**
- The skin will be smooth without thickening
- Repeated attacks of ADLA (fever, chills and pain)
- Later the swelling will become persistent, does not reverse on elevation of the limb
- Skin becomes thickened and it is **no more pitting**
- Formation of skin folds, nodules and warty changes
- The limb will attain enormous size interfering with mobility—**elephantiasis**

Q 21. What are the organisms responsible for filariasis?

1. *Wuchereria bancrofti*
2. *Brugia malayi.*

Q 22. Which organism will cause hydrocele more often?

The *Wuchereria bancrofti.*

Q 23. What are the sites of lymphdema?

Sites of lymphedema

- Lower limbs (commonest)—Unilateral or bilateral
- Upper limbs
- Male genitalia
- Breast in females.

Q 24. What are the differences between bancrofti and malayi lymphedema?

Bancrofti	*Malayi*
Involve the entire affected limb	Swelling is confined to the legs below the knee or upper limb below the elbow
Genitalia and breast are involved	No involvement of genitalia and breast
Hydrocele is common	Hydrocele is rare

Q 25. What is the clinical difference between lymphedema and venous edema?

The lymphedema will affect the toes much more than other forms of edema. Later the toes get squashed together and become squared-off.

Venous edema	*Lymphedema*
• The edema is **around the ankle,** if thrombosis is confined to the calf. It may extend to the groin, if the iliac vein is thrombosed	• The lymphedema **affects the foot**. The contour of the ankle is lost and there is infilling of the submalleolar depression. The dorsum of the foot will appear as a **buffalo hump.** The toes appear **square.** The skin on the dorsum of the toes cannot be pinched because of the subcutaneous fibrosis—**Stemmer's sign** • The lymphedema usually spreads upto the knee level but can involve the whole limb
• Edema will **pit**	• Early stages pits, later on **nonpitting**
• The skin—lipodermatosclerosis if long standing **(early stage skin is normal)**	• **Skin is hyperkeratotic** later on **nodules** and folds of skin are found. Fissuring, verrucae, **warts** (papillae) are also seen. Fungal infections of the skin and nails and chronic eczema are also seen. Dilated dermal lymphatics form blisters and are called lymphangiomas
• The muscles are **thick and woody**	• **Muscles are normal**
• Regional lymph nodes—**not enlarged**	• Lymph nodes are **enlarged** in secondary lymphedema.

Q 26. What is the dangerous complication of lymphedema?

Lymphangiosarcoma (very rare)—This condition is rapidly fatal. Lymphangiosarcoma was originally described for post mastectomy upper limb edema (**Stewart-Treves' syndrome**). It is suggested that the lymphedema leads to impairment of immune surveillance and therefore predisposes to other types of malignancy.

Q 27. What is phlegmasia alba dolens? (PG)

This results from venous thrombosis of the ilio-femoral segment. The patients present with swelling which commences below the knee and spreads to the thigh reaching upto the inguinal fold. The edema pits on pressure. The limb is pale. There is tenderness along the course of the femoral vein. The foot feels colder. The acute phase will last for 2 to 4 weeks.

Q 28. What is phlegmasia cerulea dolens? (PG)

This is due to deep vein thrombosis affecting the iliofemoral vein and it blocks all the main veins in the skin. The **skin is deeply cyanotic and blue**. The limb is greatly swollen and it feels tense. It is **difficult to feel the arterial pulsations** in the affected limb because the tissues overlying the vessels are bloated and stiff. Finally **venous gangrene** will appear.

Q 29. What is cellulitis?

Cellulitis is a spreading inflammation of the cellular tissue caused by *Streptococcus pyogenes*. This may be **superficial** or **deep**. The superficial is again classified into **cutaneous** and **subcutaneous**. The clinical features are:

- The affected parts are swollen, tense and tender.
- Later it becomes red, boggy and shiny.

Note: The classical description is:

"Swelling with no edge, no limit, no fluctuation and no pus"

Q 30. What are the investigations?

1. Night examination of the peripheral smear for microfilaria
2. ELISA test for circulating filarial antigen (**CFA**)—In the early stage CFA may be positive
3. **Lymphoscintigraphy**—is useful to differentiate primary and secondary type of lymphedema (it is performed by injecting radio labelled albumin or dextran in the web space of the toes and scanning the lymphatics **using a gamma camera**)—not routinely done
4. **USG**—will demonstrate thickening of the subcutaneous tissue in lymphatic filariasis in contrast to increase in size of the muscle compartment seen in varicose veins
5. **Doppler**—helps to confirm venous problems
6. **CT/MRI**—rarely required – reveal thickening of skin and subcutaneous tissue and **honey comb pattern in cases of lymphedema**
7. **MR Angiogram**—useful to establish the diagnosis of arteriovenous malformation.

Q 31. What are the surgical complications of filariasis?

Surgical complications of filariasis

1. Chronic lymphadenitis
2. Chronic epididymo-orchitis
3. Hydrocele—the most common feature of filariasis (40% of the hydroceles are filarial)
4. Chyluria
5. Elephantiasis:
   - Scrotum
   - Upper and lower limbs
   - Breast
   - Vulva
6. Chylous ascites
7. Chylothorax
8. Chylous diarrhea.

Q 32. What is the management of lymphedema?

The management consists of:

- Conservative management of the edema
- Drug therapy
- Surgery.

Q 33. What is the conservative management of lymphedema?

1. Prevention of infection
   - General cleanliness
   - Avoiding bare foot walking
2. Massage
3. Limb elevation
4. Exercise
5. Compression garments
6. Intermittent pneumatic external compression—the limb is enclosed in an inflatable encasing which is inflated upto 150 mm of Hg
7. Use of custom built stocking
8. Decongestive lymphedema therapy (DLT) – Intensive period of **therapist led care** and maintenance phase of **self care**

   Intensive phase: by therapist:
   - Skin care
   - MLD (**M**anual **L**ymphatic **D**rainage) – performed daily
   - MLLB (**M**ulti **L**ayer **L**ymphedema **B**andaging)—nonelastic MLLB for severe and compression type for mild
   - **S**imple **L**ymphatic **D**rainage (SLD)
   - Exercise

   Maintenance phase:
   - **S**imple **L**ymphatic **D**rainage (SLD)—daily.

Note: The pressure exerted by the lymphedema bandaging may be graduated—100% for ankle and foot, 70% for knee, 50% for mid thigh and 40% for growing.

Q 34. What is the drug therapy of lymphedema?

1. **DEC (Diethyl Carbamazine)**—DEC kills the adult worms and has no effect on microfilaria.

   Dose—6 mg/kg/day over 3 divided doses after meals for five days.

   Repeated courses may be required.

2. Combination therapy with Albendazole plus Ivermectin

   or

   Albendazole plus DEC

3. **Antibiotics** – long term benzathine penicillin has been prescribed

4. Anti-inflammatory, antihistamines and antipyretics.

Q 35. What are the surgical options for the lymphedema of limb? (PG)

Can be classified into two groups:

Drainage procedures

1. Lymphonodovenous shunt procedures
2. Direct lymphaticovenous anastomosis (technically more difficult and operating microscope is required)
3. Monofilament nylon netting—a subcutaneous web of nylon fiber is created
4. Omental transposition—a subcutaneous tunnel is made in the limb and a long mobilized length of omentum is placed for lymphatic drainage.

Excisional procedures—(debulking procedures).

Q 36. What is lymphonodovenous shunt? (PG)

- Localize the **draining nodes** by injecting patent blue in the web space
- Vertical or horizontal skin incision is made centering on the saphenofemoral junction
- Mobilize the saphenous vein for 6 to 8 cm and ligate the distal end

  (Rule out saphenofemoral incompetence)
- Identify a suitable moderate sized lymph node and make a transverse section of the node without mobilization. Discard the superficial portion of the lymph node
- Rotate the proximal end of the vein and tailor it close to the node. Now section the saphenous vein at a suitable point for anastamosis
- Anastomose the vessel wall to the lymph node capsule with six zero prolene sutures, burying the node to the vessel.

Q 37. What are the excisional procedures?

The essence of this form of treatment is to excise all or part of the involved skin and subcutaneous tissue. The cover is given by skin graft or raising flaps:

Charles procedure: The entire skin is excised and the area grafted, this is followed by pressure bandage. It is not recommended for the dorsum of the foot as it has too many tendons and very minimal deep fascia.

Thompson procedure (Swiss roll operation): He implanted the de-epithelialized dermal flaps behind the deep fascia in attempts to promote direct drainage. Necrosis of the buried portion is frequent and when it occurs the discharge almost never stops.

Case

43 Hydrocele of tunica Vaginalis Sac (Epididymal Cyst, Spermatocele, Varicocele, Hematocele, Chylocele, etc.)

Case Capsule

A 35-year-old male patient presents with increase in size of the right side of the scrotum of two years duration. He gives history of **frequency of urine and painful micturition**. On examination, the right side of the scrotum shows a swelling of **15 × 10 cm size** which is **confined to the scrotum** (**can get above the swelling**). The surface of the swelling is smooth and it is well-defined. There is no local rise of temperature. Upper **posterior part of the swelling is tender**. The swelling is **fluctuant and translucent**. It is **not reducible**. On percussion it is dull. The right testis is **not separately felt**. The skin of the scrotum over the swelling is freely mobile. The **spermatic cord** is felt above the swelling and is **tender**. The contralateral testis and genitalia are normal. There is no evidence of any mass or lymph nodes in the abdomen. There are no supraclavicular lymph nodes.

Checklist for history

1. History of **painful micturition** and frequency of urine

Contd...

Contd...

2. History of **trauma**
3. History of **pain and discomfort** in the testis
4. History of **malaise and weight loss** (tumor)
5. History of **filariasis**
6. History of tuberculosis and family history of **tuberculosis.**

Checklist for clinical examination

1. Elicit **fluctuation**
2. **Get above the swelling** or not (Flow chart 43.1)
3. Palpation of testes
4. Palpation of cord
5. Palpation of vas deferens
6. Look for **translucency**
7. **Examination of abdomen** for lymph nodes (Para-aortic nodes)
8. Look for **supraclavicular nodes**
9. Always do **ultrasound abdomen** to rule out tumor and other pathology.

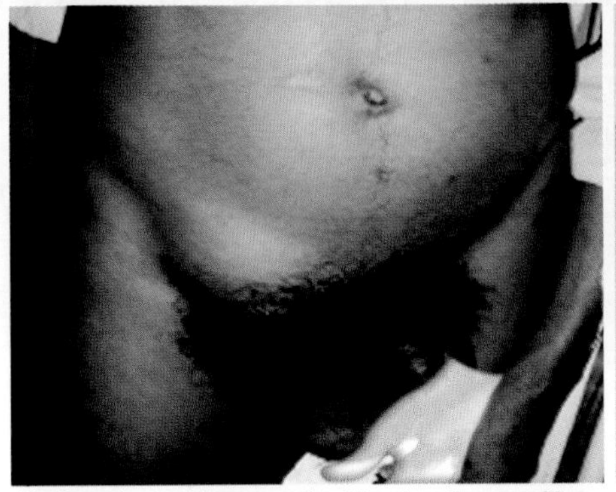

Hydrocele en bissac patient in standing position

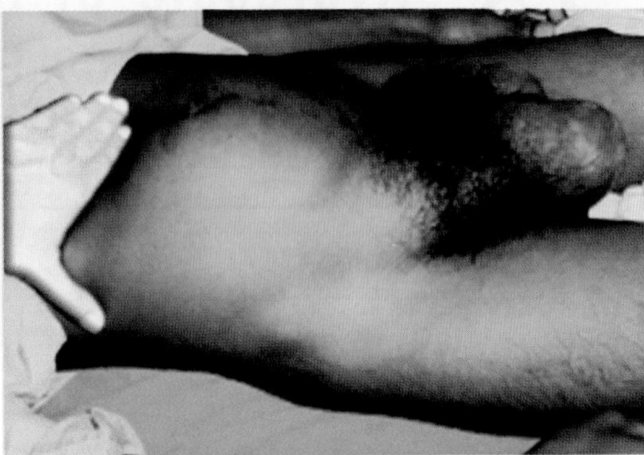

Hydrocele en bissac showing the abdominal extension

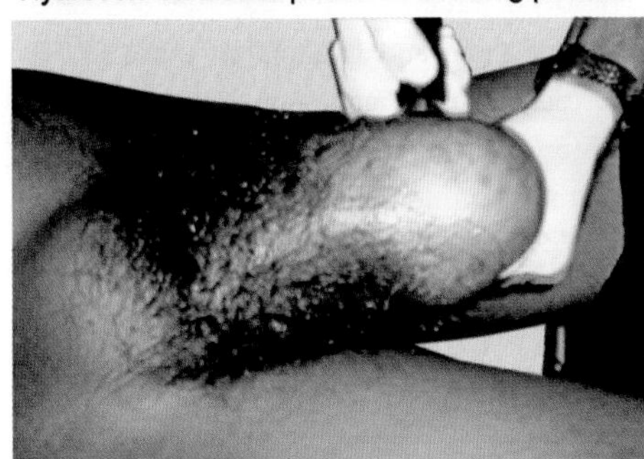

Hydrocele en bissac showing transillumination

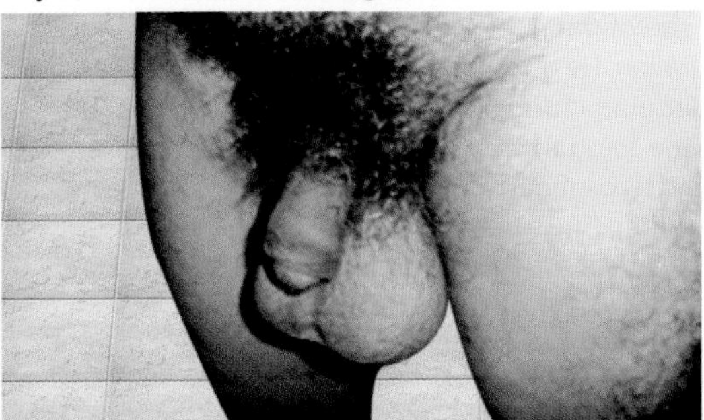

Hydrocele of Tunica vaginalis sac on left side

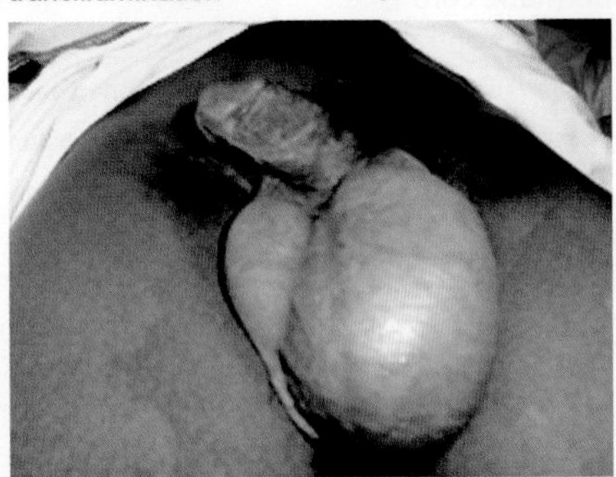

Hydrocele of Tunica vaginalis sac on left side

Flow chart 43.1: Scrotal and inguinoscrotal swellings

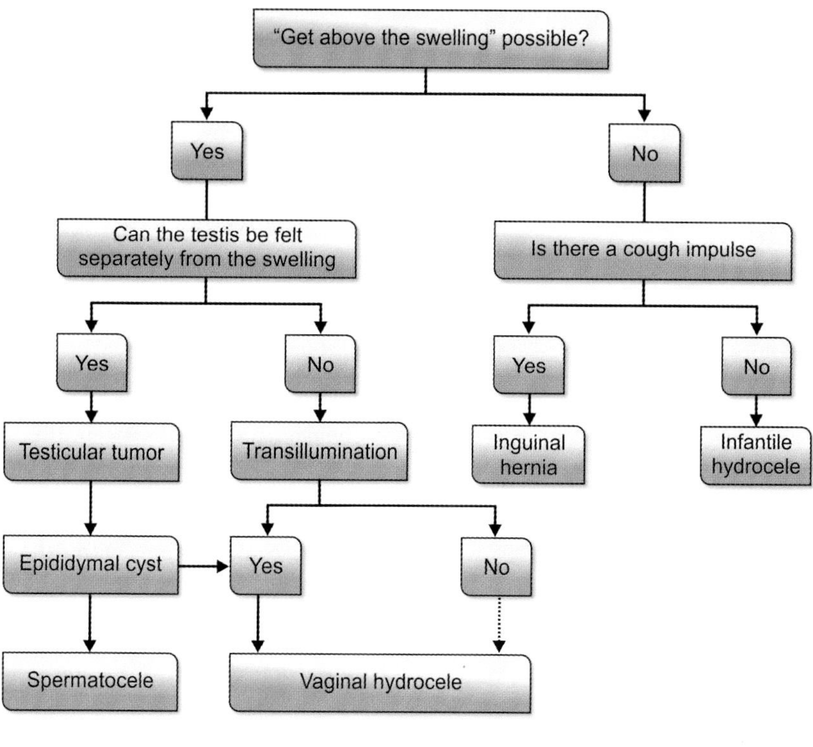

Q 1. What is the diagnosis in this case?

Hydrocele of tunica vaginalis sac (right side).

Q 2. What is the order of palpation of testis?

The order of palpation is from below upwards (Fig. 43.1):

1. Testis
2. Tunica vaginalis
3. Epididymis
4. Cord structures
5. External inguinal ring.

Q 3. Why this is hydrocele?

The points in favor of hydrocele are:

1. Can get above the swelling (purely scrotal)
2. Cystic in consistency
3. Fluctuation
4. Transillumination positive
5. Testis cannot be felt separately
6. It is not reducible usually
7. No impulse on coughing.

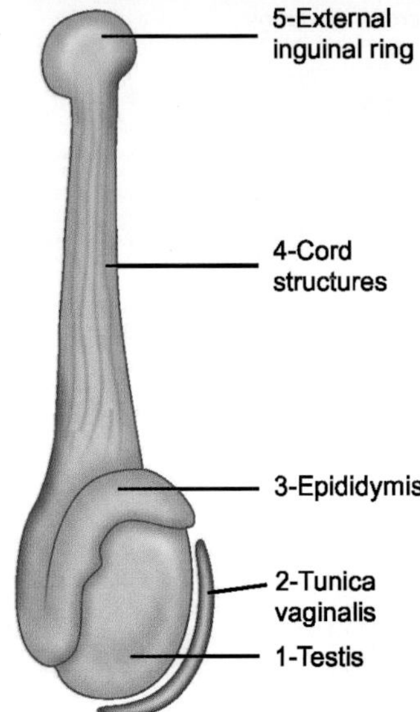

Fig. 43.1: Order of palpation of the testis (from below upwards)

Q 4.Hydrocele of what?

Hydrocele of tunica vaginalis sac [TV sac].

Q 5. What is hydrocele?

Hydrocele is an abnormal collection of serous fluid in some part of the processus vaginalis, usually the tunica.

Q 6. Can you get a hydrocele which is not transilluminant?

Yes.

The criteria for transillumination in hydrocele are:

a. Sac must be thin
b. The fluid must be clear.

When the **sac is thick** or the **fluid is not clear**, then it won't be transilluminant.

Q 7. What are the conditions in which it is not transilluminant?

a. Infected hydrocele (Pyocele)
b. Hematocele
c. Chylocele
d. Thickened and calcified sac.

Q 8. Can you get hydroceles which are inguinoscrotal?

Yes. In the following situations, it may be inguinoscrotal.

a. *Infantile hydrocele:* When the fluid collection extends from **scrotum up to the deep inguinal ring**.
b. *Congenital hydrocele:* Where the sac and the fluid are **communicating with the peritoneal cavity**.
c. *Hydrocele en bissac* [**bilocular hydrocele**]: Here the sac communicates with extension of the sac underneath the anterior abdominal wall and we can elicit cross fluctuation between the abdominal swelling and scrotal swelling.
d. *Funicular hydrocele:* Where the fluid collection is communicating with peritoneal cavity and it is coming down up to the testes **without involvement of the vaginal part**. The funicular **process is closed just above the tunica vaginalis**. The fluid collection is confined to the funicular region.
e. *Encysted hydrocele:* Where the fluid collection is confined to the cord region and the traction test will be positive.
f. *Hydrocele of hernial sac:* Where the **neck of the hernial sac** is occluded at the deep ring region by omentum and fluid accumulates distal to the sac.

Features of hydroceles presenting as inguinoscrotal swellings

Type	*Age*	*Communicationwith peritoneal cavity?*	*Cause*
a. Vaginal hydrocele	All	No	May be primary or secondary to tumor, trauma or infection
b. Congenital hydrocele	Children < 3 years	Yes	The communicating orifice is too small for the development of hernia
c. Infantile hydrocele	All age groups	No	The processus vaginalis is closed at the deep ring and as a result of incomplete absorption of fluid from the tunica vaginalis
d. Funicular hydrocele	All age groups	Yes	Processus vaginalis is closed just above the tunica vaginalis. It does not produce a proper scrotal swelling
e. Encysted hydrocele of the cord	All	No	May occur anywhere along the cord. May present as inguinal or scrotal swelling. **Traction test positive**
f. Hydrocele of the hernial sac	Older age	No	Neck of the hernial sac closed by adhesions or plug of omentum. The distal sac is filled with serous fluid secreted by the peritoneum

Q 9. What is the etiology of hydrocele?

It is produced by:

a. *Defective absorption of fluid:* This is the explanation for primary hydrocele
b. *Excessive production of fluid:* Secondary hydrocele
c. *Interference with lymphatic drainage of scrotal structures:* Filariasis
d. *By connection with peritoneal cavity:* As in congenital variety.

Q 10. What is the color of the hydrocele fluid?

Hydrocele fluid is amber-colored [color of urine].

Q 11. What are the constituents of hydrocele fluid?

It contains:

- Albumin
- Fibrinogen
- Cholesterol crystals
- Crystals of tyrosine.

Note: Because of **the presence of fibrinogen** it will clot the blood.

Q 12. What is acute hydrocele?

Sudden appearance of hydrocele in young men is associated with a testicular tumor and it is a dangerous situation.

Q 13. What is hydrocele of canal of Nuck?

It occurs in females in the inguinal region and **the cyst lies in relation to the round ligament.** It is similar to hydrocele of the cord [encysted hydrocele]. But, hydrocele of the canal of Nuck is always at least **partially within the inguinal canal.**

Q 14. What is hydrocele of Nuck?

It is nothing but lymph cyst of the neck.

Q 15. What are the types of hydrocele?

The hydrocele is classified into **congenital and acquired types.**

Four types of congenital hydroceles
a. Vaginal hydrocele
b. Infantile hydrocele
c. Congenital hydrocele
d. Hydrocele of the cord.

The acquired variety is further classified into **primary and secondary**.

Differences between primary and secondary

Primary [Idiopathic]	*Secondary*
• Most common in middle and later life	Same
• Big size	Small size
• Defective absorption of fluid	Excessive production of fluid
• Palpation of testis difficult	Testis easily palpable
• Tense cyst	Loose cyst
• Transillumination positive	May be negative

Q 16. What are the causes for secondary hydrocele?

The important causes for secondary hydrocele are:

a. Tumor
b. Tuberculosis
c. Filariasis.

Q 17. How will you rule out a tumor in a case of hydrocele?

a. By palpation of testis:
   - Testis will be separately palpable in case of tumor
   - The testis becomes relatively heavy in neoplasm (comparatively the testis is light in gumma of the testis)
   - The testicular sensation will be absent or peculiar **sickening sensation** will be felt
   - The testis will be nodular, indurated and irregular.
b. By ultrasound examination—one can rule out a mass lesion in the testis
c. By tumor markers—β hCG and α fetoprotein.

Q 18. How will you rule out tuberculosis?

Clinical features of tuberculosis of epididymis

i. Tuberculosis attacks epididymis (**syphilis attacks testis, filariasis attacks both**)
ii. Tuberculosis affects the **globus minor first**
iii. In tuberculosis, the epididymis is craggy and the vas is beaded
iv. A **posteriorly placed ulcer that is fixed to the epididymis** is a tuberculous ulcer (anteriorly placed ulcer that is fixed to the testis is gummatous ulcer).

Q 19. How will you rule out filariasis?

The cord will be tender and thickened in filariasis.

Q 20. What are the features of filarial hydrocele and chylocele?

- It accounts for 80% of the hydroceles in tropical countries
- Chylocele is because of rupture of lymphatic varix with discharge of chyle into the hydrocele
- *Wuchereria bancrofti* is the organism responsible
- The fluid may contain liquid fat and cholesterol
- Adult worms are demonstrated in epididymis removed at operation.

Q 21. What is post-herniorrhaphy hydrocele?

It is because of interruption of the lymphatic drainage of the scrotal contents as a result of inguinal hernia repair.

Q 22. What is hydrocele of hernial sac?

When the **neck of the hernial sac is plugged with omentum**, fluid accumulates in the distal hernial sac.

Q 23. What are the other differential diagnoses of a cystic swelling in this region?

Other differential diagnoses are epididymal cyst and spermatocele.

Q 24. How will you differentiate epididymal cyst from spermatocele?

Epididymal cyst	*Spermatocele*
• It is a cystic degeneration of the epididymis	• It is a **retention cyst** from some part of the sperm conducting mechanism
• Usually above and behind the body of the testes	• Situated in the head of the epididymis
• Multilocular	• Unilocular
• Usually multiple and often bilateral	• Single
• Brilliantly transilluminant [**Chinese lantern appearance**]	• **Negative**
• Fluid is **crystal clear**	• **Barley water color (contains spermatozoa)**
• Treatment is excision (excision mayinterfere with transport of sperms)	• Large ones are **aspirated or excised**

Q 25. What is the treatment of hydrocele of TV sac (Tunica vaginalis sac)?

It is mainly treated by surgery.

Q 26. What are the surgical options?

1. **Jaboulay's** procedure (Eversion of the TV sac)
2. **Lord's operation** (when the sac is thin-walled) the sac is opened and it is **plicated** around the testis. In this operation, there is minimal dissection, the chance for hematoma is reduced and there is no need for a drain.

Q 27. Can you drain the hydrocele fluid?

Drainage of hydrocele fluid is usually not done because of the fear of complications like infection and hematocele.

Q 28. What are the complications of hydrocele?

Complications of hydrocele:

a. Hematocele
b. Infection and pyocele
c. Hernia of hydrocele
d. Calcification of the sac
e. Rupture as a result of trauma or spontaneous
f. Atrophy of the testis.

Q 29. What are the causes for hematocele?

Causes for hematocele

- Tapping of hydrocele (damage to small vessels during tapping)
- Testicular trauma
- Postoperative
- Tumor.

Q 30. What is clotted hematocele?

- It is because of a spontaneous slow ooze of blood into the tunica vaginalis
- Usually it is painless
- A tumor may present as clotted hematocele.

Q 31. What is the treatment of clotted hematocele?

- Orchidectomy (It is very difficult to differentiate tumor from a benign condition like this).

Q 32. What is the most important complication of hydrocele operation?

Hematocele.

Q 33. What is varicocele?

It is a varicose dilatation of the veins draining the testis (pampiniform plexus).

Q 34. What are the signs demonstrable in varicocele?

Signs of varicocele

1. It feels like a **'bag of worms'**
2. It can only be felt with the patient standing. If the patient is asked to lie down, the **veins of the plexus will empty**
3. A **thrill is felt** while the patient is coughing
4. The **'bow' sign**: lightly hold the varicocele between the fingers and thumb. Now the patient is instructed to bow. Tension within the veins become appreciably less by this procedure
5. The **scrotum** on the affected side **hangs lower than normal**
6. The testis below a large varicocele may be **smaller and softer** than the normal side
7. After emptying the varicocele in supine position, obstruct the external ring and make the patient stand up. The varicocele will **slowly fill up from below upwards.**

Q 35. What is the incidence of varicocele?

It is seen in up to 15% of the male population.

Q 36. Which age group is affected by varicocele?

- Seen in adolescence and early adulthood
- Seen in tall thin men with pendulous scrotum (short, fat individuals are seldom affected).

Q 37. What are the symptoms of varicocele?

- Chronic dull ache in the scrotum, worse on standing for prolonged periods
- May be associated with oligospermia (the association remains unclear).

Q 38. On which side varicocele is more common and why?

- Varicocele is more common on left side because the left testicular vein enters the left renal vein at right angles (95%)
- At times the left testicular artery arches over the left renal vein to compress it
- The loaded left colon may press on the left testicular vein.

Q 39. What is the significance of recent onset of left sided varicocele?

It is associated with **left renal cell carcinoma** because of **obstruction of the renal vein** by a tumor thrombus growing through the left renal vein.

Q 40. What is the venous drainage of testis and epididymis?

The draining veins form a plexus called **pampiniform plexus** in the scrotal region. The veins become fewer as they traverse the inguinal canal. At or near the deep inguinal ring, they join to form **one or two testicular veins**. They pass upwards behind the peritoneum and join the **renal vein on left side and inferior vena cava on right side**.

Q 41. What is the peculiarity of the testicular vein?

They are having valves only at the termination which may be absent (**valve less system**).

Q 42. Is there an alternative venous drainage for the testis?

Yes. The collateral venous return from the testis is through the **cremasteric veins** which drain into the inferior epigastric vein.

Q 43. What is the relationship between varicocele and spermatogenesis?

- Normally the scrotal temperature is 2.5°C less than the rectal temperature

- The presence of unilateral varicocele interferes with the normal temperature control of the scrotum that reduces the temperature differential to (scrotum/rectum) about 0.1°C below the rectal temperature
- Since varicocele is relatively common, those who are having oligospermia with varicocele, it is tempting to blame the varicocele as the cause for infertility (not yet clinically proved).

Q 44. What are the muscles responsible for supporting the testis?

Dartos and cremaster.

Q 45. What are the actions of dartos and cremaster?

- Dartos bears the weight of the testis and acts as a kind of thermostat
- The cremaster is responsible for reflex retraction of the testis during threat of trauma and during fight.

Q 46. What is the grading of varicocele?

- Grade I: Impulse felt in the scrotum on Valsalva maneuver
- Grade II: Tortuous and dilated veins palpated without Valsalva maneuver
- Grade III: Varicocele is visible through the scrotal skin.

Note: **Sonologically:** More than two to three veins of 3 mm or greater in size are found with enlargement on standing and reflux on Valsalva maneuver.

Q 47. What is subclinical varicocele?

Those which are impalpable on physical examination are called subclinical varicocele.

Q 48. What are the indications for surgery?

3 'S'

- Symptoms
- Subfertility
- Service recruitment.

Q 49. What are the procedures available?

- Palomos operation
- Laparoscopic ligation of testicular veins
- Embolization of the testicular vein under radiographic control.

Q 50. What is Palomos operation?

- It is a ligation of the testicular veins above the inguinal ligament where the pampiniform plexus coalesce to form one or two veins.
- An incision is made 3 cm above the deep inguinal ring. The external oblique, internal oblique and transversus muscles are split and the testicular veins are ligated extraperitoneally (the alternative venous pathway for the testis is described above).
- This operation can be done laparoscopically also.

Q 51. What is "triangle of doom"?

It is a laparoscopic finding seen in hernia surgery and varicocele surgery. The triangle is formed medially by the vas deferens, laterally by the testicular vessel and an imaginary line joining these two structures. Inside this triangle the **iliac artery and vein are seen** which are likely to be injured and hence called triangle of doom.

Q 52. Will varicocele recur after surgery?

Yes. Recurrence is common after all types of varicocele surgery.

Case

44 Inguinal Hernia/Femoral Hernia

Case Capsule

A 60-year-old male patient presents with a swelling in the **right inguinoscrotal region** of 2 years duration. He also complains of dragging and aching sensation in the groin. He is a chronic smoker with bronchitis. For the last 2 years, he has **difficulty in passing water**. He has to get up 3–4 times every night for this purpose. There is no history of chronic constipation, abdominal pain or vomiting. He says the swelling is present **only during standing position** and it will disappear as soon as he lies down. On examination, there is a **large pear-shaped swelling** seen above the crease of the groin and medial to the pubic tubercle of 8 × 4 cm size. The swelling is not extending to the scrotum, but confined to the inguinal region. There is a visible **expansile cough impulse**, which is demonstrated in palpation also. One "**cannot get above the swelling**": The swelling is reducible. By applying pressure over the internal ring (**Deep ring occlusion test**), the swelling cannot be held reduced. A **defect is felt** in the abdominal wall above the pubic tubercle. The swelling is **dull to percussion**. The contralateral side is normal, so also the external genitalia. **Malgaigne's bulging** is noted on the left sided while performing head raising test. The abdominal examination revealed no scars and no mass lesions. Perrectal examination is normal.

Checklist for history

- History of **chronic cough, asthma, bronchitis**
- History of **heavy weight lifting**
- History of **constipation** (straining to pass motion)
- History of **urinary complaints:** night frequency, hesitancy-difficulty to initiate the act of micturition and urgency, etc.
- History of **pain in the groin**
- History of epigastric pain (dragging on the mesentery)
- History of **appendicectomy (damage to ilio-inguinal nerve)**
- History of **abdominal pain and vomiting.**

Checklist for clinical examination

1. Always examine the patient in **standing position**, while the examiner sits.
2. Always examine **both inguinal regions** (20% hernias are bilateral)
3. Look for visible **expansile impulse** on coughing
4. Look for palpable expansile impulse on coughing

Contd...

Contd...

5. Assess whether you can **get above the swelling** or not
6. Swelling is **reducible or not**
7. Assess the percussion note: **Resonant if the content is gut, dull if the content is omentum**
8. Always examine the **genitalia** (there may be dual pathology)
9. Feel the testis (**testis will be separate** from the swelling)
10. Locate epididymis above and posterior to the testis
11. Feel along the spermatic cord
12. Always look for abdominal scars especially **appendicectomy scar** which will injure the ilioinguinal nerve
13. Assessment of the abdominal muscle tone—head raising test. [**Malgaigne's bulgings**—minor bulging of both inguinal canal region in head raising test. This is normal and seen when the muscles are weak]
14. Examine the abdomen for visceral malignancy
15. **Examine the chest** for respiratory problems
16. **Per rectal examination** to rule out benign hypertrophy of prostate.

Finally before presenting the case, determine whether the hernia is

1. Inguinal/femoral
2. If inguinal, direct/indirect
3. Complete/incomplete
4. Determine the content—intestine/omentum
   - Soft and resonant—intestine
   - Firm, rubbery and dull—omentum
5. Complicated/uncomplicated
   - Irreducibility, obstruction, strangulation, incarceration and inflammation.

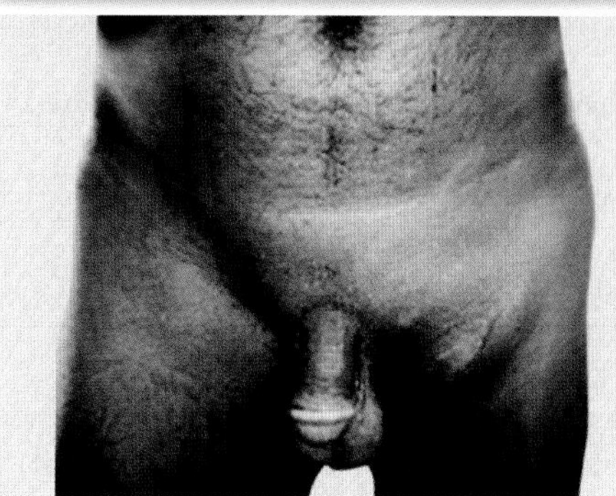

Femoral hernia

Right incomplete indirect inguinal hernia

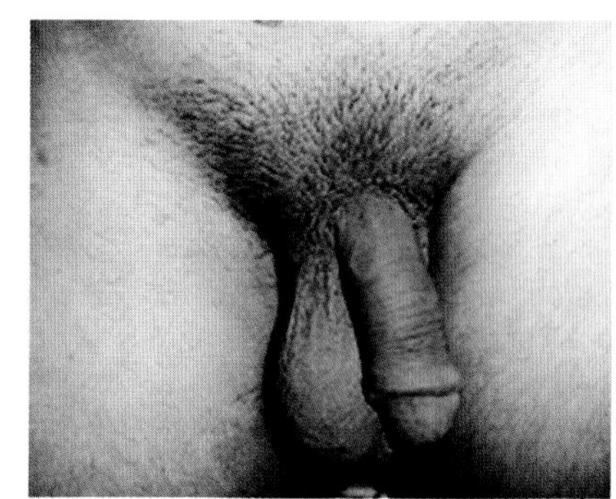

Right sided indirect inguinal hernia

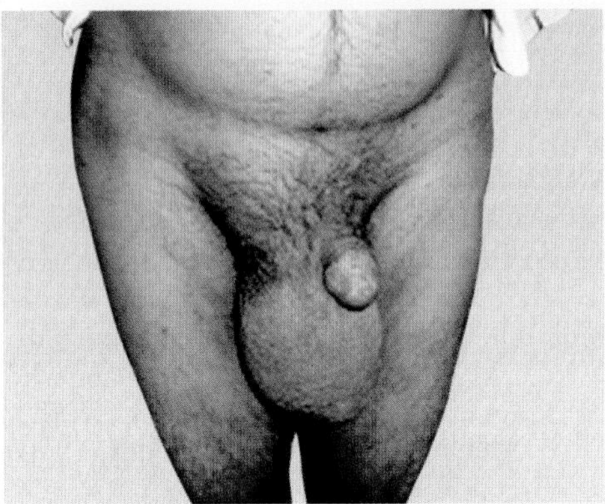
Right inguinoscrotal swelling—inguinal hernia

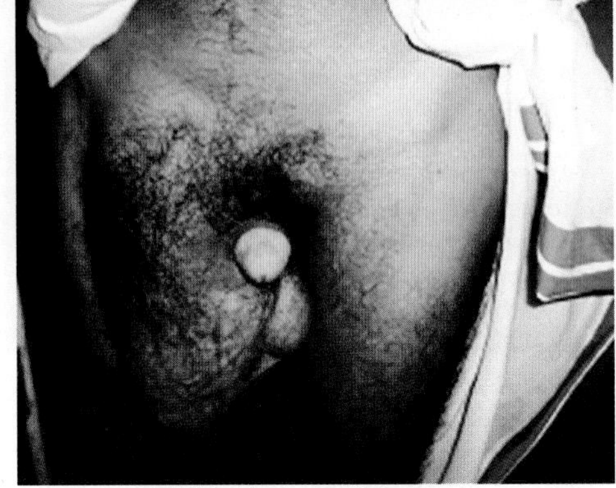
Right sided complete hernia

Q 1. Why this is hernia?

The points in favor of hernia are:

1. Inguinoscrotal swelling
2. Visible and palpable impulse on coughing [an impulse is often better seen than felt].
3. Cannot get above the swelling [inguinoscrotal]
4. Reducibility [absent in case of complication]
5. Ring occlusion test
    a. Positive in case of indirect hernia [swelling will not come out]
    b. Negative in case of direct hernia [swelling will come out].

Q 2. What is the definition of hernia?

Hernia is defined as the protrusion of a viscus in part or in whole through a normal or abnormal opening in relation to the abdomen. Exceptions are rare. For example, lung hernia, muscle hernia, internal hernia, etc.

Q 3. What are the parts of hernia?

The hernia has got a sac, coverings and content. The sac has got a neck, body and fundus. The coverings of the hernia varies depending on whether it is indirect, direct or femoral [Read Anatomy]. The contents are omentum [omentocele], intestine [enterocele] or other organs, e.g. if Meckel's diverticulum is forming the content, it is called Littre's hernia. Appendix will form a content on right side and sigmoid will form a content on left side. Urinary bladder will form content on both sides.

Q 4. What is the name of the hernia where part of the circumference of the viscus is forming the content?

Richter's hernia.

Q 5. What is the test to differentiate between direct and indirect inguinal hernia?

Deep ring occlusion test is the test of choice to differentiate these two. Before doing this, the patient should be in supine position and the hernia should be reduced. Reducibility is tested in the recumbent position. If this is not possible, flex the thigh in order to keep the pillars of the external ring relaxed.

Q 6. What is Zieman's test?

This is done in the standing position. The clinician stands behind and somewhat to the right for the right side and behind and somewhat to the left for the left side. The hand of the corresponding side is used for examination [Right hand for right side and left hand for left side]. He places his index finger over the indirect hernial site, the middle finger over the direct hernial site, and ring finger over the femoral hernial site. The patient is requested to hold the nose and blow. A peculiar gliding motion of the walls of the sac will be felt beneath the relevant finger corresponding to the type of hernia.

Q 7. What are the clinical differences between direct and indirect inguinal hernia?

Clinical differences between direct and indirect inguinal hernia

No		*Direct*	*Indirect*
1.	Extend to scrotum	Does not go down to the scrotum	Can descend into the scrotum
2.	Direction of reduction	Reduce upwards and then straight backwards	Reduce upwards, then laterally and backwards
3.	Controlled by pressure over the internal ring	Not controlled after reduction, by pressure over the internal inguinal ring	Controlled, after reduction by pressure over the internal inguinal ring
4.	Direction of reappearance after reduction	The bulge reappears outwards to original position	The bulge reappears in the middle of the inguinal region and then flows medially before turning down to the neck of the scrotum
5.	Palpable defect	Defect may be felt in the abdominal wall above the	No palpable defect as it is behind the fibers of the external oblique pubic tubercle muscle
6.	Relationship of cord to sac	Sac appears medial to the inferior epigastric artery and is outside the spermatic cord (posterior to the cord)	The sac is inside the spermatic cord

Q 8. What are the peculiarities of direct inguinal hernia?

Peculiarities of direct inguinal hernia

- Appear later in life
- Do not occur in children
- Rare in women
- Rarely strangulate

Contd...

Contd...

- Direct hernia is always acquired
- Usually seen in males
- They do not often attain large size or descend into the scrotum
- The protruding mass mainly consists of extra-peritoneal fat
- The neck of the sac is wide.

Q 9. How will you assess the content of the sac?

If it is omentum:

- It will give a doughy feel
- The first part of the hernial sac is reduced easily and the last part is difficult to reduce.

If it is intestine

- The first part is difficult to reduce and the last part is reduced easily
- It has got a characteristic gurgling sound during reduction.

Q 10. What is sliding hernia [Hernia-en-glissade]?

Sliding hernia is a condition where portion of cecum and appendix on right side, sigmoid on left side and urinary bladder on both sides will slide down behind the sac. Even though it is not inside the sac, it forms the posterior wall of the sac. If the wall of the sac is unusually thick peroperatively, one should carefully rule out a sliding hernia.

Q 11. What is Maydl's Hernia?

This is the so-called W loop hernia where the small intestine forms a W loop within the hernial sac. The importance of this type of hernia is in case of obstruction, even if the visible intestine inside the sac is viable if one is not pulling out the rest of the intestine, you are likely to miss gangrene for the rest of the bowel.

Q 12. How will you differentiate inguinal hernia from femoral hernia?

Inguinal	*Femoral*
• Above and medial to the pubic tubercle	• Below and lateral to the pubic tubercle
• Above the crease of the groin	• Below the crease of the groin
• Can be reduced completely	• Cannot be reduced completely
• Cough impulse usually present	• Many do not have cough impulse

Q 13. Why femoral hernia is usually irreducible?

The femoral hernias are having:

a. Narrow neck of the sac
b. The contents are adherent to the peritoneal sac.

Q 14. What is the direction of enlargement of femoral hernia?

It is usually downwards, forwards and upwards.

Q 15. What is the name of the triangle in which you get the direct hernia?

The direct hernia comes out through Hesselbach's triangle. It is bounded medially by the lateral border of rectus abdominis, laterally by the inferior epigastric artery and below by the inguinal ligament.

Q16. What are the differential diagnoses of inguinal hernia?

Differential diagnoses of inguinal hernia
a. Femoral hernia
b. Vaginal hydrocele
c. Undescended testis in superficial inguinal pouch
d. Hydrocele of the cord
e. Lipoma of the cord
f. Infantile hydrocele
g. Ectopic testis
h. Lipoma of the cord
i. Hydrocele of canal of Nuck
j. Psoas abscess
k. Psoas bursae
l. Sapheno-varix
m. Enlarged lymph nodes
n. Femoral aneurysm.

Note: There are two lumps which occur in the line of the spermatic cord which can pop in and out of the external ring, viz. undescended testes and hydrocele of the cord.

Q 17. What are the three types of inguinal hernia?

a. *Bubonocele:* When the hernia is limited to the inguinal canal.
b. *Funicular:* When the processus vaginalis is closed just above the epididymis. Here the contents of the sac can be felt separately from the testis.
c. *Complete:* [scrotal] In complete hernia, the testis appears to lie within the lower part of the hernia.

Q 18. What is the situation of testis in a complete (scrotal) hernia?

It is sited posteroinferior to the hernia.

Q 19. What are the etiological factors for hernia?

Etiology of hernia

a. Congenital: Preformed sac where the processus is patent
b. Acquired:
   i. Increased intra-abdominal pressure [chronic cough, straining, whooping cough, etc.]
   ii. Smokers [collagen deficiency due to smoking]

Contd...

Contd...

   iii. Intra-abdominal malignancy [acute onset of hernia]
   iv. Obesity [muscles are weak, fat separate muscle bundles and weakens aponeurosis]
   v. Multiparity [for femoral hernia—stretching of pelvic ligaments]
   vi. TA/TF deficiency—transverses abdominis, transversalis fascia deficiency
   vii. After peritoneal dialysis—previous weakness or enlargement of patent processus
c. Hereditary
d. The evolutionary factors are:
   i. Absence of posterior rectus sheath below the arcuate line
   ii. Adoption of upright position
   iii. Change from quadrapedal to bipedal locomotion [In animals, the weight of the abdominal content is directed away from the inguinal region].

Q 20. What is the definition of inguinal canal?

Inguinal canal is an **intermuscular** slit situated between the superficial and deep inguinal rings (Fig. 44.1).

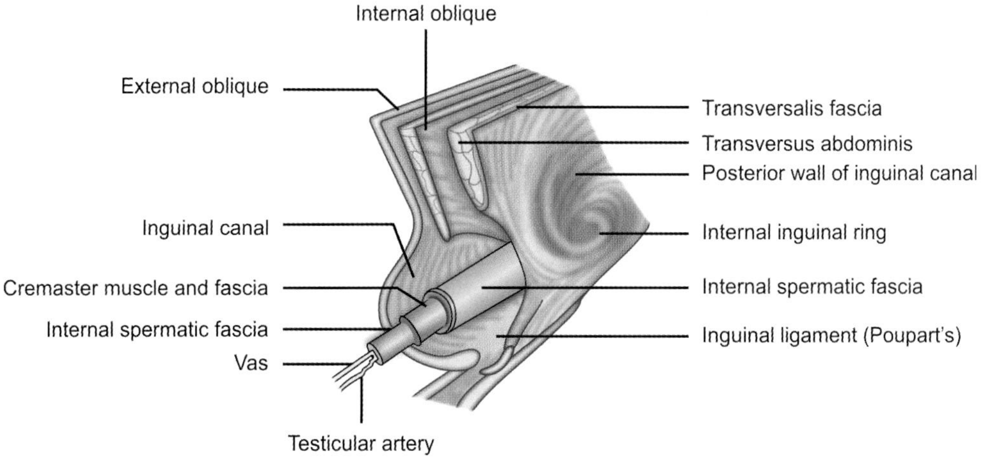

Fig. 44.1: Anatomy of inguinal canal and related structures from inside the abdomen

Q 21. What is external inguinal ring?

- It is an opening in the external oblique aponeurosis
- This is formed by the two crurae of the external oblique aponeurosis
- It lies just above and medial to the pubic tubercle.

Q 22. What is internal ring?

- It is an opening in the fascia transversalis
- This is a 'U' shaped condensation of the fascia transversalis
- It is situated ½ inch (1.25 cm) above the mid inguinal point [between the pubic symphysis and the anterior superior iliac spine]
- The inferior epigastric artery runs medially.

Q 23. What is mid point of the inguinal ligament?

- It is situated between the pubic tubercle and the anterior superior iliac spine
- It is 1–1.5 cm lateral to the mid inguinal point.

Q 24. What is Myopectineal orifice of Fruchaud?

The opening in the lower abdominal wall bounded above by the myoaponeurotic arch of the lower edge of the internal oblique and transversus abdominis muscle (conjoint tendon), below by the pectineal line of the superior pubic ramus, laterally by the iliopsoas muscle and medially by the lateral border of the rectus muscle. This serves as the passage for blood vessels, nerves, lymphatics, muscles and tendons between the abdomen and the lower limb. The space is arbitrarily divided into upper and lower halves by the lower free aponeurotic edge, viz., inguinal ligament. This space is closed off posteriorly by the transversalis fascia. This is the site for direct, indirect and femoral hernias. All the three can be repaired by a single piece of mesh by covering this orifice (Fig. 44.2).

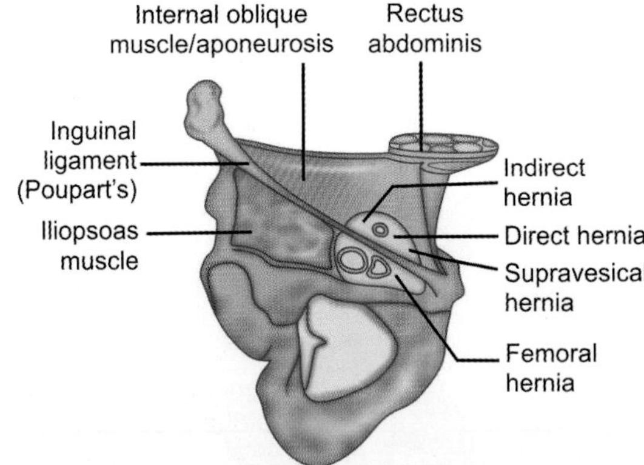

Fig. 44.2: Myopectineal orifice of Fruchaud and possible locations of hernias

Q 25. What is space of Bogros?

It is located in front of the peritoneum just beneath the posterior lamina of the transversalis fascia. For all practical purposes it is a lateral extension of the retropubic space of Retzius. The space of Bogros is used for the location of prosthesis during the repair of inguinal hernia in laparoscopic surgery.

Q 26. What is conjoined tendon?

By definition, this is the fusion of fibers of the internal oblique aponeurosis with similar fibers from the aponeurosis of the transversus abdominis muscle just as they are inserted on the pubic tubercle, pectineal ligament, and the superior ramus of the pubis. In reality conjoined tendon is present only in 5% of individuals and therefore it is considered as a myth and a better terminology is conjoined area.

Q 27. What is transversalis fascia?

The term may be restricted to the internal fascia lining the transversus abdominis muscle. In the inguinal area the transversalis fascia is bilaminar enveloping the inferior epigastric vessels.

Q 28. What is the frequency of various types of hernia?

Frequency of types of Hernia

- Inguinal—75% (indirect 65% – 55% are right sided and direct 35%)
- Femoral—20% in women and 5% in men
- Umbilical—15%
- Rarer forms—1.5%
- Bilateral—12%

Q 29. What is the frequency of direct hernia?

- About 35% of inguinal hernias are direct in males (65% indirect)
- 12% will have contralateral hernia
- About four-fold increased risk for future development on contralateral side.

Q 30. Inguinal hernia is more commonly seen on which side?

About 55% seen on right side.

Q 31. What is the frequency of direct hernia in females?

Women practically never develop a direct inguinal hernia.

Q 32. What is the sex-wise incidence of hernia?

The male to female ratio for inguinal hernia is 20:1.

Q 33. What is funicular direct inguinal hernia [prevesical hernia]?

This is a narrow necked hernia with prevesical fat and sometimes a portion of the bladder that protrudes through a small oval defect in the medial part of conjoint muscle, just above the pubic tubercle. It occurs in elderly males and occasionally becomes strangulated.

Q 34. What is dual hernia [Pantaloon, "saddle-bag"]?

This is a type of hernia where two sacs straddle the inferior epigastric artery, one sac being medial and other lateral to the artery. This is one of the causes for recurrence, if one is overlooked during surgery.

Q 35. What will be the course of action, if a patient develops sudden asymptomatic hernia?

One must search for occult intra-abdominal malignancy and ascites. Do the following tests.

- Digital rectal examination
- Fecal study for occult blood
- Sigmoidoscopy/colonoscopy
- Double contrast barium enema.

Q 36. Why must a hernia be repaired?

Because of the potential dangerous complications.

Q 37. What are the complications of hernia?

Complications of hernia
• Irreducibility • Obstruction • Strangulation • Incarceration • Inflammation.

Q 38. What is the cause for inflammation in hernia?
Inflammation will occur when the sac contain the following structures:

- Appendix
- Meckel's diverticulum
- Salpinx.

Q 39. Is it possible to get strangulation without obstruction?
Yes—in Richter's hernia.

Q 40. What is obstructed hernia?
It is a condition where constriction of the neck of the sac leads to obstruction of the loops of small bowel within it. This will produce symptoms of intestinal obstruction.

Q 41. What is strangulated hernia?
Strangulation is a condition where constriction of the venous return of the bowel occurs initially, which leads to congestion, arterial occlusion and gangrene of the bowel. When a loop of gut is strangulated there will also be intestinal obstruction.

Q 42. What is incarcerated hernia?
Here the contents are fixed in the sac because of their size or adhesions. The hernia is irreducible, but the bowel is not strangulated.

Q 43. What is the classification for hernia? (PG)
Many classifications are available. The **Gilbert's** classification with addition by—**Rutkow and Robbins** remains the most practical classification.

Type I, II and III are indirect, IV and V are direct. Type VI, both indirect and direct and Type VII femoral hernia.

Rutkow and Robbins modification of Gilbert's classification		
Type I	–	Tight internal ring
Type II	–	Moderately enlarged internal ring
Type III	–	Patulous internal ring more than 4 cm with sliding component or scrotal component which will also impinge on direct space
Type IV	–	Entire floor of the canal is defective
Type V	–	Direct diverticular defect of no more than 1 or 2 cm in diameter
Type VI	–	Both direct and indirect
Type VII	–	Femoral hernia

Q 44. What is Bendavid classification? (PG)

Bendavid classification of hernia

He proposed the Type, Staging and Dimension (TSD) classification.

There are five types of groin hernias as per this classification.

Type I:	Anterolateral (indirect)
Type II:	Anteromedial (direct)
Type III:	Posteromedial (femoral)
Type IV:	Posterolateral (prevascular)
Type V:	Anteroposterior (inguinofemoral). The three stages are:
Stage I:	Extends from the deep inguinal ring to the superficial inguinal ring
Stage II:	Goes beyond the superficial inguinal ring, but not into the scrotum
Stage III:	Reaches into the scrotum

In the TSD classification the 'D' refers to the diameter of the hernial defect at the level of the abdominal wall. The widest anterolateral measurement is recorded in centimeters.

Q 45. What is Nyhus classification? (PG)

Nyhus classification of hernia

Type I: Indirect inguinal hernia in which the internal ring is of normal size. The area of Hesselbach's triangle remains normal

Type II: Indirect inguinal hernia in which the internal ring is attenuated but does not impinge on the floor of the canal. The Hesselbach's triangle is pathophysiologically intact

Type III: Consist of three subtypes:

Type IIIA: Direct inguinal hernia

Type IIIB:

- Indirect inguinal hernia with a large dilated ring that has expanded medially and encroaches on the inguinal floor
- The hernial sac frequently reaches to the scrotum
- The sliding and pantaloon hernias are included in this group

Type IIIC: Femoral hernia

Type IV: Recurrent hernia

- Recurrent direct – IV A
- Recurrent indirect – IV B
- Recurrent femoral – IV C
- Combination – IV D

Q 46. What are the preoperative investigations in a case of inguinal hernia?

a. Chest examination and chest X-ray PA view
b. Perrectal examination to rule out prostatic hypertrophy
c. Urodynamic study in male patients above 50 years
d. Cardiac assessment [ECG]
e. Rule out diabetes—blood sugar
f. Complete blood cell count including Hb estimation.

Q 47. What is the anesthesia of choice for hernia surgery?

It can be done under local anesthesia, spinal or general anesthesia. In Shouldice Hospital in Toronto, they routinely do all hernia operations under local anesthesia. This hospital is solely dedicated for hernia surgery and the recurrence rate in this hospital is less than 1%.

Q 48. What are the advantages of local anesthesia?

Advantages of local anesthesia

a. Peroperative assessment of the hernia is possible [Peroperative cough test]
b. The repair is not done under tension
c. Postoperative pain is less
d. Postoperative retention of urine is less frequent
e. The patient can leave the hospital in the same day evening or next day [Day case surgery].

Q 49. What are the surgical procedures available (Flow chart 44.1) ?

The procedures are:

a. Herniotomy
b. Herniorrhaphy
c. Hernioplasty.

The basic procedure for any hernia repair is herniotomy. Herniotomy may be done alone or combined with either herniorraphy or hernioplasty.

Q 50. What is herniotomy?

Herniotomy is the process of identification of the sac, separation of the sac from the cord, opening the sac, reducing the content, transfixion and ligature of the neck of the sac followed by excision of the sac.

Q 51. Why herniotomy alone is done in children?

Because of the following reasons herniotomy alone is sufficient in children:

Flow chart 44.1: Management of inguinal hernia

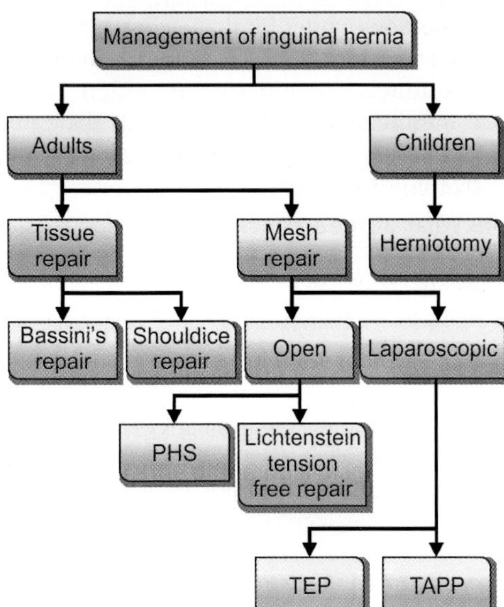

a. The obliquity of the canal is less
b. For all practical purposes the superficial and deep inguinal rings are almost superimposed and therefore there is no need for repair
c. The muscles are very strong in children.

Q 52. What is the difference between herniorraphy and hernioplasty?

In herniorrhaphy, a simple repair of the posterior wall alone is done. Examples are:

a. Shouldice's repair [Gold standard herniorrhaphy previously]
b. Bassini's repair [Time tested technique, nowadays not recommended].

In hernioplasty, some form of synthetic material is used to strengthen the posterior wall and cover the defect [polypropylene mesh].

Note: a and b are tissue repairs.

Q 53. What is Shouldice's repair?

This surgery was devised by E.E. Shouldice (1890–1965) of Toronto. This is also called Canadian Repair. The Shouldice hospital surgeons are true hernia specialists and they restrict their surgery to hernia patients.

This is a **four layer repair** using non-absorbable monofilament (polypropelene) suture material. The basic principle of Shouldice's technique is the **division of transversalis fascia obliquely**, suturing of the lower leaf of transversalis fascia to the under surface of the upper leaf (**first layer**) followed by the suturing of the lower border of transversalis fascia to the inguinal ligament (**second layer**). This is called imbrication of a double layer of transversalis fascia to the inguinal ligament. This is followed by a double layer of conjoint tendon—internal oblique muscle suturing to the inguinal ligament (**third and fourth layers**).

- In short, it is a 4 layer repair. In first layer, the lower leaf of the divided transversalis fascia is sutured first to the under surface of the upper leaf by continuous 30 polypropylene suture.
- The first layer is continued as the second layer where the lower border of the upper leaf is sutured to the inguinal ligament by the same suture material continuously. The first layer is started medially from the pubic tubercle region and goes laterally and then comes medially as the second layer.
- The third layer is started laterally at the deep inguinal ring region and comes medially and then it is continued again laterally as the fourth layer.

- The third and fourth layers are suturing of the conjoint tendon and under surface of the external oblique/inguinal ligament.

Q 54. What is Bassini's herniorrhaphy?

This is the oldest technique of hernia repair where after herniotomy the conjoint tendon is approximated to the inguinal ligament using No.1 size interrupted polypropylene sutures (synthetic nonabsorbable).

Q 55. What is the current gold standard surgery for hernia repair [hernioplasty]?

The gold standard current hernia surgery is the Lichtenstein Tension-free Hernioplasty. Here approximately 16 × 8 cm size mesh (polypropylene) is placed anterior to the posterior wall after herniotomy and overlapping it generously in all directions including medially over the pubic tubercle.

Q 56. What are the essential steps of inguinal herniorrhaphy?

- Local anesthesia/regional anesthesia/general anesthesia.
- An oblique inguinal skin crease incision approximately 1.5–2 cm above the medial two-thirds of the inguinal ligament.
- Incise the fatty and membranous layers of the superficial fascia (fascia of Camper and fascia of Scarpa).
- Ligate the superficial circumflex iliac, superficial epigastric and superficial external pudendal vessels (external pudendal may be retracted to avoid edema scrotum).
- Identify the external oblique aponeurosis and external ring. Divide the external oblique aponeurosis along the line of its fibers and turn back the edges.
- Identify the internal oblique and conjoined tendon above and the inguinal ligament below. The cord is in between.
- In indirect inguinal hernia, the sac is inside the spermatic cord and the cremaster muscle has to be divided in the line of the spermatic cord for identifying the sac. In direct hernia the sac is posterior to the cord.
- Safeguard the ilioinguinal nerve, vas deferens and spermatic artery.
- Identification of the sac and isolation of the sac from the cord (the sac is seen as pearly white structure).

Indirect inguinal hernial sac

- If the sac is small, it can be freed in toto. If it is of long and scrotal type, the fundus of the sac must not be sought (the blood supply to the testis may be compromised by such a procedure). The sac is isolated upto the neck of the sac until the parietal peritoneum can be seen on all sides and extraperitoneal fat is visualized. The inferior epigastric vessels are seen on the medial side.
- Open the sac, reduce the contents (omentum and intestines are returned to the peritoneal cavity).
- Herniotomy: The neck of the sac is transfixed as high as possible and the rest of the sac is removed.

Direct hernial sac

- In this situation there is no need to incise the cremaster muscle to identify the sac (the hernial sac is seen posterior to the cord).
- Push the direct hernial sac inwards (no need to open the sac and reduce the contents. Transfixion and ligation and herniotomy are not required).

- Interrupted polypropylene sutures are put so that the sac will remain invaginated.

Repair of both direct and indirect hernia

- The best tissue repair is the four layer repair of Shouldice (read the steps above).
- For Lichtenstein tension-free repair, the polypropylene mesh is used to reinforce the posterior wall. The mesh is sutured below to the inguinal ligament, above to the internal oblique and conjoined tendon. The mesh should overlap beyond the pubic tubercle medially. Laterally the mesh is incised to accommodate for the spermatic cord. Finally, the spermatic cord will be lying over the mesh.

Closure

- Approximate the external oblique aponeurosis
- Subcutaneous sutures are put with interrupted absorbable sutures
- Skin is closed, ideally by skin tapes.

Q 57. Can you do hernia repair by laparoscopy?

Yes.

Q 58. What are the methods of laparoscopic hernia repair? (PG)

TEP and TAPP.

TAPP: Transabdominal preperitoneal repair—Here after entering the peritoneal cavity, the peritoneum is incised cephalad to the inguinal floor and the hernia defects are dissected. Moderate sized indirect sacs are dissected and reduced. Large sacs are occasionally transected and the distal sac left in situ leading to a possible hydrocele formation avoiding hematoma. Mesh is secured to Cooper's ligament and the underside to the conjoined tendon with no staples being placed lateral to epigastric vessels.

TEP: Total extraperitoneal repair—Here the peritoneal cavity is not entered. With the help of an infraumbilical trocar, the preperitoneal space is entered using a combination of carbon dioxide and blunt dissection to expose the entire myopectineal orifice. Polypropylene mesh is then placed between the underside of the abdominal wall and the peritoneum fixing the mesh to Cooper's ligament and the aponeurotic sling.

Q 59. What are the indications for laparoscopic hernia repair? (PG)

Indications for laparoscopic hernia repair

- Bilateral inguinal hernia
- Recurrent hernia
- Femoral hernia.

Q 60. What is Stoppa groin hernia repair? (PG)

It is also called giant prosthetic reinforcement of visceral sac [GPRVS].

- This is a revolutionary and innovative bilateral properitoneal prosthetic hernioplasty. The procedure is although useful for repair of all hernias of the groin, it is mainly used to manage complex hernias at high risk for recurrence and for recurrent groin hernias.
- The essential feature of GPRVS is the replacement of the transversalis fascia in the groin by a large prosthesis that extends beyond the myopectineal orifice (MPO).
- The prosthesis envelops the visceral sac held in place by intra-abdominal pressure and later by connective tissue ingrowth.
- The mesh adheres to the peritoneum and renders it inextensible so that it cannot protrude through the parietal defect. Here the parietal defects are not closed and should not be closed. GPRVS is a suture less and tension-free repair.

Bilateral GPRVS

- Bilateral GPRVS may be achieved through a subumbilical midline or Pfannenstiel incision.
- The preperitoneal space is cleaved in all directions, exposing the space of Bogros and the space of Retzius, the superior ramus of the pubis, the obturator foramen, iliac vessels and the iliopsoas muscle.
- The elements of the spermatic cord are parietalized.
- The chevron-shaped mesh is tailored to the patient and should measure transversely 2 cm less than the distance between the anterior superior iliac spines and vertically should measure the distance between the umbilicus and the symphysis pubis.
- In obese patients, the mesh should be several centimeters wider than the interspinous dimensions.
- The repair also can be done unilaterally and the mesh implanted through a lower quadrant transverse abdominal incision or through an anterior groin incision.

Q 61. What is the management of dual hernia?

The sac should be delivered to the lateral side of the deep epigastric vessel and dealt with.

Q 62. What are the vessels likely to be injured in hernia surgery?

Vessels likely to be injured in hernia surgery

1. Pubic branch of the obturator artery
2. Aberrant obturator artery originating from the deep inferior epigastric artery—'**Artery of death**'
3. Inferior deep epigastric artery
4. Deep circumflex iliac vessel
5. Cremasteric artery
6. External iliac vessel.

Q 63. What is the course of action if a deep bite is taken through external iliac vessel?

- Remove the suture (do not tie the suture), If not the artery will blow out within 2–3 days
- Apply pressure.

Q 64. What are the nerves inside the inguinal canal?

1. Ilioinguinal nerve (T12 - L1)
   - It is in close relationship to spermatic cord
   - It is seen in the usual position only in 60% of cases
   - It may be absent
   - Innervation—base of the penis at the scrotum and adjacent side.
2. Iliohypogastric nerve (T12 - L1)
   - Seen 1 to 2 cm above the inguinal canal
   - Supplies suprapubic area
   - Injured while a relaxing incision is put over the rectus sheath.
3. Genitofemoral nerve (L1,2,3)

   Genital branch
   - Prone to injury at the internal ring
   - Penetrate the internal oblique at the origin of the cremaster
   - Motor innervation—cremaster muscle
   - Sensory innervation—to the penis and scrotum.

   Femoral branch
   - Innervation—upper thigh (less likely to be injured).

Q 65. If a nerve is cut what is the course of action? (PG)

- It may be ligated or clipped to allow closure of the neurilemmal sheath
- Repair is impossible.

Q 66. What is the blood supply to the testis?

Blood supply to the testis
a. Testicular artery (major supply)—from aorta
b. External spermatic artery—from inferior epigastric artery—also supply cremaster muscle
c. Artery to vas deferens—from superior vesical artery.

Note: There is a rich collateral existing between these three vessels. In addition the vesical and prostatic branches communicate with the above. The scrotal vessels from internal and external pudendal vessels, freely communicate with vessels in the spermatic cord external to the superficial inguinal ring.

Q 67. What will happen if testicular artery is ligated? (PG)

Ligation of testicular artery alone at the deep ring may not lead to testicular atrophy provided collateral circulation is undisturbed.

Q 68. What are the steps in surgery which will jeopardize the collateral supply to the testis? (PG)

- Removal of testis from scrotum
- Dissection of sac distal to the external ring.

Q 69. What are the complications of hernia surgery?

Complications of hernia surgery
i. Hematoma
ii. Seroma
iii. Wound infection
- Superficial incisional surgical site infection
- Deep incisional surgical site infection
iv. Infection of mesh
v. Scrotal edema
vi. Postherniorrhaphy hydrocele
vii. Recurrent hernia
viii. Ischemic orchitis
ix. Testicular atrophy
x. Chronic residual neuralgia (sensory nerve):
• Ilioinguinal neuralgia
• Genitofemoral neuralgia
xi. Obstruction of vas deferens
xii. Dysejaculation.

Q 70. What is the incidence of recurrent hernia?

1. For inguinal hernia: 2.3 to 20%
2. Femoral hernia: 11.8 to 75%

Q 71. What is the most common site of recurrence? (PG)

- Medially: The transversus abdominis tendon is inserted to the rectus sheath as much as 2 cm above the pubic tubercle. If the mesh is not reaching beyond the pubic tubercle for 1cm, there is chance for recurrence
- The second most common site is at the internal ring.

Q 72. What are the causes for hematoma after herniorrhaphy? (PG)

- Bleeding from superficial vessels (external pudendal, circumflex iliac and superficial epigastric vessels).
- On a deeper plane, during resection of the cremaster, careless ligature of the external spermatic artery can result in tense hematoma and ecchymosis that extend to the scrotum.
- Injury to the deep inferior epigastric vessel (one artery and two veins) during division of the transversalis fascia.
- Bleeding from venous circulation within the space of Bogros.
- Bleeding from iliopubic artery.

- Injury to aberrant obturator artery from the deep inferior epigastric artery when sutures are inserted to Cooper's ligament (artery of death).
- Injury to femoral vein and artery.

Q 73. How to avoid scrotal edema? (PG)

- Do not divide external pudendal vessels at the medial limit during incision
- Bilateral simultaneous herniorrhaphy will cause edema of penis and scrotum.

Q 74. What is the cause for post herniorrhaphy hydrocele? (PG)

- Overzealous skeletonization of the spermatic cord
- Severance of the lymphatic drainage.

Q 75. What is ischemic orchitis? (PG)

- Ischemic orchitis will produce swollen, painful, hard and tender spermatic cord, epididymis and testicles
- It is seen within 24–72 hours of hernia surgery
- May be associated with fever
- The pain and tenderness will last for 6 weeks
- Swelling will last for up to 5 months
- The process is sterile and there is no suppuration
- It is as a result of intense venous congestion secondary to massive thrombosis of the veins of the cord.

Q 76. What is the natural course of ischemic orchitis? (PG)

- Subsides completely

or

- Testicular atrophy as late as 12 months (no pain or tenderness).

Q 77. What are the causes for chronic residual neuralgia? (PG)

It may be due to the following reasons:

- Primary damage to the nerve—stretching, contusion, crushing and suture— compression
- Secondary damage—cicatrical compression and suture granuloma.

Q 78. What are the manifestations of chronic residual neuralgia? (PG)

- It may be a neuroma pain, referred pain or projected pain
- The pain will be out of proportion to the pathology
- Patient may be unable to return to work.

Q 79. What is the treatment of chronic residual neuralgia? (PG)

- Nerve block
- Neurectomy (division of three nerves)
- TENS
- Drugs.

Q 80. What are the causes for dysejaculation? (PG)

- It may be due to adhesion of the vas deferens
- Painful and burning sensation in the groin preceding, during and after ejaculation.

Q 81. What is the management of infected mesh? (PG)

- Infection does not necessarily imply removal of a mesh unless the mesh is sequestrated and bathed in purulent exudates.
- Usually will subside with culture and sensitivity and appropriate antibiotics and irrigation. Partial resection may be required.

Q 82. What is "metastatic emphysema of READ"? (PG)

Acquired herniation is considered as the end result of a collagen deficiency which is mentioned as metastatic emphysema of Read.

Femoral Hernia

Q 83. What are the diagnostic points in favor of femoral hernia?

- The femoral hernia is below and lateral to the pubic tubercle (inguinal hernia is above and medial to the pubic tubercle)
- The swelling is placed more laterally than the inguinal hernia
- Irreducibility is encountered ten times more frequently with a femoral hernia
- The visible impulse on coughing may be absent in the supine position.

Q 84. What are the three stages of femoral hernia?

Stage I: There is a rounded reducible swelling below the medial end of the inguinal ligament.

Stage II: The hernia after passing through the femoral canal bulges into the femoral triangle (Scarpa's triangle). Usually this variety is irreducible.

Stage III: Further expansion downward is prevented by blending of fascia, the fundus mounts upwards in front of the inguinal ligament and overlies the inguinal canal. By this time it is always irreducible. Finally, the femoral hernia takes the shape of a retort.

Q 85. Femoral hernia is more common in which sex?

- In female patients (commonest hernia in female is inguinal hernia)
- Female to male ratio is 2:1
- Elderly group is involved in female (after repeated pregnancies)
- The commonest age group in male is 30-45.

Q 86. What are the boundaries of femoral canal?

It is bounded medially by the lacunar ligament, laterally by the femoral vein, superoanteriorly by the inguinal ligament and inferoposteriorly by the Astley Cooper's ligament (pectineal).

Q 87. What are the most important problems of femoral hernia?

- It has got a very narrow neck and therefore the hernia is more prone for strangulation
- It is more likely to obstruct and strangulate than inguinal hernia
- Strangulation without obstruction is possible in femoral hernia (Richter's hernia).

Q 88. How to differentiate femoral hernia from saphenavarix?

- Saphenavarix is softer than the femoral hernia.
- Cruveilhier's sign: In the erect position when the patient coughs or blows his nose, there is a tremor imparted to the palpating fingers as though a jet of water entering and filling the pouch.
- Saphenavarix is usually associated with varicosity of the long saphenous vein.
- There will be blue discoloration of the skin over the saphenavarix.

Q 89. How to differentiate irreducible femoral hernia from enlarged lymph node (Cloquet's node)?

It is a perplexing problem. When you suspect Cloquet's node, search for a focus of infection in the following areas:

- Lower limb
- Buttocks
- Perineum
- Anus
- Genitals.

Note: Pressure by the hernial sac on the superficial epigastric or circumflex iliac vein causes distension of the superficial epigastric vein on the anterior abdominal wall (**Gaur's sign**).

Q 90. How to differentiate reducible femoral hernia and psoas abscess pointing beneath the inguinal ligament?

Cold abscess arising from tuberculous disease of the body of the lumbar vertebrae will track along the psoas sheath to the insertion of psoas major muscle

- A psoas abscess will point lateral to the femoral artery (it will be reducible and painless)
- Examination of the back will reveal evidence of tuberculosis of the spine
- There will be a swelling in the iliac fossa and cross fluctuation can be elicited between the swelling in the femoral region and iliac fossa.

Q 91. What is Laugier's femoral hernia?

This is a hernia through a gap in the lacunar (Gimbernat's) ligament. When there is unusual medial position of the femoral hernial sac, one should suspect Laugier's femoral hernia. The hernia is nearly always strangulated at the time of diagnosis.

Q 92. What is Narath's femoral hernia?

This occurs only in patients with congenital dislocation of the hip and is due to the lateral displacement of the psoas muscle. The hernia lies behind the femoral vessels.

Q 93. What is Cloquet's hernia?

This is one in which the sac lies under the fascia covering the pectineus muscle. It may coexist with usual type of femoral hernia.

Q 94. What is the ideal timing for femoral hernia surgery?

As early as possible (early surgery).

Q 95. What is the principle of repair of femoral hernia?

Suture of the inguinal ligament to the pectineal ligament after dealing with the sac.

Q 96. What are the operations available for femoral hernia?

a. **"Low" operation of Lockwood:** Here an incision is made 1cm below and parallel to the inguinal ligament. After dealing with the sac and contents (freeing the omentum, etc.), the neck of the sac is pulled down and ligated as high as possible. The femoral canal is closed by three nonabsorbable interrupted sutures by suturing the inguinal ligament to the iliopectineal line. Alternatively a role of polypropylene mesh may be kept and anchored with nonabsorbable sutures placed medially, superiorly and inferiorly.

b. **The Lotheissen's operation:** This is an inguinal approach. The transversalis fascia is divided in the line of incision avoiding injury to the inferior epigastric vessel. The sac is withdrawn upwards after releasing the adhesions and its contents are dealt with. The femoral ring is now obliterated by suturing the conjoined tendon to the iliopectineal line to form a shutter by protecting the femoral vein. Alternatively a polypropylene mesh is inserted into the preperitoneal space and anchored inferiorly to the iliopectineal line, superiorly to the Cooper's and superomedially to the rectus sheath.

c. **McEvedy's approach**: This operation may be carried out by three incisions

   i. Vertical incision (an incision extending from the femoral canal region in the thigh upwards to above the inguinal ligament)

   ii. Oblique incision

   iii. Unilateral Pfannenstiel incision: It can be made a complete Pfannenstiel if laparotomy is required.

Through the lower part of the incision the sac is dissected out and through the upper part of the incision which is going above the inguinal ligament, the upper part of the procedure is carried out.

- An vertical incision is put parallel to the outer border of the rectus muscle 2.5 cm above the superficial inguinal ring until the extra-peritoneal space is identified
- By Guaze dissection the hernial sac entering the femoral canal is identified
- If the sac is small and empty it may be drawn upwards, if large the fundus of the sac is opened below and dealt with before delivering the sac upwards.
- After freeing the sac, the neck is ligated
- The conjoined tendon is sutured to the iliopectineal ligament with nonabsorbable sutures
- Alternatively a polypropylene mesh may be kept and sutured inferiorly to the iliopectineal ligament and medially to the rectus sheath
- Advantage of this technique is that if resection of the intestine is required, it can be easily carried out.

Case 45 Incisional Hernia (Ventral Hernia, Postoperative Hernia)

Case Capsule

A 45-year-old **obese** female patient presents with **diffuse bulging of the surgical scar** of the **lower abdomen** (12 × 5 cm size). Patient gives history of **cesarean section** 10 years back. On examination there is a lower midline scar in the anterior abdominal wall. After the surgery she noticed a swelling which was **increasing steadily** and reached the present size. Initially most of the swelling used to get reduced in the supine position. Of late the swelling is only **partially reducible**. The **skin overlying the swelling is thinned out** and atrophic. **Expansile impulse** on coughing is seen at the swelling. Palpation of the abdomen **revealed a defect** in the abdominal wall of about (10 × 4 cm size). Normal peristalsis can be seen through the skin overlying the bulge. She gets **attacks of colic** for the last 3 months.

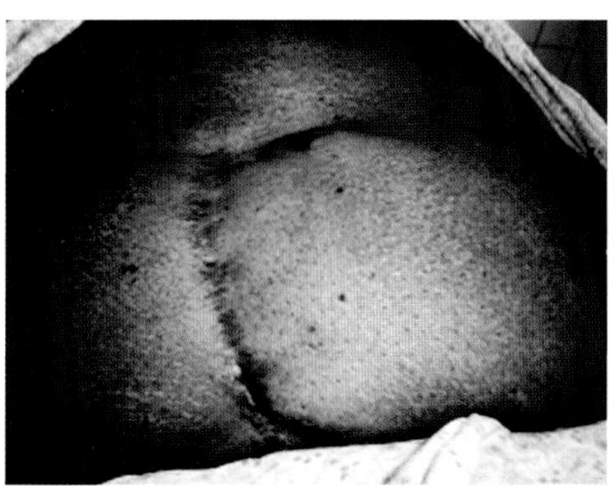

Incisional hernia to the left of the scar

Read the checklist of abdominal examination.

Checklist for history

- Verify **previous operation note**
- History of **drainage tube through the wound**
- History of **wound infection**—Deep wound infection is notorious for causing incisional hernia
- Reason for initial operation
- History of **postoperative coughing, vomiting and abdominal distension**
- History of **COPD**
- History of **steroid intake**
- History of **jaundice** in the postoperative period.

Q 1. What is the diagnosis in this case?

Incisional hernia.

Q 2. What are the diagnostic points in favor of incisional hernia?

- History of lower abdominal surgery with a lower midline scar

- The swelling is seen at the site of the scar in the abdominal wall
- The swelling is partially reducible in the supine position
- The swelling is more in the standing position
- Expansile impulse on coughing present
- Palpable defect in the lower abdomen.

Q 3. What is the most important clinical sign for incisional hernia?

- The swelling will become **more prominent in head raising test**
- Reducibility and cough impulse.

Q 4. If the lump does not reduce and does not have a cough impulse, what are the differential diagnoses?

Then it may not be a hernia. The following differential diagnoses are to be considered:

Differential diagnoses if it is not reducible
• Deposit of tumor—Desmoid tumor
• Hematoma
• Foreign-body granuloma
• Old abscess
• Lipoma.

Q 5. What is incisional hernia?

- It is a **hernia through an acquired scar** in the abdominal wall.
- An incisional hernia usually starts as a **symptomless partial disruption of the deeper layersof a laparotomy wound** during the immediate or early postoperative period, the event being unnoticed if the skin wound remains intact.

Q 6. What are the causes for incisional hernia?

Causes for incisional hernia

1. **Technique of wound closure** (**technical failure** is the most important cause for incisional hernia):
   - Selection of suture material for closure of the **fascial layer** (nonabsorbable synthetic, monofilament, No 1 size suture material is preferred for closing the fascia, e.g. Polypropylene)
   - Method of closure: Single layer mass closure with interrupted 'far and near' sutures
   - Length of suture material must be at least 4 times the length of incision but < 5 times if continuous suture is used
   - Use Jenkin's formula for closure of the fascia: The bites must be taken at least 1 cm away from the fascial edge and 1 cm apart (the reason for this is the fact that the collagenolysis will extend upto 1 cm from the fascial edge during healing)
2. **Drainage tube:**
   - Keeping drainage tubes through the wound – higher tendency to burst and later produce incisional hernia
3. **Type of incision:**
   - Midline and vertical incisions have greater tendency than horizontal wounds—more tendency to produce burst abdomen
4. **Wound infection:**
   - Following operations for peritonitis—more chance for wound infection and wound dehiscence
   - Operations on pancreas and subsequent leakage
5. **Postoperative events**—leading to wound disruption
   - Postoperative vomiting
   - Persistent postoperative cough
   - Postoperative abdominal distension—due to ileus
   - Postoperative ventilation

Contd...

Contd...

6. **Creation of stoma (colostomy, ileostomy, etc.)**
7. **Collagen deficiency—Decreased ratio of collagen I/III (increase in collagen III)**
8. **Failure to close the fascia of laparoscopic trocar sites over 10 mm size**
9. **General condition of the patient**
   - Obesity—There is increased intra-abdominal pressure in obesity—Increased incidence of seroma and hematoma in wounds
   - Jaundice
   - Cirrhosis
   - Malignant disease
   - Hypoproteinemia
   - Anemia
   - Malnutrition
   - COPD
   - Abdominal wounds in pregnancy
   - Steroids.

Note: These are the causes for wound dehiscence (Burst abdomen) also.

Q 7. Since incisional hernia is a symptomless partial disruption of the deeper layers of the laparotomy wound, it is better to know something about wound dehiscence. What is the timing of wound dehiscence and what are the manifestations?

- Between 6th and 8th day of surgery
- The initial manifestations is serosanguinous (pink) discharge from the wound which is the **pathognomonic sign of wound disruption.** It signifies intraperitoneal contents lying extra-peritoneally
- Patient may volunteer the information that they 'felt something give way'
- In revealed dehiscence the omentum and coils of intestines may be found lying outside.

Q 8. What are the three most important etiological factors?

Three most important causes for incisional hernia

- Technical failure in wound closure
- Wound infection
- Subclinical wound dehiscence in the postoperative period.

Q 9. What is ventral hernia?

The term ventral hernia should be restricted to incisional hernia arising in abdominal **midline operative wounds**.

Q 10. What is the management?

The most important investigations are:

• X-ray chest	– To rule out COPD and other pulmonary diseases
• Ultrasound abdomen	– To demonstrate the size of the defect – To rule out other intra-abdominal pathology
• Hematological examination	– To rule out anemia
• Biochemical investigation	– To rule out hypoproteinemia
• Nutritional assessment	
• Evaluation of cardiac status and renal status. After proper evaluation, surgery is recommended	

Q 11. Is there any conservative management? If so what is the indication?

- Abdominal belt is sometimes recommended especially in upper abdominal incisional hernias

- Belt is also recommended until the patient is fit for surgery.

Q 12. What are the preoperative preparations required?

- Weight reduction by dieting and exercise
- Patient is asked to stop smoking
- Treat the respiratory problems.

Q 13. What are the complications of incisional hernia?

Complications of incisional hernia
• Irreducibility • Obstruction • Strangulation (Rarely) • Ulceration of the overlying skin.

Q 14. What is large hernia?

A hernia can be considered large when the fascial edges cannot be approximated without tension (more than 4 cm).

Q 15. Which hernia is more dangerous, small or large?

Small hernias may cause bowel obstruction early and therefore more dangerous.

Q 16. In a very large hernia of long duration in which most of the intestines are in the sac, what additional precaution is taken to prevent postoperative embarrassment?

There are three important problems in this situation:

- Increased risk of **paralytic ileus** from visceral compression
- **Pulmonary complications** as a result of elevation of the diaphragm when the contents are reduced.
- Risk of failure of hernioplasty.

This may be managed by enlarging the abdominal cavity preoperatively by **prolonged pneumoperitoneum.** This is achieved by increasing the intra-abdominal pressure to 15–18 cm of water with the help of a pneumoperitoneum apparatus for several weeks preoperatively.

Q 17. What are the surgical procedures available for repair of incisional hernia?

1. Anatomical repair (primary fascial repair)—Useful only for small hernias < 4 cm size because of the high incidence of recurrence
2. Mesh repair (tension free repair)—**The gold standard treatment**
3. Autogenous repair by vascularized innervated muscle flaps—Reserved for large and recurrent hernias
4. Complex apposition (considered obsolete and is of historical importance only. Examples are: Keel's operation, Cattel's operation).

Q 18. What are the most important steps of fascial repair?

- The hernial sac is dissected
- The adherent omentum and bowel are released from the sac
- The contents are reduced
- The mouth of the sac is defined
- The layers are repaired with nonabsorbable sutures—No 1 polypropylene, first the peritoneum and then the fascial layer.

Q 19. What is mesh repair and what is the ideal plane for keeping the mesh? (PG)

- The mesh repair can be done either by **Open method or Laparoscopic method**
- The initial steps are same as the fascial repair
- For incisional hernias above the umbilicus, a sheet of polypropylene mesh is inserted between the posterior rectus sheath and muscle fibers and anchored in place **(Inlay repair)**
- For hernias below the umbilicus the mesh is placed in the preperitoneal space **(Inlay repair)**

- The mesh may also be placed as **on lay** in front of the fascia **(Inlay is superior)**
  (Here the deficiency can be bridged by sewing the mesh to the fascia on either side of the defect ensuring at least a 4 cm overlap of the fascial edges)
- Tension-free mesh repair can be undertaken **laparoscopically** apparently with good results.

Q 20. What is autogenous repair by vascularized innervated muscle flaps? (PG)

- This method is reserved for **massive midline defects and recurrent hernias**
- It is also done after removal of infected synthetic mesh
- The autogenous tissue reconstruction was introduced by **Ramirez et al**
- The technique utilizes bilateral, innervated, bipedicle, rectus abdominis—transverse abdominis—internal oblique muscle flaps, that are transposed medially to reconstruct the central defect.

Q 21. What are the complications of incisional hernia repair?

Complications of incisional hernia repair
• Wound infection • Seroma formation • Wound sinus • Enterocutaneous fistula • Recurrence • Infection of the mesh.

Case

46 Epigastric Hernia (Fatty Hernia of the Linea Alba)

Case Capsule

A 40-year-old **strong muscular laborer** male patient presents with a **mid line firm swelling** in the epigastrium of 2.5 cm size, which is associated with **epigastric pain** after a large meal, (**postprandial epigastric discomfort**) which is **relieved by lying down**. He has in addition **abdominal bloating** and occasional **nausea and vomiting**. There is **no impulse on coughing.** The swelling is not reducible. The swelling clinically appears to be parietal in nature. The hernial orifices are normal. There is no organomegaly and no other masses felt per abdomen.

Read the checklist for history and examination of abdomen.

Q 1. What is the most probable diagnosis in this case?

Epigastric hernia.

Q 2. What is the cause for postprandial epigastric discomfort in this case?

It may be because of the epigastric distension after full meal.

Q 3. What are the differential diagnoses?

a. Parietal swellings	*b. Intra-abdominal conditions*
• Subcutaneous lipoma	• Peptic ulcer
• Neurofibroma	• Gallbladder diseases
• Fibroma	• Hiatal hernia
• Divarication of rectus abdominis (Diastasis)	• Pancreatitis • Small intestinal obstruction

Q 4. What is epigastric hernia?

- Hernia through the linea alba between the umbilicus and the xiphisternum
- They develop through the opening of para-midline nerves and vessels
- 80% occur just off the midline.

Q 5. Which sex is affected more?

More common in men than women

Q. 6. What is the incidence and age group affected?

- 3 to 5% of the population.
- Age group is 20–50 years.

Q 7. What are the peculiarities of epigastric hernia?

- They are better felt than seen
- Impulse on coughing may not be there
- Reducibility is not there even in uncomplicated hernias
- Usually no peritoneal sac and no bowel content.

Q 8. What is the usual content in epigastric hernia?

Preperitoneal fat which will come out through the openings in the linea alba for vessels. Usually there is **no peritoneal sac**.

Q 9. What are the stages of the hernia formation?

- First stage it is sac less (Only preperitoneal fat protrusion)
- Second stage—A small pouch of peritoneum is drawn after it
- Last stage—Small tag of omentum gets into the sac and adherent to it.

Q 10. What are the usual symptoms and signs?

Symptoms and signs

- May be identified by routine clinical examination
- Present as painless swellings
- Mass in the epigastrium (difficult to feel in obese patients)
- Mildepigastric pain/Burning epigastric pain
- Abdominal bloating, nausea or vomiting (these symptoms may be also due to concomitant other visceral pathology)
- Symptoms may occur after a large meal followed by relief in lying down position.

Q 11. What are the complications of epigastric hernia?

- Incarceration
- Strangulation.

Q 12. What are the investigations for confirming the diagnosis?

- Ultrasound abdomen/CT to demonstrate the defect in the linea alba especially in obese patients (ultrasound will also rule out biliary pathology and other visceral causes for pain)
- Upper GI endoscopy to rule out peptic ulcer and other gastroesophageal diseases
- Assessment of the cardiac status, renal status and respiratory status before surgery
- Hemogram and biochemical investigations.

Q 13. What is the surgical management of epigastric hernia?

It is managed by epigastric hernia repair.

Q 14. What are the essential steps of epigastric hernia repair?

- Anesthesia—GA/Local (for small cases)
- Position of the patient—supine
- Drapes are arranged so that the whole of epigastric area from costal margin to just below the umbilicus is exposed for surgery
- **Incision**—Vertical/horizontal. **Vertical incision has the advantage** for ruling out more than one defects in the linea alba so that, hernia is not missed. Another advantage is that the abdomen can be opened if required
- The **herniated fat is dissected** out from the surrounding abdominal fat
- The opening in the linea alba which is usually tiny is identified and **enlarged transversally**
- The hernia is incised at the neck to determine **whether peritoneal sac is present or not**

- If sac is there, open the sac and **reduce the contents**, transfix the neck. If sac is not there, **reduce the protruding extraperitoneal fat**
- The opening in the linea alba is closed by overlapping its edges (**double breasting**) with **two rows of interrupted polypropylene**/nylon sutures. (First row of mattress sutures, and second row of simple sutures)
- Subcutaneous sutures are put with interrupted cat gut
- Skin is closed preferably with skin tapes.

Summary of epigastric hernia

- Usually no impulse on coughing
- Usually not reducible
- Smaller the hernia, greater the symptoms
- Symptoms mimic peptic ulcers
- Rule out gastrointestinal pathology like peptic ulcer by investigations before surgery
- Rule out epigastric hernia in all cases of dyspeptic symptoms
- Rule out multiple hernias which is there in 20% of patients.

Case

47 Paraumbilical Hernia, Umbilical Hernia in Adults and Children

Case Capsule

A 50-year-old **obese multiparous female** patient presents with a swelling on **one side of the umbilicus** with pain and discomfort of one year duration. She also complains of recurrent attacks of **colicky abdominal pain**. On examination, there is a swelling of about **3 cm size** which is **firm in consistency** having **expansile impulse on coughing**. The swelling is **reducible** and according to the patient at times it is not going in. Once the hernia is reduced, a firm fibrous edge of the **defect of about 2 cm size** is felt at the periphery of the umbilical cicatrix. The umbilicus is stretched into a **crescent shape**. There is no other hernia.

Read the checklist for history and examination of abdomen.

Q 1. What is the most probable diagnosis in this case?

Paraumbilical hernia.

Q 2. What is paraumbilical hernia?

It is a herniation through the linea alba just above or sometimes just below the umbilicus, sometimes on the sides (**supraumbilical hernia/infraumbilical hernia**).

Q 3. What are the differences between umbilical hernia and paraumbilical hernia?

In umbilical hernia the herniation occurs through the umbilical scar and the umbilical scar is weak. The abdominal contents bulge through the weak spot everting the umbilicus.

Differences between umbilical hernia and paraumbilical hernia

	Umbilical hernia	*Paraumbilical hernia*
1.	The abdominal contents bulge **through** the weak **umbilical scar**	Herniation **through the linea alba** just above or below the umbilicus
2.	Umbilicus is **everted**	The hernia is beside the umbilicus and push it to one side taking a **crescent shape**
3.	The entire fundus of the sac is covered by the umbilicus	Half of the fundus of the sac is covered by umbilicus and the remainder by the adjacent abdominal skin

Contd...

Contd...

4.	More common in girls than boys	5 times more seen in females
5.	May be c**ongenital or acquired**	**Always acquired**
6.	**Ascites (cirrhosis) and malignant peritoneal effusion** are predisposing factors for acquired umbilical hernia. The congenital variety is due to incomplete closure of umbilical ring at birth	**Obesity, repeated pregnancies and flabby abdominal** muscles are responsible for paraumbilical hernia
7.	Neck of the sac is wide	Neck of the sac is narrow and complications can occur early
8.	Congenital type can wait up to 4 years because spontaneous closure can occur	Always needs surgery

Q 4. What are the etiological factors for para-umbilical hernia?

- Obesity
- Flabby abdominal muscles
- Repeated pregnancy.

Q. 5 What is the content in paraumbilical hernia?

Greater omentum, small intestine and transverse colon.

Q 6. What are the clinical manifestations of paraumbilical hernia?

- Swelling/lump
- Dragging pain
- Gastrointestinal symptoms—traction on stomach and transverse colon
- Intestinal Colic and signs of intestinal obstruction.

Q 7. What are the complications of paraumbilical hernia?

- Dragging pain
- Irreducibility (omental adhesions)
- Obstruction—colic
- Strangulation—due to the **narrow neck** and the **fibrous edge** of the linea alba
  - Presence of loculi may also result in strangulation of the bowel.
- Ulceration
- Intertrigo in longstanding cases.

Q 8. What are the differential diagnoses of paraumbilical hernia?

- Lipoma
- Neurofibroma
- Desmoid tumor
- Hematoma
- Sister Joseph nodule (umbilical metastasis)
- Caput medusa.

Q 9. What are the indications for surgery in paraumbilical hernia?

Surgery is indicated in all cases.

Q 10. What are the investigations required?

- Ultrasound abdomen
  - To identify the defect
  - To rule out other pathologies
- Plain X-ray abdomen—when obstruction is suspected
- X-ray chest

- Assessment of the cardiac status
- Assessment of the renal status
- Complete hemogram.

Q 11. Any preparation required before surgery?

- If the hernia is symptomless and the patient is obese—weight reduction.
- In symptomatic patients surgery is done without weight reduction.

Q 12. What is the surgical management of paraumbilical hernia?

- Paraumbilical hernioplasty, without excision of the umbilicus (modified Mayo's repair)
- In Mayo's repair the umbilicus is excised.

Q 13. What are the indications for prosthetic mesh in paraumbilical hernia surgery?

- Very large paraumbilical hernia (fascial defect more than 4 cm size)
- Recurrent paraumbilical hernia.

Q 14. What are the essential steps of paraumbilical hernioplasty?

- A curved incision is put over the hernia depending on the situation of the hernia in relation to the umbilicus
- The hernial sac is identified and dissected all around
- After opening the neck of the sac, the contents are released and reduced
- The sac is excised
- The defect in the linea alba is closed by non-absorbable polypropylene sutures
- For larger hernias prosthetic mesh repair may be required if the surgery is elective.

Q 15. What are the causes for congenital umbilical hernia?

- It is due to incomplete closure of the umbilical ring at birth
- **Failure of complete obliteration** at the site where the **fetal umbilical vessels** (umbilical vein and two umbilical arteries) are joined to the placenta during gestation.

Q 16. What is the incidence of Congenital umbilical hernia?

- About **20% of the full-term** neonates may have incomplete closure and umbilical hernia
- **75–85% of the premature infants** (weight between 1 and 1.5 kg) show evidence of umbilical hernia at birth.

Q 17. Is there any sex/race predilection for congenital umbilical hernia?

- It is more common in girls than boys
- The incidence is higher in black children than white children.

Q 18. What is the natural course of congenital umbilical hernia?

- About 80% will decrease in size and close spontaneously by five years of age
- Congenital umbilical hernia of **more than 2 cm size** rarely close spontaneously.

Q 19. What are the complications of congenital umbilical hernia?

- Incarceration
- Small bowel obstruction (1 in 1500 umbilicus hernias)
- Spontaneous rupture (very rare in first year of life due to excessive crying) results in partial evisceration requiring urgent intervention.

Q 20. What are the indications for surgery in congenital umbilical hernia?

- Ring size of **more than 2 cm**
- Failure of closure of the umbilical ring **above 4 years.**

Q 21. What are the steps for umbilical hernia repair?

- A curved (**'smile'**) incision in the natural skin crease immediately below the umbilicus. The curved incision **should not extend beyond** 180°. It is considered important to preserve the umbilical cicatrix after excising the sac.
- The skin cicatrix is dissected upwards and the neck of the sac is isolated.
- After ensuring that the sac is empty, the defect is repaired with polypropylene sutures.

Q 22. What are the causes for adult umbilical hernia?

Adult umbilical hernia may be a manifestation of:

- Cirrhosis
- Malignant peritoneal effusion.

Q 23. What is the most important complication of adult umbilical hernia?

- Incarceration—It is a well-documented complication of effective relief of ascites following diuresis, paracentesis, peritoneo-venous shunt and TIPS (**T**ransjugular **I**ntra-hepatic **P**ortosystemic **S**hunt).

Q 24. What are the important problems in the surgical management of adult umbilical hernia?

- Cirrhotic patient may have caput medusae which may interfere with repair.
- Repair may be difficult requiring a prosthetic mesh.
- A subcutaneous suction drain should be avoided because of the increased risk of infection of the ascitic fluid.

Q 25. What is omphalocele (exomphalos)?

- It is due to **failure of all or part of the mid gut to return to the celom** during early fetal life
- There is a **midline abdominal defect**
- **Liver and bowel** are seen contained within a sac composed of **inner layer of peritoneum and outer layer of amnion** from which **the umbilical cord arises at the apex and center.**

Q 26. What are the types of omphalocele?

- *Omphalocele major*—more than 4 cm size
- *Omphalocele minor*—less than 4 cm size (herniation of the umbilical cord).

Note: A single loop of intestine in omphalocele minor may not be obvious and ligation of the umbilical cord without recognizing this fact will result in transection of the intestine. This will leave an umbilico enteric fistula.

Q 27. What are the structures seen in omphalocele major?

Structures seen in omphalocele

- Liver—Evidence of adhesions to the sac
- Spleen
- Stomach
- Pancreas
- Colon
- Bladder
- Intestine—Lies freely mobile.

Q 28. What is the incidence of omphalocele?

Occurs once in **every 6000 births.**

Q 29. What are the associated anomalies in omphalocele?

Associated anomalies are seen in **30–70% of infants** and the following anomalies are seen:

- Trisomy 13, 18, 21
- Tetralogy of Fallot
- Atrial septal defect
- Beckwith—Wiedemann syndrome (large for gestational-age baby).

Hyperinsulinism
Visceromegaly
Hepatorenal tumors
Cloacal extrophy.

Q 30. What is the management of omphalocele?

- Work up for associated anomalies
- Orogastric tube to prevent distension of abdomen
- Since there is a sac covering the viscera, **emergency operation is not necessary**
- Various surgical options are there for the management.

Q 31. What are the surgical options?

1. **Nonoperative therapy**—This is recommended for premature infants with a gigantic intact sac with associated anomalies where survival of a major operation is questionable.

   The intact sac is painted daily with desiccated antiseptic solutions (Mercurochrome) and this will allow to form an **eschar over the sac.** Granulation tissue grows from the periphery over the eschar. This will ultimately form a ventral hernia, which can be repaired later.
2. **Skin flap closure**:
   - The sac is gently trimmed
   - The skin is freed from the fascial edges and undermined laterally
   - The umbilical vessels are ligated
   - The skin flaps are approximated in the midline with simple sutures
   - The ventral hernia is repaired at a later date (months to years later).
3. **Staged closure**:
   - The sac is trimmed
   - The skin is further freed from the fascial attachment
   - Prosthetic material like **PTFE** (Polytetrafluoroethylene) is sutured with interrupted nonabsorbable sutures circumferentially to the full thickness of the musculofascial abdominal wall to form a **silo**
   - The top of the silo is gathered and **tied with umbilical tape**
   - Daily the silo is opened under strict aseptic conditions and the contents examined for infection
   - The viscera are pushed gently back into the abdominal cavity and the child is observed for signs of **raised intra-abdominal pressure**
   - The silo is tied at reduced level daily until the **sac is flush with abdominal wall**
   - The fascia may be closed with interrupted sutures at this stage
   - Skin is closed over the top.
4. **Primary closure**:
   - The sac is gently dissected away from the skin edge and underlying fascia
   - The intestine is evacuated completely of meconium and fluid distally and proximally with the help of a nasogastric tube
   - The abdominal wall is stretched gradually and repeatedly in all quadrants achieving a doubling of volume
   - The viscera are then replaced
   - The fascial layer is closed primarily under moderate tension.

Q 32. What is gastroschisis?

- **It is a defect** in the abdominal wall to the **right of the normal insertion of the umbilical cord,** without any investing sac (compare with omphalocele)
- It is seen at the site of involution of the right umbilical vein.

Q 33. What is the incidence of gastroschisis?
Twice as common as omphalocele.

Q 34. What is the cause for gastroschisis?
There is a controversy as to whether gastroschisis represents a **ruptured omphalocele sac in utero or simply a separate entity**.

Q 35. What are the differences between omphalocele and gastroschisis?

Sl. No	*Omphalocele*	*Gastroschisis*
1.	The midline abdominal defect as a result of **failure of return of the mid gut** to the celom	Defect to **the right of the normal insertion** of the umbilical cord (at the site of involution of the right umbilical vein)
2.	The bowels are contained **within a sac** composed of peritoneum and amnion	There is **no sac** covering the intestine
3.	The **umbilical cord arises at the apex** ofthe sac	There is **normal insertion** of the umbilical cord
4.	**Liver may be seen** as a content inside the sac	Liver is **not seen**
5.	The bowel is not **edematous**	**Bowel is edematous** and intestines are matted together and appears to be short
6.	Urgent **repair is not required** because of the covering sac	**Urgent repair** is required

Q 36. What are the associated anomalies in gastroschisis?

- Non-rotation of the mid gut
- Intestinal atresia.

Q 37. What is the surgical management?
Urgent primary closure.

Case

48 Desmoid Tumor, Interparietal Hernia (Interstitial), Spigelian Hernia

Case Capsule

A 30-year-old female patient presents with a **painless parietal swelling below the level of umbilicus** of 1 year duration. There is history of **cesarean** operation during her first pregnancy. She noticed the swelling **within one year of the child birth**. She also gives history of **using oral contraceptives**. There is **no history of trauma**. On examination the swelling is **hard in consistency** of about **6 × 4 cm size** overlying the upper part of the cesarean scar. The inguinal lymph node are not enlarged. The rest of the abdomen is normal. There is **no organomegaly**. The X-ray chest is normal.

Read the checklist for history and examination of abdomen.

Q 1. What is the most probable diagnosis?

Desmoid tumor (**aggressive fibromatosis**).

Q 2. What are the points in favor of a diagnosis of desmoid tumor?

- Onset of the swelling within a year of childbirth
- Use of oral contraceptives
- History of cesarean operations
- Presence of painless hard parietal swelling below the umbilicus.

Q 3. What are the types of desmoid tumor?

Classification of desmoid tumors

- Sporadic type
- Part of inherited syndrome
  - FAP (**Mesenteric Desmoids**)
  - Risk increased 1000 fold in patients with FAP

It may also be classified as:

1. Superficial (fascial)—Dupuytren's fibromatosis (they are having slow growth)
2. Deep (musculoaponeurotic)
   - Relatively rapid growth and attains large size
   - It has high rate of local recurrence
   - Involves musculature of trunk and extremities

Contd...

Contd...

Depending on the location it is classified as:
- Extra-abdominal—shoulder girdle
- Abdominal wall
- Intra-abdominal (mesenteric and pelvic desmoid).

Q 4. What is the significance of oral contraceptives and cesarean?
- There is association between the development of this neoplasm and abdominal trauma like operations
- Oral contraceptive use also has been associated with the occurrence of these tumor.

Q 5. What is the incidence of desmoid tumors?
About **2.4 to 4.3** cases/million people.

Q 6. What are the differential diagnoses?

Differential diagnoses
- Interparietal hernia
- Spigelian hernia
- Lipoma
- Neurofibroma
- Foreign body granuloma
- Suture granuloma
- Incisional hernia
- Abdominal wall sarcoma.

Q 7. What are the investigations required for further management?
- MRI—Provides information regarding the **extent of the disease and its relationship** to intra-abdominal organs
  - Homogeneous and isointense to muscle on T1 weighted images
  - Greater heterogeneity with signal less than fat in T2 weighted images.
- **Core biopsy/incisional biopsy**—Tumor composed of spindle cells with variable amounts of collagen. The fibroblasts are highly differentiated and l**ack mitotic activity**
- **Estrogen receptor** may be positive in the tumor.

Q 8. What is the most important problem of desmoid tumor after resection?
- Local recurrence even after complete resection **(40%)**.
- Multiple local recurrences are common.

Q 9. What is the surgical management of desmoid tumors?
Complete resection with a tumor-free margin.

Q 10. After complete resection with tumor free margin, there will be a big defect in the anterior abdominal wall. How to tackle the defect?
Prosthetic mesh repair is necessary after excision of the desmoid when the size of the swelling is big.

Q 11. What is the chance for systemic metastasis?
Systemic **metastases are extremely rare.**

Q 12. Is there any role for radiation therapy in the management of desmoid tumor?
The **combination of surgery and radiation therapy** improves the local failure rate.

Q 13. Is there any role for radiation alone in the management of desmoid tumor?
Radiation alone is reserved for those patients with **unresectable tumors.**

Q 14. Is there any role for drugs in the management of desmoid tumor?

Yes:

- NSAIDs
- Antiestrogens.

Note: The response rate for each of these agent is **50%.**

Q 15. Is there any role for chemotherapy in the management of desmoid tumor?

- They are reserved for **unresectable** clinically aggressive disease
- Partial response is seen with doxorubicin, dacarbazine or carboplatin.

Q 16. What is interstitial hernia?

- Here the hernial sac **passes between the layers of** the anterior abdominal wall.
- The sac may be **associated with, or communicate with**, the sac of a **concomitant inguinal or femoral hernia.**

Q 17. What are the varieties of interstitial hernia?

1. **Preperitoneal (20%)**—Usually it is a diverticulum from the femoral or inguinal hernial sac (**no swelling** is likely to be apparent in this condition).
2. **Intermuscular (60%)**—It passes between the muscular layers of the anterior abdominal wall (between external oblique and internal oblique muscles). It is usually associated with inguinal hernia.
3. **Inguinosuperficial (20%)**—The sac expands beneath the superficial fascia of the abdominal wall or thigh. It is usually associated with incompletely descended testis.

Q 18. What are the complications of interstitial hernia?

- Intestinal obstruction
- Strangulation.

Q 19. What is the treatment of interstitial hernia?

Surgical repair depending on the type of hernia.

Q 20. What is Spigelian hernia?

- This is a rare variety of interparietal hernia occurring at the level of **arcuate line.**
- The fundus of the sac clothed by the extraperitoneal fat may lie **beneath the internal oblique muscle**, and then spreads like a mushroom between the internal and external oblique muscles.
- The patient is usually above 50 years of age.

Q 21. What is the clinical presentation of Spigelian hernia?

It will present as a soft reducible mass lateral to the rectus muscle and below the umbilicus.

Q 22. How to confirm the diagnosis of Spigelian hernia?

- Ultrasound scanning—can be performed in the standing position if no defect is visible in supine position
- CT scan.

Q 23. What is the most important complication of Spigelian hernia?

Strangulation.

Q 24. What is the treatment of Spigelian hernia?

- A muscle splitting incision is put over the swelling
- Isolate the sac, reduce the contents and transfix the sac
- Transversus muscle, internal oblique and external oblique muscles are repaired by direct apposition
- Laparoscopic approach may also be used.

Case 49 Gynecomastia/Male Breast Carcinoma

Case Capsule

A 20-year-old male patient presents with **bilateral breast enlargement** that is more on right side. Right breast is 9 × 6 cm size and left breast 7 × 6 cm size. His **external genitalia are normal.** Testicular size is normal and **secondary sexual characteristics are normal**. No other abnormality detected clinically.

Checklist for history

- History of trauma
- Duration of breast enlargement
- Unilateral/bilateral
- History of breast pain
- History of drug intake
- History of sexual function
- Symptoms of hypogonadism
- Loss of libido, impotence, decreased strength
- Changes in weight
- Changes in virilization
- Symptoms of hyperthyroidism
- Symptoms of renal disease
- History of alcoholism—cirrhosis.

Checklist for examination

General

- Look for masculine features, body hair, voice, muscles, secondary sexual development
- Look for signs of hyperthyroidism

Abdominal

- Look for liver
- Abdominal mass (adrenal)

Genitalia

- Cryptorchidism
- Testicular atrophy
- Testicular tumor

Breast

- Size
- Presence of lumps
- Features of malignancy
- Nipple changes
- Ulceration
- Axillary nodes
- Unilateral/bilateral.

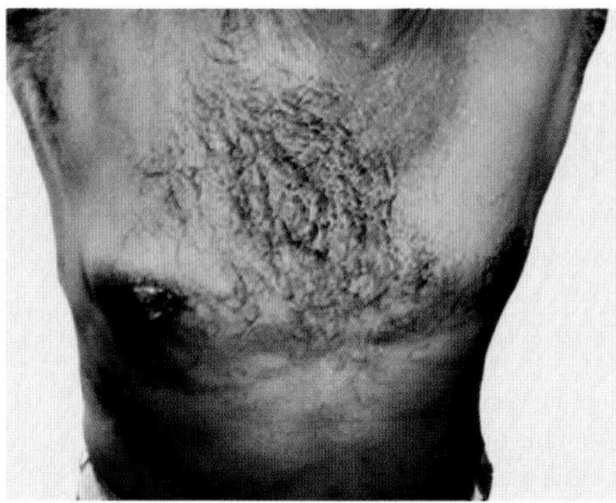

Cancer of the male breast with skin ulceration

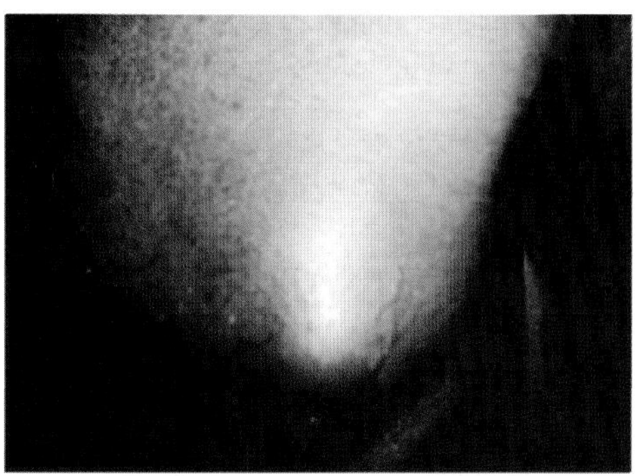

Carcinoma male breast—left side

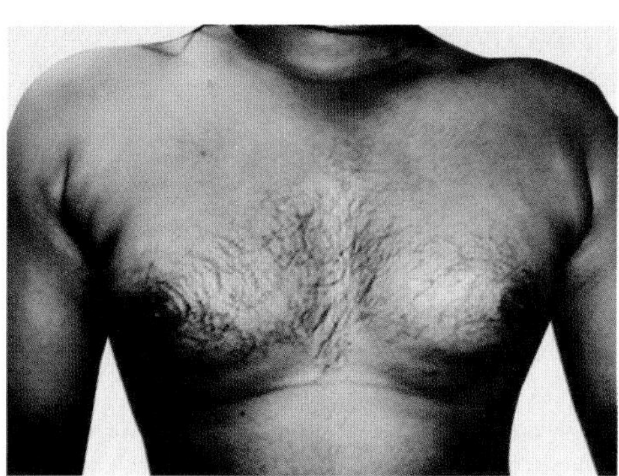

Bilateral gynecomastia

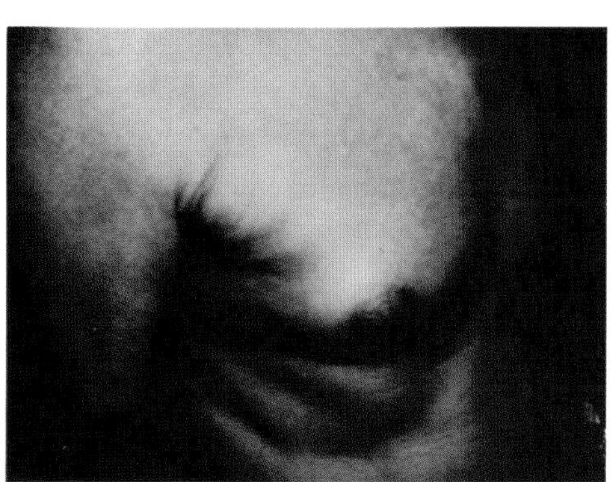

Unilateral gynecomastia with lump beneath

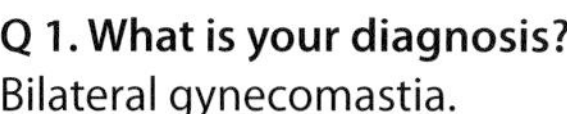

Q 1. What is your diagnosis?

Bilateral gynecomastia.

Q 2. What is gynecomastia?

It is an enlargement of the male breast, secondary to **proliferation of both epithelial and stromal** components.

Q 3. What is the word meaning of gynecomastia?

It is a Greek word meaning:

Gyne = female
Mastos = breast

Q 4. What is the clinical presentation?

It presents as **palpable or visible**, unilateral or bilateral, breast enlargement; that may or may not be tender.

Q 5. What are the causes for gynecomastia?

It is an **imbalance between** the stimulatory effects

of **estrogens** and inhibitory effects of **androgens** on the growth of breast tissue.

Causes for gynecomastia		
• Idiopathic gynecomastia	–	25%
• Pubertal gynecomastia	–	25%
• Drug-induced gynecomastia	-	25%
• Cirrhosis/malnutrition	–	8%
• Primary hypogonadism	–	8%
• Testicular tumors	–	3%
• Secondary hypogonadism	–	2%
• Hyperthyroidism	–	1.5%
• Renal disease	–	1%
• Dialysis associated gynecomastia		
• Hyperprolactinemia		
• Klinefelter's syndrome		

Q 6. What is the incidence of gynecomastia?

• Young adults	–	36%
• Older men	–	57%
• Hospitalized elderly	–	70%
• Autopsy	–	55%

Q 7. What are the peak periods for physiological gynecomastia?

There are three peak periods of physiological gynecomastia.

1. *In neonates*—transplacental transfer of maternal estrogen (regresses completely by the end of 1st year)
2. *Puberty*—transient gynecomastia occur in up to 60% of boys (regresses after 2 years)
3. *Late in life*—progressive testicular dysfunction and reduction of serum testosterone level and elevated luteinizing hormone level (LH).

Q 8. What are the causes of drug-induced gynecomastia?

Drugs causing gynecomastia with their mechanism of action	
Mechanism of action	*Drugs*
Direct breast stimulation by binding to estrogen receptor	INH Digoxin Estrogens Cannabis
Stimulation of testicular leydig cell estrogen	Human chorionic gonadotropins
Peripheral aromatization of androgens to estrogen	Testosterone
Suppression of the endogenous testosterone	Anabolic steroids
Decreased estrogen metabolism	Cimetidine
Estrogen displacement from serum human binding globulin	Spironolactone Ketoconazole
Inhibition of testosterone biosynthesis	Vincristine Methotrexate Ketoconazole Metronidazole Alcohol
Androgen receptor antagonism	Cimetidine Cyproterone acetate Cannabis
Elevated serum prolactin	Phenothiazines
Unknown mechanism	Calcium channel blockers Angiotensin-converting enzyme inhibitors Diazepam Haloperidol Phenytoin

Contd...

Contd...

	Antihypertensive: – Amlodipine – Methyldopa – Reserpine Amiodarone Metoclopramide Theophylline Ranitidine Omeprazole

Q 9. What are the causes for gynecomastia in cirrhosis?

a. Alcohol **inhibit the hypothalamic – pituitary – testicular axis** leading to low serum testosterone
b. Peripheral **aromatization of androgens** to estrogen increases in liver disease
c. Serum human binding globulin (**SHBG**) **levels** are elevated causing a further decrease in free testosterone levels
d. Some alcoholic beverages contain phytoestrogens.

Q 10. What is refeeding gynecomastia?

Significant weight loss and malnutrition are often accompanied by hypogonadism as a result of decreased gonadotropin secretion. With weight gain, gonadal function return to normal resulting in a **second puberty**.

Q 11. Hypogonadism is a cause for gynecomastia. What are the causes for hypogonadism?

A. Primary hypogonadism (congenital)
- Anorchia
- Klinefelter's syndrome
- Hermaphroditism
- Hereditary defects in testosterone synthesis

Contd...

Contd...

B. Acquired hypogonadism
- Mumps orchitis
- Trauma
- Castration
- Granulomatous disease (leprosy)
- Cytotoxic chemotherapy

C. Secondary hypogonadism
- Partial hypopituitarism will lead on to androgen deficiency.

Q 12. What is the cause for gynecomastia in hyperthyroidism?

There are two reasons:

a. The serum human binding globulin (SHBG) is increased in hyperthyroidism that attaches more testosterone to it with resultant decreased free testosterone available
b. The peripheral conversion of androgens to estrogens is enhanced in hyperthyroidism by aromatization.

Q 13. What are the estrogen producing tumors?

a. Leydig cell tumors—secrete estradiol (90% benign)
b. Estrogen producing adrenal tumors (usually malignant).

Q 14. What are the causes for gynecomastia in renal failure?

- Low levels of serum testosterone
- Raised estradiol
- Raised LH levels
- Increase in serum prolactin

Q 15. What is Simon's classification of gynecomastia?

Simon's classification of gynecomastia

- Group 1—Minor but visible breast enlargement without skin redundancy
- Group 2 A— Moderate breast enlargement without skin redundancy
- Group 2B—Moderate breast enlargement with minor skin redundancy
- Group 3—Gross breast enlargement with skin redundancy that looks such as a pendulous female breast.

Q 16. What are the differential diagnoses?

- Breast carcinoma
- Pseudogynecomastia
- Lipoma
- Neurofibroma
- Lymphangioma
- Dermoid cyst
- Hematoma.

Q 17. What is pseudogynecomastia?

Enlargement of the breast because of fat deposition rather than to glandular proliferation that is seen in obese men. There will be generalized obesity. There will not be any history of breast pain or tenderness.

Q 18. What are the investigations required in this patient?

a. **The investigations for asymptomatic group** must be kept to a minimum.
   Biochemical assessment of liver, kidney and thyroid function should be performed.
   1. LFT
   2. RFT
   3. TFT.

   If normal re-evaluation is done after 6 months.
b. Men with recent breast enlargement with breast pain and tenderness (symptomatic) do the following:
   1. Serum total and free testosterone level
   2. Luteinizing hormone
   3. FSH
   4. Estradiol
   5. Prolactin
   6. Human chorionic gonadotropins (β hCG)
   7. Urinary 17—Ketosteroids—for feminizing adrenal tumors
   8. Sex chromatin study—if Klinefelter's syndrome is suspected.
c. Imaging studies should not be ordered, unless indicated clinically or by blood results.
   1. USG/mammogram of breast
   2. FNAC/core biopsy breast
   3. Open biopsy of the breast
   4. Testicular ultrasound scan
   5. CT scan of the adrenal
   6. MRI scan of pituitary.

Q 19. What is the cause for discrepancy in size of the breast in bilateral gynecomastia?

Discrepancy in size is explained by:

a. Asynchronous growth of the two breasts
b. Differences in the amount of breast glandular and stromal proliferation.

Q 20. Mention one situation where gynecomastia predisposes to the development of carcinoma?

- Klinefelter's syndrome—phenotypic male with karyotype XXY
- Gynecomastia is seen in 80% of cases
- The increased risk for carcinoma breast is 10–20 fold greater than normal
- Patient develops lobular structure in this gynecomastia.

Q 21. What is the incidence of breast cancer in men?

About 0.2% of all malignancies in men.

Q 22. What are the histological stages in gynecomastia?

Two histological stages are seen:

a. *Proliferative stage/florid (early stage) less than a year:*
   - Ductal proliferation and ductal hyperplasia
   - Stroma is loose and edematous
   - Clinically breast pain and tenderness
   - Acinar development not seen in males because it needs progesterone
b. *Quiescent stage or inactive or asymptomatic cover 12 months (late stage):*
   - Reduction in proliferation
   - Dilatation of ducts
   - Fibrosis of stroma.

Q 23. What is the management of gynecomastia after the investigations?

It can be managed by:

a. Medical treatment
b. Surgery.

Principles of management of gynecomastia

1. Spontaneous improvement is seen in 85% without treatment
2. When gynecomastia has been present for > 2 years, medical therapy is unlikely to be effective
3. Medical therapy should be limited to only 6 months
4. Stop the drugs causing gynecomastia
5. Gynecomastia following chemotherapy will resolve spontaneously
6. Treat the hyperthyroidism
7. Surgical removal of testicular/adrenal tumors
8. Hypogonadism is treated with testosterone.

Q 24. What are the drugs used for medical management?

Drugs used for medical management of gynecomastia

I. *Androgens*
   i. Dihydrotestosterone—injection or percutaneous administration (Testosterone is aromatized to estradiol that will exacerbate the gynecomastia and therefore dihydrotestosterone is used that is nonaromatizable androgen)
      - ↓in Breast volume in 75%
      - Complete resolution in 25%
   ii. Danazol (weak androgen)—400 mg daily
      - The only licensed drug for the treatment of gynecomastia in UK
      - Complete resolution in 23%
      - Inhibits pituitary secretion of LH and FSH
      - Course of therapy is for 6 months

II. *Antiestrogens*
   i. Clomiphen citrate—response rate 36 – 95%
   ii. Tamoxifen 10 mg twice daily
      - Complete regression in 78%
      - 10 mg/day for 3 months—safe for painful idiopathic or physiological gynecomastia

iii. *Aromatase inhibitors*

Testolactone—an aromatase inhibitor is tried with good result in pubertal gynecomastia.

Q 25. What are the indications for surgery?

Indications for surgery in gynecomastia

- Social embarrassment
- Psychological trauma
- When there is no underlying treatable condition
- When trial of hormone treatment have failed.

Q 26. What are the surgical options?

1. Open subcutaneous mastectomy by a circum areolar incision extending from 3 to 9 O'clock position

2. *Endoscopic*—assisted subcutaneous mastectomy (very small distant incision)
3. *Liposuction*—assisted mastectomy (for pseudogynecomastia)
4. *Ultrasound*—assisted liposuction.

Note: In Simon's grade **I, IIA and IIB the nipple is left in its normal position**. Grade III cases require skin resection and repositioning of the nipple areolar complex. Otherwise there will be redundant skin folds and the nipple/areolar complex will be at a lower position than normal.

Q 27. What are the complications of surgery?

Complications of surgery for gynecomastia
1. Nipple/areolar ischemia
2. Nipple distortion
3. Risk of saucer deformity
4. Hematoma
5. Seroma
6. Infection
7. Skin redundancy
8. Skin necrosis
9. Breast asymmetry.

Q 28. Can you prevent iatrogenic gynecomastia?
Yes.

1. Select a drug with lowest association for gynecomastia
   Calcium channel blocker
   - Nifedipine—highest frequency
   - Verapamil—lower
   - Diltiazem—lowest association

   H_2 Receptor / Proton pump inhibitor
   - Cimetidine—highest
   - Ranitidine—lower
   - Omeprazole—lowest
2. Prophylactic breast irradiation (low dose of 900 rads) is effective in preventing gynecomastia and mastodynia in patients receiving estrogen therapy for prostate cancer.

Carcinoma Male Breast

(**Read female breast cancer**).

Q 29. What are the suspicious clinical findings for carcinoma?

Suspicious clinical findings for carcinoma of male breast
• Unilateral hard mass
• Eccentric mass rather than subareolar
• Nipple retraction
• Skin dimpling
• Nipple discharge
• Axillary lymphadenopathy.

Q 30. Is there any increased incidence of male breast cancer in patients with benign gynecomastia?
No.

Q 31. What is the incidence of male breast cancer and the mean age at diagnosis?

- < 1% (0.7%)
- Mean age at diagnosis – 65 years (5 – 10 years older than in females).

Q 32. What are risk factors for male breast cancer?

Risk factors for male breast cancer
• Radiation exposure
• Estrogen administration
• Cirrhosis of liver
• Klinefelter's syndrome
• Hepatic schistosomiasis
• Positive family history
• BRCA 2 gene.

Q 33. Why male breast cancers present as advanced malignancies?

- There is only small amount of soft tissue in the male breast and therefore, the carcinoma will infiltrate the skin and nipple early
- Early involvement of pectoral fascia and muscle because of the above reason
- Lack of awareness of male breast cancer.

Q 34. What is the prognosis of male breast cancer?

Similar to that of the female breast cancer when compared stage for stage.

Q 35. What are the prognostic factors in male breast cancer?

- Nodal status
- Tumor size
- Receptor status.

Q 36. What is the surgical management of male breast cancer?

- Modified radical mastectomy (MRM)
- Breast conservation may not be possible in most of the instances
- Radiotherapy is given because of the narrower margin of excision and locally advanced nature of the disease.

Q 37. Is there any role for tamoxifen in male breast cancer?

- Yes. It is given for ER positive patients for 5 years (20 mg daily)
- Many male breast cancers are ER positive
- It is used for the first line hormonal manipulation.

Q 38. What is the role of adjuvant systemic chemotherapy in male breast cancer?

- Same indication as in female breast cancer.

Q 39. Is there any role for orchiectomy in male breast cancer?

- No. **Orchiectomy is obsolete**
- LHRH (Luteinizing hormone releasing hormone) analog is a better option
- Orchiectomy is used as a 2nd line hormonal manipulation in metastatic male breast cancer occasionally in some centers.

Case 50 Fibroadenoma/Cystosarcoma/Breast Cyst/Fibroadenosis/Fibrocystic Disease/Mastalgia/Mastopathy/Chronic Mastitis

Case Capsule

A 20-year-old female patient presents with **two painless lumps** in her right breast of 6 months duration. There is no history of any nipple discharge. There is no family history of any breast diseases. Her menstrual history is normal. There is no history suggestive of cyclical mastalgia. On examination, two **very freely mobile rubbery hard** lumps are felt (which are **disappearing from the palpating fingers**) in the upper outer quadrant of the right breast each about 2 cm in diameter. The nipple areolar complex is normal. There is no skin involvement or fixity. There are no palpable axillary lymph nodes.

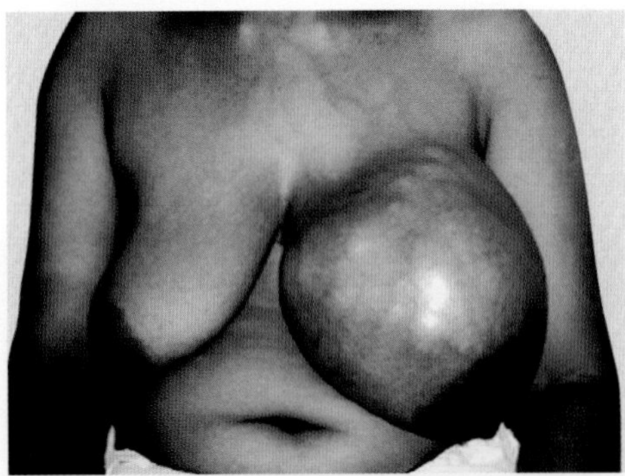

Cystosarcoma of left breast

Read the checklist for history and examination of breast in long case section.

Q 1. What is the probable diagnosis in this case?

Fibroadenoma.

Q 2. What are the clinical points in favor of fibroadenoma?

Clinical points in favor of fibroadenoma of the breast

- Painless, freely mobile, rubbery hard swellings in the breast **(Breast mouse)**
- The age group (15 to 25 years)
- No fixity to skin or deeper structures
- No axillary lymph node involvement
- Multiplicity.

Q 3. What are the causes for painless lump in the breast?

Causes for painless lump in the breast

- Fibroadenoma
- Carcinoma
- Fibroadenosis
- Traumatic fat necrosis.

Q 4. What are the causes for painful lump in the breast?

Causes for painful lump in the breast
• Mastitis • Breast abscess • Fibroadenosis • Fat necrosis.

Q 5. What are the causes for massive enlargement of the breast?

Causes for massive enlargement of the breast
• Giant fibroadenoma • Cystosarcoma phyllodes • Sarcoma of the breast • Benign hypertrophy of the breast (Diffuse hypertrophy) • Filarial elephantiasis of the breast • Colloid carcinoma of the breast.

Q 6. What are the causes for cystic swellings in the breast?

Causes for cystic swellings in the breast
• Fibroadenosis • Galactocele • Abscess • Lymph cyst • Hematoma • Parasitic cyst.

Q 7. What is fibroadenoma?

- It is hyperplasia of a single lobule where as neoplasms arise from a single cell
- It is not a benign neoplasm, but are best considered as aberrations of normal development and involution (ANDI)
- They arise in the fully developed breast during the 15 to 25 year period (after 40 years they are less common)
- They show the same hormonal dependence as the remainder of the breast, e.g. they lactate during pregnancy and involute during the perimenopausal period.

Q 8. What is the incidence of fibroadenoma?

- They account for 12% of all palpable symptomatic breast masses
- They are more frequently seen in Negro population (black races).

Q 9. How will you classify fibroadenoma?

There are four separate entities of fibroadenomas. They are:

Four types of fibroadenoma
1. Common fibroadenoma 2. Giant fibroadenoma 3. Juvenile fibroadenoma 4. Phyllodes tumor.

Q 10. What is intracanalicular and pericanalicular fibroadenoma?

- This is a conventional classification by the pathologists
- This histological distinction has no clinical relevance
- This terminology can therefore be abandoned.

Q 11. What is giant fibroadenoma?

- A fibroadenoma must measure over 5 cm in size to qualify for this definition
- They may or may not have different behavior to an ordinary fibroadenoma
- Treatment is enucleation through a submammary incision.

Q 12. What is phyllodes tumor (serocystic disease of brodie/cystosarcoma phyllodes)?

- There is stromal over growth and they are highly cellular and heterogenous
- Mitosis is seen in sarcoma
- Mammoglobin is positive
- It is a distinct pathological entity and better classified separately from fibroadenoma
- They occur in women **more than 40 years**
- Clinically they present as large **massive tumor** with an unevenly bosselated surface
- **Pressure necrosis** of the overlying skin will result in ulceration
- They are mobile despite the size
- Some of the tumors are purely benign, some are malignant with higher mitotic index
- **Cystosarcoma phyllodes are a misnomer:** usually neither cystic nor sarcomatous (sarcomatous change can occur)
- If mammogram negative—**MRI may be useful** and positive—70% pick up is there for MRI
- The malignant variety recur locally
- Malignant tumors may metastasize via the bloodstream
- Treatment for **benign variety-wide local excision, malignant need simple mastectomy.**

Note: **Phyllus means—"leaf-like"**—branching projections of tumor tissue into the cystic cavities of this neoplasm histologically.

Q 13. What are the indications for mastectomy in phyllodes tumor?

- Malignant tumor
- Massive tumor
- Recurrent tumor.

Note: Mastectomy is followed by radiotherapy. Axillary dissection is recommended.

Q 14. What are the differences between Phyllodes tumor and carcinoma breast?

Sl No.	*Phyllodes tumor*	*Carcinoma*
1.	No nipple retraction	Nipple retraction may be there
2.	Absence of skin involvement, tethering and skin fixity	Tethering, fixity and skin involvement may be there
3.	Bosselated surface	Not bosselated
4.	Warm to touch	Need not be warm
5.	No axillary node involvement	Axillary nodes present
6.	Ulceration of the overlying skin may occur due to **pressure necrosis**	Skin ulceration is due to direct skin involvement
7.	There will be a gap between the skin and the tumor when there is ulceration	The ulcer is fixed to the tumor
8.	For malignant phyllodes, simple mastectomy alone without axillary dissection	Breast conservation and axillary dissection and radiotherapy or modified radical mastectomy

Q 15. What is the natural course of fibroadenoma?

- One-third get smaller or disappear over two year period
- Less than 5% increase in size
- The reminder stay the same size, but becomes clinically less distinct with time
- There is no need for excision in below 30 years age group.

Q 16. Can fibroadenoma turn malignant?

No. Breast cancer is no more likely to develop in fibroadenoma than in any other part of the breast.

Q 17. Can fibroadenoma occur after the menopause?
No. Does not normally occur after menopause, but may occasionally develop after administration of hormone.

Q 18. What are the investigations for suspected fibroadenoma?
The triple assessment consisting of:
- Clinical examination
- Imaging—USG
- FNAC/core biopsy.

Q 19. What are the indications for surgery in fibroadenoma?

Indications for surgery in fibroadenoma
- Lump more than 3 to 4 cm in size
- Above 30 years
- Suspicious cytology
- Patient desire.

Note: If access to good quality cytology and USG is not available, it is wise to excise all fibroadenomas to be certain in that no malignancy is missed.

Q 20. What is the incision for excision of fibroadenoma?
- The lines of tension in the skin of breast (the Langer's lines) are generally concentric and parallel with the nipple areolar complex. Therefore, a curved incision that parallels the areola is cosmetically acceptable.
- Radial incisions are not recommended in the breast (except in 3 and 9 O' clock position).

Q 21. What is complex fibroadenoma?
This is a relatively uncommon pathological lesion and appear to be associated with a slightly increased risk of breast cancer (1.5 to 2 times).

Q 22. What is juvenile fibroadenoma?
They occur in adolescent girls and is rare.

Q 23. What is diffuse hypertrophy of the breast (benign hypertrophy)?
- It is due to **alteration in the normal sensitivity** of the breast **to estrogenic hormones**
- They occur in healthy **girls at puberty**
- At times they also develop during pregnancy
- The breasts attain enormous dimensions
- The treatment is reduction **mammoplasty**/ antiestrogen.

Q 24. What is breast cyst?
- They are due to **nonintegrated involution** of stroma and epithelium.
- Most commonly occur in the **last decade of reproductive life**
- Often **multiple**, may be **bilateral**
- Confirmed by **USG** and **aspiration**
- Can mimic malignancy.

Q 25. What is the management of breast cyst?

Management of breast cyst
- More than 35 years do mammogram prior to needle aspiration (1 to 3 % of patients with cysts have an incidental carcinoma)
- Aspirate the cyst to dryness with 21 gauge needle
- No need for fluid cytology unless evenly blood stained
- After aspiration examine the patient for residual mass
- If there is a residual lump do FNAC from that
- 30% of the cysts will recur and require reaspiration
- Review the patient 3 to 6 weeks after cyst aspiration to check for refilling.

Q 26. What are the indications for excision of the breast cyst?

Indications for excision of the breast cyst

- If the cysts refill more than twice
- If the fluid is blood stained
- If there is residual lump.

Q 27. What is the risk of carcinoma in breast cyst?

- The relative risk for carcinoma is 1.5 to 4 times
- The risk is greatest in young patients less than 45 years (risk may be as high as 6 times that of the general population).

Q 28.What is the management of multiple asymptomatic cyst?

- Generally no treatment is indicated for multiple cysts
- Regular USG and mammogram every 1 to 2 years
- Only symptomatic cysts are aspirated.

Q 29. What is galactocele?

- Galactocele presents as a solitary subareolar cyst and always dates from lactation
- It contains milk and in long-standing cases the walls tend to calcify
- It may reach enormous sizes.

Q 30. What are the benign diseases associated with increased risk for invasive breast cancer?

- ADH (Atypical Ductal Hyperplasia) / Lobular hyperplasia
- Gross cysts
- Moderate and florid hyperplasia
- Papilloma with fibrovascular core
- Sclerosing adenosis
- Complex fibroadenoma.

Q 31. What is fibroadenosis and what is the pathogenesis (fibrocystic disease/chronic mastitis/ mastopathy)?

- Seen in women of reproductive age group (35 to 45 years)
- The nomenclature of benign breast disease is confusing and various synonyms are used as mentioned above
- A new system has been developed and described by the Cardiff Breast Clinic terming it as ANDI (Aberration in Normal Development and Involution)
- The breast is a dynamic structure that undergoes changes throughout reproductive life in addition to the cyclical changes throughout the menstrual cycles
- ANDI involves disturbances in breast physiology extending from an extreme of normality to well-defined disease process.

Q 32. What are the pathological changes in ANDI?

Pathological changes in ANDI:

- Fibrosis—fat and elastic tissue replaced
- Adenosis
- Cyst formation
- Papillomatosis
- Epitheliosis
- Hyperplasia of epithelium lining ducts and acini.

Q 33. What are the clinical features of ANDI?

- Cyclical breast pain (mastalgia) may or may not be there
- The lump may be solid or cystic
- Multiple lumps or generalized nodularity may be there
- Increase in lumpiness and tenderness before menstrual period
- It may affect one or both breasts
- Associated nipple discharge may be there: clear, green or serous.

Q 34. What is the Bloodgood's blue domed cyst?

It is nothing but large cyst associated with ANDI.

Q 35. What is Schimmelbusch's disease?

Presence of multiple cysts in both breast seen in ANDI is called Schimmelbusch's disease.

Q 36. What is the management of fibroadenosis?

Triple assessment—(The imaging of choice less than 35 years is USG and more than 35 years mammogram) and rule out malignancy.

Q 37. What is the treatment of lumpy breast of ANDI?

Treatment of lumpy breast of ANDI

- Exclude malignancy
- Reassurance for lumpy breast
- Adequate support for the breast:
  Appropriately fitting and supporting bra should be worn throughout the day and soft bra (sports bra) worn at night
- Avoid caffeine drinks
- Pain chart—chart the pattern of pain throughout the month (to note the exacerbation of pain in the premenstrual period and the cyclical nature)
- Medications.

Q 38. What are the drugs used for the management of ANDI?

Drugs used for the management of ANDI

- Evening primrose oil, (GLA) gamma linolenic acid—dose is 6 to 8 capsules per day
- More effective for > 40 years group
- It is given for a period of 3 months (will help 50%)

Contd...

Contd...

- For intractable symptoms Antigonadotrophin - Danazol 100 mg tds.
- Prolactin inhibitor—Bromocriptine—2.5 mg twice daily, increasing the dose over 1–2 weeks (A newer antiprolactin agent, cabergoline, is now available)
- Tamoxifen 20 mg daily—Antiestrogen will deprive the breast epithelium of estrogenic drive
- LHRH agonist—not recommended for routine use.

Note: All these drugs are not given simultaneously. A planned escalation of treatment from the simple evening primrose oil to the other drugs downwards is given.

Q 39. What is the management of noncyclical mastalgia?

- Exclude extramammary causes for pain
- Biopsy on localized tender area may be required
- Identify the trigger spot
- Inject the trigger spot with local anesthetic/nonsteroidal analgesic.

Q 40. What is Tietze syndrome?

It is nothing but Tender costochondral junction (commonest cause for noncyclical mastalgia).

Q 41. What are the clinical differences between the benign lumps of the breast and malignant mass?

Comparison of clinical features of commonly seen breast lumps:

Disease	*Age group*	*Presence of pain*	*No swellings*	*Consistency*	*Surface node*	*Axillary*
Fibroadenoma	15–25 30–40	No	1 or more	Rubbery	Smooth/ bosselated	No
Fibroadenosis ANDI	35–50	Yes	1 or more or diffuse	Variable	Indistinct	No
Breast cyst	30–50	Occasional	1 or more	Tense and hard	Smooth	Normal
Carcinoma	25 +	No	1	Stony hard	Irregular	Yes

4

SECTION

Radiology and Imaging

Radiology Questions and Answers

1 – Small Intestinal Obstruction

Instructions for viewing the skiagram of the abdomen:

1. The entire abdomen should be visualized from the top of the diaphragm to the hernial orifices in the groin
2. Always take **both supine and erect films** especially when you are suspecting intestinal obstruction
3. Remember the **five basic densities**.
   a. Gas – Black
   b. Fat – Dark grey
   c. Soft tissue/fluid – Light grey
   d. Bone/calcification – White
   e. Metal intense white – Intense white
4. Look for **bones** – Spine, pelvis, chest cage and the sacroiliac joints (presence or absence of scoliosis and abnormality in bones)
5. **Look for soft tissue shadows:** The liver, spleen, kidneys, bladder and psoas muscles (liver on the right side, the left kidney higher than the right, stomach, spleen and cardiac shadow on the left side)
6. Gas shadow in the body of the stomach
7. Gas in the descending colon and inside pelvis
8. Look for radiopaque shadows
9. Look for any **abnormal soft tissue shadows**
10. Check for the 'R' marked low down on the right side (**always check left and right on every film**)

Q 1. What is your observation?

Supine abdominal film (AP view) demonstrating **jejunal loops with Valvulae conniventes** suggestive of distal ileal obstruction (Intestinal obstruction).

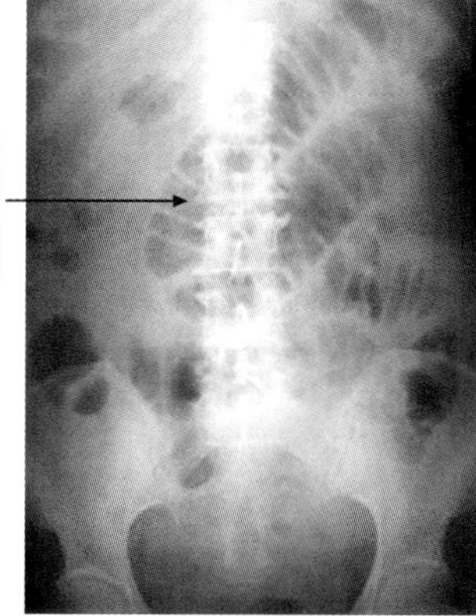

Intestinal obstruction

Q 2. Why fluid levels are not demonstrated in this film?

Fluid levels do not appear on supine AP films (the characteristic radiological feature of intestinal obstruction is demonstration of multiple fluid levels which is possible only in erect film or decubitus film). The supine film is taken for demonstration of the intestinal loops so that the level of obstruction can be ascertained.

Q 3. Why this is AP film?

Virtually every abdominal X-ray is an AP film, i.e. the **beam passes from front to back** with the film behind the patient who is lying down with the X-ray machine overhead.

Q 4. What are the characteristic intestinal patterns identified in intestinal obstruction?

1. Jejunum—**Valvulae conniventes** – coiled spring shaped folds crossing the entire lumen is seen in the jejunum when it is distended (caliber of the bowel should not exceed 2.5–3 cms, increasing distally. The folds **completely pass across** the width of the bowel, they are **regularly spaced** and gives a **concertina or ladder effect**.
2. Ileum—**Feature less** described by Wangensteen (Structure less pattern)
3. Colon—**Haustrations**: Folds of mucosa visualized across the bowel only partially. The colonic mucosal folds **do not completely cross the lumen** and they are **placed irregularly** and do not have indentations placed opposite one another.

Note: That the colon is peripheral and contains feces and the small bowel is central and contains fluid and gas).

Q 5. What is the essence of treatment of intestinal obstruction?

The three essential principles are: **Drip, suction and relief of obstruction.**

- Drip and suction (IV fluids: fluid and electrolyte replacement and nasogastric decompression)
- Relief of obstruction by surgical interference at the appropriate time
- Surgical treatment is delayed until resuscitation is complete provided there is no strangulation or closed loop obstruction
- Remember the aphorism: "The sun should not both rise and set on a case of unrelieved intestinal obstruction."

Q 6. What are the clinical features of the strangulation (which is an absolute indication for surgical relief of obstruction)?

- Continuous pain
- Tenderness with rigidity/rebound tenderness of the abdomen
- Shock

Note: Persistent pain even in the absence of tenderness and rigidity in spite of conservative management is also an indication for surgery.

2 – Intestinal Obstruction

Q 1. What is this skiagram and what is your observation?

Erect abdominal film with multiple fluid levels suggestive of **intestinal obstruction.**

Q 2. Why do you say that this is an erect film?

The **gas in the gastric fundus** is suggestive of typical erect film.

Q 3. Upto how many fluid levels are normal?

In the normal adult erect film, usually **upto 3 fluid levels** are normal. They are:

1. One at the fundus of the stomach
2. One at the duodenal cap
3. One in the terminal ileum.

Note: In infants < 1 year old a few fluid levels in the small bowel may be physiological.

Q 4. What is the cause for fluid level?

For fluid level you need fluid, gas and horizontal beam. **Without gas you won't see the fluid.** The fluid levels appear later in the course of the intestinal obstruction. It takes some time for the gas and fluid to separate.

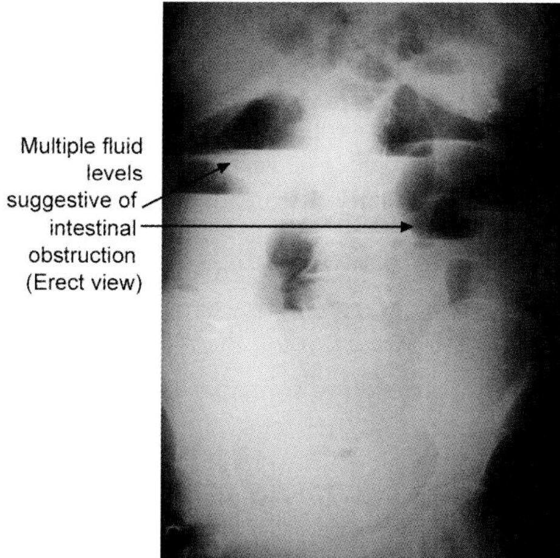

Plain radiograph—abdomen

Q 5. What is the cause for distension of abdomen in intestinal obstruction?

The distension proximal to the obstruction is produced by **gas and fluid**.

Q 6. Which is the commonest nature of gas seen in intestinal obstruction?

- Majority is made up of nitrogen (90%) and the remaining hydrogen sulphide (oxygen and carbon dioxide are reabsorbed)
- Overgrowth of aerobic and anaerobic organisms produce gas.

Q 7. What is the cause for fluid inside the intestine in obstruction?

It is constituted by 3 factors:

1. Various digestive juices
2. Absorption from the gut is retarded
3. Fluid secreted from the bowel wall.

Q 8. What is the importance of the number of fluid levels?

- When the fluid levels are more the obstruction is advanced
- The number of fluid levels are directly proportional to the degree of obstruction
- The more distal the site of the obstruction, the number of fluid level increases.

Q 9. Can you get fluid levels in non obstructing conditions?

Yes; It may be seen in the following conditions:

1. Acute pancreatitis
2. Inflammatory bowel diseases
3. Intra-abdominal sepsis.

Q 10. What is the most important differential diagnosis of small bowel obstruction?

Paralytic ileus. It is hard to differentiate between paralytic ileus and obstruction radiologically. Combined small and large bowel dilatation may form the classic radiological sign of paralytic ileus.

Q 11. What are the common causes of intestinal obstruction?

- Postoperative adhesions (upto 40% of cases)
- Internal strangulation of bowel (band or internal hernia)
- External hernia (e.g. inguinal 12%)
- Tumors (15%)
- Fecal impaction (8%)
- Pseudoobstruction (5%)
- Inflammatory bowel disease—Crohn's disease
- Intussusception – usually children; in adults often associated with a tumor. Tends to begin in the ileum
- Congenital atresias – newborns
- Gallstone ileus.

Q 12. How will you classify intestinal obstruction?

Can be classified as:

1. Depending on the mechanism: Dynamic (mechanical obstruction) and Adynamic
2. Depending on the site: Small bowel (high and low) and large bowel.
3. Depending on the intactness or compromise of the blood supply:
   Simple obstruction and strangulating obstruction (compromised blood supply affecting the viability of the intestine)
4. Depending on the cause: Intraluminal, intra mural and extramural.

Intraluminal	*Intramural*	*Extramural*
• Impaction	• Malignancy	• Adhesions/ bands
• Bezoars	• Stricture	• Hernia
• Foreign bodies		• Volvulus
• Gallstones		• Intussusception

5. Depending on whether it is acute or chronic
   - Acute obstruction (usually small intestinal)
   - Chronic obstruction (large intestinal)
   - Acute on chronic
   - Subacute – incomplete obstruction
6. Depending on whether it is **complete or incomplete.**

Q 13. What are the clinical features of intestinal obstruction?

Quartet of symptoms
• Pain
• Distension
• Vomiting
• Absolute constipation

Q 14. What is closed loop obstruction?

- When bowel is obstructed at both the proximal and distal point closed loop obstruction will occur (carcinomatous stricture of the colon with a competent ileocecal valve).
- There is no early distension of the proximal intestine
- When gangrene of the strangulated segment occurs, retrograde thrombosis of the mesenteric vessel will occur.

Q 15. What is absolute constipation?

Failure to pass neither feces nor flatus is called absolute constipation which is suggestive of complete intestinal obstruction.

Q 16. Mention a few situations where constipation may not be present in spite of intestinal obstruction?

Intestinal obstruction without constipation
• Richter's hernia
• Mesenteric vascular obstruction
• Gallstone ileus
• Partial intestinal obstruction

3 – Volvulus of the Sigmoid

Q 1. What is your observation?

a. Plain skiagram of abdomen - supine film with **pneumatic tyre** appearance: grossly distended loop of sigmoid colon extending from the pelvis to the undersurface of the diaphragm. The loop running diagonally from right to left with two fluid levels. Compression together of the two medial walls produce the **'coffee bean sign'**.

b. Barium enema picture showing the '**bird beak**' appearance: Retrograde running of contrast per rectum will show this appearance (point of convergence of the distended loops appearing as the birds beak or '**bird of pray**'.

Q 2. What is the diagnosis in this case?

Sigmoid volvulus

Q 3. What is volvulus?

Axial rotation of the bowel about its mesentery is called volvulus.

Q 4. How will you classify volvulus?

May be classified as:

- Primary – Sigmoid volvulus (the commonest spontaneous type in adults), cecal volvulus and volvulus neonatorum
- Secondary– Rotation of bowel around an acquired adhesion or stoma.

Q 5. What are the other radiological signs of volvulus sigmoid?

a. **Lack of haustration:** This as a result of enormous distension of the colon

b. **Liver overlap sign**: Indicative of the degree of distension of the colon, i.e. the colonic loop will reach the height of the liver or above it on the right side.

c. **Left flank overlap sign**: The left limb of the coffee bean overlies the descending colon.

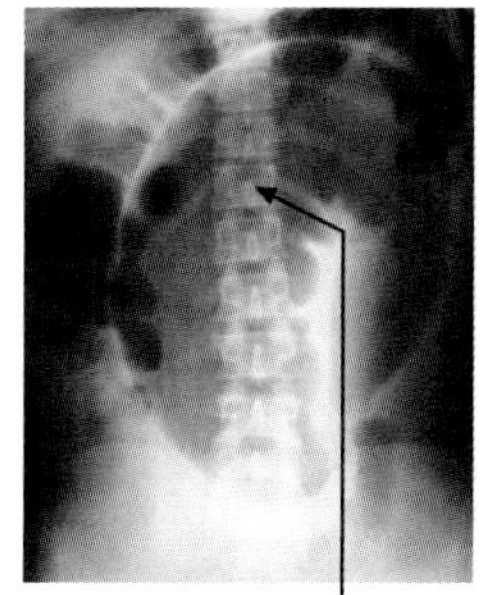

Pneumatic tyre appearance

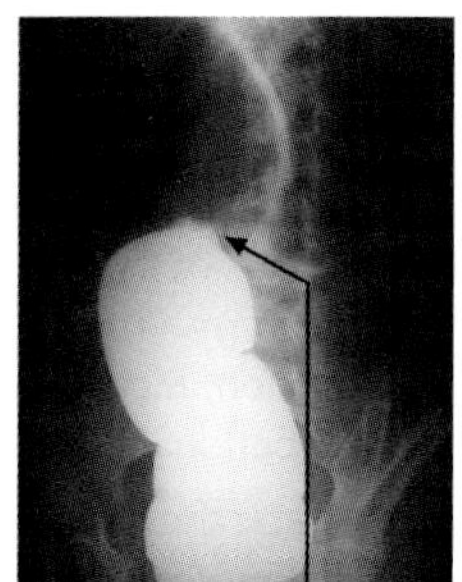

Bird beak appearance

Volvulus sigmoid—plain film and barium enema

Q 6. What are the likely symptoms?

Intermittent abdominal pain and distension along with constipation usually occurring in elderly patients. During acute presentation the patient will be severely ill with severe abdominal pain, obstipation and distension of the abdomen. Digital rectal examination will reveal an empty rectum.

Q 7. What is the direction of twist of volvulus of sigmoid?

Anticlockwise.

Q 8. What is cecal volvulus and what is the direction of twist?

The cecum folds in a cephalad direction anteriorly over the fixed ascending colon. The direction is **clockwise**.

Q 9. What are the predisposing factors for sigmoid volvulus?

- High residue diet and overloaded colon
- Chronic constipation
- Long pelvic mesocolon
- Narrow attachment of pelvic mesocolon
- Band/adhesions of the sigmoid to the parities as a result of peridiverticulitis

Q 10. What are the clinical features of sigmoid volvulus?

- Chronic type (Elderly): Intermittent large bowel obstruction followed by passage of large quantities of flatus and feces
- Acute type (Young individuals): Abdominal distension, hiccough, wretching and absolute constipation.

Q 11. What is the emergency treatment of volvulus of the sigmoid?

- Endoscopic detorsion initially with flexible sigmoidoscope (most will recover)
- Insertion of flatus tube if the above one is not available
- Resuscitation of the patient
- Definitive surgery in the form of resection of the sigmoid and restoration of the continuity of the bowel (sigmoidectomy) with or without a proximal defunctioning colostomy
- Hartmann's procedure (after sigmoidectomy the distal end is closed and left and the proximal end is brought out. This is a procedure recommended for emergency surgery when the surgeon is not experienced)
- Paul-Mikulicz procedure (not done nowadays).

Q 12. What is compound volvulus?

It is a rare condition known as ileosigmoid knotting where the long pelvic mesocolon allows the ileum to twist around the sigmoid colon resulting in gangrene of either or both segments of the bowel.

4 – Pneumoperitoneum (Gas under the Diaphragm)

Q 1. What is your observation?

Skiagram chest showing **dark crescentic area** of gas under the hemidiaphragm.

Q 2. What is the ideal skiagram for demonstration of pneumoperitoneum?

Erect Plain X-ray abdomen or erect chest film demonstrating the diaphragm.

Q 3. In seriously ill patients the use of erect films may not be possible. What is the recommended method for demonstration of pneumoperitoneum?

Decubitus films with the left side down (left decubitus) centered on the right upper flank should be taken (this is the method used for confirmation of a **small amount of free gas** and to demonstrate fluid levels in a sick patient who is too ill to sit up). A horizontal cross table beam is used rather than the vertical beam from overhead for supine films. **5 to 10 minutes are spent** with the patient in this position to allow the free gas to track up before the exposure is made.

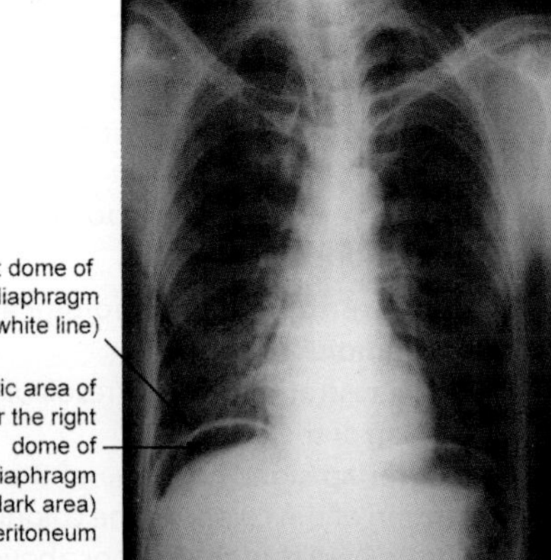

Skiagram chest

Q 4. What is the origin of the word decubitus?

The word originated from the Latin word – Decumbere meaning to lie down, like a Roman patrician lying on his side eating at a banquet.

Q 5. What are the other signs of pneumoperitoneum?

1. Double wall sign – Both sides of the wall of a loop of bowel become visible because air on the inside and air on the outside are demonstrated
2. Silver's sign – Visualization of falciform ligament
3. Football or Dome sign – with a large pneumoperitoneum the unde surface of the diaphragm may be surrounded by air giving a dark dome-like appearance in the upper abdomen (may be there even in supine film).

Q 6. What are the differential diagnoses of gas under the diaphragm?

1. Chilaiditi's syndrome – (Colonic inter- position): The incidental finding of pockets of gas beneath the right hemidiaphragm with multiple bands of mucosal folds. It may be seen with Shrunken livers (Cirrhosis), in COPD and postoperatively where the surgeon has pushed the gut out of the way.
2. Linear atelectasis:
3. Subphrenic abscess with fluid level under the diaphragm
4. Meteorism due to excessive air swallowing associated with crying in children

Q 7. What are the causes for pneumoperitoneum?

With peritonitis – hollow viscera perforation

- Perforated peptic ulcer (gastric, duodenal)
- Malignant ulcer perforation
- Appendix perforation
- Intestinal obstruction with perforation
- Ruptured diverticular disease
- Inflammatory bowel disease – Crohn's disease, ulcerative colitis
- Steroid induced perforation
- NSAIDs induced perforation
- Stress ulcers – burns, sepsis, multisystem trauma etc.
- Chemotherapy and radiotherapy

Without peritonitis

- Postlaparotomy
- Postlaparoscopy
- Peritoneal dialysis
- Tube testing for sterility
- Pneumatosis coli
- Huge pneumothorax (tracking from chest)
- Escape of air from the tracheobronchial tree in obstructive airway disease

Q 8. What are the stages of peritonitis?

1. Stage of chemical peritonitis
2. Stage of illusion
3. Stage of frank general peritonitis.

Q 9. What are the clinical findings of perforation with peritonitis?

1. Generalized tenderness
2. Generalized guarding
3. Board-like rigidity of the abdomen
4. Obliteration of liver dullness
5. Absent bowel sounds
6. Free fluid may or may not be demonstrated.

Q 10. What is the management of duodenal ulcer perforation with peritonitis?

1. Resuscitation of the patient—Nasogastric decompression, IV fluids, correction of electrolytes, and make the patient fit for surgery
2. Exploratory laparotomy

3. Identify the site of perforation, suck out the pus
4. Closure of the perforation with 3 interrupted absorbable sutures and reinforce with a patch of pedicled omentum
5. Thorough peritoneal toilet and peritoneal lavage
6. Flank drainage
7. Closure of the abdomen.

5 – Cannon Ball Lesion, Pulmonary Metastasis, Primary Malignancy of Lung

Q 1. What is your observation?

Skiagram chest showing **two types of coin shadows** in the left lung (solitary pulmonary nodule).

Q 2. What are the differential diagnosis?

1. Primary malignancy of lung (18%)
2. Metastasis lung (64%)
3. Tuberculosis
4. Fungi: Histoplasmosis, coccidiomycosis
5. Benign neoplasms: (18%) Hamartoma, hemangioma
6. Granulomatosis

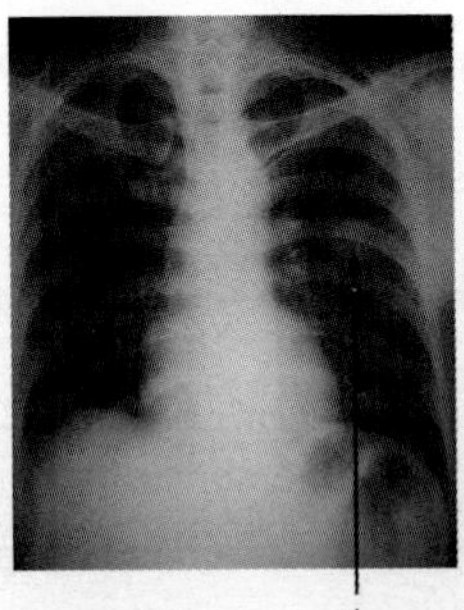

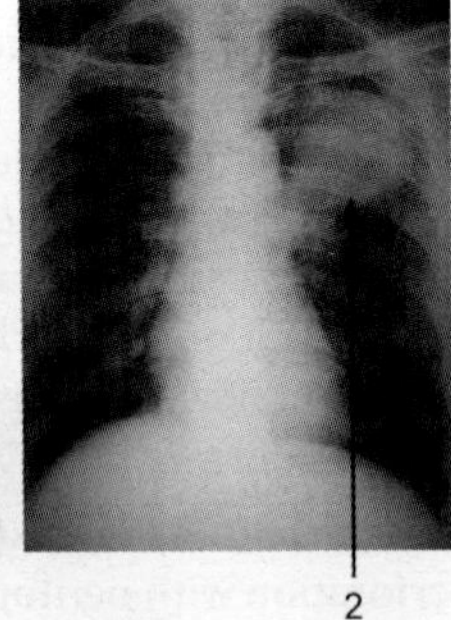

Skiagram chest showing two types of coin shadows in left lung— pulmonary metastasis

Q 3. Can you differentiate benign from malignant radiologically?

It may be difficult to differentiate. The differences between benign and malignant lesions are given below:

Benign	Malignant
• Lesions are small (< 1cm)	• Lesions are larger
• Stable for more than 2 years	• Grows rapidly
• Calcified	• Lack calcium
• Target or popcorn	• Appear speculated distribution (surface umbilication ornotching) Eccentric or excavated
• Hounsfield unit > 175 unit	• < 175 units

Q 4. What are the causes for pulmonary metastasis?

1. Head and neck malignancies
2. Carcinoma breast
3. GI malignancies (Colon, stomach and pancreas commonest)
4. Renal cell carcinoma and other genitourinary tumors)
5. Sarcomas: Osteogenic sarcoma, soft tissue sarcoma, retroperitoneal sarcoma, etc.
6. Malignant melanoma.

Q 5. What is the incidence of metastasis in the lung?

- 30% of all patients with malignancies develop pulmonary metastasis
- 1.2% have solitary lung metastasis.

Q 6. What is the classification of primary neoplasms of the lung?

- It is classified into:
  1. Small cell carcinoma (Oat cell cancer) 20%
  2. Non-small cell Lung cancer (NSCLC)
     - Adenoma carcinoma (commonest)
     - Squamous carcinoma (cavitating tumors)
     - Large cell undifferentiated (included with neuroendocrine tumors)
     - Bronchioalveolar carcinoma (Ground glass appearance on radiograph).

Q 7. What are the symptoms of metastasis in the lung?

- Cough
- Hemoptysis
- Fever
- Dyspnoea
- Pain.

Q 8. How will you proceed to investigate such a case?

1. CT of the lung: To assess the lungs for other nodules (CT can identify nodules as small as 3mm).
2. Sputum cytology
3. FNAC from the peripheral lesions
4. Bronchoscopy for central lesions
5. PET to differentiate malignancy.

Q 9. If the report is coming as adenocarcinoma metastasis, what next?

Do bone scan and CT of the head to rule out metastasis in the bone and brain.

Q 10. If the report is coming as squamous cell carcinoma and there is history of head and neck squamous cell carcinoma, what will be your inference?

Still, one should address it as a new primary.

Q 11. What is the treatment of the primary in the lung?

Lobectomy + mediastinal lymph node dissection.

Q 12. What is the surgical approach for lung resection?

- Posterolateral thoracotomy
- Anterolateral thoracotomy
- Median sternotomy.

Q 13. What are the adverse prognostic factors in metastasis?

1. Multiple or bilateral lesions
2. More than four lesions on CT
3. Tumor doubling time < 40 days
4. Short disease- free interval
5. Advanced age.

Q 14. What are the indications for resection of metastasis?

Medically fit patient with resectable disease with the following criteria

a. Primary must be controlled or controllable
b. No other sites of disease may exist
c. No other therapy can offer comparable results
d. The operative risk must be low

Q 15. What are the surgical options for resection of metastasis?

- Can be done as open procedure by thoracotomy
- Video assisted thoracoscopy (VAT) for metastatic disease.

Q 16. What is the success rate with surgical removal of pulmonary metastasis?

a. Testicular tumor - 51% 5-year-survival
b. Head and neck - 47% 5-year-survival
c. Colon cancer, renal cell carcinoma and osteogenic sarcomas – prolonged survival
d. Melanoma - 10 – 15% survival.

6 – Goiter

Q 1. What is your observation?

Skiagram of the neck lateral view showing soft tissue shadow suggestive of goiter and the trachea showing luminal narrowing.

Q 2. What is the purpose of skiagram of the neck in thyroid swellings?

Skiagram neck AP and lateral views are obtained preoperatively because of the following reasons:

- To assess the position of the trachea (this will help the anesthesiologist for intubation).
- The AP view will reveal displacement of trachea (displacement of the trachea is suggestive of retrosternal extension of the goiter).
- The lateral view will reveal luminal narrowing (chance for scabbard trachea is there)
- It will also reveal calcifications in thyroid.

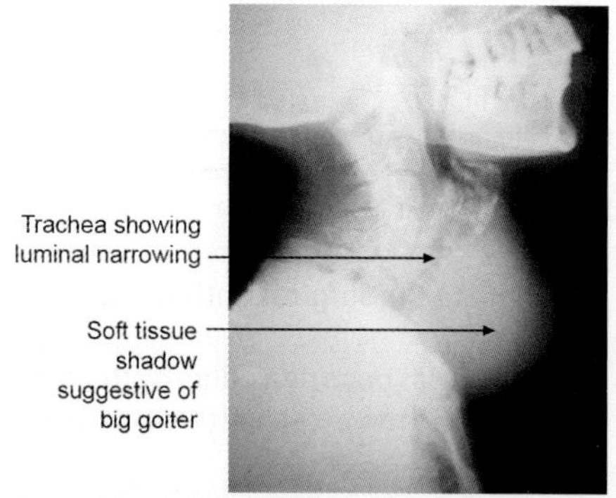

Skiagram neck—lateral view

Q 3. What type of calcification you get in long-standing goiters?

Dystrophic calcification (the types of calcifications in general are: metastatic, dystrophic, heterotopic and calcinosis).

Q 4. When do you suspect retrosternal extension radiologically?

If the soft tissue shadow is coming down below the clavicles one should suspect retrosternal extension.

Q 5. What is the investigation of choice for ruling out retrosternal extension?

CT scan.

7 – Chronic Calcific Pancreatitis, Tropical Chronic Pancreatitis

Q 1. What is your observation?

Plain skiagram of abdomen AP view showing multiple radiopaque shadows in the region of the head, body and tail of pancreas.

Q 2. What are the causes for radiopaque shadows in plain X-ray abdomen?

1. Normal calcified structures
   - Costal cartilage (mistaken for biliary, renal and splenic calcification)
   - Pelvic phleboliths – Vein stones (mistaken for ureteric and bladder calculi)
   - Mesenteric lymph nodes (calcified): They tend to be mobile and show changes in position from film-to-film.
   - Iliac arteries (calcified)
   - Aorta (calcified)
   - Splenic artery (the Chinese dragon sign): Serpiginous parallel - walled calcification
   - Curving osteophytes in osteoarthritic spine
   - Fecolith (seen in 14% of patients with acute appendicitis)

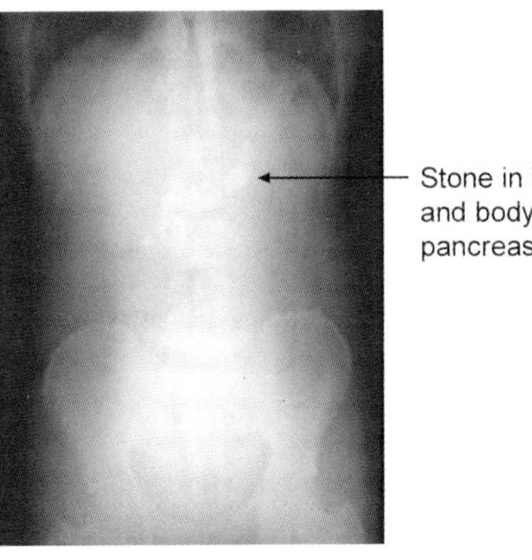

Plain skiagram abdomen

2. Abnormal calcification
   - Renal stones (85% are radiopaque)
   - Ureteric stones
   - Urinary bladder stones
   - Gallstones (only 15% are radiopaque)
   - Pancreatic stones
   - Fracture transverse process of the vertebrae.

Q 3. Why do you suspect pancreatic stones?

The stones are located at the upper lumbar spine passing upwards obliquely to the left towards the splenic hilum.

Q 4. How will you differentiate renal stones from gallstones?

This can be confirmed by taking a lateral view of the abdomen. If the stone is superimposed on the vertebrae it may be a renal stone. If it is in front of the vertebrae it may be gallstones.

Q 5. What are the conditions which will produce calcification of the pancreas?

1. Tropical chronic pancreatitis (seen in Kerala State of South India)
2. Chronic pancreatitis
3. Cystic fibrosis.

Q 6. What is the etiology of tropical chronic pancreatitis?

Etiology is unknown (alcohol ingestion do not play a part): The following factors are attributed

- Malnutrition
- Dietary
- Familial
- Genetic
- Cassava ingestion (high content of cyanide).

Q 7. What are the pathological changes?

1. Dilatation of pancreatic duct with large intraductal stones along the pancreatic duct
2. Fibrosis of the pancreas
3. High incidence of pancreatic cancer is seen.

Q 8. What are the diagnostic points of tropical pancreatitis?

1. Young patient below the age of 40 with type I diabetes having symptoms of diabetes, abdominal pain, steatorrhea and malnutrition
2. The patient looks ill and emaciated
3. Serum amylase is normal
4. Plain X-ray abdomen will show pancreatic calcification.

Q 9. What is the treatment of tropical chronic pancreatitis?

Medical treatment:

- Pancreatic enzymes
- Insulin therapy for diabetes
- Management of pain as per analgesic ladder.

Endoscopic management:

1. Small head stones can be managed by endoscopic extraction at ERCP
2. If pancreatic duct stricture is predominant with upstream dilatation, a stent can be inserted.

Surgical treatment: Done only for intractable pain

- The operations are:
  1. Extraction of pancreatic duct stones followed by longitudinal pancreatojejunostomy (**Frey procedure**)
  2. **Beger procedure** (Head coring): Duodenum preserving resection of the pancreatic head
  3. If mass lesion is there at the head of pancreas, a pancreaticoduodenectomy is done
  4. If the disease is limited to the tail of the pancreas, a distal pancreatectomy is done
  5. Intractable pain with diffuse disease: Total pancreatectomy.

8 – Gallstone

Q 1. What is your observation?

Plain radiograph of abdomen showing a radiopaque stone in the region of the gallbladder, suggestive of gallstone.

The second picture is a barium enema taken to rule out diverticulosis of the colon because of the patient's left lower abdominal complaints. There is no evidence of diverticulosis in the picture (Normal study).

Q 2. What is Saint's triad?

The association of gallstones, hiatus hernia and diverticulosis.

Q 3. How it is differentiated from renal stones?

Answer given Skiagram No:7.

Q 4. How many percentage of the gallstones are radiopaque?

10% (90% are nonradiopaque in contrast to renal stones (85% radiopaque).

Q 5. What are the types of gallstones?

1. Cholesterol stones

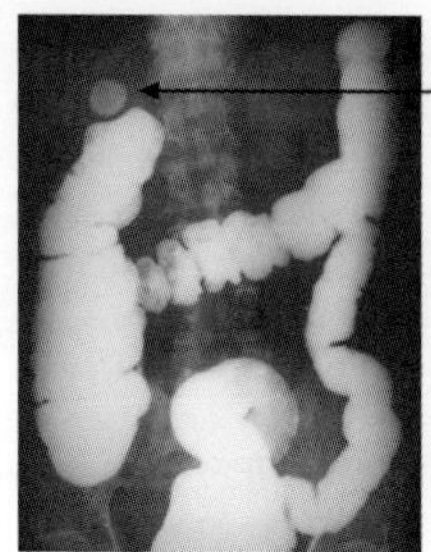
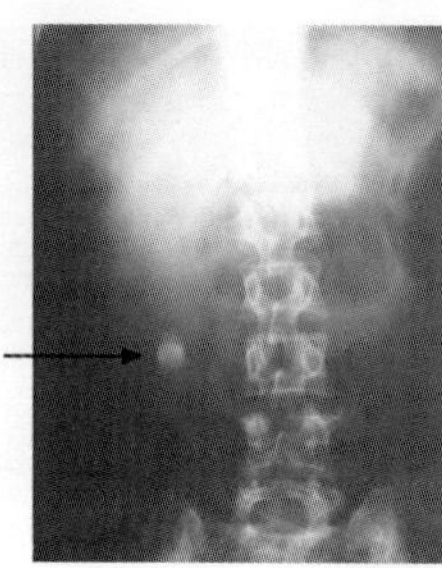

Gallstone in plain radiograph and barium enema

2. Pigment stones (**brown or black**): contain < 30% cholesterol.
   - **Black stones** are composed of insoluble bilirubin pigment mixed with calcium phosphate and calcium bicarbonate. The incidence rises with age. They are also seen in **hemolytic conditions** like hereditary spherocytosis and sickle cell disease. Therefore it is important to do a **peripheral smear** examination and **fragility test** if pigment stone is suspected. In hereditary spherocytosis in addition to cholecystectomy a **splenectomy** has to be done.
   - **Brown pigment stones:** Contain cholesterol and calcium bilirubinate, calcium palmitate and calcium stearate. They are usually seen in bile duct and related to infected bile as a result of deconjugation of bilirubin diglucuronide by bacterial beta glucuronidase. It is also associated with presence of foreign bodies and parasites.
3. Mixed stones (pure cholesterol + a mixture of calcium salts, bile acids, bile pigments and phospholipids

Note: In the West 80% are cholesterol and mixed stones.

In Asia 80% are pigment stones.

Q 6. What is Mercedes – Benz or Seagull sign?

The center of a stone may contain radiolucent gas in a triradiate or biradiate fissure giving characteristic dark shapes in radiograph. This is called Mercedes Benz sign.

Q 7. What is "porcelain" gallbladder, what is the importance of it?

Calcification of the gallbladder in plain X-ray is called porcelain gallbladder. The importance of this appearance is an association of **carcinoma in up to 25% of patients.**

Q 8. What are the complications of gall-stones?

Complications of gallstones

- Biliary colic
- Acute cholecystitis:
  Empyema of gallbladder
  Gangrene of gallbladder
  Perforation of gallbladder with peritonitis
  Mucocele of gallbladder
- Chronic cholecystitis
- Bile duct stone – obstructive jaundice
- Cholangitis – secondary to bile duct obstruction (**Charcot's triad** consisting of intermittent fever, intermittent pain and intermittent jaundice).
- Acute toxic cholangitis (**Reynold's pentad** consisting of Charcot's triad + mental obtundation + hypotension)
- Acute pancreatitis (Gallstone pancreatitis)
- Gallstone ileus (stone obstructing the bowel usually the terminal ileum)
- Gallbladder carcinoma (0.08% of symptomatic patients)

Q 9. What are the etiological factors for gall stone formation?

1. Supersaturation of bile by cholesterol or decrease in bile acid concentration and unstable unilamelar phospholipid vesicles
2. Nucleating factors: **Infection** (klebsiella, *E-coli*, Enterococci, Bacteroides and typhoid organism), mucus and glycoprotein
3. Stasis (Impaired gallbladder function): Repeated pregnancy
4. Enterohepatic circulation is not taking place. For example, Ileal resection, Cholestyramine.

Q 10. What is Moynihan's aphorism?

"Gallstone is the tomb stone erected to the memory of the organism within it" This statement was given with respect to gallstones having salmonella organism inside leading to **typhoid gallbladder**. *Salmonella typhimurium* can infect the gallbladder and produce chronic cholecystitis or acute cholecystitis and the patient will remain a typhoid carrier by excreting bacteria in the bile ("**Typhoid Mary**", a cook general who passed *salmonella typhi in* her feces and urine and was responsible for nearly twenty epidemics of typhoid in and around New York city in USA). Surgeons should not give patients their stones after surgery if there is any suspicion of typhoid.

Q 11. What is the incidence of gallstone?

10-15% of the adult population.

Q 12. What is the incidence of asymptomatic gallstone developing future symptoms?

1-2% will develop symptoms per year.

Q 13. What is the treatment of symptomatic gallstones?

Laparoscopic cholecystectomy.

Q 14. Why stone dissolution is not recommended in gallstones?

It is not recommended because of two reasons:

1. Dissolution by ESWL will result in fragmentation of the stones. They come down and produce obstructive jaundice.

2. Removing gallstones without removal of the gallbladder will lead to gallstone recurrence.

Q 15. What is the treatment of asymptomatic gallstones?

- Observation is enough
- Cholecystectomy is indicated in the following situations:
  1. Diabetic patients – chance for infection and complication
  2. Hemolytic anemias
  3. Patients undergoing Bariatric surgery for morbid obesity
  4. Calcified gallbladder wall (Porcelain gallbladder).

Q 16. What is the timing of surgery for acute cholecystitis?

1. Early laparoscopic cholecystectomy (preferred) during the golden period (72hours): The open conversion rate of laparoscopic cholecystectomy is five times higher than in the elective setting
2. Elective surgery after a period of conservative treatment for 6 weeks.

9 – Fracture of Ribs, Flail Chest

Q 1. What is your observation?

Skiagram chest showing multiple fracture ribs shown with arrows.

Q 2. What are the clinical signs of fracture rib?

- Crepitus
- Deformity
- Limitation of chest wall movement.

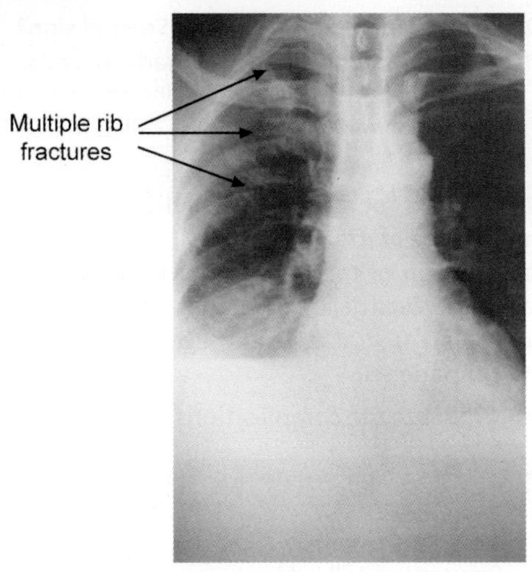

Skiagram chest

Q 3. What are the consequences of fracture rib?

- Atelectasis
- Sputum retention
- Hypoxia
- Hypercapnia.

Q 4. What are the complications of fracture ribs?

1. Intractable pain
2. Pneumothorax, tension pneumothorax
3. Hemothorax
4. Hemopneumothorax
5. Flail chest and stove in chest.

Q 5. What is flail chest?

When **three or more ribs** are fractured in **two or more places**, flail chest will occur. The diagnosis is made clinically not radiologically by observing

paradoxical movement of the chest wall at the fractured area. The affected segment of chest wall is displaced inwards on inspiration and outwards on expiration and **less air therefore moves into the lung.**

Q 6. What is stove in chest?

When there is a local indentation without any paradoxical movement as a result of multiple fractures, it is called stove in chest.

Q 7. What is the consequence of flail chest?

As a result of impaired chest wall movements, less air is entering the lung. In addition there may be voluntary splinting of the chest wall due to pain. The patient may go into **hypoxia** (in addition there may be associated lung contusion).

Q 8. What is the first aid treatment of flail chest?

Turn the patient to the side of the paradoxical movement so that this movement is prevented.

Q 9. What is the treatment of flail chest?

The treatment consists of the following:

1. Oxygen administration
2. Analgesia
3. Tube thoracostomy if required
4. Mechanical ventilation in selected cases (**PEEP**) developing respiratory failure
5. Physiotherapy.

Q 10. What is the mechanism of action of mechanical ventilation?

It is nothing but **internal splinting** of the chest until fibrous union of the broken ribs occur.

Q 11. Is there any role for operative fixation of the segment?

May be used in selected cases.

Q 12. Is there any role for strapping of fractured ribs?

No. Any sort of the splinting the chest wall will result in impaired chest wall movement and less of oxygenation.

Q 13. What is the treatment of pain of fracture ribs?

1. Analgesic (NSAIDs)
2. Intercostal nerve block by injection of local anesthetics
3. Intrapleural local analgesia if chest tube is there
4. Epidural analgesia for multiple fracture ribs with intractable pain.

Q 14. What is the significance of fracture of the first rib?

10% of fracture of the first rib are associated with **major vascular and brachial plexus injury.**

10 – Pneumothorax

Q 1. What is your observation?

Skiagram chest showing pneumothorax right side with collapsed lung border.

Q 2. What are the clinical features of pneumothorax?

- Decreased air entry on the affected sides
- Hyperresonance on percussion over the affected chest.

Q 3. What is the skiagram of choice in chest trauma?

A standard erect chest X-ray PA view and lateral view.

Q 4. What is the problem of AP supine film?

It causes apparent mediastinal widening and obscure hemothorax.

Q 5. What is the skiagram of choice in pneumothorax?

Erect expiratory chest X-ray.

Q 6. Is there any role for repeat X-ray if the initial chest X-ray appears normal?

In 10% of cases the initial chest X-ray appears normal and the pneumothorax becomes apparent over the first 8 hours and there after it should be repeated.

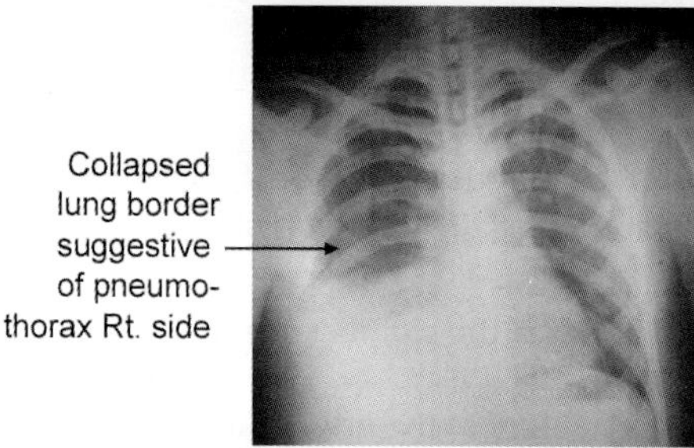

Skiagram chest

Q 7. What is the difference between simple pneumothorax and tension pneumothorax?

A pneumothorax with **mediastinal displacement** to the opposite side is called tension pneumothorax. This is manifested by **tracheal shift** to the opposite side and shift of the **apex beat**. The air is forced into the thoracic cavity without any means of escape by a **one way valve** either from the lung or through the chest wall. As a result of tension, the lung will be completely collapsed and the opposite lung will be compressed because of the mediastinal shift. This will result in decrease in the venous return.

	Simple pneumothorax	*Tension pneumothorax*
Tracheal position	Normal	Displaced
Percussion note	Normal	Increased (hyperresonant)
Jugular pressure	Normal	Elevated (unless hypovolemic)
Breath sounds	Normal (unless large)	Decreased
Respiratory distress	Variable	Severe

Q 8. What are the causes for tension pneumothorax?

1. Penetrating chest injury
2. Blunt chest injury with lung injury
3. Primary spontaneous pneumothorax
4. Secondary pneumothorax – diseases of lung (tuberculosis, cavitating lung disease)
   - necrosing tumors
   - diseases of plurae
5. Iatrogenic lung injury due to **central venous cannulation**
6. Mechanical ventilation.

Q 9. What are the clinical features of tension pneumothorax?

Clinical features of tension pneumothorax
• Acute dyspnea
• **Distended neck veins**
• Weak pulse
• Low blood pressure
• Tracheal shift
• Shifting of the apex beat
• Hyperresonance on the affected hemithorax
• Absent breath sounds on the same side

Q 10. Mention another condition where there is elevated JVP as a result of chest trauma?

Cardiac tamponade: Cardiac injury resulting in hemopericardium which may seal temporarily the bleeding from the cardiac injury.

Q 11. What is the diagnostic triad for cardiac tamponade?

Beck's triad: Elevated JVP, diminished heart sounds (Muffled) and pulse paradox (15mm of Hg fall on inspiration).

Q 12. How to confirm tension pneumothorax?

It is a clinical diagnosis and treatment must be instituted urgently without wasting time for radiology.

Q 13. What are the radiological findings of tension pneumothorax?

Radiological findings of tension pneumothorax

- The lung is completely collapsed (the collapsed lung margin can be seen, the rest of the chest cavity showing only air without any lung markings)
- The mediastinum is pushed to the opposite side
- The diaphragm is flattened and pushed down
- The spaces between the ribs are widened on the affected side (spreading of the ribs)

Q 14. What is the treatment of tension pneumothorax?

- Urgent needle thoracostomy by inserting a large bore needle into the **second intercostal space** in the midclavicular line
- This is followed by tube thoracostomy in the safe **triangle** which is connected to an underwater seal.

Q 15. Is there any role for conservative management of small traumatic pneumothorax?

- All traumatic pneumothoraces are drained to prevent tension pneumothorax
- This will encourage early lung expansion and evacuate any hemothorax
- Without drainage half of all pneumothoraces will increase over the first 24 hours.

Q 16. What is sucking wound?

It is **nothing but open pneumothorax** as a result of open defect in the chest of more than 3cm. This will lead on to hypoventilation or hypoxia.

Q 17. What is the treatment of sucking wound?

1. Closing the defect with **sterile occlusive dressing sealed on three sides** so that the air will escape but preventing the air entry
2. Tube thoracostomy
3. Formal closure of the defect may be required.

Q 18. If there is failure to expand the lung with effective drainage, how one should proceed?

This is an indication for bronchoscopy (and often thoracotomy).

11 – Surgical Emphysema

Q 1. What is your observation?

Skiagram chest showing air spaces in the subcutaneous tissue suggestive of surgical emphysema (**Subcutaneous emphysema**).

Q 2. What is surgical emphysema?

- It is the presence of air in the tissues
- It requires a breach of air containing viscus which is in communication with soft tissues and the **generation of positive pressure** to push the air along tissue planes.

Q 3. What is the physical sign of surgical emphysema?

Crepitus (a peculiar crackling sensation imparted to the examining fingers when one places the fingers fan wise on the affected area and exerts light pressure).

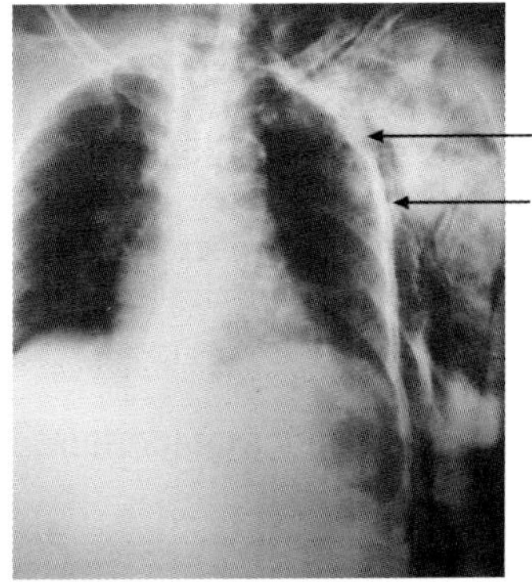

Skiagram chest

Q 4. What is the cause for crepitus?

Presence of gas in the subcutaneous tissue

Q 5. What are the causes for surgical emphysema?

Causes for subcutaneous emphysema

1. **Traumatic**: Fracture of the ribs – emphysema may extend from the ankle of the jaw to the scrotum
   Lung injury
   Bronchial injury
   Fracture of the nasal fossa
   Laryngeal injury
   Tracheostomy
   Fracture skull involving the frontal sinus
2. **Infective**: Gas gangrene
3. **Extraneous**: A poorly managed chest drain with build up of pressure
   Extravasation of fluids
   Effusion of blood
   Entrapped air during closure of surgical wound
4. **Subcutaneous emphysema complicating rupture of the esophagus** (most serious). It will also produce **mediastinal surgical emphysema**

Q 6. What is the probable cause in this case?

Lung injury, secondary to fracture ribs.

Q 7. What is the treatment of surgical emphysema?

a. If there is no respiratory distress and no pneumothorax then no treatment is required
b. If there is respiratory distress tube thoracostomy is done
c. If there is no improvement, suspect bronchial injury for which thoracotomy and closure of the bronchial injury may be required.

12 – Hemopneumothorax, Tube Thoracostomy, Safe Triangle

Q 1. What is your observation?

Skiagram chest showing hemopneumothorax with tube thoracostomy in position.

Q 2. What are the causes for hemopneumothorax?

1. Blunt chest trauma
2. Penetrating chest injury
3. Fracture ribs
4. Aspiration of hemothorax.

Q 3. What are the radiological signs of hemopneumothorax?

1. Obliteration of costophrenic angle
2. Fluid level with air shadow above
3. Collapsed lung border.

Q 4. What are the clinical features of hemothorax?

Tracheal position	–	Displaced
Percussion note	–	Decreased (dull)
Breath sounds	–	Decreased
Respiratory distress	–	Variable

Q 5. What is the minimum blood required for blunting of the costophrenic angle?

- **250-400 ml** in erect film (in supine film it is not apparent with < 1000 ml)
- In lateral decubitus film opacification is more obvious.

Q 6. What is the source of bleeding in hemothorax?

It may be from the following sites:

1. Bleeding from intercostal vessel

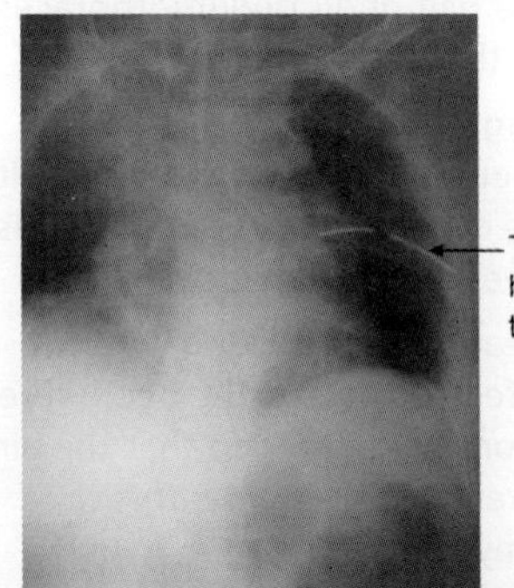

Skiagram chest

2. Bleeding from internal mammary artery
3. Bleeding from the lung.

Q 7. What is massive hemothorax?

If the **initial drainage** from the chest is more than **1500 ml** of blood or ongoing hemorrhage of more than **200 ml/hr** over 3-4 hours.

Q 8. What are the indications for thoracotomy?

Thoracotomy is required only in 10% of major injuries. The important indications are:

Indications for thoracotomy in chest trauma
1. If the **initial drainage** from the chest is more than **1500 ml** of blood or ongoing hemorrhage of more than **200 ml/hr** over 3-4 hours
2. Great vessel injury
3. Tracheobronchial rupture
4. Persistent air leak
5. Cardiac injury
6. Esophageal injury
7. Diaphragmatic injury

Q 9. What is the management of hemothorax and hemopneumothorax?

Tube thoracostomy.

Q 10. What is the safest site for insertion of chest tube?

Safe triangle.

Q 11. What are the boundaries of safe triangle?

The safe triangle bounded by:

- 5th rib below
- Posteriorly by the midaxillary line
- Anterior axillary line anteriorly (lateral to the pectoralis major muscle).

Q 12. What is the importance of this triangle?

Why safe triangle is selected
• It is important to remember that the abdominal cavity is extending upto the nipple level
• Any insertion of tube below the 5th rib is likely to enter the abdominal cavity and consequent injury to the viscera
• The thickness of the **chest wall** in this triangle is thin and constituted only by the intercostal muscles (inner and outer) and no other muscle is coming in the triangle. Therefore it is easier to insert the chest tube here
• The **interspace** is large here
• **No impairment** of accessory respiratory muscles
• Away from mediastinal structures and internal mammary artery
• Since the position of the tube is anterior, in the supine position the tube will not kink.

Q 13. What is the ideal direction of the chest tube for the purpose of draining hemopneumothorax?

- The tube should go posteriorly and upwards towards the apex of the lung **(apex for air, posteriorly for blood)**
- A drain for pleural effusion and empyema should be nearer the base.

Q 14. How will you prevent neurovascular injury during chest tube insertion?

The tube should pass over the **upper edge of the rib** to avoid neurovascular bundle.

Q 15. What are the important steps of tube thoracostomy?

1. Take sterile precautions and paint the selected area of the chest wall with antiseptics (centering the safe triangle).

2. Infiltrate local anesthesia at the site including the pleura
3. Make and skin incision in the intercostal space for about 2.5 cms
4. Blunt dissection is carried out through the intercostal muscles
5. An oblique tract is made **(the skin incision is made one interspace lower)** so as to enter the pleural cavity
6. The gloved finger is introduced into the pleural cavity and the pleural adhesions are separated
7. Sterile chest tube is introduced with the help of an artery forces in an upward and medial direction
8. See that all the side holes are inside the chest cavity
9. The tube is fixed in position with a retaining stitch and see that the retaining stitch is not obliterating the tube
10. The tube is connected to under water seal of the chest drain bottle
11. The wound is sealed
12. Take chest radiograph and see that the chest tube is in position.

Q 16. What is the daily postoperative care of the tube?

- See that the air column in the tube is moving (means, the tube is in the chest cavity. If the column is not moving, the tube is occluded or it is not in the chest cavity).
- Look for air bubbling-suggestive of air escape from the pleural cavity if there is pneumothorax.
- See that the lower end of the chest tube is below the under water seal of the draining bottle.
- Measure the total drainage of blood in the draining bottle (whenever the bottle is full, it should be emptied after clamping the chest tube).
- See that all the side holes of the chest tube are inside the chest cavity- (there should not be any air leak at the tube chest wall junction).
- Check for air entry on the side by auscultation
- Take check X-ray of the chest to look for expansion of the lungs and clearance of the costophrenic angle.

Q 17. Is there any role for applying suction to the chest drain?

No:

Q 18. When to remove the chest tube?

Indications for removal of the chest tube

- Remove the drain when it is no longer draining
- The drain should be removed when there has been no air leak for 24 hours with a fully expanded lung
- If the patient is ventilated the drain should be left until after extubation or there has been no air leak for five days

Q 19. What are the causes for failure to expand the lung?

1. Inadequate drain size
2. Position of the drain not reaching the apex
3. Kinking of the tube
4. Excessive air leak

Q 20. What are the complications of tube thoracostomy?

1. Infection – empyema
2. Danger of disconnection of the tube and siphoning of air.

Q 21. What are the radiological findings of rupture of the diaphragm?

Traumatic rupture is **commonly seen on left side**. The radiological findings are:

1. Stomach containing fluid level within the left hemithorax (the fluid level in stomach will not be completely across the hemithorax unlike hemopneumothirax)
2. Compressed lung lying above and medial to the top of the intrathoracic stomach
3. Gas shadows of intrathoracic colon if the escaping viscera is colon
4. Lateral view showing double fluid level if there is intrathoracic gastric volvulus.

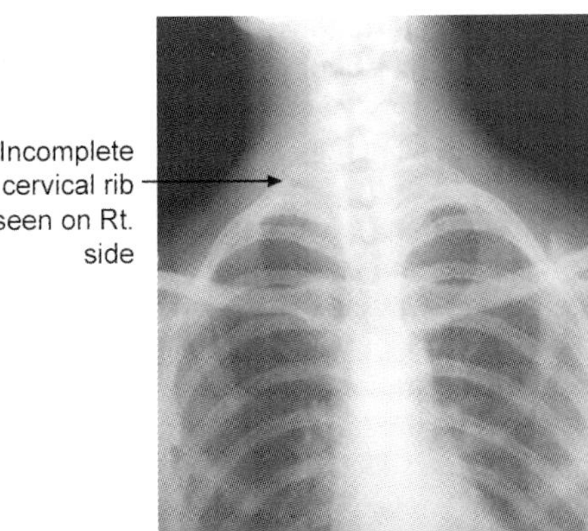

Skiagram neck

13 – Cervical Rib, Thoracic Outlet Syndrome

Q 1. What is your observation?

Skiagram neck showing **incomplete cervical rib** on right side.

Q 2. What is cervical rib?

It is an extension of costal element of transverse process of C_7 vertebra.

Q 3. What are the types of cervical rib?

1. Complete fibrous band (commonest type) from the transverse process and reaching anteriorly over the first rib or manubrium. It is not demonstrated radiologically
2. Complete bony type (radiopaque)
3. Partly bony and partly fibrous
4. Partly bony: With free end of the rib expanding as a bony mass.

Q 4. What are the various clinical syndromes associated with cervical rib?

- Cervical rib syndrome
- Thoracic outlet syndrome
- Thoracic inlet syndrome
- Scalenus anticus syndrome.

Q 5. What are the clinical features of cervical rib?

It can be classified as:

1. **Neurological symptoms**: As a result of compression of the lower trunk of the brachial plexus (C_8 and T_1) mainly T_1 resulting in **wasting of the interossei** and numbness and tingling of the little finger and medial side of the hand and forearm.

2. **Vascular manifestations**: The cervical rib causes angulation of the subclavian artery producing constriction at the level of the rib followed by a **poststenotic dilatation**, which may also produce a **thrombus** inside and **embolus** formation. It will finally produce features of ischemia in the hand and forearm and **digital gangrene**. It will also produce wasting of thenar, hypothenar and forearm muscles.
3. **Local manifestations**:
   Bony mass in the supraclavicular fossa Palpable thrill over the subclavian artery Bruit over the subclavian artery.

Q 6. What are the differential diagnoses of the above symptoms?

1. Carpal tunnel syndrome
2. Cervical disk disease.

Q 7. What is scalene triangle and what is the pathology of cervical rib?

This scalene triangle is bounded by:

Scalenus anterior	–	anteriorly
Scalenus medius	–	posteriorly
First rib	–	below

Etiopathology of cervical rib

- The subclavian artery and lower trunk of the brachial plexus crosses the first rib in the scalene triangle.
- The presence of cervical rib compress the subclavian artery and lower trunk of brachial plexus more on T1 area.
- As a result of constriction at the site of the cervical rib, the artery distally dilates (poststenotic dilatation) which may contain thrombus which leads to embolus. The vascular manifestations are as a result of the pressure from the cervical rib.
- The neurological manifestations are as a result of pressure on the lower trunk.

Q 8. What are the upper limb positions which will precipitate the symptoms of cervical rib?

1. Prolonged hyperabduction of the upper limb. For example Painters, hair dressers and truck drivers
2. Carrying heavy weight in the shoulder can also precipitate the symptoms.

Q 9. How to radiologically differentiate first rib from cervical rib?

The transverse process of the first thoracic vertebra has obliquity upwards whereas the transverse process of C7 vertebra has obliquity downwards. If a radiologically demonstrable rib arises from the latter (transverse process with obliquity downwards), then it is cervical rib.

Q 10. What are the other investigations required other than skiagram of neck and chest?

- Nerve conduction studies
- Color Doppler for vascular assessment
- Arteriogram if required (If there is a post-stenotic dilatation it is suggestive of cervical rib).

Q 11. What are the clinical tests for cervical rib?

1. Adson's test
2. Elevated Arm Stress Test (EAST)
3. Roos test
4. Tinel test.

Q 12. How Adson's test is carried out?

The patient sits and the examiner feels the radial pulse of the patient. Now the patient is instructed to take a deep breath. He holds it and turns his chin up and to the affected side. A diminution or obliteration of the radial pulse indicates the presence of scalenus anticus syndrome.

Q 13. What is Elevated Arm Stress Test?

Arm is elevated above the shoulder with the elbow stretched fully. Now ask the patient to move the fingers rapidly. Patient will feel fatigue on the affected side if cervical rib is present.

Q 14. What is Roos test?

Ask the patient to raise the arm above the shoulder. On the affected side the patient cannot hold the arm in that position and drops the hand down.

Q 15. What is Tinel test?

Light percussion over the brachial plexus in the supraclavicular fossa produces peripheral sensations and reproduces the symptoms of neurological impingement.

Q 16. What is the treatment of cervical rib?

The cervical rib may be **symptomatic or asymptomatic** (may be **unilateral or bilateral**). Asymptomatic cases are left alone. Symptomatic cases can be managed conservatively or surgically.

A. **Conservative treatment** for a period of 3-6months consisting of:
   Physiotherapy
   Postural correction.
B. **Surgery** if there is no response with conservative treatment:
   - **Resection of the first rib** which may be done either by a **supraclavicular approach** or by a transaxillary approach. It will widen the thoracoaxillary channel.
   - Anterior scalene muscle must be divided in all the procedures
   - Excise the associated fibrous band
   - Arterial stenosis may need arterial reconstruction in some cases
   - If there is associated thrombosis of subclavian vein manifested in the form of unilateral arm swelling, catheter— directed thrombolysis is carried out.

14 – Intravenous urogram, Renal and Ureteric Stones, Nonvisualization of Kidney

Q 1. What is your observation?

Intravenous Urogram (IVU or IVP – IVU is a better terminology than pyelogram) showing ureteric stone on left side with hydroureter.

Q 2. How intravenous urogram is carried out?

It is carried out by intravenous injection into a vein in the antecubital fossa of **iodine containing dye** like sodium diatrizoate (**urografin**) or meglumide (about **20 ml** of the dye). It is filtered from the blood by the glomeruli and does not undergo tubular absorption and rapidly passes through the urine.

Q 3. What is the preparation for IVU?

1. Bowel preparation in the form of laxatives on each of the two preceding nights and charcoal tablets for 48hours for absorption of gas
2. **Nothing to drink for 8 hours** before the examination (fluid restriction is contra indicated in patients who are in renal failure or myelomatosis and in infants. Dehydration is dangerous).
3. The investigation is done with an empty stomach in the morning
4. The patient is asked to void immediately before the examination
5. Diuretics are not given prior to the examination (the dye as such has got diuretic effect).

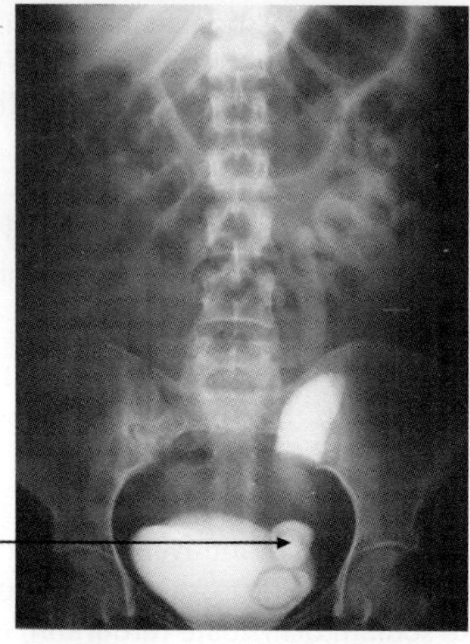

Intravenous urogram

Q 4. What are the contraindications for IVU?

The contraindications are:

1. Those who are **allergic to iodine, patients with atopy and eczema**
2. If the blood urea is **more than 60 ml**/100 ml
3. Impaired renal function
4. Anuria
5. Infants
6. Pregnant women.

Q 5. What are the types of urogram?

1. Intravenous urogram
2. Retrograde pyelography (the contrast is injected through ureteric catheter after cystoscopy
3. Antegrade pyelography (the contrast is injected to the pelvis).

Q 6. How many films are taken?

1. **Scout film** (the plain X-ray abdomen taken before injection of the dye).
2. **Nephrogram** picture at 2 minutes, when the dye is being filtered by the glomerulus – shows the renal parenchyma opacified by contrast medium. A delayed nephrogram on one side indicates functional impairment.
3. **Serial films** thereafter at **5, 10, 15, 20 and 30 minutes** after the injection of the dye (the contrast is **excreted into the collecting system** opacifying the renal pelvis and calyces).
4. Another film at 1 hour followed by another at 2 hours.
5. The patient is asked to void urine and a post micturition film is taken to show the **details of the bladder area**.
6. If there is poor functioning of kidney, films are taken after 8-hours.

Q 7. What are the indications for IVU?

With the introduction of CT scan the indications are becoming less and less.

The indications are:

1. To demonstrate **stones** within the urinary tract which are not visualized in ultrasonography.
2. To demonstrate **tumors** which will distort the pelvicalyceal system.
3. Hydronephrosis.
4. To show details of **abnormal anatomy** (horse - shoe kidney, bifid pelvis, bifid ureter and ectopic kidney).
5. In cases for **trauma** for extravasation of the dye and nonvisualization of the kidney.
6. To demonstrate tumor infiltration from elsewhere of the kidney, ureter and bladder areas.

Q 8. If pelvicalyceal system on one side is not visualized what is the inference?

- That side the kidney is not functioning.

- If there is delay of appearance of the dye on one side the inference is there is poor functioning on that side.

Q 9. What are the causes for nonvisualization of the kidney?

When 90-95% of the parenchymal function is lost the kidneys are nonvisualized. In such cases radioisotope study using DTPA labelled with technetium 99m can be used.

1. Gross hydronephrosis with no function
2. Tumors
3. Trauma
4. Tuberculosis
5. Congenital absence of one kidney.

Q 10. Can you visualize the entire length of ureter in a single film?

No. Because of the ureteric peristalsis, the entire ureter may not be visualized (The entire ureter is visualized only when the ureter is diseased as in the case of tuberculosis).

Q 11. What are the changes of hydronephrosis in IVU?

Calyceal changes: Normally the calyces are cup-shaped. In hydronephrosis the following changes are seen.

- Loss of cupping
- Flattening and
- Clubbing of the calyces.

Q 12. What is the appearance of the pelvi- calyceal system in tumor?

Spider leg deformity of the pelvicalyceal system (distortion).

Q 13. What is double dose IVU?

When 2 ampoules (40ml) of the dye is used for delineation of the nonfunctioning side, it is called double dose IVU.

Q 14. What is infusion pyelogram?

When six ampoules (120ml) are put in a bottle and given as infusion, it is called infusion pyelogram.

Q 15. How many percentage of the renal stones are radiopaque?

85-90%. Owing to the calcium content.

Q 16. What is staghorn calculus?

It is a calculus filling the entire pelvicalyceal system consisting of **triple phosphate** or struvite (calcium, ammonium and magnesium phosphate). It is smooth and dirty white in color, seen to grow in **alkaline urine** in the presence of **urea splitting proteus organism.** They are radiopaque.

Q 17. What are the types of renal stones?

1. Oxalate calculus
2. Phosphate (triple phosphate)
3. Uric acid and urate calculi
4. Cystine calculus
5. Xanthine calculus.

Q 18. What is the treatment of staghorn calculus?

1. PCNL (**P**ercutaneous **N**ephrolithotomy)
2. ESWL (**E**xtracorporeal **S**hock **W**ave **L**ithotripsy)
3. Silent Staghorn Calculus in the elderly is treated conservatively.

Q 19. Which side is operated first in cases of bilateral renal stones?

Kidney with better function is treated first unless the other kidney is more painful or infected.

Q 20. What is the treatment of ureteric stones?

1. Conservative: Calculi smaller than 0.5 cm pass spontaneously (larger stones, impacted stones and infection in the upper urinary tract are indications for intervention)

2. Ureteroscopic stone removal (URS): Ureteroscope is a long, thin **endoscope passed transurethrally** across the bladder into the ureter for removal of the **impacted stones.**
3. Push bang: Stone in the middle or upper part of the ureter is flushed back into the kidney using a ureteric catheter and treated with ESWL later.
4. Open surgery: Ureterolithotomy.

15 – Hydronephrosis

Q 1. What is your observation?

Intravenous urogram showing dilatation of the calyces and delayed excretion of dye on right side suggestive of **hydronephrosis**.

Q 2. What are the changes suggestive of hydronephrosis?

See Question 11 of Skiagram No:14.

Q 3. What is hydronephrosis?

Aseptic dilatation of pelvicalyceal system due to **partial or intermittent** obstruction. When there is infection it is called pyonephrosis. Complete and continuous obstruction may not produce hydronephrosis.

Q 4. What is Dietl's crisis?

It is nothing but intermittent hydronephrosis. The patient will present with loin mass and renal pain. After a few hours the pain is relieved and the **swelling disappears following the passage of large volume of urine.**

Q 5. What are the causes for hydronephrosis?

Hydronephrosis may be **unilateral or bilateral.** The most common cause for unilateral hydronephrosis are **idiopathic pelvi – ureteric junction obstruction and calculus.**

Causes for hydronephrosis	
Causes for unilateral hydronephrosis	*Causes for bilateral hydronephrosis*
Causes inside the lumen • Stones • Sloughed papillae **Causes in the wall** • Idiopathic pelviureteric junction obstruction • Ureterocele • Stricture of the ureter • Tumors of the ureter • Bladder cancer involving ureteric orifice **Causes outside the wall** • Carcinoma of the colon, cecum, rectum, uterus, prostate, etc. • Retroperitoneal sarcomas • Retroperitoneal fibrosis	**Congenital** • Posterior urethral valve • Urethral atresia **Physiological** • Pregnancy **Acquired** • Benign prostatic enlargement • Carcinoma of the prostate • Bladder neck obstruction • Urethral stricture • Phimosis

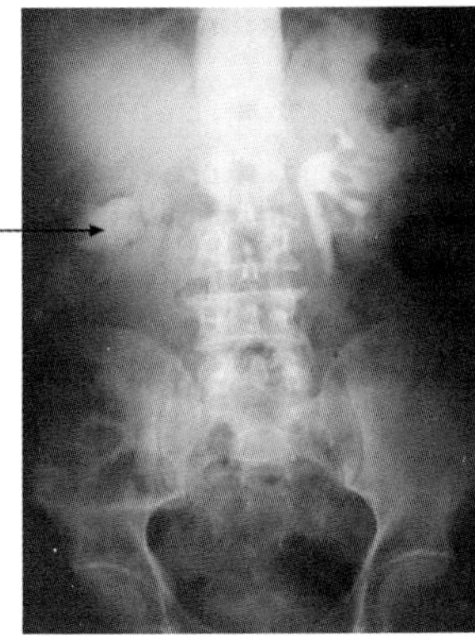

Intravenous urogram (IVV)

Q 6. What happens to the renal parenchyma in hydronephrosis?
The renal parenchyma is destroyed by pressure from the dilated calyceal system.

Q 7. What is Whitaker test?
Percutaneous puncture of the kidney through the loin and fluid infusion at constant rate with monitoring of intrapelvic pressure is the basis of this test. Abnormal rise in pressure is suggestive of obstruction.

Q 8. What are the indications for surgery?
- Increasing hydronephrosis
- Infection
- Pain
- Parenchymal damage.

Q 9. What is the surgical treatment of idiopathic pelvi – ureteric junction obstruction?
Anderson-Hynes pyeloplasty (provided reasonable functioning parenchyma remains). A 'V' segment is excised from the stenotic area and repair is done so that the narrowed area is widened. Another operation is V-Y plasty.

Q10. Is there any endoscopic procedure available?
Yes: Endoscopic pyelolysis by passing a balloon up the ureter and disrupting the pelvi ureteric junction.

Q 12. What is the role for nephrectomy?
The basic aim of the treatment is to conserve the kidney. Nephrectomy is done only when the renal parenchyma is grossly destroyed.

16 – Barium Swallow, Achalasia Cardia

Q 1. What is your observation?
a. Skiagram chest showing mediastinal widening
b. Barium swallow showing '**smooth pencil-shaped' narrowing** at the lower end of esophagus ("**bird's beak**" appearance).
   - **Widening of the mediastinum** is as a result of large fluid-filled esophagus (soft tissue shadow with air **fluid level just to the right of the atrium).**
   - The barium swallow shows smooth pencil-shaped narrowing distally with proximal dilatation of the esophagus. Being a benign condition of long duration there is enough time for proximal dilatation to occur in the esophagus in achalasia. The **narrowing in carcinoma is irregular** and described as 'rat tail appearance'. In carcinoma of the esophagus, the patient may not be alive in majority of cases by the time the esophagus dilates proximally.

The probable diagnosis in this case is achalasia cardia.

Q 2. What is achalasia?
The word meaning is 'a chalasia' (Greek): Failure to relax:

It is due to the loss of ganglion cells in the myenteric plexus (Auerbach's plexus).

Q 3. What are the etiological factors for achalasia?

- Chagas' disease: Destroys parasympathetic ganglion cells
- Infection: Herpes zoster of neurons
- Degenerative disease of the neurons.

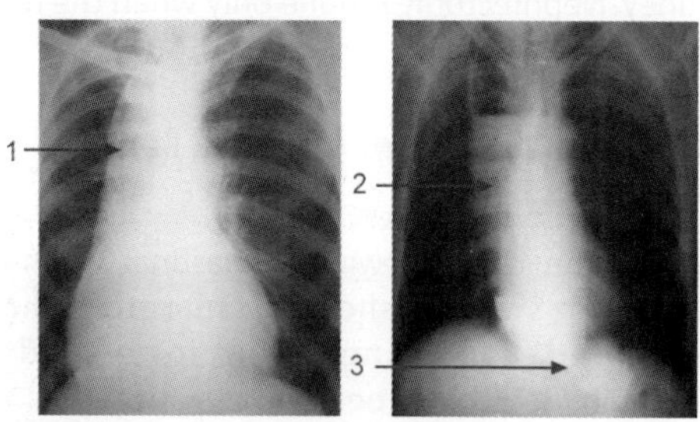

Dilated sigmoid esophgus presents as widening of the mediastinum which is demonstrated in barium swallow. Also shows smooth pencil shaped narrowing at the lower end of esophagus

Skiagram chest and barium swallow

Q 4. How it differs from Hirschsprung's disease?

In Hirschsprung's disease the dilated colon contains normal ganglion cells, whereas in achalasia there are no ganglion cells in the dilated segments.

Q 5. What are the physiological abnormalities in achalasia cardia?

They are:

- Loss of peristalsis in the body of the esophagus
- Nonrelaxation of the lower esophageal sphincter
- Dilatation and tortuosity of the lower esophagus – **mega esophagus** and **sigmoid appearance**
- Stasis of food and fluid – **retention esophagitis**
- The emptying of esophagus takes place by hydrostatic pressure of the content
- Absent fundal gas in the stomach.

Q 6. What are the clinical features of achalasia cardia?

- Pain (early stages)
- Dysphagia (**more for liquid than for solid in contrast to carcinoma**)
- Regurgitation of food (Recurrent pneumonia is seen)
- Aspiration at night.

Q 7. What is the endoscopic finding in achalasia cardia?

- Dilated tortuous esophagus
- Food residue and fluid in the esophagus
- Tight cardia
- Evidence of esophagitis.

Q 8. What is the confirmatory test for achalasia cardia?

Esophageal manometry: Raised resting pressure in the esophagus.

Q 9. What is pseudoachalasia?

- This is produced by adenocarcinoma and benign tumors of the esophagus
- Cancers outside of the esophagus, e.g. bronchus can also produce pseudoachalasia.

Q 10. What are the treatment options in achalasia cardia?

- Pneumatic dilatation
- Heller's myotomy
- Injection of botulinum toxin into the lower esophageal sphincter with temporary effect for a few months (has to be repeated)
- Drugs will give only transient relief
  Sublingual Nifedipine
  Calcium Channel Antagonists.

Q 11. What is pneumatic dilatation?

- The dilatation of the cardia was originally described by Plummer using **Plummer's hydrostatic bag**.

- This is now replaced by pneumatic dilatation using **plastic balloons** of sizes **30-40 mm** diameter which are introduced over a guide wire.
- Progressive dilatations are carried out over a period of weeks.
- Perforation is the most important complications.

Q 12. What is Heller's myotomy?

This can be carried out either by **open method or laparoscopic method**. In this procedure a **longitudinal incision is made** in the anterior aspect of the **lower esophagus and cardia** to divide the muscles of the narrow segment without injuring the mucosa so that the mucosa will pout.

Q 13. What is the most important complication of Heller's myotomy?

Gastroesophageal Reflux.

Most surgeons therefore perform a **partial anterior fundoplication.** This is called **Heller – Dor's** operation .

17 – Barium Swallow, Carcinoma of the Esophagus

Q 1. What is your observation?

Barium swallow picture showing narrowing at the lower end of the esophagus having the typical **'rat tail appearance'** suggestive of '**carcinoma of the lower end of esophagus**'.

Q 2. What are the pathological types of carcinoma of the esophagus?

- Squamous cell carcinoma – affects the upper two – thirds (most common type)
- Adenocarcinoma – affects the lower third.

Q 3. What are the etiological factors for carcinoma of the esophagus?

Etiological factors for carcinoma of the esophagus

- Tobacco
- Alcohol
- Fungal contamination of the food
- Nutritional deficiencies
- Barrett's esophagus
- GERD (Gastroesophageal reflux disease)
- Hot liquids
- Poor oral hygiene
- Achalasia
- Plummer-Vinson syndrome

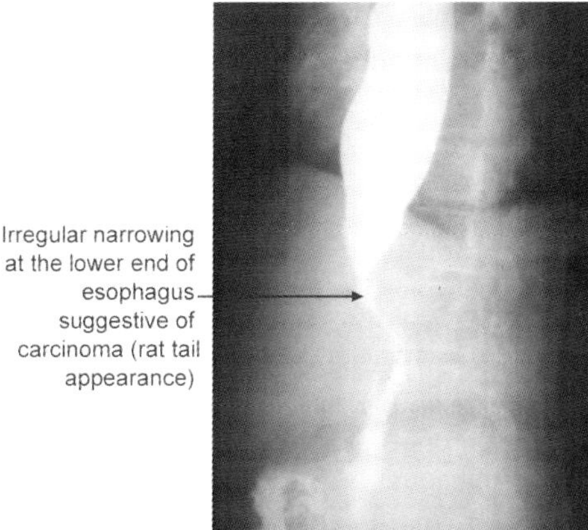

Barium swallow

Q 4. What are the clinical features of carcinoma of the esophagus?

Clinical features of carcinoma of the esophagus

- Dysphagia
- Regurgitation
- Vomiting
- Odynophagia
- Weight loss

Q 5. What are the clinical features suggestive of advanced malignancy?

Clinical features suggestive of advanced malignancy

- Enlarged supraclavicular lymph nodes
- Horner's syndrome
- Recurrent laryngeal nerve palsy (Hoarseness — Incurable disease)
- Diaphragmatic paralysis

Q 6. In which country you get the highest incidence of carcinoma of the esophagus?

Linxian in Henan Province **in China**.

Q 7. What are methods of spread of carcinoma of the esophagus?

- Longitudinal spread (via the submucosal lymphatics)
- Horizontal spread (laterally through the layers of esophagus)
- Lymphatic spread (**commonest—predominantly caudal spread**) Any node from superior mediastinum to the celiac axis may be involved
- Blood stream spread (liver, lungs, brain, bones)
- Transperitoneal – for the intraabdominal part of the esophagus.

Q 8. What is the significance of supraclavicular lymph nodes in carcinoma of the esophagus?

Supraclavicular lymph nodes are **suggestive of metastasis** (**M1**). So also celiac node involvement in distal esophageal tumor.

Q 9. What are the most important investigations in carcinoma of the esophagus?

1. Endoscopy and biopsy for confirmation of the diagnosis.

Staging investigations

2. **Endoscopic ultrasound** is the most important staging investigations—for depth of tumor, invasion of the adjacent organs and for metastasis to lymph nodes
3. **Chest radiography** for pulmonary metastasis
4. Liver function tests (**LFTs**)—Abnormal LFTs are suggestive of liver metastasis. Normal LFT does not rule out liver metastasis.
5. **Ultrasound abdomen**—to rule out liver metastasis.
6. **Bronchoscopy** (for middle and upper thirds).
7. **Laparoscopy**—for carcinoma arising from the abdominal esophagus-abdominal and hepatic metastasis
8. **Spiral CT**—for local spread and lymph node assessment (also for assessment of metastasis).
9. **MRI** – Magnetic Resonance Imaging
10. **PET** (**P**ositron **E**mission **T**omography) – combined with CT.

Q 10. What are the most important bad prognostic factors in carcinoma of the esophagus?

- Depth of tumor penetration
- Regional lymph node involvement.

Q 11. What is the management of carcinoma of the esophagus?

1. If the patient is **unfit for surgery** or metastasis or adjacent organ invasion or peritoneal spread—**palliation for dysphagia,** e.g. chemo radiotherapy and endoscopic palliation.
2. If fit for surgery and **there is no lymph node metastasis** – surgery alone (radical oesophagectomy).
3. If **lymph node metastasis** is present **multimodal therapy** – neoadjuvant treatment, chemo radiotherapy.
   - Radical esophagectomy for curative treatment with **10 cm clearance above** the macroscopic tumor and **5 cm distally.**

- Adenocarcinoma involving gastric cardia need some degree of gastric resection.

Q 12. How many percentage of the carcinoma of the esophagus are operable?

Above two-thirds of the tumors at the time of diagnosis are inoperable and only **one-third is operable**.

Q 13. What are the most important factors to be considered before deciding surgical option if it is operable?

1. General condition of the patient
2. Tumor location
3. Endoscopic appearance
4. Nodal status.

Q 14. What is the incision of choice for radical surgery?

- **For lower third growth: Left thoracoabdominal** incision for carcinoma of the lower end of the esophagus below the aortic arch (esophagogastrectomy – part of the upper stomach is removed followed by esophago gastric anastomosis).
- **For middle third growth:** If the tumour is above the level of aortic arch, the **two phase Ivor Lewis** operation along with two field **lymphadenectomy** (abdominal and mediastinal nodes) by an **initial laparotomy** for construction of a gastric tube followed by a **right thoracotomy** for resection of the tumor and esophagogastric anastomosis.
- **For upper third growth:** McKeown operation for carcinoma of the **upper thoracic esophagus:** It is a three phase operation with three field lymphadenectomy: Here a third incision is put in the neck for removal of the nodes there and creating the cervical anastomosis.

Q 15. What are the viscera used for inter- position as a substitute for esophagus?

They are placed in the substernal space and the following viscera are used.

- Stomach (commonly used)
- Jejunum
- Colon.

Q 16. What is the blood supply of the transposed stomach into the chest cavity?

Right gastroepiploic and right gastric vessels.

Q 17. What are the complications of surgical treatment?

Complications of surgical treatment
• Anastomotic leakage • Respiratory complications • Recurrent laryngeal nerve injury • Chylothorax • Reflux: It can be avoided by subtotal esophagectomy and making the esophagogastric anastomosis high up in the chest

Q 18. What is transhiatal esophagectomy?

- This was devised by **Orringer** for the removal of Chagasic mega esophagus
- This is a useful procedure for the lesions of the **lower esophagus, but dangerous for the middle third lesion**
- The stomach is mobilized through an abdominal incision
- The cervical esophagus is mobilized through a cervical incision
- The diaphragm is opened from the abdomen and the posterior mediastinum entered
- The tumor and lower esophagus are mobilized under vision

- The upper esophagus is mobilized by blunt dissection
- Total esophagectomy is done and esophago-jejunostomy is carried out in the neck.

Q 19. What is the role of neoadjuvant treatments?
Neoadjuvant therapy for **adenocarcinoma** is using platinum is based is chemotherapy.

Q 20. What is the role of chemoradiation?
It is indicated for squamous cell carcinoma of the esophagus in patients who are unfit for surgery.

Q 21. What is photodynamic therapy?
This is an endoscopic technique for treating **early esophageal cancer** and dysplasia of **Barrett's esophagus** for patients who are unfit **or unwilling for surgery.** Here a photozensitizer is administered which is taken up preferentially by dysplastic and malignant cells which is followed by exposure to laser light. The main disadvantages is skin photosensitization.

Q 22. What are the palliative procedures?

1. Intubation - Self-expanding metal stents (**SEMS**): They are inserted under radiographic or endoscopic control. This will produce wider lumen for swallowing than the old conventional rigid plastic and rubber tubes. The risk for injury to the esophagus is also less in this case.
2. Intubation with plastic and rubber tubes (Mousseau—Barbin tube—this requires laparotomy).
3. **Endoscopic laser**—It is useful for recanalization of the obstructed growth and also for canalizing occluded stent. It has to be repeated.
4. Bipolar **diathermy** endoscopically.
5. Argon - beam plasma **coagulation.**
6. Alcohol injection.
7. Brachytherapy: Intraluminal radiation is given by an introduction system.

Q 23. What are the terminal events of carcinoma esophagus?

- Tracheo-esophageal fistula
- Severe respiratory infection and sepsis
- Cancer cachexia
- Immunosuppression.

18 – Barium Meal, Carcinoma of the Stomach

Q 1. What is your observation?
This is a **barium meal picture** showing a **persistent** (for a lesion to be designated as persistent, the observer needs more than one film or watch the fluoroscopy) **irregular filling defect** in the antral region towards the greater curvature side suggestive of carcinoma of the stomach.

Q 2. What is the difference between barium meal and barium swallow?

- Both investigations are done by using **barium sulphate**
- Both are done under fluoroscopy
- Both are done on empty stomach
- In barium swallow a **thick solution of barium** sulphate is given to the patient for swallowing. This is mainly done for the study of esophagus and pharynx
- For barium **meal a dilute solution** of barium sulphate is used (**about 500 ml is given orally**)
- Microcrystallized barium sulphate solutions are available which gives better images
- When you take a sequential films of the small intestine after barium meal, it is called barium meal follow-through.

Q 3. Why barium sulphate is used?

- Barium is radiopaque and in sulphate form it is not absorbed
- Barium is stable in acidic medium
- **Barium phosphate is a poison** and therefore cannot be used.
- For identification of leaks and perforation water soluble contrast materials like **gastrograffin** may be used

Q 4. For delineation of the mucosa what technique is used?

Double contrast barium meal is done—by giving **effervescent tablets** along with barium. This will give the double contrast picture.

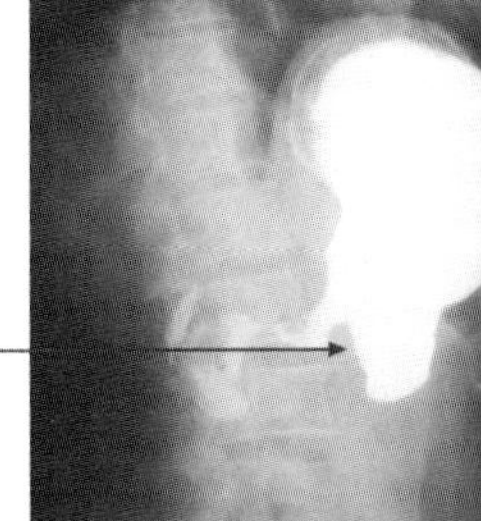

Barium meal

Q 5. What are the radiological signs of carcinoma stomach in barium meal?

- Persistent mucosal irregularity (early stages)
- Persistent loss of peristalsis in a particular segment
- Persistent irregular filling defect.

Q 6. What is the difference between benign and malignant ulcer in barium meal?

- In benign ulcer, the ulcer protrudes outside beyond the stomach margin and is seen in the lesser curvature usually.
- In benign ulcer radiating mucosal folds will be demonstrated towards the border of the ulcer.
- In benign ulcer, the ulcer is demonstrated as a **niche in the lesser curvature** and a **notch in the greater curvature**.
- The malignant ulcer will appear as though it is sitting inside the stomach and the mucosa surrounding the ulcer will not show mucosal folds.

Q 7. What are the disadvantages of barium meal examination?

- In barium meal examination we see the shadow of the lesion
- We are not directly visualizing the lesion
- Biopsy cannot be taken from the lesion
- It **cannot be used in perforation** since it can cause peritonitis.

Note: With the introduction of fiberoptic endoscopes, now-adays **upper GI endoscopy** and biopsy is the preferred investigation for carcinoma of the stomach.

Q 8. When such a lesion is identified in Barium meal what is the investigation of choice?

Upper GI endoscopy and biopsy.

Q 9. Is it an early lesion or an advanced lesion?

Advanced gastric carcinoma.

Q 10. What is the likely clinical presentation in this case?

Features of carcinoma stomach like:

- Loss of appetite

- Loss of weight
- Epigastric pain
- Epigastric mass

Since it is a big tumor occupying the antrum it is likely to produce **features of gastric outlet obstruction** like:

- Vomiting
- Visible gastric peristalsis
- Succussion splash
- Electrolyte abnormalities: **Hypochloremic alkalosis** (The acid - base disturbance is less pronounced in malignancy than benign and there is relative hypochlorhydria found in gastric cancer).

Q 11. Is it likely to be operable? Is there any role for surgery in this case?

- Unlikely to be operable
- Since it is obstructing the pylorus, **palliative intubation or a palliative gastrojejunostomy** (Anterior, antecolic, long loop, gastrojejunostomy and jejunojejunostomy– not a good operation) may be required for this patient. Another option is a **palliative gastrectomy**
- **Laser recanalization** is a better option.

Q 12. What is the normal capacity of the stomach and what is the length of the stomach?

- 40 ounces (40 × 30 = 1200 cc)
- 12 inch long (30 cm).

Q 13. What is linitisplastica and what is the capacity of the stomach in linitisplastica?

Linitisplastica or leather—bottle stomach

- Linitis means woven linen
- It is **diffuse type of carcinoma** involving the entire stomach
- There is thickening of the entire wall of the stomach with great contraction of the lumen
- It is also called **leather - bottle stomach**
- The capacity of stomach is reduced 4 ounces (120 cc) and the length of the stomach may be as small as 4 inches (10 cm)
- Endoscopy and ordinary biopsy may be normal and deep punch biopsy is required

Read for Details of Carcinoma Stomach, Refer Section 2, Long Case No:7

19 – Barium Meal, Gastric Outlet Obstruction

Q 1. What is your observation?

Barium meal picture showing the following findings:

1. Gastric outlet obstruction
2. Dilatation of the stomach
3. The barium is not going to the duodenum and duodenum is not demonstrated
4. The stomach has got **mottled appearance** which is due to the retained food particles inside.

Q 2. What are the causes for gastric outlet obstruction?

Causes for gastric outlet obstruction

1. Duodenal ulcer with **pyloric stenosis** (common)
2. Antral gastric carcinoma (common)
3. Congenital hypertrophic pyloric stenosis (**Ramstedt's pyloromyotomy** is the treatment)
4. Adult type of pyloric stenosis (**Pyloroplasty** is the treatment)
5. Pyloric mucosal diaphragm (Excision of the diaphragm)
6. Gastric Bezoar (Vegetable matter taking the shape of the stomach called **phytobezoar** and if it is hair it is called **trichobazoar)**
7. Lymphoma
8. Gastritis
9. Crohn's disease
10. Tuberculosis

Note: Gastric outlet obstruction should be considered malignant until proven otherwise.

Q 3. Is pyloric stenosis a correct terminology?

It is a **misnomer**. The stenosis is found in the first part of the duodenum if it is due to duodenal ulcer. True pyloric stenosis is seen only in a pyloric channel ulcer.

Q 4. Is barium meal indicated if you suspect gastric outlet obstruction?

Should not be performed until the stomach is emptied.

Q 5. What are the clinical features of benign gastric outlet obstruction?

Clinical features of benign gastric outlet obstruction
• Peptic ulcer pain of long duration • Vomitus lacking bile and containing food material taken several days previously • Loss of weight • Dehydration • Distended stomach • Visible gastric peristalsis • Succussion splash

Q 6. What are the metabolic abnormalities of benign gastric outlet obstruction?

Metabolic abnormalities of benign gastric outlet obstruction
• **Hypochloremic alkalosis** (Sodium and potassium are normal initially) • Urine initially has low chloride and high bicarbonate (**Alkaline urine**) • Bicarbonate is excreted along with sodium resulting in **hyponatremia** • Dehydration leads to sodium retention and potassium and hydrogen ions are excreted in urine in turn producing **paradoxical aciduria** • **Hypokalemia** • Alkalosis leads to hypocalcemia and **tetany**

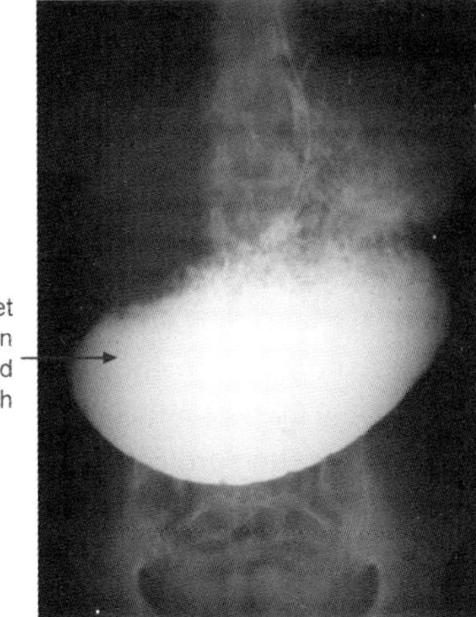

Barium meal

Q 7. What is the normal emptying time of the stomach?

3 to 4 hours.

Q 8. What is Saline Load Test?

It is an objective test for assessing the degree of pyloric obstruction.

Through a nasogastric tube, **700 ml of normal saline** (at room temperature) is infused over 3 to 5 minutes and the tube is clamped. **Thirty minutes later**, the stomach is aspirated and the residual volume of saline is recorded. Recovery of more than 350ml indicates obstruction.

Q 9. How to proceed in such a case?

Upper GI endoscopy is indicated to rule out an obstructing neoplasm.

Q 10. What is the preoperative preparation?

1. Nasogastric decompression

2. Gastric lavage with saline until the effluent is clear. This will allow the **pyloric edema and spasm to subside**
3. Repeat the saline load test after 72 hours and check whether there is improvement
4. If there is improvement and if malignancy can be ruled out patient can be managed medically, slowly starting liquid diet followed by solid diet
5. If there is no improvement, patient needs surgery depending on the pathology on endoscopy.

Q 11. What is the surgical treatment of severe gastric outlet obstruction secondary to duodenal ulcer?

- Gastrojejunostomy and truncal vagotomy
- Endoscopic balloon dilatation in early cases.

20 – Barium Meal, Duodenal Deformity

Q 1. What is your observation?
Barium meal picture showing duodenal deformity (**trefoil deformity**) suggestive of cicatrizing **duodenal ulcer**.

Q 2. What is duodenal cap?
The first 2.5 cm of the first part of the normal duodenum which is radiologically demonstrated is called duodenal cap (it is roughly triangular in shape).

Q 3. What are the radiological findings of duodenal ulcer?

1. Deformed duodenal cap
2. Nonvisualization of the duodenal cap
3. Trefoil deformity (also called **trifoliate** deformity).

Q 4. What is the cause for trefoil deformity?
It is due to secondary diverticulum formation at the duodenal cap region.

Q 5. What is the cause for non visualization of the duodenal cap?
It is due to the spasm of the first part of the duodenum.

Q 6. What are the complications of duodenal ulcer?

• Acute complications	Perforation (anterior ulcers) Hemorrhage (posterior ulcers)
• Subacute complications	Residual abscess formation
• Chronic complications	Pyloric stenosis Penetration to pancreas Intractability

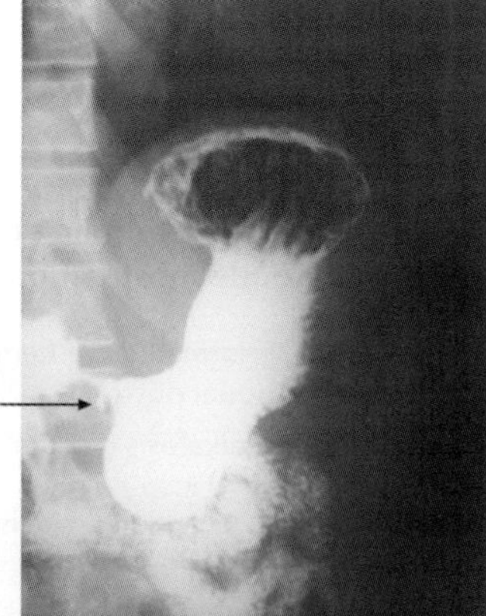

Barium meal

Q 7. What is kissing ulcer?
When there is both posterior and anterior duodenal ulcers it is called kissing ulcers.

Q 8. Erosion of which artery is responsible for hemorrhage?

Gastroduodenal artery.

Q 9. Can duodenal ulcer turn malignant?

No.

Q 10. What are the common sites of peptic ulcers?

- First part of the duodenum
- Stomach (**lesser curvature**)
- Lower end of the esophagus
- Meckel's diverticulum having **ectopic gastric epithelium**
- Gastro jejunal stoma (**Stomal ulcer**) – on jejunal side

Q 11. What are the etiological factors for peptic ulcers?

Etiological factors for peptic ulcers

- It is an imbalance between the aggressive factors (acid) and defensive factors (mucosal protective factors – including the mucus)
- "No acid no ulcer" is still true (Normal or low level of acid in gastric ulcer)
- Infection with H. pylori (most important)
- Genetic factors
- Blood group - common in O group patients
- Cigarette smoking
- Alcohol
- Drugs - NSAIDS, Steroids
- Hyperparathyroidism

Q 12. What is the treatment of duodenal ulcer?

Duodenal ulcer is a medical problem and is treated by:

- H2 – receptor antagonists and proton pump inhibitors
- Eradication of Helicobacter pylori (Proton pump inhibitor + Metronidazole and Amoxycillin).

Q 13. What are the indications for surgery?

Indications are complications:

- Perforation
- Stenosis.

Q 14. What is the surgical procedure of choice for stenosis?

- Truncal vagotomy and gastrojejunostomy is the operation of choice
- Pyloroplasty is contraindicated when there is cicatrization of the duodenum
- HSV (Highly Selective Vagotomy) alone is contraindicated since there is duodenal obstruction. It can be done in early cases of stenosis provided **dilatation of the duodenum** can be successfully carried out.

21 – Double Contrast Barium Enema, Carcinoma Cecum

Q 1. What is your observation?

Double contrast barium enema showing **irregularity of the mucosa** of the cecum suggestive of carcinoma.

Q 2. What is double contrast barium enema?

In addition to the barium sulphate solution given as enema, air is injected so that the mucosa will be delineated.

Q 3. What is the preparation for barium enema?

- Low residue diet for 3 days before the examination
- Patient is given laxatives at bed time for two days
- Liquid diet for 24 hours
- The **colon must be empty**. This can be achieved by enema and colon washout
- The patient must be undressed completely (wearing an open - backed gown).

Q 4. What is the position of the patient for barium enema?

The patient is initially in the **left lateral** position and followed by **prone** position.

Q 5. What is the procedure?

1. About **1 liter of barium sulphate** is introduced per anally using an enema tube from the enema can
2. A Foley's catheter with inflated bulb is used in children
3. The procedure is done under fluoroscopy
4. X-ray is taken after completely filling the colon
5. Air is insufflated to delineate the mucosa (**Double contrast**)
6. Finally a post evacuation film is taken (Patient is asked to evacuate the barium).

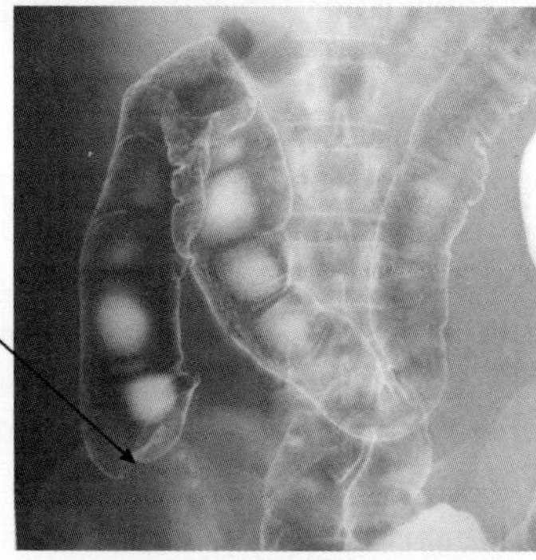

Barium enema—double contrast shows mucosal pattern

Q 6. What are the precautions to be taken when it is carried out for Hirschsprung's disease?

1. Saline is used instead of water for diluting the barium
2. Prior enemas may deflate the mega colon and distend the aganglionic segment
3. Foley's catheter is not used to avoid false negative study.

Q 7. What further investigations are carried out in this case?

1. Colonoscopy and biopsy
2. CEA level for getting the baseline value
3. X-ray chest to rule out metastasis in the lung
4. Ultrasound abdomen to rule out free fluid and metastasis liver
5. CT of the abdomen to find local invasion.

Q 8. What are the possible radiological findings in carcinoma of the colon?

- Apple core deformity with shouldering on both sides
- Irregular filling defect
- Irregularity in the mucosa
- Annular lesions and strictures on left side
- Synchronous polyps and multiple carcinomas (5%).

Q 9. What are the likely clinical presentations in carcinoma of the cecum?

1. Mass in the right iliac fossa
2. Anemia
3. Symptoms of intermittent obstruction when the growth forms the apex of the intussusception.

Q 10. What is the treatment of carcinoma of the cecum?

Right hemicolectomy.

(Read section on long cases no:10).

22 – Barium Enema, Apple Core Deformity of the Ascending Colon

Q 1. What is your observation?

Barium enema showing the typical **apple core deformity** with shouldering on either side in the ascending colon suggestive of carcinoma.

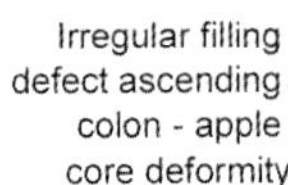
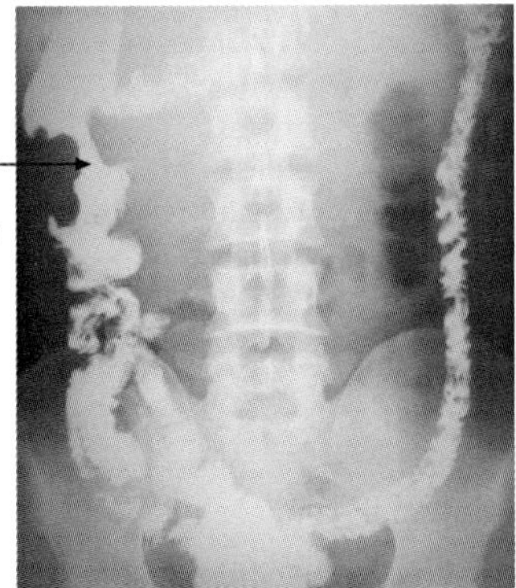

Barium enema

- **Read skiagram No: 21**
- **Read section on long cases No:10.**

23 – Barium Enema, Ileocecal Tuberculosis

Q 1. What is your observation?

1. The **cecum is pulled up** and is seen in the subhepatic region. Normally the cecum should be at the level of iliac bone.
2. **Obtuse ileocecal angle.** Normally the ileum joins the cecum at right angles.
3. The terminal ileum is narrow–**napkin lesion.**
4. Narrow terminal ileum with wide open ileocecal valve is called **Fleischner sign.**
5. **Sterlin sign** – Fibrotic terminal ileum opening into contracted cecum.

All these findings are suggestive of **ileocecal tuberculosis.**

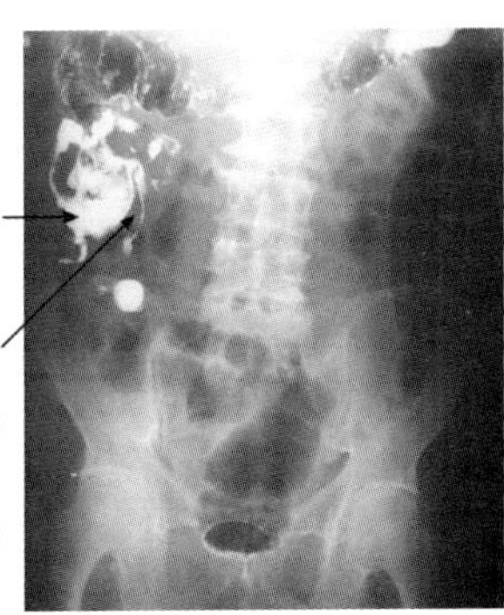

Barium enema showing cecum

Q 2. What are the likely clinical features?

- General symptoms like: weight loss, malaise, evening rise of temperature, etc.
- Alternating constipation and diarrhea
- Mass in the right iliac fossa
- Features of distal small bowel obstruction – abdominal pain, distension and vomiting.

Q 3. What are types of small intestinal tuberculosis?

Ulcerative type and hyperplastic type.

Q 4. What are the differences between ulcerative type and hyperplastic type?

No	*Ulcerative*	*Hyperplastic*
1.	Secondary to pulmonary tuberculosis	Primary
2.	Primary tuberculosis in the chest	No primary in the chest
3.	The virulence of the organism outstrips the resistance of the host	The host resistance is stronger than the virulence of the organism
4.	Patient is very ill	Not very ill

5.	Multiple transverse ulcers in the ileum, the overlying serosa studded with tubercles	Thickening of the intestinal wall and narrowing of the lumen
6.	Clinical presentation is diarrhoea and bleeding per rectum	Mass right iliac fossa
7.	Gross caseation is seen	Absence of gross caseation

Read section on long cases No: 9 for management

24 – Barium Enema, Carcinoma of the Descending Colon

Q 1. What is your observation?

It is a barium enema picture showing filling defect in the descending colon suggestive of **carcinoma of the descending colon.**

Q 2. What is your differential diagnosis?

The filling defect may also be due to a **pericolic abscess.**

Q 3. How to confirm your diagnosis?

Colonoscopy and biopsy.

Q 4. How many percentage of carcinomas are seen in descending colon?

4%.

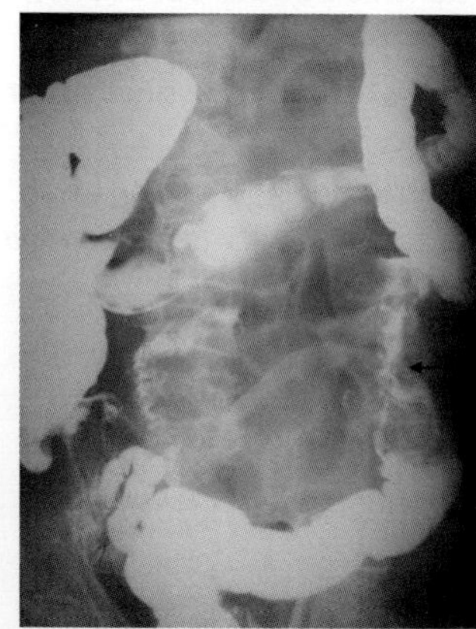

Barium enema

Q 5. What is the most important clinical feature of left sided colonic malignancy ?

Alternating constipation and diarrhea and colicky abdominal pain.

Q 6. What is the cause for alternating constipation and diarrhea?

The left sided growths are of the stenotic variety which leads to **constipation**. This in turn will produce **stercoral enteritis.** Enteritis leads on to diarrhea. This is again followed by constipation forming a vicious cycle.

Q 7. What are the most important complications of descending colon growth?

- Large bowel obstruction (commonest)
- Perforation.

Q 8. What is the site of perforation in such a case?

It can perforate in 3 situations:

a. At the site of the growth
b. Proximal to the growth at the site of stercoral ulcer.
c. Perforation of the cecum if the ileocecal valve is competent.

Q 9. What is the surgical procedure of choice for this lesion?

- **Left hemicolectomy** (mid transverse colon to upper sigmoid is removed)
- In this procedure the left colic artery is ligated preserving the inferior mesenteric artery
- Subtotal colectomy and ileosigmoid or ileo rectal anastomosis is another option.

25 – Barium Enema, Intussusception

Q 1. What is your observation?

1. Barium enema picture showing nonfilling of the colon beyond the hepatic flexure
2. The typical "**claw sign**" of **intussusception** is demonstrated. The barium is seen as a claw around a **negative shadow of intussusception**. It is also called **pincer** shaped filling defect (**Coil spring appearance**).

Q 2. What is the definition of intussusception?

Telescoping of proximal into the distal intestine is called intussusception.

Q 3. What is the age group commonly affected?

Infancy (**5-10 months**).

Q 4. What are the causes for intussusception?

Causes for intussusception
1. Idiopathic (hyperplasia of the **Peyer's patches** in the ileum during **weaning period**) Upper respiratory tract infection and gastroenteritis may precede the intussusception
2. Meckel's diverticulum acting as a lead point
3. Polyps
4. Submucosal lipoma
5. Carcinoma
6. Henoch - Schönlein purpura
7. Appendix – acting as a lead point
8. Peutz - Jeghers syndrome

Q 5. What are the common causes in adults?

The adult causes for lead point are:

- Tumor (carcinoma)
- Polyp
- Submucosal lipoma.

Q 6. What are the parts of intussusception?

- Inner tube or entering layer
- Middle tube or returning layer
- Outer tube or the sheath (**intussuscepiens**).

Note: The inner tube and the middle tube together are called **intussusceptum**).

The part that advances is called apex

The neck is the junction of the entering layer with the mass.

Q 7. What are the types of intussusception depending on the location?

Anatomical types of intussusception
1. Ileocolic (**commonest variety**)
2. Ileocecal – ileocecal valve forming the apex
3. Ileo Ileocolic
4. Ileoileal
5. Colocolic
6. Multiple
7. Jejunogastric

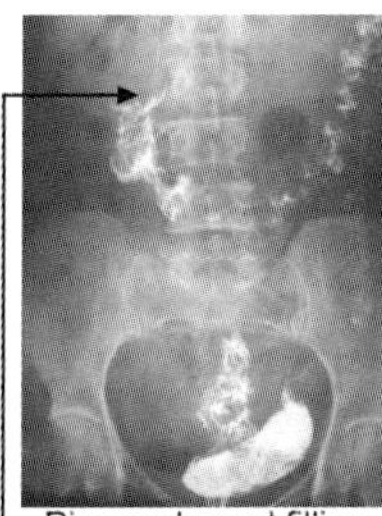

Pincer-shaped filling defect (Claw sign)

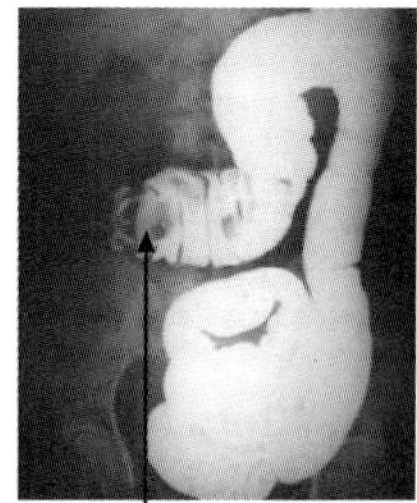

Coil spring appearance

Barium enema—Intussusception

Q 8. What is retrograde intussusception?

Telescoping of the distal intestine into the proximal is called retrograde intussusception. The typical example is a jejunogastric intussusception seen after a gastrojejunostomy.

Q 9. What type of intestinal obstruction is produced in intussusception?

Strangulating obstruction (the blood supply of the inner layer is usually affected).

Q 10. What are the diagnostic clinical features and important diagnostic signs?

Clinical features of intussusception

- Colicky abdominal pain (screaming and drawing up of the legs in infants)
- "**Redcurrant jelly**" stool (initially the stool may be normal)
- Vomiting is a later event (Milk followed by bile)
- Dehydration
- Abdominal distension
- **Sausage – shaped mass** with concavity towards the umbilicus which harden on palpation (**Disappearing mass**)
- Sign de-dance (Emptiness of right iliac fossa)
- Blood - stained mucus on rectal examination
- Palpable **mass per rectum** (apex of the intussusception)
- The finger can be introduced between the mass and anal verge in intussusception which is not possible in prolapse rectum

Q 11. What is the ultrasound finding in intussusception?

Doughnut appearance of concentric rings in transverse section.

Q 12. What is the nonoperative management?

Nonoperative management consists of:

- Resuscitation – IV fluids (fluid and electrolyte correction)
- Nasogastric decompression
- **Hydrostatic reduction** – Using barium enema or air (**pneumatic reduction**).

Q 13. What is successful hydrostatic reduction?

- Free reflux of barium or air into the small bowel is suggestive of successful reduction
- Resolution of symptoms and signs.

Q 14. What are the contraindications for non operative management?

Contraindications for nonoperative management

- Signs of peritonitis
- Perforation
- Shock

Q 15. What is the recurrence rate of non operative management?

10%.

Q 16. What are the indications for surgery?

Indications for surgery

- Contraindications for nonoperative reduction
- Failure of pneumatic or hydrostatic reduction
- Suspected pathological lead point
- Gangrene

Q 17. What is the operative method of reduction?

- Laparotomy is done initially (transverse right sided incision for children)
- **Manual reduction** – gently compress the most distal part of the intussusception towards its origin (don't pull)
- After reduction check for viability of the bowel
- If irreducible or gangrenous do **resection and anastomosis.**

26 – T-Tube Cholangiogram

Q 1. What is your observation?

It is a T-tube cholangiogram showing the **normal CBD** (Common Bile Duct) with the horizontal limb of the T-tube inside the CBD and the vertical limb coming outside the body. The dye is coming down the CBD and filling the duodenum. There is **no evidence of any obstruction or residual stone** in the CBD. This is a **normal study**.

Q 2. What is the purpose of T-tube?

- The T-tube is put inside the bile duct after exploration of the bile duct (**choledochotomy**) for removal of stones (**choledocholithotomy**).
- After clearing the stones there will be some **papillary edema and spasm** and therefore the **dye may not come to the duodenum** after the **peroperative cholangiogram.** Therefore a T-tube is put for **drainage of the infected bile**. This tube is later utilized for T-tube cholangiogram after **7 to 10 days.**

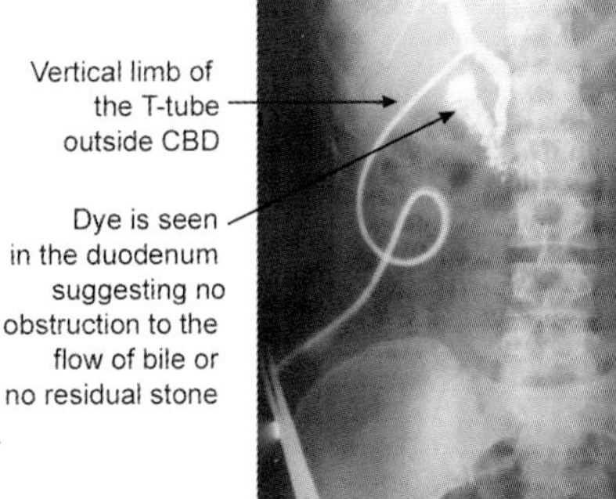

T-tube cholangiogram

- The T-tube is then connected to a **drainage bottle** and the 24 hour measurements are taken daily. As the edema and spasm of the papilla disappear, the quantity of bile coming to the bottle will decrease gradually over a period of one week. It allows time for relief of the papillary spasm.
- This tube can also be used for **T-tube cholangiogram postoperatively** for demonstration of residual stones.

Q 3. What is the incision in the CBD for choledochotomy?

- A **longitudinal incision** in the supraduodenal part of the CBD
- After removal of the stones the T-tube is inserted and the duct closed around it.

Q 4. What is the timing of T–tube cholangiogram?

- **Usually 7-10 days** after surgery. by that time the papillary edema and spasm will disappear and the bile will become clear.
- The quantity of bile draining to the bottle will come down as the natural passage to the duodenum becomes patent.

Q 5. What is the purpose of T–tube cholangiogram?

1. To look for **residual and retained stones** in the CBD - identified as **negative shadows** (radiolucent) inside CBD
2. To look for **free flow** of the bile **into the duodenum.**

Q 6. How will you differentiate air and radiolucent shadow of residual stone?

If it is air, change of position of patient will result in change of position of the shadow.

Q 7. How can you avoid air?

The T – tube is **initially flushed with 20 ml of normal saline** so that the air bubble is removed before injecting the dye.

Q 8. What dye is used and how much quantity?

Iodine containing dye usually **urograffin 3 ml** is injected into the T-tube.

Q 9. Is there any role for clamping the T-tube before removal?

- T – tube is clamped for increasing periods of time for 2-3 days before removal (8hours, 12hours, and 24 hours).
- If there is residual stone and **obstruction to the flow** of bile to the duodenum, it will produce **pain, jaundice and leak along the side of the T-tube.**

Q 10. When is the T – tube removed?

If there are no residual stones and there is free flow of bile into the duodenum then the T tube is removed usually **around 10 days.**

Q 11. What is the technique of removal of T- tube?

It is removed by gentle traction.

Q 12. If residual stones are found, what is the management?

- The T-tube is left in place for 6 weeks, so that a mature tract is formed. There is a chance that the stone may pass to the duodenum mean while.
- The stone can be later removed percutaneously by an interventional radiologist (**Burhenne technique**).

Q 13. What are the indications for choledochotomy?

Indications for choledochotomy

1. Radiologically demonstrated stone (In per-operative cholangiogram)
2. Sonologically demonstrated stone in the CBD
3. Palpable stone in the CBD
4. CBD diameter more than 1cm (More than 6mm sonologically)
5. History of obstructive jaundice
6. Abnormal LFT (Raised bilirubin and alkaline phosphatase)
7. Multiple faceted stones in the gallbladder

Q 14. What is the alternative for choledocholithotomy?

- **Endoscopic sphincterotomy** and stone extraction using **Dormia basket** (Open choledochotomy is used less nowadays which is replaced by minimally invasive techniques).

27 – Percutaneous Transhepatic Cholangiogram (PTC) for Obstructive Jaundice

Q 1. What is your observation?

It is a picture of Percutaneous transhepatic cholangiography (**PTC**) showing;

1. Dilatation of intrahepatic biliary radicle
2. Obstruction to the passage of dye beyond the Common Hepatic Duct (**CHD**).

The findings are suggestive of **obstructive jaundice** probably cholangiocarcinoma at the junction.

Q 2. What are the indications for PTC?

1. It is usually done in cases of **obstructive jaundice** when the level of obstruction is at the level of confluence and CHD region. It will **delineate the proximal limit of the lesion** and the nature of the lesion.
2. For **external biliary drainage** in obstructive jaundice with cholangitis as a preoperative measure.
3. For **insertion of indwelling stents** to bypass the obstruction in inoperable cases of obstructive jaundice.

4. The drainage catheter can be left in place for a number of days and then the tract can be dilated so that a **flexible choledochoscope** can be introduced for the diagnosis of stricture of biliary duct. A **biopsy** also can be taken with choledochoscope.

Q 3. What are the precautions to be taken before PTC?

1. Check the coagulation profile and correct the prothrombin time before doing this **invasive procedure** by administering **vitamin K_1 10 mg IV daily for 3 days**
2. Give **prophylactic antibiotics**
3. The injection needle is introduced under **fluoroscopic control or ultrasound or CT guidance**
4. If surgery is contemplated, it is preferable to do it in the morning of the day of surgery.

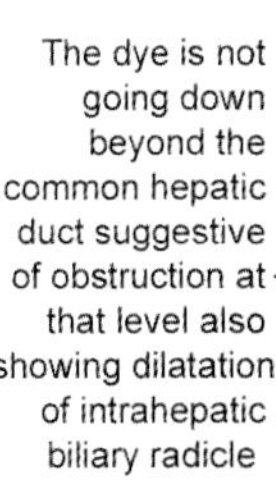

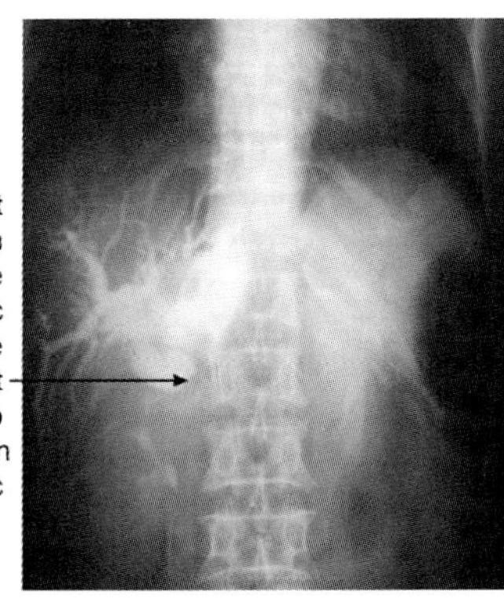

Percutaneous transhepatic cholangiogram (PTC)— for obstructive jaundice

Q 4. What is the procedure?

1. After giving local anesthesia the **Chiba or Okuda needle** is introduced into the liver through the 8th intercostal space in mid- axillary line.
2. Needle is placed in a dilated biliary radicle under sonological guidance or fluoroscopy.
3. The bile is under tension and it is aspirated and sent for culture and cytology.
4. Water-soluble contrast medium is then injected into the biliary system and multiple images are taken to visualize the area and nature of obstruction.
5. A catheter is introduced into the biliary system if external biliary drainage is required.

Q 5. What are the complications of PTC?

1. The bile is under tension and it will **leak** into the peritoneal cavity producing **biliary peritonitis**
2. Bleeding
3. Infection
4. Septicemia.

28 - Ultrasound Abdomen – Intussusception, B-mode and Real Time Ultrasonography

Q 1. What is your observation in the ultrasound picture of the abdomen?

The ultrasound showing the typical doughnut appearance of concentric rings is suggestive of **intussusception.**

Q 2. What is ultrasonography?

- Ultrasound is energy in the form of mechanical vibrations, the frequency of which is in **excess of that to which the human ear is sensitive,** i.e. greater than 20,000 Hz.

- Ultrasound makes use of high frequency sound waves generated by a transducer containing the **piezoelectric material.**
- The sound waves are reflected by tissue interfaces (as the sound energy passes through various tissues of the body, it interacts by **reflection, refraction, defraction, scattering and absorption.**
- The echoes vary depending on the tissue type.
- The frequencies in the range of 3 to 20 MHz are used (1 MHz being equal to 1000,000 Hz).
- For abdomen **3 to 7 MHz** transducer is used
- Low frequency waves have greater penetrating powers than high frequency waves, but produce less definition. (For superficial structures higher frequency transducers are used).

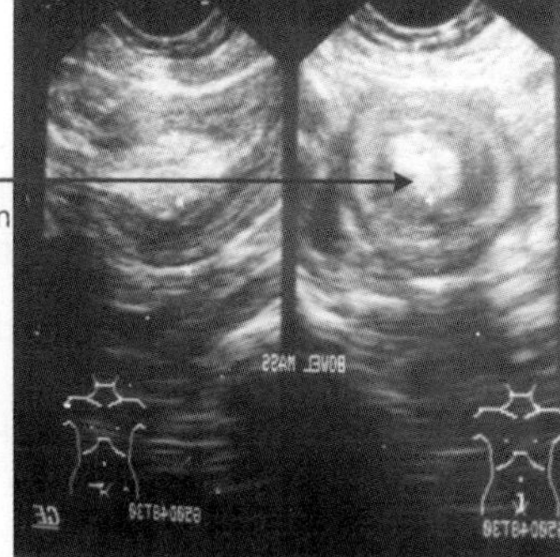

USG—abdomen

Q 3. What is piezoelectric effect?

It is the process of conversion of **electrical to mechanical energy**.

Q 4. What are the examples of piezoelectric materials?

- Quartz
- Lithium sulphate
- Synthetic ceramic lead zurconate tinanate (PTZ): most commonly used

Q 5. What is B- mode ultrasound?

This is the primary display mode introduced in 1972. It is called B-mode or **brightness mode display** which gives two dimensional cross- sectional representation of the tissues under examination on horizontal and vertical axes while encoding echo amplitude information in gray levels of 1 and 14.

Q 6. What is real time ultrasonography?

This is the universally accepted method which produces about **40 B - scan images per second.** This is above the **flicker rate of the eye** (**16-18 images/ second**) and the examiner perceives a continuum of motion like the systolic dilatation and diastolic diminution of the diameter of the aorta.

Q 7. What are the uses of ultrasonography?

Use of ultrasound in surgery

1. It can differentiate solid and cystic lesions
2. Vascular system can be assessed (by Doppler study)
3. Guided biopsies are possible
4. Can differentiate benign and malignant lesions
5. First - line investigation of choice of the liver: For hepatic tumors, metastasis, abscess formation, cystic diseases, etc.
6. First-line investigation of choice of the biliary system: Intrahepatic biliary radicle dilatation, assessment of the CBD size, identification of the stones, assessment of the wall thickness of gall bladder, etc.
7. First-line investigation of choice of the renal tract.
8. Fluid collection in the peritoneal cavity, pleural cavity and pericardial cavity can be identified
9. Can identify lesions in other solid organs like spleen

10. Pancreatic diseases: Difficult to visualize distal body and tail. Head and proximal body can be visualized by making use of the acoustic window of the liver
11. Lesions of thyroid can be assessed
12. Breast lesions can be ascertained in young patients < 35 years
13. Testicular lesions.
14. Imaging method of choice in obstetrics and gynecology
15. Endocavitary ultrasound is possible.

Q 8. What are the advantages of ultrasound?

1. It is noninvasive
2. No radiation hazard
3. Inexpensive
4. Interaction with patient is possible.

Q 9. What are the disadvantages of ultrasound?

- It is operator dependent
- Little information is gained in tissues beyond bone and air-filled structures like viscera
- Pulmonary and skeletal system cannot be assessed.

Read the management of intussusception **skiagram No:25**

29 - Ultrasound Abdomen, Gallstone

Q 1. What is your observation?

Ultrasound examination of the gallbladder area showing a gallstone casting an **acoustic shadow** at the neck of the gallbladder (posterior acoustic shadows are suggestive of stones).

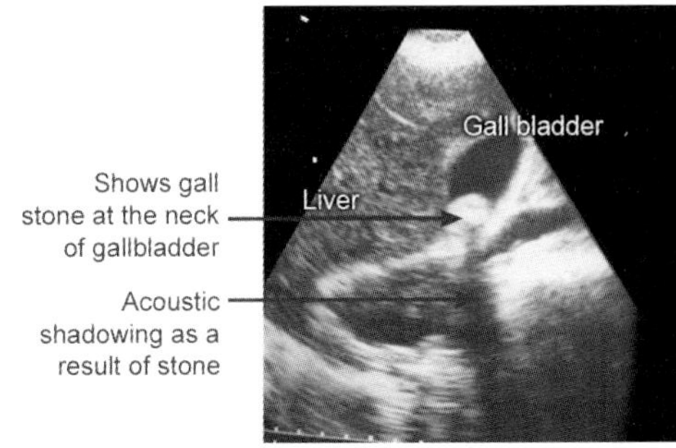

USG—abdomen

Q 2. What further sonological assessment of the biliary system is required when stone is identified?

1. Gall-bladder thickness (If thick it is suggestive of previous inflammation).
2. Pericholecystic collection.
3. Size of cystic duct – if wide possibility of stone slipping to the CBD is there.
4. Intra hepatic biliary radicle dilatation suggestive of obstruction to the flow of bile
5. Size of the CBD (Upper limit 6mm sonologically. More than 6mm suggestive of obstruction of the bile duct).
6. Look for stones in the CBD.

Read Skiagram No:8 for gallstones and cholecystitis

30 – CT Brain, Extradural and Subdural Hematoma

Q 1. What is your observation?

Axial Computerized Tomography (CT scan) of the brain showing **right sided hyperdense lesion** suggestive of **subdural** hematoma (**Concave**

appearance in contrast to the biconvex appearance of the extradural hematoma) with mass effect with midline shift to the opposite side.

Q 2. What is CT scan?

- It was introduced by **Godfrey Newbold Hounsfield** in 1963 (British Engineer - Awarded Nobel prize in 1979).

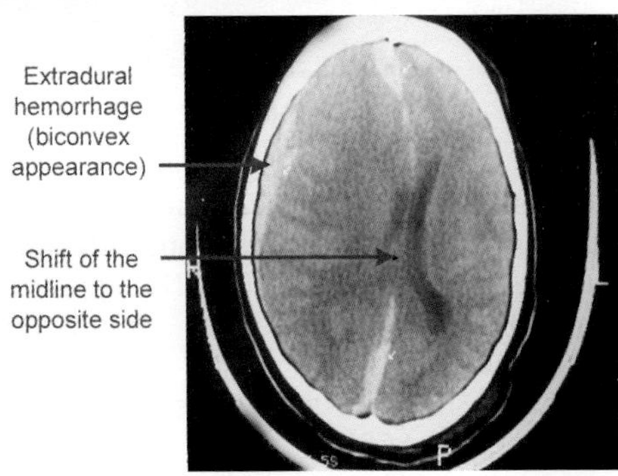

CT— Brain

- It consists of a **gantry** containing the X-ray tube where the patient is placed, **filters and detectors** which revolve around the patient, acquiring the information at different angles and projections which is **mathematically reconstructed** to produce a 2 dimensional gray scale image by a computer.
- It can **pass through air and bone.**
- The entire body can be studied in a **series of cross sections** and therefore called **tomogram**
- Resolution is very high and can be increased by using contrast medium.

Q 3. What is Hounsfield unit?

The **attenuation value** of tissues obtained in the gray - scale image is **related to that of water,** which is given a CT number of **zero Hounsfield Unit** (HUs). The Hounsfield units of various tissues are given below:

Hounsfield units of various tissues	
• + 1000 HUs	– Bone
• Zero HUs	– Water
• Minus 100 HUs	– Fat
• Minus 1000 HUs	– Air

Other tissues come in between bone and air.

Q 4. What is the difference between conventional CT and Helical/Spiral CT and multislice CT?

- In conventional CT the individual scans are acquired during **suspended respiration.**
- In spiral CT because of the continuous rotation of the X-ray tube with the **beam tracing a spiral path** around the patient, during a single breath hold for 30seconds, 3cm or more of tissues can be covered.
- Rapid acquisition of image is therefore possible in spiral CT.
- Imaging arterial and venous phase is possible in spiral CT.
- Three dimensional analysis is possible in spiral CT.

Q 5. What are the advantages of CT scan?

Advantages of CT scan
• Highest resolution than plain radiograph
• 1 to 2mm sections are possible
• Radiation exposure is less

- Images of the chest, abdomen and pelvis is possible under 20seconds in new generation machines (**Multislice CT Scanner**)
- High resolution CT (**HRCT**) is used to for lung diseases
- The natural contrast of the tissues can be **enhanced with the use intravenous contrast medium**
- Scanning during **arterial phase and venous phase** is possible which may aid in characterization of lesions
- **CT guided biopsies** are possible
- Improved spatial resolution has resulted in the development of **CT angiography, virtual colonoscopy and virtual bronchoscopy**
- Three dimensional images can be reconstructed

Q 6. What are the disadvantages of CT scan?

- High dose of ionizing radiation
- Increased cost
- Availability of the equipment
- Radiological expertise required for interpretation.

Q 7. What is the reason for concave appearance in the given CT?

In subdural hematoma the blood spreads across the surface of the brain. Since there is less resistance to blood moving through the subdural space than through the extradural space, it takes the concave shape (In **extradural** hematoma a **lentiform or lens-shaped or biconvex** hyperdense lesion is seen).

Q 8. What are the types of hemorrhages in relation to the brain?

1. Extradural (outside dura, associated with fracture skull and more common in the young).
2. Subdural – **acute subdural** and **chronic subdural.**
3. Subarachnoid hemorrhage.
4. Intracerebral hemorrhage.
5. Intraventricular hemorrhage.

Q 9. Which type of hematoma is more common — extradural or subdural?

Subdural is more common **(5:1).**

Q 10. What are the differences between extradural and acute subdural hematoma?

Differences between extradural and acute subdural hematoma

	Acute subdural	*Extradural*
Cause	Need not be associated with fracture of the skull	Always associated with skull fracture
Cause	Injury to the cerebral veins	Arterial injury (major dural venous sinus possible)
Age group	Any age	Younger age
Location	Space between **dura and arachnoid.** Depends on the area of bleeding	Space between **bone and dura** Usually temporal region.
Mass effect and midline shift	Less common and late since it is venous	More common and early since it is arterial
Conscious level	Impaired conscious level from the time of injury	Conscious level normal initially
Lucid interval	Not present	Present

Brain damage	Extensive damage (laceration) may be seen	**No primary damage or minimal**
March of paralysis	May occur on both sides	Typical paralysis on the opposite side
CT appearance	Hyperdense diffuse and **concave** appearance	**Lentiform** or biconvex hyperdense lesion with or without mass effect or midline shift
Treatment	Evacuation via craniotomy. Small hematomas may be managed conservatively	Immediate surgical evacuation via craniotomy
Mortality rate	40%	2 to 18%

Q 11. Which artery is involved in extradural?

Tearing of meningeal artery: The largest **meningeal artery is the middle meningeal artery** which is involved in trauma to the temporal region (P**terion** is the **thinnest part of the skull** overlying the meningeal artery).

Q 12. What is the nature of paralysis on the contralateral side in extradural hemorrhage?

The paralysis is seen in descending manner starting from face, arms, body, legs, etc.

Q 13. What is Hutchinson's pupil?

This is a clinical finding in **extradural hemorrhage.**

1. Initially the pupil on the **side of injury contracts** due to irritation of the oculomotor nerve and the contralateral pupil remains normal
2. The pupil on the **injured side becomes dilated** due to paralysis of the oculomotor nerve while the **contralateral pupil contracts** as a result of irritation by mass effect and shift of midline
3. Finally the pupils of **both sides become dilated** and fixed which is **a grave sign.**

Q 14. What is lucid interval?

It is the period following head injury when the patient complains of headache, is fully alert and oriented with no focal deficits. This is followed after minutes or hours by rapid deterioration in conscious level, contralateral hemiparesis and the classical Hutchinson's pupil.

31- CT Scan Abdomen, HCC, Metastasis, Focal Nodular Hyperplasia, Hepatic Adenoma, Hemangioma

Q 1. What is your observation?

CT scan section of abdomen showing a well-encapsulated lesion in the right lobe of liver with lack of enhancement in the central part of the lesion.

Q 2. What are the possible differential diagnoses?

Differential diagnoses are:

1. Focal nodular hyperplasia
2. Hepatic adenoma
3. Metastasis
4. Hepatocellular carcinoma.

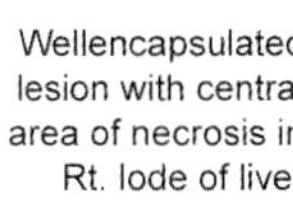

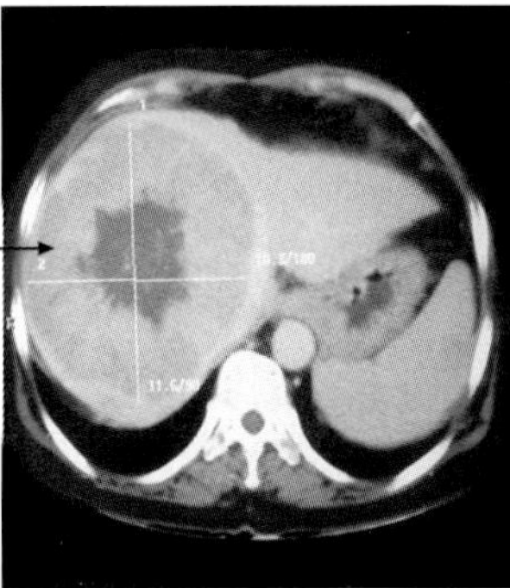

CT-scan— Abdomen

Q 3. What are the characteristics of focal nodular hyperplasia (FNH)?

The contrast CT in FNH may show **central scarring** and well-vascularized lesion. A **sulphur colloid liver scan** can differentiate from other lesions. The FNH contain both **hepatocytes and Kupffer cells**. The Kupffer cells take up the sulphur colloid, whereas **Kupffer cells are absent in adenomas, primary and metastatic tumors**.

Q 4. What are the features of hepatic adenoma?

- They are well-circumscribed vascular solid tumors.
- **Angiography** will show **well-developed peripheral arterialization**
- They have got malignant potential
- They are associated with sex hormones and oral contraceptives
- Withdrawal of hormones is associated with regression of the lesion
- Resection is recommended.

Q 5. What are the features of hepatocellular carcinoma (HCC)?

- Contrast enhancing lesion in the CT (**Early arterial phase enhancement** is suggestive of HCC whereas delayed contrast enhancement or slow contrast enhancement is seen in hemangioma).
- **Lipiodol uptake is seen in HCC** after administering poppy seed oil (Lipiodol) into the hepatic artery at selective mesenteric angiogram and doing CT scan of the liver after 2 weeks.

Q 6. What are the features of metastatic lesion?

Lack of enhancement of the mass lesion in the liver after IV contrast is suggestive of metastasis.

Note: In summary early arterial enhancement and Lipiodol uptake are suggestive of **HCC**, non enhancement of the lesion is suggestive of **metastasis**, sulphur colloid uptake is suggestive of **focal nodular hyperplasia** and slow and late enhancement is suggestive of **hemangioma** of liver.

Read section on Liver malignancy - Long case no:8

32 – Mammogram, Carcinoma Breast and Benign Lesions

Q 1. What is your observation?

1. Oblique view of mammogram showing irregular calcified lesion in the breast
2. Four axillary lymph nodes of different sizes.

Q 2. What is mammography?

It is nothing but plain X-ray of the breast using low voltage and high amperage X-rays.

Q 3. What are the views recommended for mammography?

1. Craniocaudal view: This will be marked in the film as CC for craniocaudal
2. Oblique view.

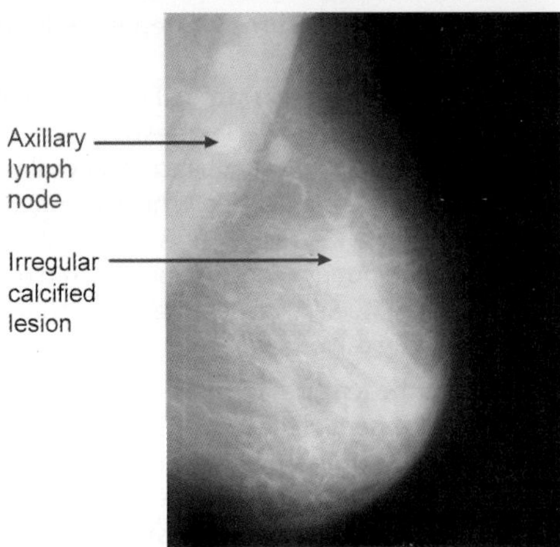

Mammogram—carcinoma breast and bengin lesions

Q 4. What is the radiation dose of mammography?

Less than 0.1cGY is standard (each chest X-ray delivers 1/4th of this radiation volume).

Q 5. Can you image the breast by mammography in all age groups?

Mammography is **rarely of value** in women **aged under 35years** because breasts are **relatively radiodense** and low sensitivity for the procedure in this age group. Therefore ultrasound is used for imaging in this age group.

Q 6. What are the indications for mammography?

Indications for mammography

1. For **screening** women above 50 years
2. Screening asymptomatic women **above 35 years** who have a **high risk of cancer**
3. Women with previously diagnosed **atypical ductal hyperplasia.**
4. To differentiate **benign from malignant lesions**
5. To identify **multicentricity** when carcinoma is diagnosed.
6. For assessment of the **size of the lesion before chemotherapy** so that the response of the lesion can be assessed.
7. For assessment of the **axilla for nodal enlargement.**
8. For assessment of the **contralateral breast.**
9. **Surveillance of the breast** following conservative surgery.
10. Evaluation of the breast **following augmentation** mammoplasty: To diagnose disease in the breast surrounding the prosthesis and complications related to prosthesis.
11. Investigation of suspicious **breast lump in males.**

Q 7. What are the guidelines for evaluation of mammography?

The following criteria should be looked for:

1. Mass lesion: Margin and density
2. Architectural distortion
3. Asymmetric density
4. Calcification.

	Malignant	Benign
Margin of mass lesion	**Spiculated mass** lesion with ill - defined margin (commonest finding of invasive carcinoma)	**Well circumscribed** mass lesion
Density	**High density** increases the probability of malignancy	Relatively **low density**

Architectural distortion	**Stellate lesion**: Numerous straight lines radiating towards the central area	No architectural distortion
Asymmetric density	With associated microcalcification, spiculation and architectural distortion	Can occur in normal involution of glandular tissue, hormone replacement therapy and trauma
Calcification	**Clustered microcalcification** with variable shape and size: Granular, branching, rod-shaped, bizarre micro-calcifications are suspicious (tight clusters >1 cm^2 area is highly suggestive)	**Scattered and rounded** calcification with relatively uniform size and density • **Popcorn calcification** – fibroadenoma • Teacup calcification – fibrocystic disease • Needle-like calcification – duct ectasia

Q 8. What are the secondary signs of malignancy?

- Skin changes – thickening, retraction and dimpling
- Nipple retraction, flattening of the nipple
- Focally dilated duct
- Increased vascularity
- Axillary lymphadenopathy.

Q 9. What are the disadvantages of mammography?

1. It is painful.
2. It is expensive.
3. Requires high technology machinery.
4. Requires special film and processing.
5. Requires highly trained radiologists.

Q 10. What is the reason for recommending screening the breast between the age group of 50 to 70 years by mammography?

- Current available data indicate that the reduction in mortality is maximal between the age of 50 to 70years (25 to 30% reduction in mortality).
- In age group of 40 to 49years the reduction in mortality is only 7 to 8%.
- However screening mammography is recommended starting from 3**5 years** who have a high risk of developing breast cancers.

Q 11. What is the frequency of screening mammography?

- The optimum frequency for screening is probably 2 years
- Annual screening is certainly too frequent.

Q 12. What are the mammographic views recommended?

- Two views at the first screen (craniocaudal and oblique)
- Only one view subsequently (oblique).

Q 13. What is the false-negative rate of mammography?

6 to 8%.

Q 14. Can you miss the presence of carcinoma in mammogram?

- Yes. About 5% of breast cancers are missed in mammographic screening programmes
- A normal mammogram does not exclude the presence of carcinoma.

Q 15. What is BI-RADS?

Breast **I**maging **R**eporting **A**nd **D**ata **S**ystem is a quality assurance tool devised for the standardization of mammographic reporting.

BI-RADS classification of mammographic abnormalities	
Category	**Assessment**
1.	Negative
2.	Benign finding
3.	Probably benign finding
4.	Suspicious abnormality
5.	Highly suggestive of malignancy

Q 16. What is digital mammography?

Here the images are obtained in computer which are then magnified so that computer aided diagnosis is possible.

Q 17. What are the currently recommended methods of screening?

1. Clinical breast examination (**CBE**).
2. Mammographic screening.
3. Breast self-examination (**BSE**).

Note:A combination of CBE and mammography is better.

Q 18. Which is the imaging of choice for recurrence in breast?

MRI.

Q 19. What are the advantages of MRI?

1. It can differentiate scar from recurrence
2. It is the imaging of choice in breasts with implants
3. Abnormal enhancement is seen after radiotherapy and therefore it is not used within 9 months of radiotherapy.

5

SECTION

Important Tables and Charts

General

1: Universal Precautions

- All hospital staff must adhere rigorously to protective measures which minimizes exposure to the diseases transmitted through blood, blood products and body fluids
- It is based on the concept that all persons are potential sources of infection independent of diagnosis or perceived risk
- The use of universal precautions involve placing barriers between staff and all blood and body fluids.**The Universal precautions**
    1. Wearing protective gloves (Ideally double gloves during surgery)
    2. Wearing protective eyewear (Preferably goggles during surgery)
    3. Wearing mask, protective apron and gown
    4. Wearing boots for covering the foot and lower leg during surgery
    5. Washing hands after removal of the gloves
    6. Washing hands between patients
    7. Always use gloves for handling blood, blood products and body fluids
    8. Undertaking hepatitis-B vaccination
    9. Covering open wounds
    10. Staff with infected wounds and active dermatitis must stay off work
    11. Using safe sharp instrument handling techniques consisting of the following:
        a. Never recap a hollow needle after use
        b. Sharp instruments should not be passed between surgeon and nurse
        c. The sharp instruments are placed into a bowl or tray, which can then be used to transfer
        d. Only one sharp instrument be placed in the tray at a time
        e. When two surgeons are operating each surgeon will have their own sharp tray
        f. Used needles and other disposable sharps are discarded into an approved sharp container

2A: Karnofsky Index of Performance Status (KPS) Karnofsky (KPS) Scale

Category	Score	Description
A. Able to carry on normal activity, no special care needed	**100**	Normal, no complaints, no evidence of disease
	90	Able to carry on normal activity, minor signs or symptoms of disease
	80	Normal activity with effort, some signs or symptoms of disease
B. Unable to work, able to live at home, cares for most personal needs; a varying amount of assistance is needed	**70**	Cares for self, unable to carry on normal activity or to do active work
	60	Requires occasional assistance but is able to care for most of his need
	50	Requires considerable assistance and frequent medical care
C. Unable to take care of self; requires the equivalent of institutional or hospital care; disease may be progressing rapidly	**40**	Disabled; requires special care and assistance
	30	Severely disabled; hospitalization is indicated, although death is not imminent
	20	Very sick; hospitalization necessary, active supportive treatment is needed
	10	Moribund, fatal processes rapidly progressing
	0	Dead

Note: It indirectly indicates how the body and its various systems have been affected by the cancer. It also helps in prognostication of the disease. Performance status is given during presentation of the cancer patients.

2B: WHO Criteria - Performance Status

0. Able to carry on normal activity
1. Patient able to live at home. Tolerable tumor manifestations
2. Patient with disabling tumor manifestations but < 50% of time in bed
3. Patient severely disabled and > 50% of time in bed but able to stand up
4. Patient very sick
5. Dead

3A: Evidence-based Classification of Medical Literature (Agency for Health Care Policy and Research)	
Class I Evidence	**Prospective, randomized controlled trials** – the gold standard of clinical trials. Some may be poorly designed, have inadequate numbers, or suffer from other methodologic inadequacies and thus may not be clinically significant
Class II Evidence	Clinical studies in which the data were collected **prospectively and retrospective analyses** that were based on clearly reliable data. These types of studies include observational studies, cohort studies, prevalence studies, and case control studies.
Class III Evidence	Studies based on **retrospectively collected data**. Evidence used in this class includes clinical series, databases or registries, case reviews, case reports, and expert opinion

3B: Categorization of Strengths of Recommendations for Evidence- Based Practice	
Level I	This recommendation is **convincingly justifiable** based on the available scientific information alone. It is usually based on class I data; however, strong class II evidence may form the basis for a level I recommendation, especially if the issue does not lend itself to testing in a randomized format. Conversely, weak or contradictory class I data may not be able to support a level I recommendation.
Level II	This recommendation is **reasonably justifiable** by available scientific evidence and strongly supported by expert critical care opinion. It is usually supported by class II data or a preponderance of class III evidence.
Level III	This recommendation is supported by available data, but **adequate scientific evidence is lacking**. It is generally supported by class III data. This type of recommendation is useful for educational purposes and in guiding future studies.

4A: Grading of Pulses – Traditional	
4 +	Normal
3 +	Slightly reduced
2 +	Markedly reduced
1 +	Barely palpable
0	Absent

4B: Grading of Pulses - Basic

2 +	Normal
1 +	Diminished
0	Absent

5: Medical Research Council (MRC) Grading System for Motor Power

- 0 – No contraction
- 1 – Flicker or trace of contraction
- 2 – Active movement in a plane perpendicular to gravity
- 3 – Active movement against gravity
- 4 – Active movement against gravity and resistance
- 5 – Normal power

6: MRC Classification of Sensory Nerve Dysfunction

Grade	*Clinical features*
S0	No sensation
S1	Deep pain sensation
S2	Skin touch, pain and thermal sensation, i.e. protective sensation
S3	S2 also with accurate localization but deficient stereognosis. Cold sensitivity and hypersensitivity are often present
S3 +	Object and texture recognition, but not normal sensation. Good but not normal, two – point discrimination
S4	Normal sensation

7: Classification of Wounds Based on Contamination

Type of surgery	*Infection rate (%)*
Clean (no viscus opened)	1 – 2
Clean contaminated (viscus opened, minimal spillage)	< 10
Contaminated (open viscus with spillage)	15 – 20
Dirty (perforation of viscus or presence of pus)	< 40

8: Cell Cycle

1. M - Mitosis – Usually accomplished in 1 hour
2. G_0 phase – Resting phase of variable duration
3. G_1 phase – Prolonged phase upto 30 hours (unidentified processes are occurring)
4. S phase – (Synthetic phase) – DNA synthesis is occurring (Normally between 6 and 8 hours)
5. G_2 phase – Short phase in which unidentified processes are occurring (between 2 and 4 hours)

Note:

a. As many as 90% of the total population of tumor cells may be in the G_0 phase

b. The doubling time of a tumor may vary between 4 and 500 days, being most rapid for leukemias and slowest for solid tumors.

9: Nutritional Assessment Methods

1. Anthropometry
   - Body weight and body mass index (Weight in kilograms divided by height in meters squared) A BMI of < 18.5 indicates nutritional impairment
   - Fat stores – Triceps skin fold thickness
   - Muscle stores – Hand grip strength, mid arm muscle circumference (MAMC)
2. Biochemical
   - Serum albumin
   - Serum transferrin
   - Retinol binding protein
   - Thyroxine binding prealbumin
3. Immunological
   - Lymphocyte count
   - Skin hypersensitivity
4. Malnutrition Universal Screening Tool (MUST)

10A: Local Anesthetic Drugs for Infiltration and the Dosage

Drug	*Maximum dose without epinephrine (Adrenaline)*	*Maximum dose with epinephrine*
Xylocaine	4 mg/kg	7 mg/kg
Bupivacaine	3 mg/kg	
Safe volume for 0.5% of xylocaine	40 cc	100 cc
Safe volume for 1% of xylocaine	20 cc	50 cc
Safe volume for 2% of xylocaine	10 cc	25 cc

10B: Complications of Xylocaine

- Circumoral numbness (earliest manifestation)
- Muscle twitches
- Convulsions
- Followed by CNS depression which is followed by
- Cardiovascular depression (Hypotension and cardiac arrest)
- Respiratory depression

10C: Kern's Rule for Finding Out the Drug in Milligram per cc if the percentage is known

Percent of drug × 10 = mg of drug per cc
As per this formula 1 cc of 2% solution of Xylocaine contain 20 mg of the drug

11: Contraindications for Partial Thickness Skin Grafting

1. Gross infection with *Streptococcus pyogenes* or pseudomonas
2. Bone denuded of periostium.
3. Tendons denuded of paratenon
4. Cartilage denuded of perichondrium
5. Areas denuded of skin cover by previous irradiation

12: Lymphatic Drainage of Fingers

1. Little finger and ring finger	Epitrochlear nodes
2. Middle finger	Supraclavicular nodes
3. Index finger and thumb	Axillary nodes

13: Classification of Dermoids		
Type	*Origin*	*Examples*
Congenital	Arises in the line of embryonic fusion They lie deep to the skin and not attached to the skin	1. External angular: Line of fusion between frontonasal process and maxillary process 2. Postauricular: Line of fusion of the mesodermal hillocks which form the pinna 3. Sublingual: Below the tongue in the midline
Implantation dermoid	Develops after a puncture injury in which epithelial cells are implanted into the subcutaneous tissue	Found on the fingers or hand and toes
Sequestration dermoid	Formed by the inclusion of epithelial nests beneath the surface	Branchial cysts
Teratomatous dermoids	Malignant change can occur which may be carcinomatous/and sarcomatous	Found in the ovary, testis, retroperitoneum, superior mediastinum and presacral area

14: Differences between Transudate and Exudates		
Transudate	*Exudates*	
Protein	Low—most of which is albumin < 25g/L	High— > 25g/L High content of fibrinogen
Specific gravity	< 1.012	> 1.020
Glucose content	Same as plasma	Low < 60 mg/dL
pH	> 7.3	< 7.3
LDH	Low	High
Cellular debris	Few cells	More cells
Cause	Obstruction to the venous outflow from liver (ultrafiltrate of blood plasma and results from imbalance across the vascular endothelium). Permeability of endothelium—normal	Inflammatory extravascular fluid formed by the escape of fluid, proteins and blood cells from the vascular system into the interstitial tissue or body cavities due to increased vascular permeability
SAAG—(Serum Ascites albumin gradient)	> 1.1 (Ascitic fluid has less albumin than serum)	< 1.1 (Ascitic fluid has more albumin than serum)

15: Systemic Inflammatory Response Syndrome (SIRS)

(Two of the following criteria must be there)

- Hyperthermia - > 38°C or hypothermia <36°C
- Tachycardia > 90/min (no β blockers) or tachypnea >20/min
- White cell count > 12 × 10^9 or < 4 × 10^9

16: Differences between Hemangioma and Congenital Vascular Malformation

Hemangioma	*Vascular malformation*
1. Usually not present at birth	All lesions present at birth, not necessarily apparent
2. Rapid postnatal growth and slow evolution	Commensurate growth, may expand
3. Female to male 3 to 5 : 1	1:1
4. Endothelium hyperplastic	Flat endothelium
5. Increased mast cells	Normal mast cells
6. Multilaminated basement membrane	Thin unilaminated basement membrane
7. Primary platelet trapping (Kasabach – Merritt syndrome)	• Primary venous stasis • Local/disseminated intravascular coagulopathy
8. Infrequent pressure of adgacent bones	Defects with AV fistula: Hypertrophy of bones
9. Rarely overgrowth	Defects without AV fistula: Atrophy

17: Tumors Producing Hypoglycemia

1. Insulinoma
2. Hemangiopericytoma
3. Fibrosarcoma
4. Leiomyosarcoma
5. Hepatoma
6. Adrenocortical carcinoma

Trauma

18: Triage – ICRC Guidelines

- French "Triager" **to sort**
- Principle of "Best for Most"
- Categorization into three groups
- Marked in the forehead in Roman numerals

I - Urgent surgery
II – No surgery – (minor + very severe with little chance of survival)
III – Nonurgent surgery

19: Prevention of Trauma

- **Primary Prevention** – Antidrink driving, speed limit
- **Secondary** – Active – Helmet, Seat belts – Passive – ABS, air bags
- **Tertiary** – Minimize the effects of injury by improving health care delivery

20: Three Most Important X-Rays in Multisystem Trauma

- Lateral cervical spine
- Upright chest
- Pelvis

21: Trimodal Distribution of Death by *Donald Trunkey*

- Immediate death – 50% (within first few minutes)
- Early death (***GOLDEN HOUR*** and preventable death) – 30% (within first few hours)
- Late death – 20% (days or weeks after)

22: Dangerous Injuries

- Fall from height of 20 ft or more
- Crash greater than 20 miles/hr
- 20 inch impingement on the passenger compartment
- Ejection of the patient
- Roll over
- Death of another person

23: Advanced Trauma Life Support (ATLS) System (American College of Surgeons Committee on Trauma)

A Advanced
T Trauma
L Life
S Support
James Styner (1970) – Orthopedic Surgeon

24: Four Stage Approach (ATLS)

- Primary survey
- Resuscitation
- Secondary survey
- Definitive care
- It is a continuous process

25: Primary Survey (60 Sec Exam)

- **A** — AIRWAY
- **B** — BREATHING
- **C** — CIRCULATION
- **D** — DISABILITY
- **E** — EXPOSE, ENTRY

26: A– Airway Control

1. **Basic airway techniques**
   — Modified jaw thrust maneuver
   — Oral/nasopharyngeal airway
2. **Advanced Airway Techniques**
   — Oral or nasal intubation
   — Surgical/needle (13G) **cricothyroidotomy**

27: Indications for Ventilation in Chest Injury

- Tachypnea above 40
- PaO_2 below 60mm of Hg or less
- $PaCO_2$ above 45mm of Hg
- Progressive fall in PaO_2
- Extensive pulmonary contusion or diffuse infiltrative change on X-ray
- Severe flail chest — >8 Unilateral fractures of rib
- More than 4 bilateral — rib fractures

28: Life-threatening Chest Injuries

- Airway obstruction
- Tension pneumothorax
- Open pneumothorax
- Massive hemothorax — >1500 ml blood
- Flail chest
- Cardiac tamponade

29: C – Circulation

- **Radial pulse** is palpable with BP of 80mm of Hg
- **Femoral pulse** is palpable with BP of 70mm of Hg
- **Carotid pulse** is palpable with BP of 60 mm of Hg

30: The Tennis Score Classification of Hemorrhage

Hemorrhage	*% blood loss*	*Vol. of blood loss (mL)*	*Pulse rate*	*BP*	*Pulse pressure*	*Respiratory rate*
Class 1	Upto 15	Upto 750	< 100	Normal	Normal or increased	14-20
Class 2	15-30	750-1500	> 100	Normal	Decreased	20-30
Class 3	30-40	1500-2200	> 120	Decreased	Decreased	30-40
Class 4	> 40	> 2000	> 140	Decreased	Decreased	> 35

31: Five Places where Patient can Lose Large Volume Blood (Blood on the floor and four more)

- Externally
- The chest
- The abdomen
- The retroperitoneum
- Into muscle compartment

32: D—Disability (Glasgow Coma Scale)

Response	*Details*	*Score*
Eye opening	Spontaneous	4
	Speech	3
	Pain	2
	None	1
Verbal response	Orientated	5
	Confused	4
	Inappropriate words	3
	Incomprehensible sounds	2
	None	1
Best motor response	Obeys commands	6
	Localizes pain	5
	Withdrawal from pain	4
	Flexion to pain	3
	Extension to pain	2
	None	1

33: Resuscitation Phase

- Secure large bore IV access
- Shock therapy
- Continuous EKG monitoring
- Blood samples – CBC, electrolytes, glucose, coagulation studies, ABG, cross matching
- **NG tube (Nasogastric)**
- **Foley's catheter**

34: Poiseuille's Law

- Flow is proportional to the fourth power of the radius of the cannula and inversely related to it's length
- 14G two peripheral IV lines are better than the central cannula
- 14G 2 ¼" length – flow of 200cc/min
- 16G 8" length – central cannula;flow rate – 150cc/min

35: Contraindications for Nasogastric Tube and Foley's Catheter

Contraindications for NG Tube in Trauma

- Fracture of the cribriform plate

Contraindications for Foley's

- Rupture urethra—Blood at the meatus

If urethral trauma is suspected—Urethrogram

36: Avoid Hypothermia in Trauma

- All IV fluids stored at 39°C
- PRC reconstituted by warm saline
- Fluid warmer
- Warm blankets
- Warm irrigating fluids

Hypothermia Produces

- Cardiac irritability
- Coagulopathy
- Enzyme impairment

37: Bloody Vicious Cycle in Trauma

- Metabolic acidosis
- Profound hypothermia
- Coagulopathy

38: Autotransfusion—Not Recommended

- Consumptive coagulopathy
- Platelet dysfunction
- These risks may outweigh the benefits of autotransfusion

39: Secondary Survey

- Head to toe examination
- Look, listen and feel
- **High yield X-rays**
  - Cervical lateral
  - Upright chest
  - Pelvis
- **Rule out intra-abdominal bleeding** in all cases of multisystem trauma

40: Secondary Survey AMPLE History

- **A** — Allergy
- **M** — Medication
- **P** — Past medical history
- **L** — Last meal
- **E** — Events of the incident

41: Rule Out Intra-abdominal Bleeding in Every Patient

- CT scan/USG
- Physical examination
- Serial hematocrit
- FAST – Focused assessment with sonography for trauma
- DPL (diagnostic peritoneal lavage)

42: Tertiary Survey

- 15% incidence of clinically significant injuries diagnosed after initial resuscitation
- Tertiary survey – Physical examination
- Review of results
- Early detection of all clinically significant injuries

43: Damage Control in Surgery (Three Phase Surgical Approach)

Phase 1 - Control hemorrhage, contain contamination
Phase 2 - ICU – Restore normal physiology
Phase 3 - Definitive surgery

44: Monson's Zones for Penetrating Neck Injuries

- Zone 1 – Structures at the thoracic outlet (below a horizontal line inferior to the cricoid cartilage)
- Zone 2 – Between zone 1 and the angle of the mandible (between the angle of the mandible and above the horizontal line inferior to the cricoid cartilage)
- Zone 3 – From the angle of the mandible to the base of the skull (between the angle of the mandible and the base of the skull)

Note: Zone 1 – Are liberally explored
Zone 2 and 3 – With clinical evidence of vascular and visceral injuries–exploration
Without clinical evidence of vascular and visceral injuries – four vessel angiogram, esophagogram and esophagoscopy are done and depending on the finding operative exploration is done.

45: Classification of Retroperitoneal Hematoma

Zone 1	Central medial – extends from the diaphragmatic hiatus to the sacral promontory	All penetrating injuries and all Zone 1 hematomas are explored
Zone 2	Flank retroperitoneal hematoma	• All penetrating injuries explored • Blunt injury with hematomas contained in Gerota's fascia and not expanding are managed conservatively • Blunt injury with expanding hematomas are explored
Zone 3	Pelvic retroperitoneal hematoma	• Not explored • Therapeutic embolization is the treatment of choice

Burns

46: Classification of Burns			
Degree of burns	*Involvement of skin*	*Characters*	*Resolution*
First degree	Epidermis alone	Erythema	Resolves in 48 – 72 hrs Heals uneventfully No scarring
Second degree (partial thickness) two types: **superficial and deep**	**Epidermis plus some part of dermis** • **Superficial second degree**: injury to the epidermis and superficial dermis • **Deep second degree**: deep dermal involvement	• **Blister** for superficial, weepy and painful • **Reddish** for deep, decreased sensation	• Superficial heal with minimal scarring in 10 – 14 days • Deep takes 25-35 days for healing, produces hypertrophic scar and **skin grafting may be required**
Third degree (full thickness)	Full thickness involving the subcutaneous fat	• White, waxy appearance • Lack of sensation • Leathery texture • Lack of capillary refill	No potential for reepithelialization Need skin grafting
Fourth degree	Underlying muscles, tendons, bone and brain are involved		

47: Rule of Nine of Wallace		
Each upper limb	–	9% of TBSA (Total Body Surface Area)
Each lower limb	–	18% of TBSA (9% for anterior half and 9% for posterior half)
Head and neck	–	9% of TBSA
Front and back of trunk	–	18% each
Genitalia	–	1%

Note: The patients whole hand (digit and palm) represents 1% of TBSA
In children the area of head and neck is amended to 18% and the lower limb to 12%

48: Parkland Formula for Resuscitation of Burns
4ml/kg per percentage TBSA burn (TBSA × weight in Kg × 4 = volume in ml)

Note:
- This calculates the fluid to be replaced in the first 24 hours
- Half of this volume is given in the first eight hours and the second half is given in the subsequent 16 hours
- The fluid is given as Ringer's lactate
- IV resuscitation is required for children with a burn greater than 10% of TBSA
- IV resuscitation is required for adults with a burn greater than 15% of TBSA
- If oral fluids are used, salt must be added

49: Types of Burns

1. Flame burns – Damage from super heated oxidized air (mixed deep dermal and full thickness)
2. Scald – Damage from hot liquids (superficial, with deep dermal patches – may be deep in young infant)
3. Fat burns – Damage from hot oil (Deep dermal)
4. Chemical – Contact with alkali and acids and other chemicals (weak concentration of chemical produces superficial dermal and strong concentration produces deep dermal)
5. Electric burns – Conduction of electrical current through tissues (Full thickness burns)
6. Contact burns – Contact withhot solid material

50: Complications of Burns

1. **Immediate complications**
   a. Infection
      - *Clostridium tetani*
      - Streptococcal infection
      - Pseudomonas
   b. Duodenal and gastric ulceration
      - **Curling's ulcer**
      - Erosions in stomach and duodenum
   c. Renal failure
   d. Liver necrosis
   e. Pulmonary complications
      – pulmonary edema and atelectasis
   f. Burn encephalopathy in children (Cerebral edema)
2. **Intermediate complications**
   a. *Pseudomonas septicemia*
   b. Pneumonia
   c. Decubitus ulcers
   d. Constricting eschar
   e. Embolic lung phenomena
3. **Late complications**
   a. Contractures
   b. Hypertrophic scar
   c. Pruritus

51: Differences between Hypertrophic Scar and Keloid

	Hypertrophic scar	*Keloid*
Relationship with the original wound	Rises above the skin level but stays within the confines of the original wound	Rises above the skin level, extends beyond the border of the original wound
Regression	Regress over time	Rarely regress spontaneously
Familial	Not familial	May be familial, autosomal dominant
Race	Not race related	More in black than the white (15 times)
Sex	Men and women equally affected	Women > men

Contd...

Contd...

	Hypertrophic scar	*Keloid*
Age group	Children	10 – 30 years
Site	Areas of tension and flexor surfaces which tend to be at right angles to joints/skin creases	Sternum, shoulder, face, skin of ear lobe, deltoid and upper back regions
Cause	Related to tension	Unknown: can result from surgery, burns, skin inflammation, acne, chicken pox, zoster, folliculitis, lacerations, abrasions, tattoos, vaccinations, injections, ear piercing, etc. or spontaneously
Histology	Collagen bundles are flatter, more random and in a wavy pattern	Collagen bundles are virtually nonexistent and fibers arranged haphazardly and are larger and thicker
Immune system	Higher T lymphocyte and Langerhans cell content	Antinuclear antibody (ANA) against fibroblast, epithelial cells and endothelial cells present

Note: Clinically keloid is itching, spreading, tender and vascular.

Neck

52: WHO Grading (1994) of Goiter

Grade 0 : **No palpable / visible** goiter
Grade 1 : A thyroid that is **palpable** but **not visible** when the neck is in normal position
Grade 2 : An enlarged thyroid that is **visible with** the neck in normal position

53: Surgical Causes for Horner's Syndrome

1. Extracapsular invasion of cervical node
2. Extralaryngeal involvement of laryngeal cancer
3. Cervical sympathetic involvement in lung cancer
4. Cervical sympathetic involvement in carcinoma thyroid

54: Half-life of Radio Isotopes Used in Thyroid

Isotopes	*Half life*	*Route of administration*	*Rays*	*Comment*
I^{123}	13 hrs	Oral	γ rays	Will not detect nodules < 1 cm size
I^{131}	8 days	Oral	γ and β rays	Too much irradiation for diagnostic scanning
I^{132}	2.3 hrs	Oral	""	
TC^{99}	6 hrs	IV	""	

Breast

55: Reporting of Fine Needle Aspiration Cytology (FNAC) Results	
Grade	*Result*
AC0	No epithelial cells present
AC1	Scanty benign cells
AC2	Benign cells
AC3	Atypical cells present—may need a biopsy if clinically or radiologically suspicious
AC4	Highly suspicious of malignancy
AC5	Definitely malignant

56: Reporting of Core Biopsy Results	
Grade	*Result*
B1	Normal breast tissue
B2	Benign lesion
B3	Hyperplastic lesion present
B4	Severe atypia or carcinoma or carcinoma *in situ* requiring excision
B5	Malignant lesion

57A: Bloom Richardson Grading of Carcinoma Breast

1. Tumor tubule formation
   - > 75% of tumor cells arranged in tubules - score 1
   - > 10% and < 75% - score 2
   - < 10% - score 3
2. Number of mitoses
   - < 10% mitoses in 10HPF (high power field) - score 1
   - > 10% mitoses and < 20 mitoses - score 2
   - > 20 mitoses per HPF - score 3
3. Nuclear pleomorphism
   - Cells nuclei are uniform in size and shape, **relatively smal**l, without prominent nucleoli - score 1
   - Cell nuclei are somewhat pleomorphic, have nucleoli and are **intermediate in size** - score 2
   - Cell nuclei are **relatively large,** have **prominent nucleoli** / multiple nucleoli, coarse chromatin pattern and vary in size and shape - score 3

57B: Bloom Richardson Combined Scores: (BR Grade)

BR grade 3, 4, 5	-	Well-differentiated (**low grade**)
BR grade 6. 7	-	Moderately differentiated (**intermediate grade**)
BR grade 8, 9	-	Poorly differentiated (**high grade**)

58: Nottingham Prognostic Index (NPI)

Nottingham Prognostic Index (NPI)

NPI = (0.2 x size in cm) + grade + stage

Good < 3.4, **Moderate** 3.4 – 5.4, **Poor** > 5.4

59: WHO Definition of Objective Response to Anterior Chemotherapy

Complete clinical response	**Disappearance** of palpable disease
Partial response	**Decrease of ≥ 50%** in total size of tumor
No change	**Decrease of < 50%** or increase of < 25% in total size of tumor at 6 months
Progressive disease	**Increase of ≥ 25%** in total size of palpable lesion

60: Van Nuys Prognostic Index for DCIS (Ductal Carcinoma *in Situ*)

The factors responsible for local recurrence after wide local excision in DCIS are:

- Disease extent
- Excision margin
- Histological type

By scoring **three major predictors** for recurrence, a prognostic index has been developed.

Van Nuys prognostic index for DCIS (Ductal carcinoma *in situ*)

	Score
Disease extent	
• 15 mm	1
• 15 – 40 mm	2
• > 40 mm	3
Margin	
• < 10 mm	1
• 1 – 9 mm	2
• 1 mm	3
Histological type	
• Nonhigh grade	1
• High grade, no necrosis	2
• High grade + necrosis	3

- It is suggested that patients with score of **3, 4 and 5** be treated by **wide local excision**
- **6 and 7** by wide local excision and radiotherapy
- **8 and 9** by mastectomy.

61: Indications for Radiotherapy after Mastectomy in Carcinoma Breast

1. Large tumors (> 4 cm)
2. High grade tumors (Bloom Richardson grade 3)
3. Node positive tumors (4 or more nodes positive) and extranodal disease
4. Node negative tumors with widespread vascular/lymphatic invasion

62: Complications after Mastectomy

1. Seroma
2. Infection
3. Flap necrosis
4. Injury to neurovascular structures
5. Pneumothorax
6. Lymphedema
7. Frozen shoulder
8. Lymphangiosarcoma (late)

63: Causes for Nipple Retraction

1. Congenital
2. Acquired (Slit-like appearance)
   - Carcinoma
   - Duct ectasia
   - Periductal mastitis
   - Tuberculosis

Abdomen

64: Causes for Dysphagia

Lesions in the wall of the esophagus

1. Stricture
   A. Posttraumatic
   B. Corrosives
2. Benign tumors
3. Malignant neoplasms (carcinoma)
4. Acute and chronic esophagitis
5. Crohn's disease
6. Esophageal diverticulum – congenital, pulsion, traction or pseudodiverticula
7. Scleroderma
8. Abnormalities of esophageal contraction
   A. Achalasia
   B. Diffuse esophageal spasm
   C. Cricopharyngeal spasm
9. Medical conditions
   A. Bulbar paralysis
   B. Cerebrovascular accidents
   C. Tetanus
   D. Myasthenia gravis
10. Postvagotomy
11. Globus hystericus (Dysphagia occurring in moments of tension)

Lesions outside the wall of the esophagus

- Thyroid swellings
- Retrosternal goiter
- Pharyngeal pouch

Contd...

Contd...

- Aortic aneurysm
- Abnormal aortic arch
- Mediastinal tumors and lymph nodes
- Paraesophageal hiatus hernia
- Dysphagia Lusoria (Vascular ring): Anomalous aortic arch leaving a vascular ring containing the trachea and esophagus
- Tight repair of hiatus hernia

Lesions in the lumen of the esophagus

- Foreign bodies: Fish bones, coins, pins, and dentures
- Webs
- Schatzki's rings – Circumferential Web-like Obstruction at the lower esophagus in association with hiatus hernia
- Sideropenic dysphagia (Plummer - Vinson syndrome): The web is situated in the postcricoid region (**Tongue devoid of papillae, koilonychia and angular stomatitis or cheilosis**)

65: Endoscopic Grading of Esophageal Varices

Grade 1 – visible, nontortuous
Grade 2 – tortuous, nonprotruding
Grade 3 – protruding (normal mucosa in between the columns)
Grade 4 – like grade 3, no normal mucosa in between

66: Difference Between Duodenal and Gastric Ulcer

	Duodenal ulcer	*Gastric ulcer*
Age group	25 – 50	Late middle age and elderly (55 – 65)
Sex	Male preponderance	Sex incidence equal
Socioeconomic status	Higher socioeconomic group	Lower socioeconomic group
Location	Duodenopyloric junction	Anywhere along the lesser curvature. Near incisura angularis
Location of pain	Epigastrium	Epigastrium
Hunger pain	Present, and relief with food	Absent, food aggravates pain and afraid to eat

Contd...

Contd...

	Duodenal ulcer	*Gastric ulcer*
Weight gain/loss	Likely to be overweight	Weight loss
Nausea, vomiting	Not usually a feature unless obstructed	More commonly seen
Periodicity	Remitting disease characterized by: Periodicity of activity and quiescence	Periodicity not observed
Malignant change	Never	May turn malignant (0.5%)
Helicobacter pylori infection	90% of duodenal ulcer cases	75% infected
Parietal cell mass	Increased	Not increased

67: Classification of Gastric Ulcers

Type I	Ulcer in the antrum (antral ulcers)
Type II	Combined gastric and duodenal ulcer
Type III	Prepyloric ulcer (In the pyloric canal)

68: Causes of Gastric Outlet Obstruction

- Peptic ulcer disease in distal stomach/duodenum with scarring
- Gastric carcinoma in antrum
- Congenital hypertrophic pyloric stenosis
- Annular pancreas
- Bezoar (furball, vegetable matter)
- Lymphoma
- Gastritis
- Crohn's disease (stomach or duodenum)
- TB
- Impacted foreign bodies
- Metastases

69: Forrest's Classification for Activity of Bleed in Upper GI Endoscopy

Grade Ia:	Spurting vessel at base of lesion
Grade Ib:	Ooze of blood from lesion
Grade 2a:	Nonbleeding visible vessel at base of lesion
Grade 2b:	**S**tigmata of **R**ecent **H**emorrhage (SRH): adherent clot, black spot
Grade 3:	Lesion seen but no evidence of recent bleed

70A: Child - Turcote - Pugh Classification of Functional Status in Liver Disease

Parameter	*Numerical score* *1* *Class - A* *Risk – Low*	*2* *Class - B* *Risk – Moderate*	*3* *Class - C* *Risk – High*
Ascites	Absent	Slight to Moderate	Tense
Encephalopathy	None	Grade I – II	Grade III – IV
Serum Albumin (g/dL)	> 3.5	2.8 to 3.5	< 2.8
Serum Bilirubin mg/dL	< 2	2.0 – 3.0	> 3.0
Prothrombin time (Seconds above control)	< 4.0	4.0 – 6.0	> 6.0

70B:

Total score	*Child – Turcote – Pugh classification*	*Risk*
5 – 6	A	Low risk
7 – 9	B	Moderate risk
10 – 15	C	High risk

71: UICC Staging of Gallbladder Cancer

Stage I	Confined to the mucosa/submucosa
Stage II	Involvement of the muscle layer
Stage III	Serosal involvement
Stage IV	Spread to the cystic node
Stage V (advanced carcinoma)	Invasion of the liver and adjacent organs

72: Bismuth Classification of Bile Duct Strictures

Type I	Low common hepatic duct stricture – hepatic duct stump > 2 cm
Type II	Mid common hepatic duct stricture – hepatic duct stump < 2 cm
Type III	Hilar stricture with no residual common hepatic duct – hilar confluence intact
Type IV	Destruction of hilar confluence – right and left hepatic ducts separated
Type V	Involvement of the aberrant right sectoral duct alone or along with the common hepatic duct

73: Bismuth Classification of Perihilar cholangiocarcinoma

Type I	Confined to the common hepatic duct
Type II	Involves bifurcation without involvement of secondary intrahepatic ducts
Type IIIa and b	Extend into either the **right or left** secondary intrahepatic ducts respectively
Type IV	Involve the secondary intrahepatic ducts on both sides

74: Todani Classification of Choledochal Cyst

Type I (**50%**)	Fusiform or cystic dilatation of the extrahepatic biliary tract
Type II	Saccular diverticulum of extrahepatic bile duct
Type III	Bile duct dilatation within the duodenal wall (**choledochocele**)
Type IV (**35%**)	Cystic dilatation of both intrahepatic and extrahepatic biliary tract
Type V	Intrahepatic cysts (**Caroli's disease**)

75a: Ranson's Prognostic Signs for Gallstone Pancreatitis

Admission	*Initial 48 hours*
Age > 70 years	Hct fall > 10
WBC > 18,000/mm^3	BUN elevation > 2 mg/100 ml
Glucose > 220 mg/100 ml	Ca^{2+} < 8 mg/100 mL
LDH > 40 IU/l	Base deficit > 5 mEq/L
AST > 250 U/100 ml	Fluid sequestration > 4L

75b: Ranson's Prognostic Signs for Nongallstone Pancreatitis	
Admission	*Initial 48 hours*
Age > 55 years	Hct fall > 10
WBC > 16,000/mm^3	BUN elevation > 5mg/100ml
Glucose > 200 mg/100 ml	Ca^{2+} < 8mg/100ml
LDH > 350 IU/l	Pao_2 < 55 mm Hg
AST > 250 U/100 ml	Base deficit > 4 mEq/l
	Fluid sequestration > 6l

Note:

- Patients with fewer than 3 of the prognostic criteria can be expected to have a mild attack
- 3 or more criteria suggest bad prognosis
- 5 or 6 signs require ICU care

76: Glasgow Scoring System (Prognostic Score) for Acute Pancreatitis	
On admission	*Within 48 hours*
Age > 55 years	Serum albumin < 3.2 gm
WBC > 15,000/mm^3	Ca^{2+} < 8 mg/100 ml
Glucose > 200 mg/100 ml	LDH > 600 IU/l
Serum urea > 5 mg% (no response to IV fluids)	AST/ALT > 600 U/100 ml
Arterial oxygen saturation < 60 Mm Hg	

77: Anatomical Difference Between Jejunum and Ileum		
Sl. No:	*Jejunum*	*Ileum*
1.	Large circumference	Smaller circumference
2.	1 – 2 vascular arcades in the mesentery	4-5 vascular arcades
3.	Long vasa recta from the arcade	Shorter vasa recta
4.	Thick wall	Thin wall

78: Positions of Appendix

Retrocecal (65%)	12 O' clock position
Splenic	2 O' clock position
Promontoric	3 O' clock position
Pelvic (30%)	4 O' clock position
Mid inguinal	6 O' clock position
Paracolic	11 O' clock position

79: Alvarado Score (Mantrels)

	Score
Symptoms	
• Migratory RIF pain	1
• Anorexia	1
• Nausea and vomiting	1
Signs	
• Tenderness (RIF)	2
• Rebound tenderness	1
• Elevated temperature	1
Laboratory	
• Leukocytosis	2
• Shift to left (increase in the number of immature neutrophils) or banded forms	1
Total score	**10**

Note: A score of 7 or more is strongly predictive of acute appendicitis.

80: Classification of Acute Diverticulitis (Hinchey)

Stage 1	Pericolic abscess or phlegmon
Stage 2	Pelvic or intra-abdominal abscess
Stage 3	Nonfeculent peritonitis
Stage 4	Feculent peritonitis

81: Grading of Severity of Ulcerative Colitis

1. Mild	Rectal bleeding or diarrhea with four or fewer motions without systemic signs
2. Moderate	> 4 motions per day. No systemic signs of illness
3. Severe	> 4 motions per day with 1 or more signs of systemic illness

82: Signs of Systemic Illness of Ulcerative Colitis

- Fever over 37.5°C
- Tachycardia > 90/min
- Hypoalbuminemia < 3 gm/liter
- Weight loss > 3 kg

83: Comparison of Ulcerative Colitis and Crohn's Disease

Symptoms, signs, radiology, pathology, natural history and treatment	*Ulcerative colitis*	*Crohn's disease*
Diarrhea	Marked	Less severe
Gross bleeding	Characteristic	Infrequent
Perianal lesions	Infrequent and mild	Frequent and complex
Toxic dilatation	Present in 3 – 10%	Present in 2 – 5%
Perforation	Free	Localized
Systemic manifestations	Common	Common
Radiology	Confluent, diffuse	Skip areas
	Loss of haustration and lead pipe appearance	Cobble-stone appearance
	Coarse mucosa	Longitudinal ulcers and transverse ridges
	Concentric involvement	Eccentric involvement
	Internal fistula rare	Internal fistula common

Contd...

Contd...

Symptoms, signs, radiology, pathology, natural history and treatment	*Ulcerative colitis*	*Crohn's disease*
	Only colonic involvement, except back wash ileitis	Any portion of the intestine involved
Gross morphology	Confluent involvement Rectum usually involved Mesocolon not involved No thickening of bowel wall	Segmental, with skip areas Rectum often not involved Thickened mesocolon Thickened bowel wall due to transmural inflammation
	No mesenteric fat advancement	Mesenteric fat advancement towards antimesenteric border
	Widespread superficial ulcers	Longitudinal ulcers and transverse fissures
	Inflammatory polyps common (pseudo polyps)	Not prominent
Microscopic	Inflammation limited to mucosa and submucosa (crypt abscess)	Chronic inflammation of all layers of bowel wall
	Muscle coat involved in severe cases only	Muscle coat damaged usually
	Granulomas rare	Granulomas frequent
Natural history	Exacerbations and remissions, may be explosive and lethal	Indolent and recurrent
Response to medical treatment	Good response in 85%	Difficult to evaluate, less well-controlled
Type of surgical treatment	Proctocolectomy with ileoanal anastomosis	Segmental colectomy, total colectomy + ileorectal anastomosis Recurrence common

84: Differences between Ulcerative and Hyperplastic Type of Intestinal Tuberculosis

Sl.No.	Features	Ulcerative	Hyperplastic
1.	Primary/Secondary	Secondary to pulmonary tuberculosis	Primary (ingestion of milk)
2.	Virulence of the organism	Virulence outstrips the resistance of the patient	Resistance of the patient is high and virulence of the organism is low
3.	Associated pulmonary tuberculosis	Primary in the chest demons-trated (PT)	No primary in the chest
4.	Clinical presentation	Patient is very ill	Not very ill
5.	""	Diarrhea/bleeding	Mass right iliac fossa
6.	Gross pathology	Multiple transverse ulcers in the ileum	Thickening of the intestinal wall, narrowing of the lumen
7.	Pathology	Caseation present	Absence of gross caseation

85: Risk Stratification of Gastrointestinal Stromal Tumor (GIST) NIH Consensus

Risk	Size	No. of mitoses/50 HPF
Very low	< 2 cm	< 5
Low	2 – 5 cm	5 – 10
Intermediate	5 – 10 cm	10
High risk	> 10 cm	-

86: Radiographic or Endoscopic Features Suggesting Malignancy in GIST

1. Invasion to surrounding structures
2. Evidence of dissemination
3. Size > 5 cm
4. Lobulated border
5. Heterogeneous enhancement
6. Mesenteric fat infiltration
7. Ulceration
8. Presence of regional adenopathy
9. Exophytic growth pattern
10. Hemorrhage
11. Necrosis
12. Cyst formation

87: Bad Prognostic Factors in GIST

- Male gender
- Incomplete resection
- Nongastric tumor
- High tumor cellularity
- High Ki-67 count

88: Staging of Desmoid Tumors of Abdomen with its Management (SCNA June 2008)

Stage I	Asymptomatic not growing	• Simple observation • Nontoxic Therapy (NSAIDs) • Resection if found incidentally during surgery
Stage II	Symptomatic, < 10 cm in maximum diameter Not growing	• Resection • Tamoxifen + NSAIDS if unresectable
Stage III	Symptomatic, 10-20 cm in maximum diameter Asymptomatic and slowly growing	• Active treatment • NSAIDs • Tamoxifen/relaxifen • Vinblastine/Methotrexate • Adriamycin/dacarbazine
Stage IV	Symptomatic, > 20cm or Rapid growing or Complicated	• Urgent therapy – major surgery +· • Antisarcoma chemotherapy +· • Radiation

SCNA – Surgical Clinics of North America.

Vascular

89: ABI (Ankle Brachial Index) and Symptoms of Vascular Disease

ABI	*Symptoms*
> 0.9	None
0.5 to 0.8	Claudication
0.3 to 0.5	Rest pain
< 0.3	Gangrene

90: Differences between Acute Thrombosis and Embolism

Feature	*Embolism*	*Thrombosis*
• Source	• Cardiac source (60-70%) • Noncardiac source (15-20%): e.g. aneurysms, poststenotic dilatation	• Atherosclerotic stenosis (no distant source) • Hypercoagulable states • Iatrogenic (angiography and catheterization) • Trauma
• History of claudication	None	Usually present
• Onset	Sudden	Usually gradual, unless traumatic
• Contralateral pulse	Normal	May be absent
• Loss of function	Rapid	Gradual (because of the presence of collaterals)

91: Wagner's Classification of Diabetic Foot

Grade 0	High risk and no ulceration
Grade I	Superficial ulcer
Grade II	Deep ulcer (Cellulitis)
Grade III	Osteomyelitis with ulceration and abscess
Grade IV	Gangrenous patches/partial foot gangrene (fore foot)
Grade V	Gangrene of the entire foot

92: Staging of Pressure Sores (American National Pressure Ulcer Advisory Panel)

Stage 1	Nonblanchable erythema without a breach in the epidermis • Color - red/blue/purple • Consistency - firm/boggy
Stage 2	Partial thickness skin loss involving the epidermis and dermis
Stage 3	Full thickness skin loss extending into the subcutaneous tissue but not through the underlying fascia
Stage 4	Full thickness skin loss through fascia with extensive tissue destruction, may be involving muscle, bone, tendon or joint

93: Shamblin Classification of Carotid Body Tumor

Group I: The tumor can be easily removed from the carotids

Group II: Subadventitial dissection of the vessel is required

Group III: Arterial excision and grafting are required

94: Deep Vein Thrombosis (DVT) Abnormalities of Thrombosis and Fibrinolysis Responsible for DVT

Congenital

- Antithrombin III deficiency
- Protein C deficiency
- Protein S deficiency
- Resistance to activated Protein C (due to factor V Leiden)
- Increased factor VIII
- Factor VII deficiency
- Factor XII deficiency
- Disorders of the fibrinolytic system
- Mutation in prothrombin

Acquired

- Antiphospholipid syndrome
- **Lupus anticoagulant**
- Hyperhomocysteinemia
- Secondary causes of hypercoagulability
- Hyperviscosity syndrome
- Nephrotic syndrome
- Malignancy
- Diabetes
- Sepsis
- Stroke
- Pregnancy

95: Virchow's Triad for Development of Venous Thrombosis

- Endothelial damage
- Stasis of blood flow
- Hypercoagulability (Thrombophilia)

96: Risk Assessment Protocol from the THRIFT (Thromboembolic Risk Factors) Consensus Group

Risk Level	*Group*	*Suggested Prophylaxis*
Low	Minor surgery **Major surgery < 40 years** Minor trauma Minor medical illness	Leg elevation and early mobilization
Moderate	**Major surgery > 40 years** Major trauma or burns Major medical illness Minor surgery and risks Inflammatory bowel disease	As low risk + Antiembolism hosiery **or** Subcutaneous heparin Mechanical calf compression
High	Hip, pelvis, knee **fracture** Major **cancer surgery** Surgery and thrombophilia Surgery and previous thrombosis Acute lower limb paralysis Illness and thrombophilia Illness and previous thrombosis	Both antiembolism hosiery and subcutaneous heparin Mechanical calf compression

97: Risk Factors for Venous Thromboembolism

Patient factor	*Disease or surgical procedure*
Age > 60 years	**Trauma or surgery**, especially of pelvis, hip, lower limb
Obesity	**Malignancy**, especially pelvis, abdominal metastatic
Immobilization	**Recent myocardial infarction**
Varicose veins	**Heart failure**
Pregnancy	Paralysis of lower limb (s)
Puerperium	Inflammatory bowel disease
High dose **oestrogen therapy**	Nephrotic syndrome
Previous deep vein thrombosis or pulmonary embolism	Polycythemia
Thrombophilia [see previous chart]	Paraproteinemia Behçet's disease Infection

98: Diagnosis, Management and Complications of DVT

1. **Diagnosis of DVT**
   a. D-dimer assay
   b. Compression ultrasonography (Duplex ultrasonography of the deep veins)
   c. Ascending venography (rarely required)
2. **Treatment** of established DVT – **Low Molecular Weight Heparin (LMWH) f**or **5 days** and **Warfarin** for 6 months.
3. **Complications** – **Pulmonary embolism**
   – **Triad of** tender calves, pleural pain and hemoptysis
   – Sudden collapse followed by death in 20%
   – Other symptoms are central chest pain, tachypnea, cough, cyanosis
   – **CT scanning of the pulmonary arteries** show **filling defect**

Limbs

99: Causes of Unilateral Lower Limb Edema

1. Cellulitis
2. Lower limb edema from lymphatic causes
   - **Primary Lymphedema**
     a) **lymphedema congenita – onset < 2 years (more common in males Sporadic and Familial** (Milroy's Disease)
     b) **lymphedema praecox –** 2 to 35 **years, more common in females** (sporadic or familial). **The familial is called** Meige's disease**.**
     c) **lymphedema tarda –** after 35 **years (associated with obesity – the nodes are replaced with fibrofatty tissue)**
   - **Secondary Lymphedema**
     - Lymphatic filariasis
     - Other infections – Tuberculosis, lympho-granuloma inguinale
     - Tumors of the pelvic floor (prostate cancer)
     - Surgical dissection of lymph nodes (block dissection)
     - Orthopedic surgery

   Radiation therapy for malignant tumors
     - Advanced intrapelvic and intraabdominal tumors
     - Recurrent soft tissue infections
     - Podoconiosis (cutaneous absorption of mineral particles)
3. **Lower limb edema due to venous causes**
   - Chronic venous insufficiency
   - Postthrombotic syndrome
   - Deep vein thrombosis
   - Phlegmasia alba dolens **(white leg or milk leg)**
   - Phlegmasia cerulea dolens
   - Varicose vein stripping
   - Vein harvesting

Contd...

Contd...

4. Arterial causes: Arteriovenous malformation
   Aneurysm
   Ischemia - reperfusion (following lower limb revascularization)
5. Edema secondary to congenital vascular anomalies
   - Lymphatic angiodysplasia syndrome
   - Klippel – Trenaunay's syndrome
   - Hyperstomy syndrome
6. **Posttraumatic**: Sympathetic dystrophy
7. **Obesity**: Lipodystrophy. Lipoidosis
8. Gigantism
9. **Retroperitoneal fibrosis**: Causes arterial, venous and lymphatic abnormalities
10. **Hansen's disease**
11. **Dermal leishmaniasis**
12. **Mycetoma**
13. **Allergic disorders** – Angioedema

100a: Grading of Lymphoedema (Brunner)

Subclinical	Excess interstitial fluid is present with histological abnormalities in lymphatics and lymph nodes. No clinically apparent lymphedema
Grade I	Edema pits on pressure-Swelling largely/completely disappears on elevation/bed rest
Grade II	Nonpitting edema. Does not significantly reduce upon elevation
Grade III	Nonpitting edema associated with irreversible skin changes, i.e. fibrosis, papillae, etc.

100b: Another Grading of Lymphoedema

Mild	< 20% excess limb volume
Moderate	20 – 40 % excess limb volume
Severe	> 40% excess limb volume

101: Lymphangiographic Patterns of Lymphedema

• **Congenital hyperplasia** (Congenital) – Males more affected Unilateral/bilateral Involving the whole leg Progressive	• Lymphatics are increased in number, although functionally defective • Increased number of the lymph nodes are seen • May have chylous ascites, chylothorax and protein-losing enteropathy
• **Distal obliteration** (Puberty) – Females more affected Often bilateral Ankle and calf	• Absent or reduced distal superficial lymphatics • Also termed aplasia or hypoplasia
• **Proximal obliteration with distal hyperplasia** Any age, equal sex incidence, whole leg affected, usually unilateral	• There is obstruction at the level of aortoiliac or inguinal nodes • The patient may benefit from lymphatic bypass operation because of the hyperplasia
• **Proximal obliteration without distal hyperplasia**	• Cannot do lymphatic bypass operation

102: Zones of Hand (Verdan's)

Zone I	Distal to the insertion of flexor digitorum superficialis
Zone II	From distal palmar crease to flexor digitorum superficialis insertion
Zone III	Distal to transverse carpal ligament to distal palmar crease
Zone IV	Area of transverse carpal ligament
Zone V	Proximal to transverse carpal ligament

103: Seddon's Classification (1942) - Types of Nerve Injury

Neurapraxia	:	Axons are intact. Spontaneous recovery is complete
Axonotmesis	:	Axons divided. Connective tissue intact. Wallerian degeneration occurs. Axons then regenerate slowly
Neurotmesis	:	Whole nerve severed. Recovery may occur if cut ends are apposed

104: Sunderland's Classification

Sunderland grade	*Axon*	*Endoneurial tube*	*Perineurium*	*Epineurium*	*Comparison With Seddon's*
First degree	+	+	+	+	Neurapraxia
Second degree	–	+	+	+	Axonotmesis
Third degree	–	–	+	+	
Fourth degree	–	–	–	+	Neurotmesis
Fifth degree	–	–	–	–	Neurotmesis

+ Intact, – severed.

105: Complications of Amputations

Skin complications

1. Delayed healing
2. Wound infection (Staphylococcal)
3. Ulceration
4. Sinus formation

Bone complications

1. Spur formation
2. Osteomyelitis with sequestrum formation and sinus
3. Bone end may perforate in growing child
4. Cross union between two bones

Muscle complications

1. Contracture and deformity
2. Fixed flexion and abduction deformity in above knee amputation
3. Fixed flexion deformity in below knee amputation

Nerve complication

1. Painful neuroma

Idiopathic complications

1. Phantom limb
2. Painful phantom
3. Causalgia

106: Site of Election for Above Knee and Below Knee Amputation

Above knee – 10 – 12 inches (25-30 cm) below the greater trochanter

Below knee – 5½ inch (14 cm) below the tibial plateau

Anorectal

107: Degree of Hemorrhoids

• First degree	• Bleed
• Second degree	• Bleed and prolapse (Reduce spontaneously)
• Third degree	• Bleed and prolapse (Require manual reduction)
• Fourth degree	• Prolapsed, cannot be reduced • Permanently outside anus • May strangulate

108: Park's Classification of Anal Fistula

Intersphincteric fistula (45%)	• Do not cross the external sphincter except the most distal subcutaneous fibers • Run directly from the internal to the external opening
Transsphincteric fistula (40%)	• Primary track crosses both internal and external sphincters, the latter at various levels and cross the ischiorectal fossa to reach the skin of the buttock • May have secondary tracks, rarely passing through the levators to the pelvis
Suprasphincteric (Very rare)	Thought to be iatrogenic and difficult to distinguish from high transsphincteric
Extrasphincteric	Usually as a result of pelvic diseases or trauma

109: Sites of Pilonidal Sinus

1. Natal cleft (commonest)
2. Axilla
3. Umbilicus
4. Between fingers
5. Genitalia
6. Amputation stump

110: Causes for constipation

A. GI causes

1. Dietary – lack of fiber and or fluid intake
2. Structural causes
   - Colonic carcinoma
   - Hirschsprung's disease
   - Diverticular disease
3. Obstructed defecation (Painful conditions)
   - Anal fissures
   - Hemorrhoids
   - Crohn's disease
4. Motility disorders
   - Irritable bowel syndrome
   - Slow transit constipation
   - Drugs – Analgesics, opiates, antidepressants, iron, anticholinergic, antacids, etc.
   - Pseudoobstruction
5. Immobility – Elderly
6. Social – Irregular work pattern, hospitalization, travel (long flights)
7. Psychological – Institutionalized individuals/depression
8. Postoperative – Child birth, Pelvic floor repair

Contd...

Contd...

B. Nongastrointestinal disorders

1. Neurological
   - Paraplegia (Autonomic dysfunction)
   - Cerebrovascular accidents
   - Parkinsonism
   - Multiple sclerosis
2. Metabolic/endocrine
   - Hypothyroidism
   - Diabetes mellitus
   - Pregnancy
   - Hypercalcemia
3. Chagas's disease
   - Trypanosomiasis with megacolon

INDEX

D

E

F

G

H

I

J

K

L

M

N

O

P

R

S

T